Sixth Edition

VOICE THERAPY

CLINICAL CASE STUDIES

Sixth Edition

VOICE THERAPY

CLINICAL CASE STUDIES

Joseph C. Stemple, PhD, CCC-SLP, ASHAF
Edie R. Hapner, PhD, CCC-SLP, ASHAF
Lauren Timmons Sund, BM, MS, CCC-SLP

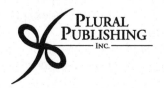

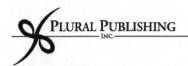

9177 Aero Drive, Suite B
San Diego, CA 92123

Email: information@pluralpublishing.com
Website: https://www.pluralpublishing.com

Copyright © 2026 by Plural Publishing, Inc.

Typeset in 10.5/13 Minion by Flanagan's Publishing Services, Inc.
Printed in the United States of America by Hatteras.

All rights, including that of translation, reserved. No part of this publication may be reproduced, stored in a retrieval system, or transmitted in any form or by any means, electronic, mechanical, recording, or otherwise, including photocopying, recording, taping, web distribution, or information storage and retrieval systems without the prior written consent of the publisher.

For permission to use material from this text, contact us by
Telephone: (866) 758-7251
Fax: (888) 758-7255
email: permissions@pluralpublishing.com

Every attempt has been made to contact the copyright holders for material originally printed in another source. If any have been inadvertently overlooked, the publisher will gladly make the necessary arrangements at the first opportunity.

Library of Congress Cataloging-in-Publication Data:
Names: Stemple, Joseph C., editor. | Hapner, Edie R., editor. | Timmons
  Sund, Lauren, editor.
Title: Voice therapy : clinical case studies / [edited by] Joseph C.
  Stemple, Edie R. Hapner, Lauren Timmons Sund.
Description: Sixth edition. | San Diego, CA : Plural Publishing, Inc.,
  [2026] | Includes bibliographical references and index.
Identifiers: LCCN 2025009055 (print) | LCCN 2025009056 (ebook) | ISBN
  9781635507317 (paperback) | ISBN 9781635504743 (ebook)
Subjects: MESH: Voice Disorders--therapy | Case Reports
Classification: LCC RF510 (print) | LCC RF510 (ebook) | NLM WV 500 | DDC
  616.85/5606--dc23/eng/20250430
LC record available at https://lccn.loc.gov/2025009055
LC ebook record available at https://lccn.loc.gov/2025009056

Contents

Foreword	*xiii*
Preface	*xv*
Acknowledgments	*xvii*
About the Authors	*xix*
Contributors	*xxi*
A Tribute to Our Prior Contributors	*xxiii*
Video Contents	*xxv*

1 The Voice and Upper Airway Evaluation
Edie R. Hapner and Lauren Timmons Sund

1 The Voice and Upper Airway Evaluation	**1**
A Brief History of the Voice and Upper Airway Evaluation	1
Models of Care	3
The Importance of an Accurate Laryngeal Diagnosis	4
Who Is Responsible?	4
Laryngeal Diagnosis Informs Treatment Decisions	4
Components of the Voice and Upper Airway Evaluation	5
The Physician's Medical Examination	5
The Speech-Language Pathologist's Assessment	7
The Case History	7
Patient-Reported Outcome Measures (PROMs or PRO measures)	7
Auditory-Perceptual Assessment	11
Visual-Perceptual Assessment	12
Cranial Nerve Examination	13
Motor Speech Assessment	13
Manual Assessment	16
Instrumental Assessment	18
Laryngeal Imaging	18
Acoustic Assessment	21
Aerodynamic Assessment	22
Stimulability	23
Documentation	24
Conclusions	24
References	25

2 From Evaluation to Intervention
Edie R. Hapner and Lauren Timmons Sund

2 From Evaluation to Intervention	**29**
Is Voice Therapy an Appropriate Treatment for the Presenting Problem?	29

vi   Voice Therapy: Clinical Case Studies

Is the Person a Good Candidate for Therapy?	31
Options for Care: Where Does Voice Therapy Fit?	33
Are You the "Right" Clinician?	33
Treatment Option Summaries by Disorder: Selected Examples	34
Treatment Options for Muscle Tension Dysphonia (MTD)	34
Treatment Options for Vocal Fold Motion Impairments	35
Treatments Options for Laryngeal Dystonia and Voice Tremor	36
Decision Making in Therapy Planning: What Therapy to Use?	37
Recalibration Strategies	38
Exuberant Strategies	39
Indirect and Augmentative Strategies	40
Decision Making in Voice Therapy Planning: How Much, How Long, and How Intense?	40
Putting It All Together in Decision Making: The Silent Factors	41
Conclusions	42
References	42

3   Phonotrauma   47

Introduction   47
Ryan C. Branski

Case Studies   48

Case Study 3.1. Conversation Training Therapy (CTT) to Treat an Adult   48
With Benign Midmembranous Lesions
Jackie L. Gartner-Schmidt and Amanda I. Gillespie

Case Study 3.2. Treating a Child With Dysphonia Using Concepts   55
From "Adventures in Voice"
Rita Hersan

Case Study 3.3. Multimodality Voice Therapy to Treat an Adult Female   61
Opera Singer With a Vocal Fold Pseudocyst
Christine Murphy Estes

Case Study 3.4. Perioperative Therapeutic Care for an Adult With a
Vocal Fold Cyst   71
Austin Collum and Megan Lee

Case Study 3.5. Multidisciplinary Treatment for an Adult With Vocal   79
Process Granulomas After TBI
Heather Starmer

Case Study 3.6. Vocal Function Exercises to Treat an Adult With   85
Undifferentiated Phonotrauma
Joseph C. Stemple

Case Study 3.7. Lessac-Madsen Resonant Voice Therapy to Treat an   93
Adult With Vocal Fold Nodules
Diana Marie Orbelo, Nicole Y. K. Li-Jessen, and Katherine Verdolini Abbott

References   101

Contents **vii**

4   Muscle Tension Dysphonia **107**
Nelson Roy
Introduction 107
Case Studies 109

Case Study 4.1. Manual Circumlaryngeal Techniques to Treat an Adult 109
With Primary Muscle Tension Dysphonia
Nelson Roy

Case Study 4.2. Boot Camp Voice Therapy for an Adult With 116
Functional Dysphonia
Claudio F. Milstein and Michelle Adessa

Case Study 4.3. Flow Phonation to Treat a Teenager With Primary 120
Muscle Tension Aphonia
Jackie L. Gartner-Schmidt

Case Study 4.4. Multimodality Voice Therapy for an Adult With 127
Vocal Fatigue
Chaya Nanjundeswaran

Case Study 4.5. Intensive Voice Therapy for a Teenager With Mutational 133
Falsetto (Puberphonia)
Lisa Fry

Case Study 4.6. Postsurgical Voice Therapy for a Child With Recurrent 140
Respiratory Papillomatosis and Ventricular Phonation
Maia Nystrum Braden

Case Study 4.7. Interprofessional Assessment and Treatment for an Adult 147
With Muscle Tension Dysphagia
Christina Kang Rosow

References 154

5   Glottal Gaps **159**
Introduction 159
Aaron Ziegler
Case Studies 161

Case Study 5.1. Inspiratory Muscle Strength Training to Augment Vocal 161
Function Exercises in an Adult With Presbyphonia
Heather Bonilha and Maude Desjardins

Case Study 5.2. Phonation Resistance Training Exercises (PhoRTE®) to 169
Treat an Adult With Presbyphonia
Aaron Ziegler and Edie R. Hapner

Case Study 5.3. Expiratory Muscle Strength Training and PhoRTE® to 179
Treat an Adult With Presbyphonia
Adam Lloyd and Maria Murljacic

Case Study 5.4. Postoperative Voice Therapy to Treat an Adult With 185
Unilateral Vocal Fold Paralysis
Maria Dietrich

viii Voice Therapy: Clinical Case Studies

Case Study 5.5. Interprofessional Treatment for an Adult With 192
Unilateral Vocal Fold Paresis
Desi Gutierrez and Matthew Hoffman

Case Study 5.6. Multimodality Teletherapy for an Adult Avocational 199
Singer With Unilateral Vocal Fold Paresis
Lauren Timmons Sund

Case Study 5.7. Interprofessional Treatment for an Adult With 207
Sulcus Vocalis
Amanda I. Gillespie and Clark A. Rosen

References 214

6 Movement Disorders Affecting the Voice 221

Introduction 221
Katherine L. Marks

Laryngeal Dystonia 221
Vocal Tremor 222
Parkinson's Disease 223

Case Studies 224

Case Study 6.1. Medical and Behavioral Management for an Adult With 224
Laryngeal Dystonia–Adductor Type
Edie R. Hapner and Michael M. Johns III

Case Study 6.2. Voice Therapy Without Medical Management for an 232
Adult With Adductor Spasmodic Dysphonia
Joseph C. Stemple

Case Study 6.3. Teletherapy Without Medical Management for an Adult 236
With Abductor Laryngeal Dystonia and Vocal Tremor
Lauren Timmons Sund

Case Study 6.4. Reducing Voicing Duration to Treat an Adult With 242
Vocal Tremor
Julie Barkmeier-Kraemer

Case Study 6.5. Multimodality Voice Therapy for an Adult Classical 255
Singer With Vocal Tremor
Kristen Bond

Case Study 6.6. The SLP's Role in Deep Brain Stimulation for Vocal Tremor 261
Elizabeth DiRenzo

Case Study 6.7. Maintaining Gains From Voice Therapy Using the 267
SpeechVive for an Adult With Parkinson's Disease
Jessica Huber

References 274

7 Upper Airway 281

Introduction: Refractory Chronic Cough 281
Laurie Slovarp

Contents   **ix**

Case Studies   284

Case Study 7.1. Behavioral Cough Suppression Therapy (BCST) for an   284
Adult With Chronic Refractory Cough
Lisa Zughni

Case Study 7.2. Using the Chronic Cough Clinical Checklist With an   290
Adult With Irritant-Induced Chronic Cough
Mariah Morton-Jones

Case Study 7.3. Behavioral Cough Suppression Therapy for an Adult   297
With Underlying Respiratory Disease
Laurie Slovarp

Case Study 7.4. Interprofessional Use of SLN Injection and BCST for an   305
Adult With Chronic Refractory Cough
Edie R. Hapner and C. Blake Simpson

Case Study 7.5. Interprofessional Use of Neuromodulators and BCST for   316
an Adult With Chronic Refractory Cough
Juliana Litts and Daniel Fink

Introduction: Inducible Laryngeal Obstruction (ILO)   322
Mary J. Sandage

Case Study 7.6. Long-Term Management of PVFM in an Adult Following   325
an Environmental Fume Exposure
Carissa Maira

Case Study 7.7. Treating Irritable Larynx in an Adult Within the   333
Framework of Central Sensitivity Syndrome
Linda Rammage

Case Study 7.8. Behavioral Management for Exercise-Induced Laryngeal   341
Obstruction (EILO) in a Collegiate Swimmer
Mary J. Sandage

Case Study 7.9. EILOBI Techniques to Treat an Adolescent Nordic Skier   346
With EILO
Emily A. Nauman

References   354

8   Performance Voice   **361**

Introduction   361
Marina Gilman

Case Studies   363

Case Study 8.1. Multimodality Voice Therapy for an Adult Voice   363
Actor/Singer With a Translucent Polypoid Lesion
M. Eugenia Castro and Megan Urbano

Case Study 8.2. Onsite Voice Therapy for an Adult Theater Actor With   371
Vocal Injury During Preparation and Performance
Debra Phyland

x Voice Therapy: Clinical Case Studies

Case Study 8.3. Myofascial Release for an Adult Touring Musical Theater 380
Performer With Vocal Fatigue
Wendy LeBorgne

Case Study 8.4. Voice Recalibration With the Cup Bubble Technique for 388
an Adult Country Singer With Chronic Phonotrauma
Jenny C. Muckala

Case Study 8.5. Timing Multimodality Voice Therapy to Treat an Adult 394
Singer With a Vocal Fold Polyp and Mild Atrophy
Juliana Codino

Case Study 8.6. Perioperative Voice Therapy for an Adult Praise and 403
Worship Leader With Phonotraumatic Lesions
Marina Gilman

Case Study 8.7. Perioperative Voice Therapy for a High School Music 409
Teacher With a Vocal Fold Polyp
Maurice Goodwin

Case Study 8.8. Perioperative Management for an Adult Jazz Singer 415
With a Vocal Fold Cyst
Sarah L. Schneider and Mark S. Courey

Case Study 8.9. Multimodality Voice Therapy for a Prepubescent Singer 423
With Vocal Nodules
Patricia Doyle and Starr Cookman

References 430

9 Gender Affirming Voice Care 437

Introduction 437
Sandy Hirsch

Case Studies 439

Case Study 9.1. Using Acoustic Assumptions in Gender Affirming 439
Voice Care for an Adult Transgender Woman
Sandy Hirsch

Case Study 9.2. Pitch-Elevation Surgery and Perioperative Voice Care 446
for an Adult Transgender Woman
Wynde Vastine and Katherine C. Yung

Case Study 9.3. Manual Therapy in Gender Affirming Voice Care for a 453
Transmasculine Adult on Hormone Replacement Therapy (HRT)
Daniel P. Buckley and Felicia A. François

Case Study 9.4. Developing a Gender Affirming Voice in a 461
Nonbinary Adult
Desi Gutierrez

Case Study 9.5. Gender Affirming Voice Care for an Adolescent 468
AC Goldberg

Case Study 9.6. Gender Affirming Voice Care via Teletherapy for a
Transmasculine Nonbinary Singer   475
Ruchi Kapila
References   483

Index   *487*

Foreword

Thirty-one years ago, as a young clinician in a dedicated "voice center," I nervously asked one of the giants of our field, G. Paul Moore, to write a foreword for the first edition of *Voice Therapy: Clinical Case Studies*. Not only was Dr. Moore a pioneer in the field of voice disorders, but he was also one of the kindest and most sharing gentlemen in our profession, always strongly encouraging to the next generation. Now, here we are, five editions later and I am the one being asked to write the foreword to this enduring text; and in so doing, I am passing the baton to the next generation who, through their contributions, continue to define and describe the remarkable growth of the profession I love.

For the first edition, Dr. Moore wrote,

> . . . the basic books usually classify deviant voices and briefly describe diseases, structural abnormalities, emotional problems, and behavioral variations that cause the vocal disorders. These texts also customarily recommend general remedial measures for recognized voice problems; however, the authors never intended their limited presentations to prepare the speech clinician to manage remedial programs expertly. Consequently, many clinicians find themselves unprepared to handle voice problems.

Indeed, the first edition of *Voice Therapy: Clinical Case Studies* was born of the frustration of writing a voice disorders survey textbook that lacked the space to fully describe the treatments available for the many voice disorders. Thus, in 1993, with the contributions of 25 master voice clinicians, physicians,

and voice pedagogues, detailed case studies explicitly and realistically presented remedial approaches used to treat voice disorders. The evolution of this text has followed the remarkable evolution of our profession with each new edition reemphasizing foundational clinical knowledge through classic cases and introducing new and exciting approaches to treatments resulting from evidence-based research, behavioral research, basic science research, advances in technology, and societal changes. The cases presented in each new edition demonstrate the immense positive impact that those who treat voice disorders have on the lives of individual patients.

This sixth edition of *Voice Therapy: Clinical Case Studies* continues the tradition of providing expert, detailed instruction to those with the privilege of providing care to individuals with voice disorders. My role in this edition has been purely ceremonial as the heavy lifting has been shared by my friends and colleagues Edie Hapner and Lauren Timmons Sund. In their hands, I am supremely confident that the intent of this text will endure. It is my desire that you will find guidance and inspiration as you study the cases presented in this book and that your patients will benefit from your dedication to learning.

With joy and contentment, *"give me now leave to leave thee."*—Hamlet, Act 1, Scene 5

Joseph C. Stemple
Professor Emeritus
College of Health Sciences
Department of Communication
   Sciences and Disorders
University of Kentucky

Preface

The sixth edition of *Voice Therapy: Clinical Case Studies* is a reenvisioning of the text that mirrors the growth of the field of voice care. An updated chapter on the voice and upper airway evaluation details the contemporary vision and purpose of the evaluation as not simply a mandatory step in the care process, but rather as a method to develop a grounded clinical hypothesis about the behavioral aspects of the voice in collaboration with our laryngology, otolaryngology, pulmonology, neurology, and gastroenterology partners. This text diligently guides the clinician through an evaluation process informed by current trends in the use of patient-reported outcome measures, advanced instrumental procedures, and the all-important stimulability testing that steers a process we refer to as the "Decision-Making Step," where the clinician feels empowered to determine if voice and upper airway therapy will play a role in the patient's care. Speech-language pathologists are independent providers and, as such, this book empowers the clinician to be a partner in care provision rather than a technician to carry out a plan prescribed by a physician or advanced practice provider. In every chapter and case, this updated text highlights the specific physiological underpinnings of treatment that might support a return to full voice; improved vocal health to reduce the incidence of phonotrauma; enhanced efficiency of voice production; reduction/elimination of activity-limiting dyspnea; and improved voice sense of self based on the results of the voice and upper airway evaluation, the clinician's understanding of cause and medical care of pathologies, and the vast appreciation of the person's needs and desires for their voice.

The coeditors of this text hope to enhance patient care by bolstering the confidence of clinicians providing voice and upper airway treatment. To this end, each case begins with authentic medical documentation including the history of present illness, perceptual assessment, instrumental assessment, and stimulability testing followed by sections on impressions and plan of care that include the frequency, intensity, and duration of care. Importantly, each case includes a section on decision making for a peek into the minds of our master clinicians and why they do what they do. The intervention section of each case is designed to walk the reader through the therapy process, step by step and session by session. Every case, new and old, has been revamped to provide a level of detail that is new to the sixth edition. Perhaps the most exciting addition to this text is the 30+ cloud-based therapy demonstrations. The coeditors have diligently inserted the video links throughout the text so the reader can quickly and easily watch the author do the therapy described in each case.

Also new to this text, the introductions to each chapter have been rewritten to reflect advances in care since the publication of the fifth edition. Updated language and understanding of voice and upper airway disorders is used in each chapter, but especially in the movement disorders (e.g., laryngeal dystonia) and upper airway chapters (e.g., inducible laryngeal obstruction). The use of telehealth is now infused throughout the book as an option for improving access to care rather than as a novelty. This sixth edition also boasts an entire chapter on gender-affirming voice care, whereas the previous edition included only two cases. We have invited our laryngology collaborators to coauthor cases with our master speech-language pathology clinicians to demonstrate all the permutations of interprofessional care that improves treatment outcomes. Within the cases, the coeditors use gray "call-out" boxes to highlight important concepts, provide additional information on controversies, offer suggestions for additional reading, or give a simple explanation for why a phrase or concept might be of the utmost importance to care.

The sixth edition of *Voice Therapy: Clinical Case Studies* honors the giants in voice and upper airway care that have come before us, especially those that have played such a pivotal role in prior editions. We particularly honor Dr. Joseph Stemple, a trailblazer in our field who has graciously passed the torch to us for this sixth edition to continue his tradition of generous teaching, mentoring, and making voice care easy and accessible to all clinicians.

We believe the sixth edition in its new format is a stand-alone text providing guidance to all clinicians for current evidence-based, effective voice and upper airway care for patients across the life span. We are so grateful to our authors for their generous cases that teach us how to be better clinicians and to the 30 authors of our videos that literally *show* us how it is done. We thank Plural and our editors for their support during the journey to reenvision this sixth edition of *Voice Therapy: Clinical Case Studies*.

We are so proud of this edition and look forward to sharing it with you.

Respectfully,
Edie and Lauren

Acknowledgments

The gargantuan task of editing a textbook is made possible through the support of many people behind the scenes. First, thank you to all of our contributors across the globe. Learning from you along the way was a delightful privilege. We are humbled by your generosity of time and talent to share cases and to put your decision making and masterful experience onto the page for the sole purpose of helping your colleagues navigate the tricky and rewarding waters of voice therapy.

Thank you to our speech pathology colleagues at the University of Alabama, Birmingham: Duane Trahan, Caitlin Stone, Sarah Hoch, Jacob Wright, Will Boswell, Melissa Tucker, and Amalee Smith PA, and to our speech pathology colleagues at the University of Southern California: Eugenia Castro, Felicia François, and Kacie La Forest. Your friendship keeps our work joyful and your collaboration elevates all that we do. Each of you has allowed us to share our attention and lightened our load to allow this text to come to fruition.

Thank you to our laryngology partners who have taught us the intricacies of the larynx "beyond the book" to make us better diagnosticians and better clinicians. Michael M. Johns III, MD, has been a partner and friend to both of us. His incredible surgical skill, clinical acumen, and ability to navigate almost any situation have been inspiring and fulfilling. It is and was an honor to share his clinical space and his unwavering support. Thank you to C. Blake Simpson, MD, a visionary, skilled, and thoughtful clinician and most notably a consummate teacher, for his partnership and for allowing me, Edie Hapner, to feel the absolute unexpected exhilaration of building a third voice center late in my career side by side, day by day, accom-

plishment by accomplishment. Thank you to Karla O'Dell, MD, and Elizabeth Shuman, MD, for their daily teamwork at USC and for making me, Lauren Timmons Sund, a better clinician.

Thank you to some very special colleagues who have helped me, Edie Hapner, continue to love and cherish the work we do over the last 44 years: Dee Nikjeh, Jackie Gartner-Schmidt, and Julie Barkmeier-Kraemer. But most especially, thank you to Lauren Timmons Sund for nearly a decade of allowing me to be a part of your successes and your joys, and for sharing this journey with me to develop a resource for our world of voice and upper airway and to always support the next generation of our colleagues.

Thank you to my (Lauren's) mentor, Edie Hapner. You took me under your wing as a new clinician, and you continue to lift me up and propel me forward. I am endlessly grateful for your devoted mentorship and friendship. Thank you to SLP friends near and far who make this work so fun and so meaningful—especially Daniel Buckley, Austin Collum, Mariah Morton-Jones, and Lisa Zughni.

Thank you to our students and fellows for keeping us on our toes, inspiring us to ask deeper questions and, as a result, providing the highest level of patient care. There is no greater joy than guiding a novice clinician in developing their confidence as a clinician and seeing them grow into a teacher themselves. Likewise, thank you to all of our mentors over the years. We stand on the shoulders of giants, and our work is possible because of those who came before us and poured into our cups. Thank you to Joe for originating this masterpiece and shepherding five editions. Thank you for entrusting us to carry on the legacy. Your work

xvii

in the field of voice disorders is incomparable and invaluable. It is a privilege for us all to continue to learn from you.

Thank you to our publishers at Plural Publishing, especially Valerie Johns, for guiding this publication to the finish line.

And thank you to our patients who give us purpose—all of this is for them.

The greatest thanks go to our ever-patient families for their love and support. A ginormous thanks to our husbands, Howard Hapner and Chase Sund, for providing unwavering support no matter our antics. To Howard for his sound advice and to Chase for his foray into medical illustration (Figure 5–4). Thank you to Edie's daughter, Brittany Hapner, for allowing her home to be our Los Angeles office and to Stephanie Hapner Petron for her 5 AM daily advice and support. Thank you to Lauren's mom, Linda Timmons, for cross-country treks to babysit during long work weekends. And no book of ours would be complete without a nod to the new members of our families who came to Earth during the writing of this text. The most special love to Kieran Sund, Lucas Petron, and Leo Petron. You are our true joy and make us stop in our tracks and marvel at the joys of all the little things.

With immeasurable gratitude,
Edie and Lauren

About the Authors

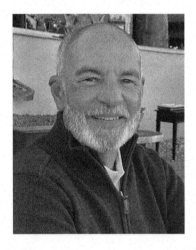

Joseph C. Stemple, PhD, CCC-SLP, ASHAF is Professor Emeritus, Department of Communication Sciences and Disorders, College of Health Sciences, University of Kentucky. Prior to his academic career he was the founder and director of the Blaine Block Institute for Voice Analysis and Rehabilitation, Dayton, Ohio and the Professional Voice Center of Greater Cincinnati. As co-director of the UK Laryngeal and Speech Dynamics Lab, his research focused on understanding voice disorders, specifically cell to society translational research. The overarching research goal was to enhance vocal function in those with voice disorders. He is a Fellow and Honors recipient of the American Speech Language Hearing Association.

Edie R. Hapner, PhD, CCC-SLP, is the George W. Barber Junior Endowed Professor of Otolaryngology at the University of Alabama at Birmingham where she also serves as the Co-Director of the UAB Voice Center and the Director of Hearing and Speech. She is a fellow of the American Speech Language and Hearing Association and Associate Fellow of the American Laryngological Association. Dr. Hapner has served on the Board of Directors for the American Speech Language and Hearing Association as the Vice President of Planning, Coordinator of the SIG 3 Voice and Voice Disorders and chaired the ASHA Annual Convention in both 2020 and 2022. She has served as a member of the Voice Committee for the American Academy of Otolaryngology and the Education Committee for the American Bronchoesophageal Association and served

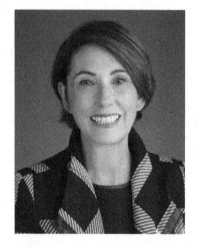

on the AAOHNS Guidelines Committee for Dysphonia. She is a founding member of PAVES, Pathway for Advanced Voice Education and Service and currently serves on the Advisory Board.

Dr. Hapner's research interests include aging voice, dystonia and adherence to voice therapy. She has co-edited Voice Therapy Clinical Case Studies Editions 4, 5 and now 6. She is co-developer of Phonation Resistance Training Exercises (PhoRTE®), an evidence-based treatment for aging voice. She developed and implemented the voice curriculum for Medbridge Inc, an online learning system for speech language pathologists. She has presented hundreds of lectures, workshops, and seminars on voice and voice disorders. She has over 70 published articles in the area of voice and voice disorders and multiple book chapters. Dr. Hapner's greatest professional accomplishment remains the mentoring of 23 consecutive voice centric clinical fellows into this incredible world of care of the voice.

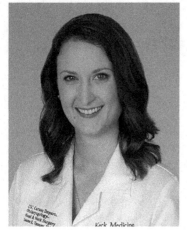

Lauren Timmons Sund, BM, MS, CCC-SLP is the Speech Pathology Director for the USC Voice Center in Los Angeles, CA. She is the Clinical Fellowship Director at the USC Voice Center and an instructor and clinical educator for the graduate SLP program at the University of Southern California.

Lauren earned her master's degree in communicative disorders from California State University, Northridge, completed a research internship at the University of Pittsburgh Voice Center, and trained as a clinical fellow in voice, upper airway, and swallowing disorders at the USC Voice Center under the mentorship of Edie Hapner, PhD. She holds a Bachelor of Music in voice performance from Illinois Wesleyan University.

Lauren specializes in the care of patients with voice and upper airway disorders with particular clinical and research interest in performance voice, aging voice, laryngeal dystonia, and interprofessional practice. She has published 20+ peer-reviewed articles and regularly presents locally and nationally. Lauren served as course co-director for the Fall Voice Conference 2024, is a past president of the Southern California Chapter of the Voice Foundation, a current committee chair for PAVES (Pathway for Advanced Voice Education and Service), and is on the Advisory Board for the Voice Foundation.

Contributors

This text is a result of the generosity of over 60 master clinicians who have selflessly shared their knowledge after committing their careers to developing the highest level of clinical acumen, clinical skill, clinical discovery, and mentorship. Their cases represent the most current evidence and practice in care of the voice and upper airway at the time of writing this text. We, the editors, thank them for their contributions and for teaching us through their research, their presentations, and certainly through these cases to be better clinicians ourselves.

Katherine Verdolini Abbott, PhD
Chapter 3

Michelle Adessa, MS
Chapter 4

Julie Barkmeier-Kraemer, PhD
Chapter 6

Kristen Bond, MM, MS
Chapter 6

Heather Bonilha, PhD
Chapter 5

Maia Nystrum Braden, MS
Chapter 4

Ryan C. Branski, PhD
Chapter 3

Daniel P. Buckley, MS
Chapter 9

M. Eugenia Castro, MS
Chapter 8

Juliana Codino, PhD
Chapter 8

Austin Collum, MA
Chapter 3

Starr Cookman, MS
Chapter 8

Mark S. Courey, MD
Chapter 8

Maude Desjardins, PhD
Chapter 5

Maria Dietrich, PhD
Chapter 5

Elizabeth DiRenzo, PhD
Chapter 6

Patricia Doyle, MA
Chapter 8

Daniel Fink, MD
Chapter 7

Felicia A. François, MS
Chapter 9

Lisa Fry, PhD
Chapter 4

Jackie L. Gartner-Schmidt, PhD
Chapter 3, Chapter 4

Amanda I. Gillespie, PhD
Chapter 3, Chapter 5

Marina Gilman, MM, MA
Chapter 8

AC Goldberg, PhD
Chapter 9

Maurice Goodwin, MS
Chapter 8

Desi Gutierrez, MA
Chapter 5, Chapter 9

Rita Hersan, MS
Chapter 3

Sandy Hirsch, MS
Chapter 9

Matthew Hoffman, MD, PhD
Chapter 5

Jessica Huber, PhD
Chapter 6

Michael M. Johns III, MD
Chapter 6

Christina Kang Rosow, MM, MS
Chapter 4

Ruchi Kapila, MS
Chapter 9

Wendy LeBorgne, PhD
Chapter 8

Megan Lee, MS
Chapter 3

Nicole Y. K. Li-Jessen, PhD
Chapter 3

Juliana Litts, MA
Chapter 7

Adam Lloyd, SLP-D
Chapter 5

Carissa Maira, MS
Chapter 7

Katherine I. Marks, PhD
Chapter 6

Claudio F. Milstein, PhD
Chapter 4

Mariah E. Morton-Jones, PhD
Chapter 7

Jenny C. Muckala, MS
Chapter 8

Maria Murljacic, MS
Chapter 5

Christine Murphy Estes, MM, MA
Chapter 3

Chaya Nanjundeswaran, PhD
Chapter 4

Emily A. Nauman, MA
Chapter 7

Diana Orbelo, PhD
Chapter 3

Debra Phyland, PhD
Chapter 8

Linda Rammage, PhD
Chapter 7

Clark A. Rosen, MD
Chapter 5

Nelson Roy, PhD
Chapter 4

Mary J. Sandage, PhD
Chapter 7

Sarah L. Schneider, MS
Chapter 8

C. Blake Simpson, MD
Chapter 7

Laurie Slovarp, PhD
Chapter 7

Heather Starmer, PhD
Chapter 3

Megan E. Urbano, MS
Chapter 8

Wynde Vastine, MA
Chapter 9

Katherine C. Yung, MD
Chapter 9

Aaron Ziegler, PhD
Chapter 5

Lisa A. Zughni, MS
Chapter 7

A Tribute to Our Prior Contributors

The profession of speech-language pathology reaches its 100th anniversary in 2025 and this text, *Voice Therapy: Clinical Case Studies*, approaches its 30th anniversary. With each edition, master clinicians have contributed their expertise in care of the voice and upper airway. With each edition, the text grows and changes to reflect the dynamic nature of our profession and our knowledge and skills. Each edition of this text is possible because of the contribution of teaching cases from the giants in our field. We honor their dedication to the field and to teaching us. We would not be where we are today without their work, and though their cases may no longer be featured in this text, they will never be forgotten. We are honored to stand on the shoulders of these giants.

Prior Editors

Edition 1	Joseph C. Stemple
Edition 2	Joseph C. Stemple
Edition 3	Joseph C. Stemple and Lisa Thomas
Edition 4	Joseph C. Stemple and Edie R. Hapner
Edition 5	Joseph C. Stemple and Edie R. Hapner

Prior Contributors

Richard D. Andreatta, PhD

Moya Andrews, PhD

Mary V. Andrianopoulos, PhD

Vrushali Angadi, PhD

Susan Baker Brehm, PhD

Mara Behlau, PhD

Alison Behrman, PhD

Andrew Blitzer, MD

Gordon W. Blood, PhD

Osiris Brasil, MD

James Case, PhD

Janina K. Casper, PhD

Kimberly Coker, MS

Lyn Tindall Covert, PhD

Daniel Croake, PhD

Ilter Denizoglu, MD

Kate DeVore, MA

Eileen M. Finnegan, PhD

Cynthia Fox, MA

Bernice S. Gerdeman Klaben, PhD

Leslie Glaze, PhD

Shirley Gherson, MS

Laureano A. Giraldez-Rodriguez, MD

Jack Gluckman, MD

Stephen J. Gorman, PhD

Rebecca Hancock, MEd

Sara Harris, FRCSLT

Marc Haxer, MA

Leah Helou, PhD

Douglas M. Hicks, PhD

Robert E. Hillman, PhD

Henry Ho, MD

Bari Hoffman Ruddy, PhD

Celia R. Hooper, PhD

John Hufnagle, PhD

Krzysztof Izdebski, PhD

Barbara H. Jacobson, PhD

Lisa N. Kelchner, PhD

Thomas J. Kereiakes, MD

Aliaa Khidr, MD, PhD

Mary McDonald Klimek, MM, MS

Danna Koschkee, MA

William Kramer, PhD

Ann W. Kummer, PhD

Linda Lee, PhD

Jeffrey Lehman, MD

Dawn B. Lowery, PhD

Glaucya Madazio, PhD

Stephen C. McFarlane, PhD

Murray Morrison, MD

Thomas Murray, PhD

Gisele Oliveira, MSc

Bryn Olson-Greb, MS

Rita Patel, PhD

Robert Peppard, PhD

Madeleine Pethan, MA

Brian Petty, MA

Bruce Poburka, PhD

Christine Ray, PhD

Sharon Radionoff, PhD

Lorraine Ramig, PhD

Bonnie Raphael, PhD

Brienne Ruel, MA

Stephen Salloway, MS, MD

Christine Sapienza, PhD

Sandy Schwartz, MS

Susan Shulman, MS

Erin Silverman, PhD

JoAnna Sloggy, PhD

Martin Spencer, MA

Tara Stadelman-Cohen, MS

Celia Stewart, PhD

R. E. (Ed) Stone, Jr., PhD

Edie Swift, MA

Robert Thayer Sataloff, MD, DMA

Jennifer Thompson, MA

Michael Towey, MA

Michael D. Trudeau, PhD

Eva van Leer, PhD

Jarrad Van Stan, PhD

Shelley Von Berg, PhD

Miriam van Mersbergen, PhD

Barbara D. Weinrich, PhD

Richard Zraick, PhD

Video Contents

 This book comes with videos on a PluralPlus companion website. Look for this icon throughout the text to identify where a corresponding video is available. (Instructions for accessing the website are on the inside front cover.)

VIDEO #	CASE	TITLE	AUTHOR
Video 1	3.1	Mapping Speech Sound Sensations	Jackie Gartner-Schmidt
Video 2	3.1	Clear Speech and Negative Practice	Amanda Gillespie
Video 3	3.3	Physical Rolldown Stretch	Christine Murphy Estes
Video 4	3.3	Labio-Lingual Trills (Raspberries)	Christine Murphy Estes
Video 5	3.6	Vocal Function Exercises	Joseph Stemple
Video 6	4.2	Gargling as a Facilitating Technique	Claudio Milstein
Video 7	4.3	Flow Phonation	Jackie Gartner-Schmidt
Video 8	4.6	Lip Trills	Maia Braden
Video 9	4.6	Inspiratory Phonation	Maia Braden
Video 10	4.6	Straw Bubbles	Maia Braden
Video 11	4.7	Resonant Voice Concepts	Christina Kang Rosow
Video 12	5.1	Inspiratory Muscle Strength Training	Heather Bonilha
Video 13	5.2	Developing Proper Form for PhoRTE	Edie Hapner and Aaron Ziegler
Video 14	5.3	Using the EMST 150 Device	Adam Lloyd
Video 15	5.6	Anchoring and Twang to Reduce Vocal Effort	Lauren Timmons Sund
Video 16	6.4	Shortened Voicing Duration for Vocal Tremor	Julie Barkmeier-Kraemer
Video 17	6.5	Contrasting Glottic Onset Types	Kristen Bond
Video 18	6.7	Calibrating the SpeechVive	Jessica Huber
Video 19	7.1	Throat Clearing Reduction Strategies	Lisa Zughni
Video 20	7.3	Relaxed Throat Breathing	Laurie Slovarp
Video 21	7.3	Box Breathing	Laurie Slovarp

continues

xxvi Voice Therapy: Clinical Case Studies

Video Contents. *continued*

VIDEO #	CASE	TITLE	AUTHOR
Video 22	7.9	Tooth Variant EILOBI Breathing Technique	Emily Nauman
Video 23	8.1	Twang for Sustainable Character Voices	Megan Urbano
Video 24	8.1	Cup Phonation	M. Eugenia Castro
Video 25	8.2	Modified Accent Method	Debra Phyland
Video 26	8.3	Myofascial Release	Wendy LeBorgne
Video 27	8.4	Cup Bubble Facilitator	Jenny Muckala
Video 28	8.5	Straw Phonation in Water Hierarchy	Juliana Codino
Video 29	8.6	/s/ Pulse and /wu/ Hierarchy	Marina Gilman
Video 30	8.8	Tongue Stretches	Sarah Schneider
Video 31	8.9	Ball Blower Semi-occluded Vocal Tract Exercise	Patricia Doyle
Video 32	9.1	Hirsch's Acoustic Assumptions	Sandy Hirsch
Video 33	9.1	Shaping Non-Speech Vocalizations	Sandy Hirsch
Video 34	9.2	Increasing Loudness After Pitch-Elevation Surgery	Wynde Vastine
Video 35	9.3	The Voice Puzzle in Gender-Affirming Voice Care	Felicia François
Video 36	9.3	Laryngeal Massage and Resposturing to Lower Pitch	Daniel Buckley
Video 37	9.4	Modifying Tongue Height to Alter Resonance	Desi Gutierrez

1

The Voice and Upper Airway Evaluation

Edie R. Hapner and Lauren Timmons Sund

A Brief History of the Voice and Upper Airway Evaluation

To understand the role of the voice and upper airway evaluation and its components, it seems fitting to first explore the history of voice care in the United States and the giants on whose shoulders we stand. The story of clinical voice and upper airway care is a fascinating one, beginning with the inception of the American Academy of Speech Correction in 1925, now the American Speech-Language-Hearing Association (ASHA). The earliest speech-language pathologists (SLPs) emerged from members of the National Association of Teachers of Speech, with a desire to infuse science into traditional speech and voice care, but with little interest in voice disorders themselves and more interest in stuttering and articulation.[1] While several prominent clinicians, namely Fairbanks and van Riper, wrote about voice care,[2,3] the treatment of the impaired voice remained primarily the purview of teachers of singing in the early years of speech pathology and continued in this context without substantial scientific underpinnings. However, during these early years, research on the science of voice care was being conducted in the lab by speech scientists such as G. Paul Moore, PhD, who defended his dissertation on laryngeal videostroboscopy[4] at Northwestern University's Speech Communication Department in 1936.[5] Around this same time, Friedrich Brodnitz, Emil Fröschels, and Paul J. Moses—prominent European phoniatricians displaced to the United States due to the antisemitic Nazi regime during World War II—advanced the collective interest and understanding of voice disorders.[6] And while we assume the interprofessional voice center began in the 1990s, Moore and Hans von Leden, MD, in fact started the first multidisciplinary voice care team at Northwestern University in 1951.

Clinical work in upper airway disorders came into the purview of the laryngologist and SLP in the 1930s and 1940s.[7] However, much of the early work in upper airway care centered around invasive methods of measuring respiratory function through tracheal punctures and esophageal balloons. The 1960s saw the initial attempts at noninvasive methods to measure respiratory and phonatory functions, and 20 years later, Smitheran and Hixon discovered that respiratory pressures could be measured at the lips as a surrogate for subglottal pressures.[8,9] The ability to noninvasively measure respiratory-phonatory function ushered in our current methods of evaluating the voice and upper airway in a clinical setting.

In the late 1980s and early 1990s, less invasive instrumental assessment of the voice became more widely available for clinical use. In the 1980s, physicians began using flexible laryngeal endoscopy as a clinical diagnostic tool to grossly examine the vocal folds, observe abduction and adduction, and determine the presence of larger lesions.[10] However, it was the introduction of laryngeal videostroboscopy that allowed the clinician to observe vocal fold pliability, glottal closure, and the finer details of the laryngeal mucosa.[11] This development shifted the theoretical underpinning of voice therapy from symptomatic to physiologic.[12] Voice clinicians could now see the vocal folds, understand their movement, and observe changes that occurred in response to treatment, thereby allowing them to understand why a patient presented with a particular symptom and thus target the root cause of the problem. Improvements in acoustic and aerodynamic assessment tools further helped clinicians understand the physiological functioning or malfunctioning of respiration, phonation, and resonance[13,14] and further advanced the field. Alongside these advances in voice care, in the early 1980s, the National Jewish Hospital in Denver began reporting on functional disorders of the vocal folds that symptomatically seemed to mimic asthma. SLP Florence Blager began publishing and presenting on the treatment of this "factitious asthma" called vocal cord dysfunction or paradoxical vocal fold motion, which could be treated with respiratory retraining by a qualified SLP.[15] More recently, this upper airway disorder has been described as inducible laryngeal obstruction (ILO).[16] Episodes of ILO are often triggered by strong odors, smoke, noxious smells, and other environmental triggers, and when symptoms are triggered by physical activity, it is known as exercise-induced laryngeal obstruction (EILO). Sandage et al (2024) published a systematic review about methods used by SLPs to treat ILO and EILO; however, this research unfortunately demonstrated a lack of consistency in the literature on types of treatment and metrics used to assess treatment outcomes.[17] Work continues in this area, and the cases in this text represent the most current thinking by master researchers and clinicians.

Another upper airway disorder, "chronic habit cough" was described in the 1980s and used respiratory retraining therapy as the treatment of choice.[18] Chronic cough was recognized as notably debilitating, reducing participation in social activities and sometimes causing secondary problems such as emesis, broken ribs, and urinary incontinence. The evidence base suggests a central sensitivity disorder as the etiology, with therapeutic interventions used by SLPs effective in treating what is now known as chronic refractory cough (CRC).[19] Research for how to best manage ILO, EILO, and CRC continues, with SLPs importantly involved in collaboration with pulmonologists, allergists, and otolaryngologists and with medications more recently added as complementary to the therapeutic process.

This brief history is intended to acquaint the reader with the advances in voice and upper airway care over the past 100 years and to illustrate how increased access to instrumental assessment has refined our diagnostic accuracy and advanced our treatments. Effective voice and upper airway care is preceded by a comprehensive, skilled evaluation and interpretation of findings. The remainder of this chapter first explores models of care for the evaluation and then the component parts of the evaluation. The evaluation is not simply the first step of care mandated by insurance companies and licensing boards, but an opportunity for the clinician to truly discover the source of a patient's voice or breathing condition and how voice or breathing function may improve if the patient is taught to use the mechanism differently.

Models of Care

The SLP is an integral member of the voice and upper airway care team, which is most often composed of the otolaryngologist (or laryngologist) and SLP, and in some cases, a neurologist or pulmonologist. In the realm of voice and upper airway rehabilitation, practice standards necessitate a multidisciplinary approach with more than one clinical specialty involved,[20] but there is variability in the way the care team collaborates across different models of practice. In the traditional model of care, the otolaryngologist sees the patient first and completes the medical history, head and neck examination, and likely a flexible endoscopic evaluation of the vocal folds or mirror examination. They may or may not complete laryngeal videostroboscopy. The physician determines whether to refer to the SLP for voice therapy, and the SLP may see the patient at a later date. Referrals to the SLP may come in the form of a written piece of paper, an electronic message, or perhaps a phone call. If the physician completes the laryngeal videostroboscopy, the SLP should ideally receive a video copy of the exam,[21] though it is not uncommon to receive only a still image or no image

at all. At times, the SLP may receive a vague diagnosis of "dysphonia."

This traditional model of care is known to have communication barriers between the physician and SLP. Even in the most collaborative of cases, it takes considerable time beyond direct patient care for clinicians to achieve optimal communication. More importantly, patient care is impacted. Studies have shown that only 53% of patients referred to therapy in this traditional model make it to the initial therapy appointment,[22] and up to 74% of referrals in this model are inappropriate referrals for behavioral management (ie, medical management would be a more appropriate first-line treatment, perhaps with therapy to follow).[23]

In contrast, in the interprofessional model of care, both the physician and the SLP see the patient on the same day or even at the same time. There are established roles for each member of the team during the assessment, including history taking, head and neck examination, clinical voice assessment, completion of patient-reported outcome measures, voice recording, laryngeal videostroboscopy, acoustic and aerodynamic assessment, and stimulability for behavior change. The appointment usually includes shared decision-making regarding the plan of care by the physician and SLP, and either one or both professionals discuss treatment options with the patient.[24] There have been several published reports on the benefits of interprofessional care in voice, including improved treatment plans, better therapy attendance, and greater improvement in voice quality of life from pre- to posttreatment,[25-27] as well as reducing lost revenue by minimizing missed appointments.[27]

In Chapters 3 through 9, you will read cases that span a variety of care models. Regardless of the model of care, you will notice the multidisciplinary theme of collaboration between SLP and physician and how different teams communicate to share information.

The Importance of an Accurate Laryngeal Diagnosis

Who Is Responsible?

As previously described, the voice and upper airway care team is most often composed of the otolaryngologist (or laryngologist) and SLP. In some cases, a neurologist or pulmonologist may be the primary physician working with the SLP. In rare cases, a primary care physician or physiatrist may refer patients to the SLP.

The SLP's referral source is relevant since different medical specialties approach clinical problems through varying lenses and testing, impacting the final differential diagnosis.

The differential diagnosis drives treatment decisions and therefore treatment outcomes. The diagnosis is generally determined following, at a minimum, a medical history, clinical medical head and neck assessment, and laryngeal imaging. When the referral source does not conduct laryngeal imaging as part of their practice, as in the case of a neurologist or primary care physician, it is within the scope of practice for the SLP to complete laryngeal videostroboscopy. However, the SLP cannot render a laryngeal diagnosis and should therefore share the results with the referring physician for diagnosis.

Does the neurologist possess thorough knowledge of laryngeal disease for diagnosis? Does the primary care physician, physiatrist, or pulmonologist? While they are experts within their own specialties, they do not have expertise in diseases and disorders of the larynx. To render an accurate diagnosis and therefore an effective treatment plan, the most specifically qualified physician, the otolaryngologist, should review the laryngeal imaging examination. Incidental, or unexpected, findings may be uncommon, but they are possible. Unfortunately, each of the editors has seen tragic cases of malignant cancers inappropri-

ately treated with antireflux medication or even voice therapy. These situations can arise when the laryngeal exam is not reviewed by a qualified examiner. Though the SLP can complete the laryngeal videostroboscopy, the editors strongly encourage making an otolaryngologist a member of *any* voice care team. Diagnosis is not within the scope of practice of the SLP, and best practice should keep laryngeal diagnosis within the purview of the otolaryngologist.

Laryngeal Diagnosis Informs Treatment Decisions

It is necessary to separate laryngeal diagnosis from disease diagnosis. A disease diagnosis, such as Parkinson's disease (PD), may be generally associated with a voice disorder, but there may be specific laryngeal findings to be addressed as well. In the case of PD, the voice disorder is typically due to a combination of glottal insufficiency, reduced respiratory support, and an impaired auditory feedback loop. Hypophonia associated with PD is often amenable to voice therapy, but there is a growing body of literature supporting the use of injection augmentation and medialization laryngoplasty in people with PD in addition to voice therapy.[28] Laryngeal imaging is necessary to assess glottal configuration and determine candidacy for such procedural interventions. Even treatments that have been researched with a particular population, such as LSVT LOUD® or Speak Out! for PD hypophonia or PhoRTE® for age-related voice changes, should not be applied prior to a comprehensive evaluation including laryngeal videostroboscopy and differential diagnosis from the otolaryngologist.

An accurate diagnosis aids the clinical decision of *if* and *when* to do voice therapy. If the voice problem is expected to recover with behavioral intervention, then voice therapy plays an important role in treatment.[21,29] If the problem is not expected to resolve with behavioral intervention as a first-line treatment, then a procedure or surgery may be suggested, potentially with therapy to follow. In some cases, a malignant diagnosis is identified and immediate medical intervention is required. While patients who are status post treatment for laryngeal cancer can benefit from voice therapy to manage treatment-related sequelae, voice therapy is not a primary treatment for any malignant laryngeal condition. It is important to note there are some situations where the laryngeal diagnosis suggests that a particular behavioral therapy is contraindicated. For example, PhoRTE®, an effective therapy developed for patients with presbyphonia, is not an appropriate treatment for a patient with a primary diagnosis of phonotraumatic lesion(s) and could harm a patient if applied inappropriately.

Though an accurate diagnosis informs decision making and prognosis to a certain extent, the SLP treats voice *function* rather than laryngeal diagnosis, and it is worth reiterating that diagnosis does not dictate treatment. Voice function arises from the interaction of all voice subsystems (respiratory, phonatory, resonatory) and not the vocal folds alone. Frequently, the SLP will treat a patient with a voice disorder secondary to a condition that is not "cured" by voice therapy, though voice production can be optimized through voice therapy. For example, recurrent respiratory papillomatosis is often treated with multiple surgeries, and voice therapy would not be effective in treating these lesions. However, undergoing multiple papilloma resections may lead to vocal fold scarring and a subsequent voice decline. In these situations, voice therapy might be applied to optimize voicing efficiency, reduce vocal effort, and/or improve endurance. Each patient case is different, and the comprehensive voice evaluation provides the information needed to determine candidacy for behavioral intervention and what might be targeted and achieved in voice therapy.

Components of the Voice and Upper Airway Evaluation

The comprehensive evaluation consists of 11 component parts that clinicians use to develop a working hypothesis of the cause of the voice or upper airway problem, prognosis, and potential treatment plans. Table 1–1 outlines the recommended component parts of the evaluation and the responsible member of the care team.

The Physician's Medical Examination

When a new patient presents to an otolaryngologist's office with a voice or upper airway concern, the physician must complete a detailed medical history of the presenting problem and a comprehensive physical examination including inspection of the ear canal, nasal cavity, and oral cavity with particular attention to the tongue, buccal cavity, gums and palate, and palpation of the neck to look for larger lymph nodes and thyroid nodules. The physician is required to clearly document the examination findings and indicate those findings that guide their medical decision making about treatment, including the impact of medical comorbidities, the need for further testing, and the risks, benefits, and alternative treatment options associated with their recommendations.

Ideally, the referring physician also completes and documents a brief neurological examination (cranial nerve evaluation, primarily), especially in someone who presents with a neurologically based voice disorder, such as vocal fold paralysis or paresis, laryngeal dystonia, or voice disorders associated with progressive neuromuscular diseases such as PD or amyotrophic lateral sclerosis (ALS). While the otolaryngologist may be one of the first professionals to recognize a neuromuscular disease, essential tremor, or movement disorder due to the patient presenting with a primary voice or

Table 1–1. Components of the Comprehensive Voice Evaluation

Component	Responsible Party
Medical Examination	Physician
History of the Problem	Physician and SLP
Clinical Perceptual Evaluation	SLP; often used by physician to rate voice quality
Patient-Reported Outcome Measures	Provided by MD and/or SLP and completed by the patient
Visual Assessment of Soft Signs	Physician and SLP
Cranial Nerve Examination	Physician; often also completed by SLP
Motor Speech Testing	SLP
Manual Laryngeal Palpation	Physician for thyroid gland assessment, SLP for laryngeal height and paralaryngeal tension
Stimulability for Voice Change	SLP
Acoustic and Aerodynamic Assessment	SLP
Laryngeal Imaging: Diagnostic Laryngoscopy and Laryngeal Videostroboscopy	Diagnostic laryngoscopy: Physician Videostroboscopy and interpretation: Physician and/or SLP

swallowing concern, it should be noted that the otolaryngologist is not the primary physician who manages these conditions. Patients with concerning neurological findings should be referred to a neurologist for further evaluation and potential treatment, which may be complementary to the options offered by the otolaryngologist and SLP. The otolaryngologist should examine the base of tongue, hypopharynx, and larynx of anyone complaining of voice or upper airway problems. This might include indirect laryngoscopy with the use of a laryngeal mirror, flexible endoscopy, or videostroboscopy. The *Guidelines for the Treatment of Hoarseness: Dysphonia* state that the physician should share the findings from their method of laryngeal imaging with the SLP, beyond a written diagnosis.[21] This would ideally be a video recording of the evaluation, but if not available, static pictures of the vocal folds should be provided at a minimum. In patients who present with upper airway complaints like dyspnea or stridor, the physician should attempt to examine the subglottis to carina (bifurcation of the trachea to the left and right bronchial tubes). Often, patients with dyspnea are sent to the otolaryngologist prior to seeing pulmonary medicine. In these cases, it is appropriate to refer patients to a pulmonologist to determine if pulmonary disease plays a role in their dyspnea. Pulmonary function tests (PFTs) are diagnostic for restrictive and obstructive pulmonary disease and guide the pulmonologist on treatment. Chronic cough or ILO/EILO can be isolated conditions, or they can co-occur with asthma, chronic obstructive pulmonary disease (COPD), or bronchiectasis, which can be treated with medications.

People with stridor may have subglottic stenosis (SGS) or posterior glottic stenosis (PGS), which is managed by the otolaryngologist, but this does not rule out other problems such as rheumatological disease, and these patients sometimes benefit from referral to both pulmonology and rheumatology.

Referral to gastroenterology can also be part of the assessment algorithm for some patients with voice and upper airway symptoms. For many years, acid reflux has been blamed as the origin of a variety of voice and upper airway disorders, but current research does not support reflux as a common primary contributor to laryngological disease.[30,31] A comprehensive assessment of the literature and current understanding of gastroesophageal reflux disease (GERD) and its role in voice and upper airway disorders is beyond the scope of this chapter. It is important to note, however, that laryngeal endoscopy is not a diagnostic tool for confirming laryngopharyngeal reflux (LPR) or GERD, as interrater and intrarater reliability are both poor for identifying supposed laryngeal findings of acid reflux.[32] Further, the American Academy of Otolaryngology–Head and Neck Surgery's (AAOHNS) clinical practice guidelines for dysphonia state that acid reflux treatments should not be applied for isolated dysphonia without appropriate workup.[21] If a patient has symptomatic complaints of GERD, a referral to gastroenterology is appropriate. The editors advise the SLP to defer counseling for issues such as esophageal diseases, diet considerations, and reflux medication to the GI physician as the most qualified clinician for such matters.

The Speech-Language Pathologist's Assessment

The Case History

Given the SLP's background in speech, voice, cognition, language, and factors that impact treatment adherence, they are well qualified to assess a patient's potential to participate in therapy independently or with support, as well as whether patients are stimulable for changing voice production or maladapted habits that propagate upper airway disorders like chronic cough. To make these determinations, the SLP must not only understand the health condition, but also become familiar with the patient's communication demands and their specific difficulties based on their activities, their environment, and personal factors. In addition, they must assess any facilitators or barriers to the patient achieving communication, voice, and/or upper airway goals. To this end, Table 1–2 lists some questions to guide the initial conversation about the patient's voice or upper airway complaint.

Patient-Reported Outcome Measures (PROMs or PRO measures)

Patient-reported outcome measures (PROMs) include any number of assessments or questionnaires completed by the patient regarding their health condition without interpretation of their responses by the clinician or any other person.[33] PROMs are a useful method of measuring the patient's perspective of the impact of their voice or upper airway disorder. Objective measures are an important part of the comprehensive voice evaluation, but no objective measure supersedes the importance of the patient's perspective about their condition, and no objective measure to date reliably correlates with patient perception of the voice disorder as measured by a PROM.[34] Because of their importance to the evaluation, PROMs have proliferated over the past 20 years, yet many lack the necessary methodological rigor needed for development.[34] The clinician should review the development papers for their chosen PROMs, as not all measures have been validated on all populations. Table 1–3 is a nonexhaustive list of commonly used PROMs in the voice and upper airway clinic.[35–46] These PROMs are used throughout the text.

Table 1–2. A Noncomprehensive List of Questions for History Taking

Questions	Potential Follow-Up Questions
When did this problem start?	What else was going on when the problem started? Were you ill? Did the problem start suddenly or gradually?
How is your problem now compared to how it was when it started?	Is today a good day, bad day, or normal day for your problem?
What makes your problem better? Have you had any medical or therapeutic interventions to make it better? What makes it worse?	Tell me about that treatment. Did it help? How long and how often did you do it? When did you stop doing it?
What are some things you are unable to do because of your problem?	Tell me more about how the problem is impacting you. Do you miss ___?
Are you having any other medical problems?	How is your swallowing/eating? Have you lost any weight?
	How is your breathing? What makes it better? What makes it worse?

Table 1–3. Commonly Used Voice and Upper Airway Patient-Reported Outcome Measures

Patient-Reported Outcome Measure	Specific Measure of Perception	Citation
Voice Handicap Index (VHI)	30-item patient perception of the impact of the voice disorder on their functional, emotional, and social lives	Jacobson BH, Johnson A, Grywalski C, Silbergleit A, Jacobson G, Benninger MS. The Voice Handicap Index (VHI): Development and validation. *Am J Speech Lang Pathol.* 1997;6(3):66-69. doi:10.1044/1058-0360.0603.66
Voice Handicap Index–10 (VHI-10)	10-item short version of the VHI measuring patient perception of the impact of the voice problem on quality of life	Rosen CA, Lee AS, Osborne J, Zullo T, Murry T. Development and validation of the Voice Handicap Index-10. *Laryngoscope.* 2004;114(9 I):1549-1556. doi:10.1097/00005537-200409000-00009
Voice-Related Quality of Life (VRQOL)	10 items measuring patient perception of the impact of the voice problem on quality of life	Hogikyan ND, Sethuraman G. Validation of an instrument to measure voice-related quality of life (V-RQOL). *J Voice.* 1999;13(4):557-569. doi:10.1016/S0892-1997(99)80010-1

Table 1–3. *continued*

Patient-Reported Outcome Measure	Specific Measure of Perception	Citation
Dyspnea Index (DI)	10 items measuring the patient's perceived impact of shortness of breath on quality of life	Gartner-Schmidt JL, Shembel AC, Zullo TG, Rosen CA. Development and validation of the Dyspnea Index (DI): A severity index for upper airway-related dyspnea. *J Voice.* 2014;28(6):775-782.
Cough Severity Index (CSI)	10 items measuring the patient's perceived impact of cough on quality of life	Shembel AC, Rosen CA, Zullo TG, Gartner-Schmidt JL. Development and validation of the Cough Severity Index: A severity index for chronic cough related to the upper airway. *Laryngoscope.* 2013;123(8):1931-1936.
Communicative Participation Item Bank (CPIB)	10 items measuring participation and barriers to participation because of communication issues	Baylor C, Yorkston K, Eadie T, Kim J, Chung H, Amtmann D. The Communicative Participation Item Bank (CPIB): Item bank calibration and development of a disorder-generic short form. *J Speech Lang Hear Res.* 2013;56(4):1190-1208. doi:10.1044/1092-4388(2012/12-0140)
Voice Problem Impact Scales (VPIS)	4 independent equal-interval scales measuring the patient's perceived impact of the voice problem on their lives overall, their work or daily activities, their home life, and their social life	Castro ME, Sund LT, Hoffman MR, Hapner ER. The Voice Problem Impact Scales (VPIS). *J Voice.* 2024;38(3):666-673. doi:10.1016/j.jvoice.2021.11.011
Voice Catastrophization Index (VCI)	A 13-item survey querying the patient's anxiety about their voice problem	Shoffel-Havakuk H, Chau S, Hapner ER, Pethan M, Johns MM III. Development and validation of the Voice Catastrophization Index. *J Voice.* 2019;33(2):232-238.
Singing Voice Handicap Index (SVHI)	36-item questionnaire based on the VHI and asking questions about the patient's perception of the impact of their voice problem on singing	Cohen SM, Jacobson BH, Garrett CG, Noordzij JP, Stewart MG, … Cleveland TF. Creation and validation of the Singing Voice Handicap Index. *Ann Otol Rhinol Laryngol.* 2007;116(6):402-406. doi:10.1177/000348940711600602

continues

Voice Therapy: Clinical Case Studies

Table 1–3. *continued*

Patient-Reported Outcome Measure	Specific Measure of Perception	Citation
Singing Voice Handicap Index–10 (SVHI-10)	10-item questionnaire based on the SVHI with questions about the patient's perception of the impact of their voice problem on singing	Cohen SM, Statham M, Rosen CA, Zullo T. Development and validation of the Singing Voice Handicap-10. *Laryngoscope.* 2009;119(9):1864-1869. doi:10.1002/lary.20580
Vocal Fatigue Index (VFI)	19-item questionnaire with 3 subscales regarding vocal fatigue: (1) tiredness of voice and voice avoidance, (2) physical discomfort associated with voicing, and (3) improvement of voice symptoms with rest	Nanjundeswaran C, Jacobson BH, Gartner-Schmidt J, Verdolini Abbott K. Vocal Fatigue Index (VFI): Development and validation. *J Voice.* 2015;29:433-440.
Glottal Function Index (GFI)	4 items measuring the patient's perceived impact of glottal insufficiency on quality of life	Bach K, Belafsky P, Wasylik K, Postma G, Koufman J. Validity and reliability of the Glottal Function Index. *Arch Otolaryngol Head Neck Surg.* 2005;131:961-964. doi:10.1016/j.jvoice.2024.04.004
Vocal Tract Discomfort Scale	Patient perception of throat tightness, dry throat, sore throat, itchy throat, sensitive throat, throat irritation, and lump in the throat on a 0-6 scale of frequency and intensity of symptoms	Mathieson L. Vocal tract discomfort in hyperfunctional dysphonia. *J Voice.* 1993;2:40-48.

Vocal fatigue and vocal effort are two of the most often heard complaints by people with voice and upper airway issues. Vocal fatigue and effort are related, but they are not the same. Vocal *fatigue* manifests as reduced vocal capacity or endurance, with changes in voice quality, pitch, and/or loudness, and it is believed to be the biomechanical effect of extended voice use.[47] Vocal *effort* is the patient's perception of the amount of muscular work they must exert during a vocal task.[48] Both voice fatigue and vocal effort can and should be measured. The Vocal Fatigue Index (VFI),[44] referenced in Table 1–3, is a validated tool to measure the result of extended voice use. The OMNI Vocal Effort Scale (OMNI-VES) is a validated 11-point equal interval scale with pictures and words to help the patient identify the level of vocal effort needed for a vocal task.[49] Throughout the cases in this text, the reader should note the choice of PROMs for different patient populations, how these tools inform treatment, and how they are used as outcome measures.

Auditory-Perceptual Assessment

The voice represents a collective picture of everything that must occur for sound to be made and shaped into meaningful units. The respiratory system or power source (the lungs), the phonatory system or sound system (the vocal folds), the resonatory system or filter (the vocal tract beginning just above the vocal folds to the lips), and the articulatory system (eg, lips, tongue, teeth, and palate) work in concert to generate sound and shape it into verbal communication. Verbal communication can be single sounds of acknowledgement; noises that indicate pain, distress, or happiness; or connected speech. No matter the final unit of communication to be heard and understood, verbal communication requires voice.

It has often been said that the clinician's assessment of the quality, flexibility, stability, loudness, and intelligibility of voice and speech is the gold standard of assessment over instrumental testing, as human perception is the true metric of communicative ability to effectively relay information. Prior to the 1990s, when instrumental assessments became more available to clinicians, the methods to assess voice were purely listening and rating the parameters of voice for their ability to produce near-normal effective communication. Today, perceptual measures continue to be paramount in the overall assessment of voice and upper airway disorders.

Many early tools to qualify the aberrant parameters of voice[50] were self-developed rating scales describing the voice with a variety of abstract phrases, such as "bacon frying in a pan" or a "stick gliding across a picket fence."[51] In 1981, Hirano described a more standardized assessment system whereby the clinician rated the voice quality on a 0–3 scale (0 being a voice without aberrant characteristics and 3 being the most severely aberrant voice quality) on the parameters of Grade (overall impairment), Roughness, Breathiness, Asthenia, and Strain.[52] The GRBAS is still used in many places today. However, the GRBAS has some limitations in that it only has a few severity options and only four aberrant parameters to rate. In 2002, the Consensus Auditory-Perceptual Evaluation of Voice (CAPE-V), a 100-mm visual analog scale for the auditory-perceptual assessment of voice by the clinician, was published. A consensus conference of experts including voice clinicians, voice scientists, and test development experts created the CAPE-V to provide a simple tool with 100 severity data points, a standard set of stimuli to assess voice quality, and several predetermined aberrant voice qualities like roughness and breathiness, as well as to allow the clinician to self-determine additional aberrant features, such as vocal tremor or spasm. The tool was revised and validated in 2009.[53] Most cases in this text use the CAPE-V as the tool of choice in the auditory-perceptual assessment of voice quality. The CAPE-V protocol is available for download at no cost on the ASHA website, and there are several references that describe the development, validation, and translation of the CAPE-V into other languages.

Voice quality is connected to the underlying physical impairments of the vocal mechanism, and the clinician can begin to develop hypotheses about laryngeal and respiratory function based on the sound of the voice. For example, a breathy voice is associated with glottal incompetence and a rough voice is related to aperiodicity of vocal fold vibration. However, instrumental assessment, specifically laryngeal imaging, is necessary to determine a reason for those phenomena, eg, what is causing the glottal incompetence or aperiodic vibration? A variety of instrumental assessments will be discussed later in this chapter.

In upper airway disorders, two other aberrant perceptual characteristics are important to describe: cough and breathing. The clinician should assess both cough strength and frequency, as well as any signs/symptoms/complaints of respiratory diseases. To assess cough, the clinician can observe spontaneous coughing or ask the patient to cough and throat clear. A strong cough is truly a lifesaving maneuver and is an indirect measure of the ability of the vocal folds to close and generate sufficient subglottal air pressure to support effective airway clearance of unwanted food, mucus, saliva, or any foreign object. Vocal fold paralysis, paresis, overall frailty, and underlying respiratory diseases can impair the strength of a cough, which can in turn impair pulmonary clearance. If accompanied by dysphagia of the pharyngeal stage of the swallow, this can lead to aspiration pneumonia. Noting the quality of the cough is also essential, ie, productive or wet versus nonproductive or dry. Often, a productive cough is connected to acute illness or underlying pulmonary disease, which warrant further physician workup. Regardless of cough quality, it is standard for the *physician* to order a chest x-ray in cases of chronic cough (cough lasting greater than 8 weeks).

The sound of respiratory difficulties and complaints of dyspnea (shortness of breath) with exertion, at rest, or with speaking should be noted in any voice and upper airway assessment. Dyspnea with speaking can be a sign of glottal incompetence with increased loss of air at the vocal folds due to incomplete closure of the vocal folds during each cycle of vibration. Aerodynamic assessment, discussed later in this chapter, can quantify this increased mean airflow rate. Dyspnea with exertion can be a sign of respiratory diseases like asthma. However, there are two laryngocentric respiratory disorders that are often misdiagnosed as asthma, and it is important to be aware of these conditions: (1) ILO and EILO caused by adduction of the vocal folds during inspiration and (2) posterior glottal stenosis (PGS) (vocal folds prevented from fully abducting) and subglottal stenosis (SGS) or tracheal stenosis, a narrowing at the subglottis or trachea,

respectively. Both ILO/EILO and stenosis of the upper airway can be associated with inspiratory stridor. Note: it is important to differentiate inspiratory stridor from expiratory wheeze, which is characteristic of asthma. Inspiratory stridor can be episodic, as in the case of ILO and EILO, or it can be more chronic, as in some cases of static airway narrowing. Prolonged intubation, autoimmune disorders, traumatic intubation, inhalation injuries, and even idiopathic causes have been linked to PGS, SGS, and tracheal stenosis. As discussed earlier, assessment for the cause of dyspnea/stridor/wheezing or breathy phonation with short phrases should be assessed in the physician's medical examination. However, if the SLP notes any of these symptoms or if the patient complains of dyspnea and it is not addressed in the medical note shared with the SLP, it is important to follow up on the symptoms, query when it happens, and share that information with the referring physician.

Visual-Perceptual Assessment

Visual observation of the patient provides valuable insight for the assessment of a voice and upper airway disorder. When watching the patient walk into the exam room, observe for signs of neurological impairment such as problems with balance or stability. When talking with the patient, observe their face for ptosis, symmetry of their smile, and drooling or difficulty with saliva management, as these are clues to an impairment of the peripheral nervous system. Observing tremor in the hands, head, or jaw, either at rest or when completing an action (eg, writing or reaching), can suggest a central neurological impairment. A slight head turn to one side or the other or chronic/tonic tension in the muscles of the neck and head may indicate cervical dystonia. Presence of any of these signs should be noted in the SLP's evaluation and warrant a referral to the neurologist.

For all patients, the SLP should also observe respiratory patterns. In the absence of pathology, many individuals demonstrate a pattern of abdominal-thoracic expansion on inhalation. Some may demonstrate a pattern primarily of thoracic expansion on inhalation. Notable engagement of the strap muscles, resulting in shoulder movement (ie, clavicular engagement), is inefficient and is sometimes seen in patients with voice and upper airway disorders. Sometimes, patients demonstrate rigidity of the abdomen or a paradoxical pattern of expansion on exhalation and abdominal engagement toward the spine on inhalation. Such abnormal breathing patterns can be the cause or a result of a voice or upper airway disorder and correcting these abnormal patterns may be treatment targets.

Cranial Nerve Examination

The cranial nerve assessment takes only moments and requires few tools to complete but can give the clinician insight into any underlying neurological or neuromuscular concerns that may be related to the patient's voice complaint. Table 1–4 lists 6 cranial nerves involved in voice and swallowing, with a quick guide to testing the nerves' viability. While some SLPs work side by side with a physician who completes the cranial nerve examination as part of their medical examination, not all do, and not all physicians adequately test the nerve or communicate that information with the SLP. We encourage the clinician to complete their own testing as part of the comprehensive voice and upper airway examination.

Motor Speech Assessment

Beyond the cranial nerve assessment, it is important for the clinician to assess for the possible presence of dysarthria or apraxia of speech as a sign of an underlying neurologic concern. A brief assessment of the symmetry, strength, speed, and coordination of the muscles used to produce speech can be incorporated into the comprehensive voice evaluation when any neurological compromise is suspected.[54] Dysarthria is characterized by speech abnormalities of speed, steadiness, range, or accuracy of movement with neurologic etiology, while apraxia of speech is characterized by impairment of motor planning or programming.[55] Most of the dysarthrias have imprecise articulation, aberrant rate of speech, and impaired diadochokinesis as cardinal signs of an underlying neuromuscular condition. Apraxia of speech can be characterized by consonant and vowel distortions, distorted substitutions, prolongations, and changes in rate of speech.[55]

Motor planning and coordination can be assessed through examining overall communication effectiveness or intelligibility, speaking rate, and diadochokinesis.[56] While testing rate of speech, or words per minute, is rarely discussed as an assessment modality in the voice and upper airway evaluation, examining words per minute (wpm) and the breakdown of words per minute over time can offer clues to neurologic impairment and serve as an outcome measure pre- and posttreatment. Words per minute can be measured in unfamiliar semantic contexts, such as in the long version of the Grandfather Passage,[57] a passage loaded with all the phonemes of the English language. The passage takes about 30 to 45 seconds to read on average, and having the patient read it through twice to obtain 1 full minute of reading is recommended. The expected average rate in reading is 183 wpm,[58] but older adults, children, second-language learners, and people with dystonia and tremor may be slower. While measuring speaking in conversation is a much more ecologically valid method to determine rate of speech, it requires transcribing minutes' worth of speaking, and it is thus, far more burdensome for the clinician. Determining speech deterioration over time can be achieved by prompting the patient to talk about a topic of their interest for 2 to 4 minutes. During this extemporaneous monologue, the clinician can assess for deterioration

14   Voice Therapy: Clinical Case Studies

Table 1–4. The Cranial Nerve Examination

Cranial Nerve	Primary Motor Function	Exam Tasks
CN V—Trigeminal	• Jaw opening, closing, lateralization	• Clench teeth (observe symmetry and palpate for symmetrical muscle bulk) • Open and close mouth (observe symmetry) • Open/close jaw against resistance
CN VII—Facial	• Lips • Cheeks • Upper face (bilateral UMN innervation) • Lower face (contralateral UMN innervation)	• Observe for symmetry and drooling (labial seal) • Show teeth (smile) and pucker • Puff cheeks (labial seal) • Raise eyebrows (wrinkle forehead) • Close eyes tightly
CN IX—Glossopharyngeal	• Stylopharyngeus • Sensory information for pharynx and tongue	• Elevate pharynx/larynx during swallowing • Gag reflex
CN X—Vagus	• Larynx • Pharynx • Soft palate (velum)	• Listen for weak or breathy voice quality, weak voluntary cough, pitch control • Palatal elevation during sustained vowel; listen for hypernasality
CN XI—Accessory	• Sternocleidomastoid • Trapezius muscles	• Rotate head against resistance • Shrug shoulders against resistance
CN XII—Hypoglossal	• Tongue movement	• Observe for asymmetries, atrophy, fasciculations • Protrude, retract, raise, lower, lateralize tongue

of speech rate, voice quality, and overall speech intelligibility over time.[20]

Alternate motion rate (AMR) and sequential motion rate (SMR) testing are diadochokinetic tasks used to measure the speed, precision, and coordination of the speech musculature. AMR tasks include quickly repeated syllables such as /pʌ/, /tʌ/, and /kʌ/, while SMR tasks involve sequencing, eg, /pʌtʌkʌ/, generally produced in a fixed period of time for measurement, eg, the clinician counts the number of productions of an AMR or an

SMR in 5 seconds. While age and cognition can impact the overall speed and precision of the task, it is generally assumed that adults are able to produce 5 to 6 repetitions of an AMR in 5 seconds.[59] Kent et al (2022)[60] describe a method to characterize productions beyond simple counting:

0 = all productions in a sample were inaccurate and not consistent, or unable to compete the task

1 = poor accuracy and consistency, with articulation errors ≥7

2 = medium accuracy and consistency, with articulation errors ≥4 and ≤6

3 = good accuracy and consistency, with articulation errors ≤3

4 = accurate and consistent productions of all targets, with flawless performance

Laryngeal diadochokinesis is a generally lesser-known task and involves the use of rapid repetition of /ʔʌ/ and /hʌ/ to assess adductory and abductory vocal fold movements, respectively. Completion of these tasks offers insight into laryngeal neuromotor function, and there are norms for ages 20 to 80 years. Most adults without neurologic impairment can produce about 5 repetitions of the task in 5 seconds, with advanced age yielding a slightly slower rate of repetition.[61]

Testing for Laryngeal Dystonia and Vocal Tremor

Laryngeal dystonia and vocal tremor are two voice disorders that are classified as motor speech disorders. Diagnosis of laryngeal dystonia is primarily auditory-perceptual and accomplished by assessing the production of phonemically loaded sentences, counting, sustained vowels and conversation, changing pitch and loudness in voiced tasks, and finally vegetative voice sounds. Vocal tremor can be similarly assessed through auditory perception, but tremor can also be visually assessed on laryngeal exam. Table 1–5 lists the phonemically loaded sentences often used to differentiate adductor and abductor laryngeal dystonia.[62] People with adductor type laryngeal dystonia will experience greater vocal effort with adductor laryngeal spasms in all-voiced contexts, while individuals with abductor type laryngeal dystonia will experience more vocal effort and demonstrate breathy voice breaks in contexts with voiceless phonemes, particularly when moving from a voiceless to a voiced

Table 1–5. Phonemically Loaded Sentences for Differential Diagnosis of Laryngeal Dystonia

Voiced Phoneme Phrases: Assessing for Adductor Laryngeal Dystonia	*Voiceless Phoneme Phrases: Assessing for Abductor Laryngeal Dystonia*
The dog dug a new bone.	Sam usually takes coffee with sugar.
We mow our lawn all year.	Put the cookies in the tin.
The waves were rolling along.	Keep Tom at the party.
We rode along Rhode Island Avenue.	Peter will keep at the peak.
Early one morning a man and a woman were ambling along Rainy Island Ave.	He saw half a shape mystically cross 50 or 60 steps in front of his sister Kathy's house.

phoneme, eg, "Peter." Additional speech tasks to assist with differential diagnosis include:

1. Counting from 60 to 65 and 80 to 85, with people with adductor laryngeal dystonia demonstrating more difficulty with counting from 80 to 85 and people with abductor laryngeal dystonia having more trouble with 60 to 65.
2. Changing pitch and increasing loudness may, in some cases, produce a temporary improvement in voice quality. This is because of "geste antagoniste," a sensory trick that temporarily reduces the impact of dystonia.
3. Whispering should eliminate the impact of the dystonia, while loud talking may improve abductor type laryngeal dystonia and increase the vocal spasms in adductor type laryngeal dystonia. However, it may not be as simple as this—sometimes louder talking can cause abductor laryngeal dystonia voice to worsen or cause adductor laryngeal dystonia voice to improve in quality with reduced spasms.
4. Vegetative tasks like coughing and throat clearing should result in a normal sound. Laughter is often more normal than connected speech.
5. Higher pitch in falsetto register can reduce adductor spasms in adductor laryngeal dystonia, as there is less engagement of the adductor muscles and more engagement of the cricothyroid muscles.

Sustained phonation of a vowel is a useful task that amplifies the presence of vocal tremor in the voice. Asking the patient to produce a vowel at a comfortable pitch and conversational loudness allows the clinician to perceive the rhythmic oscillations of the sound due to neurologically based tremor in one or more of the vocal tract structures (palate, pharynx, supraglottis, and/or vocal folds). However, the severity of vocal tremor should also be assessed in running speech by having the patient read aloud and engage in a short conversation about a topic familiar to them (avoid the stress of unfamiliar topics that can increase the severity of the tremor). The Voice Tremor Scoring System (VTSS) is a validated tool that can be used during laryngeal imaging to document the site of tremor and severity of vocal tremor in the vocal mechanism (palate, base of tongue, pharyngeal walls, supraglottis, and vocal folds).[63]

The SLP has a long history of helping identify motor speech disorders and, for many years prior to the use of MRI, neurologists relied on the SLP's assessment of communication symptoms to determine the location of the lesion in the brain and the type of dysarthria.[64] Table 1–6 lists the types of dysarthria and their signs and symptoms.[55] Further reading of dedicated motor speech texts is recommended for more in-depth education on dysarthria and apraxia of speech and their causes, treatments, and prognoses as related to treatment modalities.

Manual Assessment

Manual palpation of the paralaryngeal musculature, or "strap" muscles, is another essential piece of the voice and upper airway assessment. Many voice disorders are believed to be related to a muscular imbalance in these muscles as either a primary cause of the dysphonia or secondary cause in the presence of an organic impairment. Secondary muscle tension is believed to be caused by the need for extra muscular effort to sustain phonation when a primary voice pathology is present, such as in glottic insufficiency, loss of vocal fold pliability, or presence of vocal fold lesions. Pain, tenderness, and generalized discomfort in the thyrohyoid space or in the neck itself are frequent complaints because of strap muscle tension. Identifying the level of pain/discomfort/tenderness and the location is pivotal for treatment.

Table 1–6. Types of Dysarthria, Sites of Impairment, Associated Conditions, Signs/Symptoms

Type of Dysarthria	Anatomic Site of Impairment	Associated Conditions (Nonexhaustive)	Signs and Symptoms (Nonexhaustive)
Flaccid	Lower motor neuron	Degenerative diseases (eg, motor neuron disease); iatrogenic (eg, surgical injury); tumors	Dependent on site of LMN damage and can be quite isolated; weakness, atrophy, fasciculations, imprecise articulation, slow rate of speech, hypernasality, reduced range of motion, facial droop
Spastic	Upper motor neuron	Stroke, cerebral palsy, pseudobulbar palsy, primary lateral sclerosis	Dependent on site of UMN damage (eg, pyramidal, extrapyramidal); multiple sites of speech deficit due to UMN involvement, slow rate of speech, hypernasality, imprecise articulation, strained/strangled quality to voice, excess and equal stress during running speech, monopitch and monoloudness
Ataxic	Cerebellar control circuit	Stroke, cerebellar degeneration, TBI, tumor	Slow rate of speech, excess and equal stress, imprecise consonants, distorted vowels, irregular articulatory breakdowns
Hypokinetic	Basal ganglia control circuit	Parkinson's disease, progressive supranuclear palsy	"Blurred" speech AMRs, increased rate of speech and/or short rushes of speech, monopitch, reduced loudness, inappropriate silences
Hyperkinetic	Basal ganglia control circuit	Laryngeal dystonia, essential voice tremor, oromandibular dystonia, tardive dyskinesia	Abnormal and involuntary movements, myoclonus, strained/strangled voice, distorted vowels, variable speech rate and loudness, irregular articulatory breakdowns
Unilateral Upper Motor Neuron	Upper motor neuron	Stroke, iatrogenic (eg, surgical), CNS lesion	Imprecise articulation, slow rate, unilateral lower face weakness
Mixed	Mixed	Amyotrophic lateral sclerosis, multiple system atrophy, multiple strokes	Any combination of symptoms seen in the other dysarthrias

The Laryngeal Palpation Pain Scale (LPPS) is one of the few validated assessment tools for laryngeal palpation.[65] The LPPS identifies 13 areas bilaterally over the larynx to palpate and rate on a 10-point scale. As manual therapy has become more and more popular over the past decade as a treatment for extralaryngeal muscle tension,[66] it is important to document site and degree of tension and pain, both at the evaluation as a baseline measure and then following therapy to document improvement. Throughout the cases in this text, you will see a variety of methods used to quantify and qualify sites of tension and discomfort.

Instrumental Assessment

The instrumental assessment of voice and upper airway contains three primary component parts: (1) laryngeal imaging using diagnostic laryngoscopy for airway and videostroboscopy for voice, (2) acoustic assessment of the voice, and (3) aerodynamic assessment of voice and upper airway. The *Recommended Protocols for Instrumental Assessment of Voice: American Speech- Language-Hearing Association Expert Panel to Develop a Protocol for Instrumental Assessment of Vocal Function*[67] in the *American Journal of Speech-Language Pathology*, a journal available to all SLPs who are members of ASHA, is a comprehensive tutorial with recommended protocols for all three instrumental assessments of the voice and upper airway. For any clinician completing voice and upper airway evaluations, it is prudent to be familiar with these consensus guidelines.

Laryngeal Imaging

Laryngeal imaging is a critical component of the comprehensive voice assessment and should be completed in conjunction with the referring physician, an otolaryngologist or laryngologist. For the purposes of this discussion, the reader should assume that a knowledge-able and skilled SLP with expertise in endoscopic examination of the vocal mechanism will complete the videostroboscopy on the referral of a physician and in conjunction with an otolaryngologist/laryngologist for diagnosis of laryngeal or upper airway disease.

Mastering the technical components of completing the laryngeal examination is key to obtaining a clear image of the vocal folds from anterior commissure to the respiratory glottis (posterior to the vocal processes). The image should be centered to avoid the visual misperception of size or motion differences (due to a skewed image), sufficiently illuminated and magnified to allow for visualization of the fine details of the laryngeal mucosa, and comprehensive enough to give multiple examples of a variety of vocal tasks. The SLP is encouraged to develop a standard protocol for both the rigid and flexible examinations so that repeated examinations can easily be played side by side and compared for changes.

Selecting the most appropriate scope, rigid or flexible, is also important for obtaining relevant clinical information. When it is most important to assess the vocal fold mucosa, such as when suspicion for benign vocal fold lesions or changes in vocal fold pliability are suspected based on case history and perceptual evaluation, then a rigid scope typically offers a closer, clearer picture. The following tasks are recommended at a minimum for laryngeal videostroboscopy with a rigid scope: sustained vowels at modal pitch (typically /i/), high and low pitch, soft and loud phonation, and inhalation phonation when possible. The clinician should view the valleculae, pyriform sinuses, epiglottis and, if possible, the infraglottis/subglottis during complete abduction. When it is important to assess vocal fold motion or phonation during connected speech, singing, or even wind instrument playing or during all airway evaluations, the flexible scope offers the opportunity to view phonation in contexts beyond sustained vowels and is typically a more appropriate choice.[68] The following items and tasks are recommended for laryngeal videostroboscopy with a flexible scope:

1. View the nasal cavity and the soft palate at rest and in action while the patient repeats "kit-kat," while holding their breath, and while sustaining vowels, especially if any hypernasality is identified when speaking with the patient prior to the examination
2. View the symmetry and structure of the pharyngeal walls at rest and when saying /wi/ at high pitch to observe symmetry of pharyngeal contraction
3. Observe the valleculae, base of tongue, and the pyriform sinuses bilaterally
4. Observe the larynx and subglottis during rest breathing
5. Observe the motion of the vocal folds during repeated sniff /i/ alterations
6. Observe vocal fold vibration during sustained vowels at modal pitch, high and low pitch, soft and loud phonation, and inhalation phonation.

The clinician should describe vocal fold motion (abduction/adduction), contour of the vocal fold free edge, supraglottic activity, and vibratory parameters seen only on videostroboscopy, including glottal closure, mucosal wave, phase symmetry, amplitude of lateral excursion, periodicity, and any focal areas of stiffness. Describing the vibratory parameters is essential to understanding the integrity of structures for phonation, and these parameters must also be documented for billing/reimbursement purposes. Clinicians may use informal or published rating systems. Poburka and colleagues (2017) published a validated rating tool, the Voice-Vibratory Assessment With Laryngeal Imaging (VALI), that has clinician-friendly ratings, descriptors, images, and a comprehensive assessment of all videostroboscopy parameters.[69] Many cases in this text utilize the VALI to describe the laryngeal imaging results. No matter the tool used, when assessing videostroboscopy for purposes of voice, the clinician should comment on each vocal fold independently, ie, right side and left side, and should include all the parameters described in Table 1–7, in addition to documentation of any lesions observed anywhere in the vocal tract and the color of the vocal fold mucosa.

Laryngeal imaging is also an important component of the upper airway evaluation. Often, dysphonia co-occurs with complaints of dyspnea and/or chronic cough. If dysphonia is a concern, the examination should include videostroboscopy. If the clinician does not perceive dysphonia *and* the patient does not have any complaints of dysphonia, videostroboscopy may not be necessary. The complaint of episodic dyspnea with exercise/exertion or with other triggers mandates the clinician's attempt to observe the larynx and vocal fold movement during an episode to visualize the aberrant airway diameter. A newer technique that has gained popularity is called continuous laryngoscopy with exercise (CLE).[70] During CLE, the patient is generally exercising on a recumbent bike or treadmill while the larynx is simultaneously visualized with a flexible endoscope and the patient is being monitored for any drop in oxygen saturation. In some centers, the patient is also monitored for cardiopulmonary fitness at the same time as the CLE. During the examination, the larynx is first visualized at rest to assess for complete adduction and abduction during inspiration and, if possible, a view of the subglottis is obtained to determine presence of SGS. The patient then begins exercising at a slow speed and low exertion level before gradually increasing the degree of exercise, whether through increased speed or increased incline/resistance or both, while the examiner continues to observe the larynx during inspiration and expiration. Oxygen saturation is monitored for any drops that might indicate a cardiopulmonary problem, and an immediate referral to cardiology/pulmonology can be made as needed. The patient is

Table 1–7. Stroboscopic Parameters That Should Be Rated in Any Videostroboscopic Assessment

Stroboscopic Parameter	Descriptor	VALI Rating
Glottal Closure	The shape of the glottis (space between the vocal folds) during the most closed phase of the vibratory cycle	Rated at normal pitch and loudness: complete, anterior gap, posterior gap, hourglass, spindle gap, irregular, and incomplete
Amplitude	Magnitude of lateral movement of the free edge of the vocal fold during the open phase of the vibratory cycle	Rate both right vocal fold and left vocal fold independently. Rated as percent 0%-100%.
Mucosal Wave	Magnitude of lateral movement of the vocal fold mucosa (epithelial layer and superficial lamina propria) during the vibratory cycle	Rate both right vocal fold and left vocal fold independently. Rated as percent 0%-100%.
Nonvibrating Portion	Any areas on the vocal fold surface that appear stiff, adynamic, or nonvibratory	Rate both right vocal fold and left vocal fold independently. Rated as percent 0%-100%. There are 10 ovals on each vocal fold that represent 10% of the vocal fold.
Supraglottic Activity	Indication of any muscle tension or constriction of tissue above the vocal folds, which may obscure visualization of the vocal folds	Rate in the anteroposterior and mediolateral planes. Rated on a 0-5 scale with 0 being "full visualization" and 5 being "nearly complete obscured visualization" of the vocal folds at rest and/or during phonation. Comment on when rating and if anteroposterior or mediolateral.
Free Edge Contour	The straightness of the free edge of the vocal fold	Rate both right vocal fold and left vocal fold independently. Rated as normal, convex, concave, irregular, or rough.
Vertical Level of Approximation	The vertical alignment of the vocal folds during the closed phase of the vibratory cycle	Rated as on-plane, off-plane left lower, or off-plane right lower
Phase Closure	A cycle of vocal fold vibration in modal pitch is marked by opening phase, open phase, closing phase, and closed phase, with each phase nearly equal	Rate globally as to what phase predominates most of the cycles of vibration. Rated as nearly equal, open phase predominates, or closed phase predominates.

Table 1–7. *continued*

Stroboscopic Parameter	Descriptor	VALI Rating
Phase Symmetry	The extent to which the left and right vocal folds vibrate as mirror (opposite) images of each other, ie, if the right vocal fold is opening, the left vocal fold should be opening at the same point in the cycle	Globally rate the percent of time the vocal folds are moving at the same place in the cycle from 100% (symmetrical)-0% (asymmetrical)
Regularity	The consistency of each cycle of vibration or periodicity	Rate globally and as a percent of the time that vocal fold vibration is visible with good stroboscopic tracking. When the vocal fold cycles are not regular, the image will be blurred, and the rater will not be able to visualize the mucosal wave.

asked to indicate when they begin to feel dyspneic, and the larynx is observed for reduced abduction during inspiration that might indicate EILO.

If the complaint of dyspnea is associated with fragrance triggers like perfumes, cleaning products, or smoke, a similar flexible laryngeal examination should be completed, first examining the larynx without the triggers, then exposing patients to subtle scents when possible. It is important prior to completing this examination or CLE that there are safety measures in place that might include medical intervention if needed and, at minimum, teaching the patient rescue breathing techniques to use during the examination to stop the aberrant laryngeal postures interfering with inhalation and the sense of dyspnea.

Acoustic Assessment

Acoustic assessments are generally gathered to help quantify the perceptual characteristics of the voice perceived by the examiner. Recommended as important reading in an earlier section, the *Recommended Protocols for Instrumental Assessment of Voice: American Speech-Language-Hearing Association Expert Panel to Develop a Protocol for Instrumental Assessment of Vocal Function*[67] in the *American Journal of Speech-Language Pathology* provides a comprehensive tutorial on current thinking in the use of acoustic assessment of voice. There is some controversy about the various tools to use when instrumentally assessing the acoustics of sound production, and voice centers in Europe, Latin America, and the United States use different methods. For the purposes of this text, we will discuss the importance of standardizing the acoustic assessment, accepted instrumental tests at the time of this writing in 2025, and some less expensive alternatives for those who do not have the clinical budgets for higher-tech instrumentation.

Currently, the following acoustic measures have gained consensus for use as core measures in voice evaluation:[67]

1. Conversational loudness; loud voice and softest voice (not in a whisper) with

calculated intensity range of phonation measured in dB SPL

2. Speaking fundamental frequency measured in Hz
3. Standard deviation of speaking fundamental frequency measured in Hz
4. Physiologic frequency range of phonation measured as highest frequency of voice and lowest frequency of voice, not including vocal fry, measured in Hz
5. Cepstral peak prominence (CPP) measured in dB

Instrumentation to acquire this information ranges from more expensive, user-friendly systems to less expensive but perhaps more user-intensive. The more expensive systems typically include all of the necessary hardware and software to acquire the data, rapidly process it, and produce analysis reports. Less expensive systems are valid and reliable but may require more work to analyze the acoustic signal. However, this can also allow for greater flexibility in the methods used to analyze the signal, which is sometimes desired, especially by researchers. It is important to note that many of these systems require the user to purchase a laptop or desktop computer to run the programs, as well as a microphone and amplifier. The clinician with a less robust budget for acoustic analysis may want to investigate any of the following options available at the time of publication:

1. Pratt (https://www.fon.hum.uva.nl/praat/): Free software
   a. Phonanium (https://www.phonanium.com/): Software and training
2. Voice EvalU8 (https://mobilevoiceapps.com/voiceevalu8): Yearly subscription, run on iOS devices
3. A sound level meter with a C-weighting meeting ANSI standards, which can be used for measuring vocal intensity

No matter the system used to acquire the signal to be analyzed, it is imperative that the clinician standardize the method of signal acquisition. This includes:

1. A quiet room should be secured with attention to acoustic integrity for data acquisition. The clinician should measure the noise floor prior to data acquisition to ensure that the noise level in the room is at least 10 dB SPL lower than the quietest sound to be gathered. Air conditioning units, fluorescent lights, and noise from outside the room can all interfere with data acquisition.
2. The microphone should always be the same distance from the mouth—4 to 10 cm away at a 45- to 90-degree angle. A head-mounted omnidirectional microphone is preferred to maintain a standard distance, but a handheld microphone on a stand can also be used.
3. The same reading passages should be used for each task and directions standardized to ensure the patient comprehends the expected voice production.

Aerodynamic Assessment

Aerodynamic assessment is a noninvasive method of estimating vocal fold integrity for voice and cough production through surrogate measures. In other words, we assess airflow at the level of the mouth rather than airflow at the level of the larynx, and we use these measures to infer information about glottal closure. When mean airflow through the glottis is increased, we suspect that glottal closure is not complete and/or that the open phase predominates. Similarly, subglottal pressure, the force used to set the vocal folds into vibration, is estimated from pressure at the lips and used to infer information about vocal fold vibration. A measure of true subglottal pressure can be achieved with a tracheal puncture, but this is invasive, not within the scope of practice for the SLP, unpleasant for the patient, and unnecessary when oral pressures can be used to accurately estimate subglottal pressure. Estimated subglottal pressure is collected during repeated productions of the syllable /pi/. The occlusion for /p/ generates a stable pressure in the vocal tract, measured in cmH_2O, while the opening for the /i/ vowel brings the pressure back to 0 cmH_2O (since the vocal tract is open). In this way, the pressure peaks for /p/ can be measured. Increased subglottal pressure is related to increased perception of vocal effort and can be indicative of issues with vocal fold vibration, such as loss of pliability or a mass effect from a lesion. Stiff vocal folds require more force to be set into vibration, and this can be seen as increased subglottal pressure.

Contrary to acoustic assessment, aerodynamic measures require more advanced technology. Measures such as mean airflow rate and subglottal pressure require a pneumotachograph with a facemask. The most commonly used clinical system is the Phonatory Aerodynamic System (PAS) by Pentax. Some measures can be obtained using a portable spirometer, including vital capacity, phonation quotient (PQ), FEV1/FVC for the presence of asthma, and flow volume loops for the presence of ILO or EILO. FEV1/FVC is a ratio of the forced expiratory volume in 1 second (FEV1) to the forced vital capacity (FVC). While clinicians can be trained in using portable spirometers for these measures, it is imperative that the clinician also be trained to interpret the readings and practice only within their scope (ie, the SLP does not diagnose respiratory conditions). Alternatively, most hospitals are equipped to complete PFTs in a pulmonary lab, which is noninvasive and quickly acquired for a relatively low cost. The clinician may want to work with the pulmonary functions lab at their institution to gather this information. Measures of s/z ratio and maximum phonation time (MPT) are not instrumental assessments of phonatory aerodynamics or pulmonary function, and should not be used as such, though they may be used for other purposes.[71] Joshi (2020) found little agreement between s/z ratio and instrumental assessment of airflows, capacities, and pressures.[72] Johnson and Goldfine (2016) found significant variability across MPT trials and, like previous studies, found that MPT is not a reliable measure of phonatory airflow.[73] While the editors have read of clinicians using these measures as surrogates for aerodynamic assessment, their lack of validity and accuracy negate their use in this context.

Peak flow or peak expiratory flow is the measurement of how fast and forcefully one can expel all the air in the lungs. It has been used as a noninvasive assessment of airway status in asthmatics and more recently has been used in dysphagia to measure cough strength, known as peak cough flow. In peak flow measurements, a peak flow meter paired with a one-way single use valve is used to measure the strength and velocity of expired air by asking the patient to take a deep breath and blow as hard and fast as possible 3 times. The highest measure is used to indicate that day's maximum peak flow. In cough peak flow, the patient is asked to engage in the same deep inhalation, but this time, the patient is asked to cough as hard and fast as possible into the peak flow meter. Peak flow meters are also gaining more notoriety in measuring change in the treatment of SGS and PGS with surgical intervention or serial steroid injections. In either case, this simple noninvasive task can differentiate changes in glottal closure.[74]

Stimulability

Voice stimulability testing is a practice in which the clinician uses a series of demonstrations, cues, or therapeutic strategies to assess an individual's ability to change the sound and/ or feel of their voice, as well as their awareness of any changes. General stimulability testing is used across subspecialties within the speech-language pathology field, and the concept of testing an individual's potential for change dates back at least to the 1930s in a text by pioneer speech pathologist Lee Edward Travis (as cited in Powell & Miccio, 1996).[75] In the voice and upper airway subspecialty, clinicians widely agree that stimulability testing should be included in the comprehensive evaluation to assess patient awareness, inform prognosis, and identify potential training gestures.[76] However, the content of such testing is not well-defined. Most clinicians will trial elements of resonant voice therapy (eg, hums or sustained fricatives) or semi-occluded vocal tract exercises (eg, lip trills, straw phonation),[76] in addition to other tasks dependent on the patient in front of them. Stimulability testing with cues for "clear speech" with "crisp, clear consonants" and pitch inflection, as used in Conversation Training Therapy, has been shown to yield changes in the sound or feel of the voice in many patients.[77] The results of stimulability testing can directly influence which voice therapy techniques may be successfully utilized in therapy.[78]

Documentation

The adage "If it isn't documented, it wasn't done" applies in the medical field. Documentation can be a time-intensive task for any SLP. This text aims to support the reader in augmenting their documentation skill by providing 60 examples of documentation for the voice and upper airway evaluation. Each case in this text begins with a sample evaluation document, and all cases follow a similar format with slight variations at the discretion of the authors, reflective of their typical clinical flow. For further guidance on documentation requirements to meet CMS and other insurance standards, the reader is guided to ASHA resources, including a 2008 document titled *Documentation That Works*.[79] At the time of writing this edition of the text, AI-generated documentation is beginning to be tested to reduce clinician burden and improve accuracy and consistency of clinician documentation. While some health systems have begun to implement AI documentation, there is not a universally available HIPAA-compliant AI documentation system at this time, so the use of AI-generated documents is not presented in this edition.

Conclusions

The voice and upper airway evaluation offers the clinician the benefit of time for observation and perceptual assessment paired with instrumental assessment. In sum, the comprehensive evaluation allows the SLP to form a hypothesis regarding the cause and potential treatments for the voice and upper airway disorder. Chapter 2 guides the reader through the process of clinical decision making. The evaluation is the initial step toward developing a strong treatment plan, but using the information gleaned from the evaluation to craft an actionable plan is what we refer to as clinical decision making, and this completes the comprehensive assessment of voice and upper airway.

In this text, we have asked all 60+ contributors to start their cases with a voice or upper airway evaluation that is written as a medical document. This offers the reader an opportunity to develop their *own* hypotheses about the cause of the problem and potential care of the patient based on the expert evaluation. Subsequently, the reader is guided through the master clinician's decision making, taken through the actual treatment steps, and provided the outcomes of treatment. The reader is encouraged to reflect on their own thoughts compared to the master clinician as a learning opportunity. In all cases presented in this text and in life, the intersection of communication science and art of human interaction offers more than one evidence-based way to approach a clinical problem.

References

1. Boone DR. A historical perspective of voice management: 1940-1970. *Perspect Voice Voice Disord.* 2010;20(2):47-55. doi:10.1044/vvd20.2.47
2. Fairbanks G. *Voice and Articulation Drillbook.* Harper & Row Press; 1940.
3. Van Riper C. *Voice and Articulation.* Prentice Hall; 1957.
4. Moore G. Vocal fold movement during vocalization. *Speech Monogr.* 1937;4:44-55.
5. Brown WS, Hicks DM, Murry T. In memoriam: G. Paul Moore, Ph.D. *J Voice.* 2008;22(3):257. doi:10.1016/j.jvoice.2008.04.001
6. Von Leden H. Pioneers in the evolution of voice care and voice science in the United States of America. *J Voice.* 1990;4(2):99-106.
7. Christopher K, Wood R, Eckert C, Blager F, Raney R, Souhrada J. Vocal-cord dysfunction presenting as asthma. *N Engl J Med.* 1983;308(26):1566-1570.
8. Smitheran JR, Hixon TJ. A clinical method for estimating laryngeal airway resistance during vowel production. *J Speech Hear Disord.* 1981:138-147.
9. Hixon T, Smitheran J. A reply to Rothenberg. *J Speech Hear Disord.* 1981;47:220-223. doi:10.1044/jshd.4702.220
10. Rosen CA, Murry T. Diagnostic laryngeal endoscopy. *Otolaryngol Clin North Am.* 2000;33(4):751-757.
11. Casiano R, Zaveri V, Lundy D. Efficacy of videostroboscopy in the diagnosis of voice disorders. *Otolaryngol Head Neck Surg.* 1992;107(1):95-100.
12. Boone DR. Expanding perspectives in care of the speaking voice. *J Voice.* 1991;5(2):168-172. doi:10.1016/S0892-1997(05)80180-8
13. Titze IR. Acoustic interpretation of resonant voice. *J Voice.* 2001;15(4):519-528.
14. Verdolini K. Resonant voice therapy. In: Stemple J, ed. *Voice Therapy: Clinical Studies.* 2nd ed. Singular Publishing; 2000:46-62.
15. Blager FB. Paradoxical vocal fold movement: Diagnosis and management. *Curr Opin Otolaryngol Head Neck Surg.* 2000;8(3):180-183. doi:10.1097/00020840-200006000-00009
16. Halvorsen T, Walsted ES, Bucca C, et al. Inducible laryngeal obstruction: An official joint European Respiratory Society and European Laryngological Society statement. *Eur Respir J.* 2017;50(3). doi:10.1183/13993003.02221-2016
17. Sandage MJ, Morton-Jones ME, Hall-Landers RJ, Tucker JG. Treatment and outcome metrics for speech-language pathology treatment of upper airway disorders: A systematic review. *J Speech Lang Hear Res.* 2024;67(11):4391-4410. doi:10.1044/2024_JSLHR-24-00396
18. Gay M, Blager F, Bartsch K, Emery CF, Rosenstiel-Gross AK, Spears J. Psychogenic habit cough: Review and case reports. *J Clin Psychiatry.* 1987;48(12):483-486.
19. Vertigan A, Gibson P, Theodoros DG, Winkworth AL. The role of sensory dysfunction in the development of voice disorders, chronic cough and paradoxical vocal fold movement. *Int J Speech Lang Pathol.* 2008;10(4):231-244. doi:10.1080/17549500801932089
20. ASHA practice portal. American Speech-Language-Hearing Association. https://www.asha.org/practice-portal/
21. Stachler RJ, Francis DO, Schwartz SR, et al. Clinical practice guideline: Hoarseness (dysphonia) (update). *Otolaryngol Head Neck Surg.* 2018;158(suppl 2):S1-S42. doi:10.1177/0194599817751030
22. Hapner E, Portone-Maira C, Johns MM. A study of voice therapy dropout. *J Voice.* 2009;23(3):337-340. doi:10.1016/j.jvoice.2007.10.009
23. Rivers NJ, Maira C, Wise J, Hapner ER. The impact of referral source on voice therapy. *J Voice.* 2023;37(2):297.e7-297.e13. doi:10.1016/j.jvoice.2020.12.051
24. Gutierrez D, Simpson C, Hapner E. Exploring models of interprofessional voice care. Poster presented at: The Fall Voice Conference; 2022; San Francisco, CA.
25. Litts JK, Abaza MM. Does a multidisciplinary approach to voice and swallowing disorders improve therapy adherence and outcomes? *Laryngoscope.* 2017;127(11):2446. doi:10.1002/lary.26756
26. Starmer HM, Liu Z, Akst LM, Gourin C. Attendance in voice therapy: Can an interdisciplinary care model have an impact. *Ann Otol Rhinol Laryngol.* 2014;123(2):117-123. doi:10.1177/0003489414523708

27. Litts JK, Gartner-Schmidt JL, Clary MS, Gillespie AI. Impact of laryngologist and speech pathologist coassessment on outcomes and billing revenue. *Laryngoscope*. 2015;125(9):2139-2142. doi:10.1002/lary.25349

28. Garabedian M, Keltz A, Lerner MZ, Brackett A, Leydon C. Glottal insufficiency and Parkinson's disease: A scoping review of vocal fold medialization procedures. *J Voice*. 2024:1-14. doi:10.1016/j.jvoice.2024.09.034

29. Verdolini K, Rosen C, Branski R. *Classification Manual of Voice Disorders-I*. Lawrence Erlbaum; 2006.

30. Sulica L. Hoarseness misattributed to reflux: Sources and patterns of error. *Ann Otol Rhinol Laryngol*. 2014;123(6):442-445. doi:10.1177/0003489414527225

31. Todd Schneider G, Vaezi MF, Francis DO. Reflux and voice disorders: Have we established causality? *Curr Otorhinolaryngol Rep*. 2016;4(3):157-167. doi:10.1007/s40136-016-0121-5

32. Branski RC, Bhattacharyya N, Shapiro J. The reliability of the assessment of endoscopic laryngeal findings associated with laryngopharyngeal reflux disease. *Laryngoscope*. 2002;112(6):1019-1024. doi:10.1097/00005537-200206000-00016

33. Guyatt G, Schunemann H. How can quality of life researchers make their work more useful to health workers and their patients? *Qual Life Res*. 2007;16(7):1097-1105. doi:10.1007/s11136-007-9223-3

34. Francis DO, Daniero JJ, Hovis KL, et al. Voice-related patient-reported outcome measures: A systematic review of instrument development and validation. *J Speech Lang Hear Res*. 2017;60(January):62-88.

35. Jacobson BH, Johnson A, Grywalski C, et al. The Voice Handicap Index (VHI): Development and validation. *Am J Speech Lang Pathol*. 1997;6(3):66-69. doi:10.1044/1058-0360.0603.66

36. Rosen CA, Lee AS, Osborne J, Zullo T, Murry T. Development and validation of the Voice Handicap Index-10. *Laryngoscope*. 2004;114(9 I):1549-1556. doi:10.1097/00005537-200409000-00009

37. Hogikyan ND, Sethuraman G. Validation of an instrument to measure voice-related quality of life (V-RQOL). *J Voice*. 1999;13(4):557-569. doi:10.1016/S0892-1997(99)80010-1

38. Gartner-Schmidt JL, Shembel AC, Zullo TG, Rosen CA. Development and validation of the Dyspnea Index (DI): A severity index for upper airway-related dyspnea. *J Voice*. 2014;28(6):775-782. doi:10.1016/j.jvoice.2013.12.017

39. Shembel AC, Rosen CA, Zullo TG, Gartner-Schmidt JL. Development and validation of the Cough Severity Index: A severity index for chronic cough related to the upper airway. *Laryngoscope*. 2013;123(8):1931-1936. doi:10.1002/lary.23916

40. Baylor C, Yorkston K, Eadie T, Kim J, Chung H, Amtmann D. The Communicative Participation Item Bank (CPIB): Item bank calibration and development of a disorder-generic short form. *J Speech Lang Hear Res*. 2013;56(4):1190-1208. doi:10.1044/1092-4388(2012/12-0140)

41. Castro ME, Sund LT, Hoffman MR, Hapner ER. The Voice Problem Impact Scales (VPIS). *J Voice*. 2024;38(3):666-673. doi:10.1016/j.jvoice.2021.11.011

42. Cohen SM, Jacobson BH, Garrett CG, et al. Creation and validation of the Singing Voice Handicap Index. *Ann Otol Rhinol Laryngol*. 2007;116(6):402-406. doi:10.1177/000348940711600602

43. Cohen SM, Statham M, Rosen CA, Zullo T. Development and validation of the Singing Voice Handicap-10. *Laryngoscope*. 2009;119(9):1864-1869. doi:10.1002/lary.20580

44. Nanjundeswaran C, Jacobson BH, Gartner-Schmidt J, Verdolini Abbott K. Vocal Fatigue Index (VFI): Development and validation. *J Voice*. 2015;29(4):433-440. doi:10.1016/j.jvoice.2014.09.012

45. Bach K, Belafsky P, Wasylik K, Postma G, Koufman J. Validity and reliability of the Glottal Function Index. *Arch Otolaryngol Head Neck Surg*. 2005;131:961-964. doi:10.1016/j.jvoice.2024.04.004

46. Mathieson L. Vocal tract discomfort in hyperfunctional dysphonia. *J Voice*. 1993;2:40-48.

47. Solomon NP. Vocal fatigue and its relation to vocal hyperfunction. *Int J Speech Lang Pathol*. 2008;10(4):254-266. doi:10.1080/14417040701730990

48. Morton-Jones ME, Timmons Sund L, Castro ME, Hapner ER. Adult normative data for the OMNI-Vocal Effort Scale (VES). *Laryngoscope*. 2024;134(8):3726-3731. doi:10.10 02/lary.31464

49. Shoffel-Havakuk H, Marks KL, Morton M, Johns III MM, Hapner ER. Validation of the OMNI Vocal Effort Scale in the treatment of adductor spasmodic dysphonia. *Laryngoscope*. Published online October 12, 2018. doi:10.1002/lary.27430

50. Hammarberg B, Fritzell B, Gaufin J, Sundberg J, Wedin L. Perceptual and acoustic correlates of abnormal voice qualities. *Acta Otolaryngol*. 1980;90(1-6):441-451. doi:10.31 09/00016488009131746

51. Kreiman J, Gerratt BR. Sources of listener disagreement in voice quality assessment. *J Acoust Soc Am*. 2000;108(4):1867-1876. doi:10.1121/1.1289362

52. Hirano M. "GRBAS" scale for evaluating the hoarse voice & frequency range of phonation. *Clin Exam Voice*. 1981:83-84.

53. Kempster GB, Gerratt BR, Abbott KV, Barkmeier-Kraemer J, Hillman RE. Consensus Auditory-Perceptual Evaluation of Voice: Development of a standardized clinical protocol. *Am J Speech Lang Pathol*. 2009;18(2):124-132. doi:10.1044/1058-0360(2008/08-0017)

54. Sonies BC, Weiffenbach J, Atkinson JC, Brahim J, Macynski A, Fox PC. Clinical examination of motor and sensory functions of the adult oral cavity. *Dysphagia*. 1987;1(4):178-186. doi:10.1007/BF02406914

55. Duffy J, ed. *Motor Speech Disorders: Substrates, Differential Diagnosis, and Management*. 4th ed. Elsevier; 2019.

56. Yorkston K, Beukelman D. Communication efficiency of dysarthric speakers as measured by sentence intelligibility and speaking rate. *J Speech Hear Disord*. 1981;46(3):296-301.

57. Reilly J, Fisher JL. Sherlock Holmes and the strange case of the missing attribution: A historical note on "The Grandfather Passage." *J Speech Lang Hear Res*. 2012;55(1):84-88. doi:10.1044/1092-4388(2011/11-0158)

58. Brysbaert M. How many words do we read per minute? A review and meta-analysis of reading rate. *J Mem Lang*. 2019;109(August): 104047. doi:10.1016/j.jml.2019.104047

59. Lancheros M, Friedrichs D, Laganaro M. What do differences between alternating and sequential diadochokinetic tasks tell ts about the development of oromotor skills? An insight from childhood to adulthood. *Brain Sci*. 2023;13.

60. Kent RD, Kim Y, Chen LM. Oral and laryngeal diadochokinesis across the life span: A scoping review of methods, reference data, and clinical applications. *J Speech Lang Hear Res*. 2022;65(2):574-623. doi:10.1044/2021_jslhr-21-00396

61. Lombard L, Solomon NP. Laryngeal diadochokinesis across the adult lifespan. *J Voice*. 2020;34(5):651-656. doi:10.1016/j.jvoice.20 19.04.004

62. Cannito MP, Chorna LB, Kahane JC, Dworkin JP. Influence of consonant voicing characteristics on sentence production in abductor versus adductor spasmodic dysphonia. *J Voice*. 2014;28(3):394.e13-394.e22. doi:10.1016/j.jvoice.2013.10.010

63. Bové M, Daamen N, Rosen C, Wang CC, Sulica L, Gartner-Schmidt J. Development and validation of the Vocal Tremor Scoring System. *Laryngoscope*. 2006;116(9):1662-1667. doi:10.1097/01.mlg.0000233255.57 425.36

64. Darley FL, Aronson AE, Brown JR. Differential diagnostic patterns of dysarthria. *J Speech Hear Res*. 1969;12(2):246-269.

65. Tohidast SA, Mansuri B, Farzadi F, et al. Development and psychometric evaluation of the Laryngeal Palpation Pain Scale (LPPS). *J Voice*. 2023:1-10. doi:10.1016/j .jvoice.2023.09.025

66. Barsties V, Latoszek B, Watts CR, Hetjens S. The efficacy of the manual circumlaryngeal therapy for muscle tension dysphonia: A systematic review and meta-analysis. *Laryngoscope*. 2024;134(1):18-26. doi:10.1002/ lary.30850

67. Patel RR, Awan SN, Barkmeier-Kraemer J, et al. Recommended protocols for instrumental assessment of voice: ASHA expert panel to develop a protocol for instrumental assessment of vocal function. *Am J Speech Lang Pathol*. 2018:1-19.

68. Boles RW, Gao WZ, Johns MM, et al. Flexible versus rigid laryngoscopy: A prospective,

blinded comparison of image quality. *J Voice.* 2023;37(3):440-443. doi:10.1016/j.jvoice.2021.02.010

69. Poburka BJ, Patel RR, Bless DM. Voice-Vibratory Assessment With Laryngeal Imaging (VALI) form: Reliability of rating stroboscopy and high-speed videoendoscopy. *J Voice.* 2017;31(4):513.e1-513.e14. doi:10.1016/j.jvoice.2016.12.003

70. Heimdal J, Roksund O, Halvorsen T, Skadberg B, Olofsson J. Continuous laryngoscopy exercise test: A method for visualizing laryngeal dysfunction during exercise. *Laryngoscope.* 2009;116:52-57.

71. Gilman M. Revisiting sustained phonation time of /s/, /z/, and /ɑ/. *J Voice.* 2021; 35(6):935.e13-935.e18. doi:10.1016/j.jvoice.2020.03.012

72. Joshi A. A comparison of the s/z ratio to instrumental aerodynamic measures of phonation. *J Voice.* 2020;34(4):533-538. doi:10.1016/j.jvoice.2019.02.014

73. Johnson AM, Goldfine A. Intrasubject reliability of maximum phonation time. *J Voice.* 2016;30(6):775.e1-775.e4. doi:10.1016/j.jvoice.2015.11.019

74. Dion GR, Achlatis E, Teng S, et al. Changes in peak airflow measurement during maximal cough after vocal fold augmentation in patients with glottic insufficiency. *JAMA Otolaryngol Head Neck Surg.* 2017;143(11):1141-1145. doi:10.1001/jamaoto.2017.0976

75. Powell TW, Miccio AW. Stimulability: A useful clinical tool. *J Commun Disord.* 1996; 29(4):237-253. doi:10.1016/0021-9924(96)00012-3

76. Toles LE, Young ED. Understanding the use and importance of voice stimulability assessment among speech-language pathologists who treat voice disorders: An international survey. *J Voice.* Published online January 28, 2023. doi:10.1016/j.jvoice.2023.01.007

77. Gartner-Schmidt J, Gherson S, Hapner ER, et al. The development of conversation training therapy: A concept paper. *J Voice.* 2016;30(5):563-573. doi:10.1016/j.jvoice.2015.06.007

78. Shelly S, Rothenberger SD, Gartner-Schmidt J, Gillespie AI. Assessing candidacy for conversation training therapy: The role of patient perception. *J Voice.* 2023. doi:10.1016/j.jvoice.2023.02.008

79. Hapner ER. Documentation that works. *Perspect Voice Voice Disord.* 2008;18(1):33-42. doi:10.1044/vvd18.1.33

2

From Evaluation to Intervention

Decision Making in Voice Therapy

Edie R. Hapner and Lauren Timmons Sund

Is Voice Therapy an Appropriate Treatment for the Presenting Problem?

Voice clinicians must make a variety of evidence-based decisions when treating their patients. The most important decision that must be made when receiving a referral from a physician (or self-referral) is whether voice therapy is an appropriate treatment for the voice problem presented by the patient. This decision is driven by the multifactorial interplay of information obtained in the comprehensive voice evaluation, an overall understanding of laryngeal biomechanics and how medical interventions impact them, a grasp of wound healing, and knowledge of how various voice pathologies respond to therapy. To determine if you should recommend voice therapy, begin by considering the following:

1. Is the cause of the presenting problem something that can be resolved or improved with voice therapy?
2. If the goal of voice therapy is not to resolve a lesion or a behavior, is it perhaps for the purposes of conducting preoperative voice therapy to provide education about what to expect following surgery and how to utilize the voice in those important first weeks after surgery?
3. Perhaps the voice or upper airway disorder cannot be surgically or medically resolved. Is the goal of voice therapy to improve quality of life by optimizing communication using strategies for reducing vocal effort, increasing vocal endurance, or even improving room acoustics to aid communication? Is there a role for the speech-language pathologist (SLP) to help the patient adapt to a chronic condition through patient

education, counseling, and/or connection to appropriate support resources?

4. Perhaps the voice or upper airway disorder is also being treated medically. Is the goal of voice therapy to (1) work with medical/pharmaceutical therapies to optimize dosing or increase the duration between botulinum toxin injections in someone with laryngeal dystonia or voice tremor, (2) optimize vocal demands via patient education of Parkinson's disease (PD) drug maximum effect time, or (3) understand how neuromodulators/ superior laryngeal nerve injections may impact sensory neuropathic cough?

If the answer to any of these questions is yes, then the person is likely moving toward candidacy for voice therapy. SLPs are communication specialists, and the goal of any therapy provided by the SLP is to improve communication, whether through voice therapy alone or in conjunction with medical, surgical/procedural, or environmental interventions.

Answering the first decision-making question, whether the problem can be resolved or improved with voice therapy, requires familiarity with the cause and expected course of vocal fold lesions, neurological voice disorders, and upper airway disorders. The Classification Manual for Voice Disorders[1] is a valuable resource for learning about the plethora of vocal fold lesions, in addition to neurologically mediated voice disorders, disorders of the upper aerodigestive tract, and/or disorders associated with muscle tension imbalances. The only vocal fold lesions expected to fully recover from voice therapy are vocal nodules; however, voice therapy can be useful in reducing the size and impact of some other lesions, such as granulomas and vocal fold polyps. Medicine continues to evolve and, as such, our knowledge of vocal fold pathologies continues to grow. One example of this is the evolution of our understanding of vocal fold cysts and polyps.[2,3] Historically, the presence of a cyst or a polyp necessitated surgery. However, both studies cited demonstrate that there is a possibility of change in size of the cyst (14%) or the smaller hemorrhagic polyp (56%) that might reduce the need for surgical intervention. Regarding neurological conditions, voice therapy does not cure progressive neurological disorders like PD or movement disorders such as essential voice tremor and laryngeal dystonia, but overall voice and communication function can be improved to a variable extent depending on the condition.

Answering yes to question 2, providing perioperative voice therapy, necessitates knowing the preferences of the referring otolaryngologist who will be operating on the patient. It also requires an understanding of the expected recovery vectors for your patient. Voice rest is commonly a part of the postoperative course after microflap excision of a vocal fold lesion, but it is also one of the most controversial and misunderstood issues in voice care. Duration of voice rest, when to use voice rest, and how to support people through voice rest are only a few of the questions that continue to plague surgeons and SLPs alike.[4-6] Aside from a limited period of complete voice rest following phonomicrosurgery, complete voice rest is rarely used in clinical practice except following an acute phonotraumatic event or vocal fold injury such as a vocal fold hemorrhage or cases of ulcerative laryngitis. Gone are the days of lengthy "no talking" time for therapeutic purposes, as we know that adherence is incredibly difficult,[7] there is evidence that low-impact vocal fold vibration promotes healing[8] and, importantly, the absence of talking does not teach a person how to use their voice more efficiently when they *do* talk. There is even evidence that suggests *not* using the voice for long periods can result in changes to the layered structure of the vocal folds[9] or, at the very least, vocal deconditioning. However, short periods of voice rest after phonomicrosurgery, followed by a gradual return to voice use, have been shown to be beneficial.[10]

Answering yes to question 3, regarding what to do when the voice or upper airway disorder cannot be cured, sometimes requires us to take off our voice clinician hat and remember that as SLPs, we are well trained and equipped to help people optimize overall communication. Despite the advances in medical and surgical care of the voice witnessed over the past 3 decades, there remain problems that do not have a solution. For example, vocal fold scar and sulcus continue be described as "challenging" with few treatment options.[11] Newer treatments, such as platelet-rich plasma (PRP) injections, are being studied and show promise in improving vocal fold pliability in the case of scar.[12-14] However, to date, there are no treatments that entirely reverse the effects of scar or sulcus.

The voice that results from vocal fold scar and sulcus is dependent on the degree of injury. However, the person may complain of limited vocal endurance, increased vocal effort to produce sound, reduced vocal loudness, and dysphonia, making it hard to talk in noisy places such as social events and restaurants. The goal of therapy is not to "fix" voice quality in this case, but to help the person reduce vocal effort, increase vocal endurance, and perhaps even adjust their environment, such as using amplification in situations that are noisy or improving room acoustics to reduce background noise. The clinician may assist with optimizing the environment where the person works or help them, along with their significant other, to optimize the couple's communication effectiveness. The patient may also benefit from receiving detailed education about their chronic condition and connection to appropriate support resources. All of these may not fall under what is historically thought to be "voice therapy," but they are communication therapy and, as such, you, the SLP, are the expert in improving communication.

Answering yes to question 4, augmenting medical treatment, means understanding the impact of medication meant to help voice or cough and knowing how behavioral voice therapy may work to optimize the effects of the medication. People with laryngeal dystonia (formerly called adductor spasmodic dysphonia [ADSD] or abductor spasmodic dysphonia [ABSD]) often undergo botulinum neurotoxin injections (eg BOTOX®, a brand name that has been genericized) approximately every 3 months as the gold standard of treatment to maintain a smoother, more fluid voice quality. Voice therapy following botulinum neurotoxin (BoNT) injection has been shown to increase the duration between injections, which may mean fewer injections needed each year.[15] SLPs may also help the patient understand the effects of BoNT injections within the context of the patient's specific voice demands. Careful consideration of the side effect and effect timeline, as well as the needs of the patient, can significantly improve the patient's quality of life. While the SLP does not make dosing decisions per se, they help the patient understand the nuance of BoNT dosing and timing and help communicate with the physician. Though results of BoNT injections are typically effective for about 3 months, this is dose dependent and follows a side effect period that can include changes to voice, such as breathiness, or changes to swallowing. With smaller doses, the duration of effect may be shorter, but the side effects may be reduced. For some patients, this is ideal and the SLP can help unearth these specific patient needs. About 25% to 30% of patients receive BoNT injections at intervals of less than 90 days.[16]

Is the Person a Good Candidate for Therapy?

The voice evaluation is the primary vehicle for determining if a patient is truly an appropriate candidate for voice therapy. As discussed in Chapter 1, the SLP will learn about the history, the course, and the cause of the voice concern, and should understand the physician's medical diagnosis as well as the expected path of recovery or continued decline. Importantly, but not always communicated, the SLP should understand the physician's Plan B if therapy does not resolve the voice problem as anticipated. This includes understanding the physician's expected time frame for therapeutic change prior to consideration of further surgical/medical/procedural options, as well as what the next steps might be in the physician's plan for the patient.

Even when the problem is amenable to voice therapy and the patient is stimulable for change, other variables can impact the outcome of voice therapy. In addition to the objective measures of vocal function, the voice evaluation can give the clinician a peek into the person's cognition, ability to follow instructions, and level of independence in completing the all-important home practice between sessions. Does the person need support from a partner or caregiver to complete home practice and, if so, how does the clinician ensure this collaborative work happens?

While much has been written about cognitive decline in aging and communication, cognitive decline with certain neurological diseases and communication, and cognitive decline post stroke or traumatic brain injury (TBI) and the impact on speech, swallowing, and overall communication, very little is written about cognition and voice. Samlan et al (2020) discuss the interaction of frailty syndrome and cognitive impairment as likely to have a greater impact on voice function than physical frailty alone.[17] It is important to consider cognition in the context of voice impairment since participation in voice therapy requires cognitive resources including attention and awareness, and when queried, patients often describe voice therapy as "hard."[18] Much of the progress seen in voice is ascribed to motor learning theory.[19] Motor learning is a complex process in the brain that results from repetition of a motor task to build motor memory such that the performance of that task becomes automatic. For example, closing the electric garage door when you pull out of the garage or locking your front door when you leave are both motor habits developed through motor learning. When you first had the opportunity to back a car out of a garage and close a garage with a button push, it was probably quite intentional. Now, it is likely so automatic that you don't think about it and later wonder after leaving, *Did I close the garage door? Did I lock the front door?* Not surprisingly, the first stage of motor learning is literally called the "cognitive stage" and requires that the learner of a new motor behavior (eg, resonant voice, flow phonation) acquire a level of consciousness to the task such that small changes in the way the voice *feels* become the hallmark of generalizing the behavior. A recent study of voice therapy and cognitive resources demonstrated, as expected, depletion of cognitive resources after initially engaging in 2 common voice therapy interventions: resonant voice therapy and Conversation Training Therapy (CTT).[20]

One barrier to successful voice therapy is adherence to treatment and home practice, because the motor learning process can only advance with motor repetitions. To maximize the benefit of voice therapy, the person must be engaged in the process and have "buy-in." That is, they must believe that voice therapy is a good option for treatment of their problem and have confidence in their ability to complete home practice or make changes to their voice use, environment, and/or vocal demands. Critically, making a change in their voice must be meaningful to the person. It is prudent to engage the patient in conversation about how important it is to them to change their voice *now* and how committed they are to making the changes necessary to achieve this. Perhaps there are other more pressing things that they must immediately attend to and just knowing that they don't have a malignancy or infection is all the information they need right now. This does not make a person "unmotivated," but it does mean that it isn't the right time in their lives to commit to therapy. In these cases, we advise the patient that our services are available if and when it is the right time to pursue therapy.

Change is hard, and especially so for changing voice behaviors. Change has been suggested to happen in stages and can move forward and backward as the circumstances of life evolve.[21] We know that adherence to voice therapy can be a problem for all these reasons, and talking with the person referred for therapy about where they are in confidence, commitment, and importance (or not) regarding engaging in therapy is an absolute must.[22] One tool to measure readiness for change is the ruler exercise[23] and is often used to open a conversation about voice therapy, concerns about what is required for progress, and confidence, commitment, and importance of doing voice therapy. Open conversations about readiness for voice therapy and the patient's personal goals also support the patient's autonomy, competence, and relatedness—3 psychological needs recognized in self-determination theory as critical to behavior change and recognized in speech pathology as relevant to culturally responsive clinical care.[24]

Options for Care: Where Does Voice Therapy Fit?

Voice therapy is one option among several for treatment of a variety of voice and upper airway disorders. As voice clinicians, we must consider where voice therapy fits in the entire treatment paradigm, which may also include medical and surgical treatments. This can be a complicated puzzle to unravel, and decisions regarding the type and order of treatment are often made by the physician/surgeon. The role of the SLP is to determine if voice therapy is a viable treatment when a patient is referred, if the patient is a good candidate for therapy, and what to do in therapy. If, however, the evidence, your experience, and/or your evalua-

tion indicate that the patient is *not* a candidate for voice therapy as an initial intervention, it is best to have a conversation with the referring physician about your findings. The same is true if you identify patients who were *not* initially referred for voice therapy but you determine that therapy *would* be of benefit to the patient. Just as the SLP is not an expert in surgery, the surgeon is not an expert in therapy. Our collaboration and communication yield the highest level of patient care.

It is incumbent on the clinician to be familiar with the evidence base and best practices to facilitate meaningful discussions with the physician. Information provided in this text reflects current knowledge and best practice. However, medical knowledge and best practices can change quickly, so it is critical to continue the journey of lifelong learning. This means staying connected to the peer-reviewed literature rather than relying solely on information from online blogs, websites, or clinician opinions. Evidence-based medicine (EBM) is the "conscientious, explicit, and judicious use of current best evidence in making decisions about the care of the individual patient. It means integrating individual clinical expertise with the best available external clinical evidence from systematic research"[25]. The American Speech-Language-Hearing Association (ASHA) has championed that SLPs should utilize EBM and provides evidence maps and access to journal articles that support evidence-based practice/treatments.[26]

Are You the "Right" Clinician?

This is a tough question, but one that every clinician must answer when we receive a referral to see a patient. SLPs are communication specialists licensed to see patients across the age continuum and the disorder spectrum. However, the breadth of our field makes it impossible to be an expert on all communication disorder subspecialties. As medicine and voice therapy evolve, we must know more and more of the intricacies of voice and upper airway disorders, behavioral interventions, and even available surgical interventions by our colleagues. It can be overwhelming to stay current. We cannot overemphasize the importance of empowering SLPs as independent providers to make informed decisions about who to treat in voice therapy and what interventions to use. We have an ethical responsibility to treat only those disorders and special populations for which we have a level of knowledge and expertise that makes us the treating clinician of choice.

> At the time of this writing, Medicare requires that a physician oversee treatment and must "sign off" on the plan of care. However, this requirement does not mean that a physician determines the therapy plan. ASHA provides many resources for SLPs and audiologists for self-learning about Medicare requirements, and the reader is encouraged to take advantage of these at https://www.asha.org/practice/reimbursement/medicare/[27]

At times, SLPs are encouraged to treat populations beyond their expertise (typically by someone unfamiliar with the complexities of providing services to patients with communication disorders). In these situations, we encourage the clinician to consider the medical model for primary care and subspecialists as a guide. Would you see a podiatrist for problems with your heart? Of course not. However, you may start with your general practitioner, who then sends you to a cardiologist. In voice therapy, we see people with rare disorders such as laryngeal dystonia and vocal tremor, athletes with inducible laryngeal obstruction who are at risk of losing their scholarships or jobs, or people who make their living with their voice and have performance demands, such as singers. These people, and others, need to see an SLP with expertise and experience in

their presenting problem. In some cases, you, as the clinician, may be similar to the general practitioner. You may be referred a patient for voice therapy because of your training as an SLP with licensure and certification that indicates you can treat people with voice disorders. However, if the person presents with a problem that you are not comfortable treating, find the person who has expertise in that area and refer the patient out. We tell our mentees to "*close the loop*" all the time. If you feel the need to refer out or collaborate with another SLP, take the time to communicate with the patient and the physician regarding your rationale. Always, our aim is to provide the highest level of care for patients, whether that be through direct treatment or connecting the patient with a more appropriate resource.

Treatment Option Summaries by Disorder: Selected Examples

SLPs do not treat diagnoses, and diagnoses do not dictate therapeutic techniques. However, as previously discussed, the diagnosis provides information about what kind of improvements can be achieved through various treatment modalities and prognoses. While we treat voice behaviors and not diagnoses, it can be useful to categorize treatment by disorder type. As such, the chapters in this text are organized by categories of voice disorder for easy navigation.

Below, we discuss the treatment paradigms for several voice disorders, but these are provided as examples and the discussion is not exhaustive. The reader is guided to the chapter introductions in Chapters 3 through 9 to learn more about the various populations we see for voice and upper airway intervention.

Treatment Options for Muscle Tension Dysphonia (MTD)

Muscle tension dysphonia is classified as primary MTD (also known as functional dysphonia) and secondary MTD.[28] Primary MTD is diagnosed when there are no underlying vocal fold lesions or motion impairments that are the cause of the dysphonia. In primary MTD, the voice can be significantly impaired without vocal fold pathology. Both direct voice therapy and augmentative treatments such as physical therapy, acupuncture, and cognitive behavioral therapy have been proposed as treatments for primary MTD.[29] No matter the augmentative therapeutic modality used, direct voice therapy is the gold standard treatment for primary MTD and should always be considered in the decision-making paradigm for this disorder.

Secondary MTD is diagnosed when there is an underlying pathological cause for the dysphonia and the person responds to the change in vocal function by adding muscle tension and effort to produce voice. Causes can include glottal insufficiency, phonotraumatic vocal fold lesions, scarring, laryngeal dystonia, and tremor, in addition to muscular permutations one might make to change the pitch of the voice associated with voice-gender incongruence. Voice therapy should always be considered in the treatment of secondary MTD. However, based on the degree of severity of the underlying pathological cause, there may be a need for medical/surgical intervention prior to therapy. For example, someone with a significant secondary MTD as a result of a large glottal gap due to vocal fold atrophy, vocal fold paralysis, or scar and who cannot maintain entrained vocal fold vibration likely needs to be considered for a surgical/procedural intervention to close the glottal gap prior to voice therapy. If the patient has a phonotraumatic lesion that is large enough that they cannot achieve glottal closure and/or if the lesion is not expected to get better with voice therapy alone,[30] voice therapy may be best used after surgical removal of the lesion. Voice therapy plays a role in all secondary MTD, but the clinician must decide, and suggest to the referring physician, the optimal time to engage in voice therapy. Perhaps a short course of voice therapy to prepare the patient for surgery and subsequent voice rest with a longer, more intense course following surgery would result in better overall outcomes for the patient.

Treatment Options for Vocal Fold Motion Impairments

Vocal fold motion impairments include vocal fold paresis and paralysis. Vocal fold paralysis can be unilateral or bilateral, can be peripherally or centrally mediated, and can involve the recurrent laryngeal nerve, superior laryngeal nerve, or both.[31] Vocal fold paralysis means there is a loss of adductory and abductory movement or elongation of the vocal fold (in the case of a superior laryngeal nerve (SLN) injury). Vocal fold paralysis can occur as a result of a mass along the course of the nerve (eg, a mediastinal mass or thyroid tumor), cardiac disease, surgical insult (iatrogenic), or even a virus. Vocal fold paralysis can resolve in some cases and is believed to take up to 9 to 12 months for resolution. Importantly, the etiology of the paralysis impacts the recovery trajectory.[32] Many believe that if no recovery occurs after 6 months, the nerve is less likely to recover function.[33]

Vocal fold paresis is a partial loss of motion, not complete lack of motion, of the vocal fold. Vocal fold paresis can be unilateral or bilateral and is generally thought to be a result of idiopathic causes, potentially virally mediated. While there is little published about the recovery from vocal fold paresis, it has logically been suggested to be similar to vocal fold paralysis with a 6- to 12-month trajectory.[34]

There are 3 primary treatments for vocal fold paralysis: voice therapy, injection augmentation, and thyroplasty.[35] Treatment should be determined by factors including size of glottal gap, secondary impairments including the presence of dysphagia and dyspnea, time since diagnosed onset, and patient preference. In general, if the glottal gap is barely perceptible on laryngeal imaging with videostroboscopy and the patient is stimulable for change, voice therapy can be the first line of treatment in vocal fold paralysis. If the glottal gap is larger, procedural or surgical intervention may be more appropriate as first-line treatment.

Injection augmentation involves use of a filler substance to "plump up" the paralyzed vocal fold to push it closer to midline. This allows the fully mobile vocal fold to approximate with the motion-impaired vocal fold, resulting in improved glottal closure and ability to generate sufficient subglottal pressure for entrained vocal fold vibration. Injection augmentation is a well-studied and well-accepted temporary method to treat vocal fold paralysis. There are many injectable materials, including hyaluronic acid (HA)-based products for shorter-term injections (3 to 12 months, dependent on the product) and calcium hydroxyapatite (CaHA) for longer duration of effect (12+ months); in general, surgeon preference determines which to use.[36] Newer injectables are also being studied at the time of writing this text. This temporary procedure can be done in the operating room or in the office. It is well tolerated for patients with little down time (1 day at most). Initially, the voice can be more dysphonic with a pressed/strained and/or rough quality due to necessary overinjection to account for early absorption of the injectable. This generally resolves in the first 1 to 2 weeks after injection and is followed by the desired effect period with better voice. Most laryngologists suggest doing this temporary procedure if it has been less than 6 to 9 months since the onset of the paralysis to allow for spontaneous recovery and to determine if the patient is happy with this augmented voice. There are minimal risks associated with the procedure, and it is not necessary to wait for potential vocal fold motion recovery to inject the patient.[37]

Thyroplasty is a permanent surgical procedure that uses a medical-grade implant (Silastic or Gore-Tex) in the vocal fold to push the paralyzed vocal fold closer to midline. Similar to injection augmentation, the goal is to improve glottal closure to allow for sufficient subglottal pressure and entrained vocal fold vibration. Thyroplasty is completed with the patient awake with a local anesthetic. The surgeon makes a small incision over the thyroid laminae and drills a window to fit and place an implant to move the paralyzed vocal fold into a static paramedian position. The patient is awake so that they can produce voice during the surgery and the surgeon can determine the size of the implant to position it to produce best voice. Thyroplasty is permanent but can be removed or revised if needed, although rate of need for revision is overall low. Voice therapy is often used following injection augmentation or thyroplasty to assist the patient with optimizing voice outcomes following the procedure or surgery. This can be explained to the patient as the surgeon repairing or modifying their "instrument" and the SLP helping the patient learn how to most efficiently "play" the new instrument, ie, optimally coordinate respiration, phonation, and resonance.

Treatment options for vocal fold paresis are similar. In general, voice therapy is the treatment of choice if glottal closure can be achieved. If there is a larger glottal gap, injection augmentation and thyroplasty are also options, often with voice therapy to follow.

Treatments Options for Laryngeal Dystonia and Voice Tremor

Laryngeal dystonia, a focal dystonia, is a centrally mediated voice disorder now believed to be related to an altered sensory system and connectivity pattern throughout the brain.[38] In adductor type laryngeal dystonia, the vocal folds adduct during voiced sound productions such as voiced consonants and vowels. The sound of the voice is often strained and rough with spasms. In abductor type laryngeal dystonia, the vocal folds abduct during production of voiceless sounds, which causes a loss of sound or hallmark "breathy breaks," often in the middle of words. Much work has been done to determine the specific cause of this disorder with limited results.[39] In general, it first appears in the fifth decade of life, occurs more often in women than men, and develops over a 6-month period with stabilization of symptoms after that time.[40] While scientists work to find better methods to treat laryngeal dystonia, BoNT injection remains the gold standard of treatment. Voice therapy is used to augment BoNT injections. Studies continue on sodium oxybate and other treatments for laryngeal dystonia with promising short-term symptomatic relief,[41,42] but at the time of writing of this chapter, they are not widely available nor widely used.

Essential voice tremor (EVT) is a neurological disease of the vocal mechanism. Onset is most often in the seventh decade of life and the condition occurs more often in women than men. There may be a familial component.[43] EVT is classified as an action tremor. Given that the vocal mechanism is always in action with its movements in breathing, when viewing the larynx with laryngeal endoscopy or videostroboscopy, the examiner will usually see some degree of tremor.[44] Isolated laryngeal tremor, ie, tremor only found in the larynx, is now believed to be a phenotype of EVT, not a separate disease state.[45,46] BoNT injections remain the primary treatment for vocal tremor when the true or false vocal folds are involved, with most studies documenting some, but limited, positive results.[47] A few studies have documented the benefit of propranolol in the treatment of vocal tremor.[48] Deep brain stimulators (DBS) are used in the treatment of limb tremor and had historically been subject to problems with speech decline. However, recent studies in DBS placements and types of stimulators have demonstrated a positive impact on vocal tremor and continue to be an area of study.[49] Injection augmentation has also been suggested as a treatment for EVT, especially in those with concurrent age-related changes to the vocal folds.[50]

Voice therapy as a stand-alone treatment for EVT has also been suggested, primarily with case study evidence.[51-53] This therapy may be useful as an adjunct to other medical treatments and should be considered in people who wish to improve the outcomes from medical treatments or in those who are unable to tolerate or do not wish to use medical intervention.

Decision Making in Therapy Planning: What Therapy to Use?

Voice therapy is not a singular entity, nor is it a series of therapy techniques applied haphazardly with hopes that something will work. Patients, voice teachers, physicians, and even clinicians often refer to "voice therapy" as if the term designates something specific and understood by all. Without further description, the term voice therapy is nonspecific, like saying, "and then we did surgery," without mentioning the type or purpose of surgery.

Voice therapy involves use of specifically applied sets of systematic vocal, respiratory, resonatory, and even articulatory tasks designed to address a specific physiological goal. For example, if you want better coordination of respiration and phonation, you might use flow phonation but likely wouldn't choose laryngeal massage, as it does not directly address the discoordination of airflow and vocal fold vibration. However, if your goal is to reduce extralaryngeal muscle tension or to lower the position of the larynx in the neck to reduce excessive muscle contractions, you could use laryngeal massage and likely not flow phonation. If your primary observation is a posterior locus of resonance, you may opt for resonant voice therapy or CTT. At its core, "*sound medical decision specifies the connection between the means and the outcome*,"[54] and voice therapy requires that the task is directly connected to the desired outcome.

In exercise science it is well known that exercise must be designed specifically to the type of outcome desired, called specificity of exercise. If one needs to train endurance, train with aerobic-based exercises, and if one needs strength, train with anaerobic-based exercises.[55] Our application of exercise science to speech pathology has advanced over time. Previously, it was thought that oral motor exercises would improve speech intelligibility,[56] but it is now well understood in the motor speech literature that this is not specific enough. If the problem is sibilant sounds, you must train sibilants. If the problem is lip closure for plosives, you must train production of plosives, not just pucker the lips and hope for transfer to producing a /b/ or /p/. There may be some occasional synergies in treatments that result in the desired outcome, but there are no studies about combining different therapies and the optimal dose of each used together.

To select appropriate therapy strategies, first consider the desired physiological outcome and which tasks are designed to meet your overarching goal. For example, if the goal is to reduce the impact of glottal contact with every cycle of vibration during phonation in someone with phonotraumatic voice disorder or perhaps with high vocal dose, the clinician might suggest using semi-occluded vocal tract exercises, which optimize vocal fold shape during phonation (a rectangular shape) with distributed impact stress and heightened interaction of the source and filter to maximize efficiency of sound production.[57] On the contrary, if the goal is to maximize glottal contact while resisting subglottal pressures with the goal of voice building, prolonged exuberant /a/ phonation might be used to maximize glottal contact and increase subglottal pressure and loudness.[58]

In recent years, classification systems have been developed to delineate the ingredients of voice therapies for the purpose of improving research and acknowledging that the "active ingredients" across individual therapies are variable. A Taxonomy of Voice Therapy, developed by Van Stan and colleagues, classifies therapies by direct versus indirect methods and by intrinsic versus extrinsic

intervention delivery method.[59] Direct methods were further described as targeting auditory, musculoskeletal, somatosensory, vocal function, or respiratory systems. In 2019, Hart and colleagues developed a classification system called the Rehabilitation Treatment Specification System (RTSS) to attempt to alleviate the "black box" phenomena across all behavioral treatment modalities, including physical therapy, occupational therapy, and speech-language pathology.[60] Elements of the RTSS and its application to voice therapy have been described, but the systematic application of the RTSS to voice therapy is currently underway. The goal is to provide a comprehensive classification of various voice therapy modalities originally in a tripartite codification of (1) the patient behavior to be changed, (2) what the clinician does to modify the target behavior, and (3) how the therapy modifies the behavior.[61] "Meta therapy," or the language the clinician uses to help shape the patient's adherence to therapy and awareness of the target of the therapy task, has been mapped to the RTSS.[62]

In this chapter, we will simplify the classification of therapies described in this text as (1) those aimed at recalibration of vocal function, (2) those aimed at increasing coordinated exuberant use of the respiratory/phonatory systems, and (3) those that are augmentative. While this seems a rudimentary classification scheme, it can be a useful initial approach for delineating which therapies are aimed to address which issues. Table 2–1 classifies therapy methods into either recalibration or exuberance. This table is not comprehensive, but rather a starting place for the clinician to begin thinking about therapy methods as they relate to various targeted outcomes. The clinician is guided to refer to the RTSS to truly begin to understand all the ingredients of therapy.

Recalibration Strategies

Recalibration is defined as "the act of resetting or fine-tuning an instrument or a device."[63]

Table 2–1. Simple Classification System for Voice Therapy Strategies

Recalibration Therapies	Exuberant Therapies	Indirect and Augmentative Therapies
Flow Phonation	Phonation Resistance Training Exercises (PhoRTE®)	Vocal health and hygiene (indirect therapy)
Semi-occluded Vocal Tract Exercises (eg, lip trills, tongue trills, fricatives, hand over mouth, straw exercises, kazoo buzzes)	Respiratory muscle strength training such as IMST and EMST	Amplification (indirect therapy)
Resonant Voice Therapy	Lee Silverman Voice Treatment (LSVT LOUD®)	Physical therapy (augmentative)
Lessac-Madsen Resonant Voice Therapy	SPEAK OUT!®	Cognitive behavioral therapy (augmentative)
Adventures in Voice for Pediatric Patients	Vocal Function Exercises	Acupuncture (augmentative)
Vocal Function Exercises		Vibrational therapies (augmentative)
Conversation Training Therapy		
Lax Vox		
Manual Therapies (laryngeal reposturing, laryngeal massage, myofascial release)		
Unilateral Ear Plug (alters auditory feedback)		
SPL Monitors like the SpeechVive™ (alters auditory feedback)		

The goal of therapies classified as methods to recalibrate the vocal mechanism can include: reducing extralaryngeal tension or high laryngeal placement in the neck, balancing subglottal pressures during sound production, correcting reduced mean flow rate, breath holding, or speaking in expiratory reserve volume, just to name a few. As discussed previously, diagnosis does not dictate the therapeutic modality, but functional problems associated with certain diagnoses may benefit significantly from recalibration therapies, such as patients with primary or secondary MTD or phonotraumatic vocal fold changes.

Exuberant Strategies

Exuberant is defined as "abounding in vitality, vigorous."[64] These therapies capitalize on longer, louder, and more effortful therapy tasks. Phonation Resistance Training Exercises (PhoRTE®), inspiratory muscle strength training (IMST), and expiratory muscle strength training (EMST) are truly exercise, meaning they are based on muscle adaptation through systematically providing the upper aerodigestive tract musculature with greater and greater vocal loads or respiratory pressures to build strength. Vocal Function Exercises, although completed quietly, can also be used as an exuberant therapy to increase vocal endurance given the use of maximum duration and pitch range tasks. People with glottal insufficiency due to presbyphonia or vocal fold paresis may benefit from these therapies. People with Parkinson's disease (PD) benefit from LSVT LOUD® (Lee Silverman Voice Treatment) and SPEAK OUT!®

Indirect and Augmentative Strategies

While the definition of augment or augmentative means to amplify or increase in strength,[63] these therapies are auxiliary and meant to increase the chances that the voice will be improved. Vocal health and hygiene is a term used to describe methods to improve the health of the vocal mechanism, such as increasing surface or systemic hydration, reducing exposure to laryngeal irritants like cigarette smoke, and managing vocal dose.[65] Attending to vocal health is unlikely on its own to be a sufficient therapeutic regimen to rehabilitate the voice.[66] Some therapeutic modalities can be provided by other health care professionals, such as physical therapy or acupuncture, and are considered augmentative in the context of treating a primary voice disorder.

It is also important to mention that exercises within a category may not be interchangeable. For example, IMST and EMST are both considered exuberant, but they target different goals. IMST targets the inspiratory musculature while EMST targets the expiratory musculature, and they are not interchangeable. The literature is abundant with articles about the benefits of EMST in the treatment of dysphagia while limited in the number of articles that support the use of EMST in voice. IMST

on the other hand has been shown in several recent studies to improve the vocal function of people with presbyphonia when combined with a systematic therapy protocol such as Vocal Function Exercises or PhoRTE®,[67] while EMST combined with these therapies may not further improve voice.[58]

Decision Making in Voice Therapy Planning: How Much, How Long, and How Intense?

The FITT Principle refers to the frequency, intensity, type, and timing of exercise for the desired outcome in biophysiological adaptation of change to improve strength or endurance.[68] In other words, *how much, how hard, what type,* and *how often* must someone complete a particular exercise to achieve the desired outcome? This is often called the "exercise (dose) prescription." This also inherently considers the doses that cause positive change and the doses that can cause harmful change. Roy (2012) discusses these dosing issues in voice therapy.[69] For example, too much exercise, perhaps in too loud of voice, even with the best of intentions (clinicians' or patients') can be harmful. Research and consensus on the frequency, intensity, and duration of voice therapy is sorely lacking. LSVT LOUD® and, to a lesser degree, SPEAK OUT!®, 2 therapies for people with PD, direct trained clinicians to do therapy 4 days a week for 4 weeks in the case of LSVT LOUD® and 12 sessions in 2 to 3 months in the case of SPEAK OUT!®.

Several studies have examined traditional voice therapy (once a week) versus intensive voice therapy, defined as either 4 times a week for 2 weeks[70] or 1 to 4 hours a day for 4 to 5 successive days with 4 to 5 different clinicians,[71] in people with primary MTD (functional dysphonia). These studies indicated that intensive therapy, in the case of primary MTD, produced better outcomes. However, this does not apply to all voice therapy, nor all vocal fold pathologies treated in voice therapy. Both Desjardins et al (2022)[72] and Gartner-Schmidt et al (2017)[73] discuss that the literature lacks consensus for the duration and intensity of voice therapy. Unlike other speech therapies that may require 12 to 24 therapy sessions to improve outcomes,[74] less therapy is required to address most common voice and upper airway disorders. Recently, 2 studies using only the experience from one voice center demonstrated that it takes on average 5.2 sessions in adults to achieve positive outcomes from voice therapy[75] and 7.5 sessions in pediatric voice patients.[76] We often tell patients to anticipate needing 4 to 6 sessions of voice therapy over the course of 2 to 3 months, based on experience in clinical practice. There may be many reasons for the need for less therapy compared to when treating other communication disorders, and one important reason is that voice therapy capitalizes on motor learning that is enhanced by early generalization of concepts to use more often throughout the day, such as in conversation. Additionally, asking the patient to go home, practice emerging skills, and explore what they feel may increase their self-efficacy by developing an internal locus of control so that they can complete the task independently.[77] The frequency of therapy sessions may be comparatively less than for some other communication disorders, but ideally, the frequency of independent practice is still daily.

Similarly, there are limited guidelines on when to discharge from voice therapy. In 2009, Hapner et al noted the lack of guidelines for voice therapy discharge and developed an operational definition of discharge criteria as when (1) the patient reached therapy goals, (2) the patient indicated satisfaction with voice quality, or (3) no additional benefit was expected from future sessions and the patient was referred to another discipline (physician, singing voice specialist, psychology, and oth-

ers).[78] In 2018, Gillespie and Gartner-Schmidt queried 50 voice specialized SLPs and found the 5 most important criteria for discharge were the patient's ability to (1) independently use a better voice, (2) function with their new voice production in activities of daily living, (3) differentiate between good and bad voice, (4) take responsibility for their voice, and (5) sound better from baseline.[79]

Given the limited guidance on not only FITT but also when to discharge, clinicians are left to base their decisions on their own clinical intuition, best available evidence from studies that have been conducted, and patient preference—the true practice of EBM.[80]

Putting It All Together in Decision Making: The Silent Factors

It is often said that there are 2 variables in successful voice therapy: the *what* and the *how*.[81] The *what* consists of the therapeutic tasks and all the decisions made regarding therapy and the *how* consists of all the components of the therapeutic alliance including building trust, relevancy, communication, and partnership. The therapeutic alliance, or the bond developed between clinician and patient, has been shown to be the most important predictor of attendance, adherence, and successful outcomes from therapy.[82] Self-Determination Theory provides a framework for building this rapport through supporting a patient's 3 psychological needs of autonomy, competency, and relatedness.[83]

Iwarsson discussed the "silent know how," or the interpersonal skills that allow a clinician to connect with a patient,[84] and Helou and colleagues postulate that meta-therapy, or the language/dialogue that clinicians use to build rapport, trust, and relevancy with their patients, is the so-called "magic" of voice therapy.[62] Iwarsson believes the "silent know how" can be taught, and Helou recommends sharing dialogues between colleagues to help the therapy process. Phrases like "I'm the facilitator, you are the implementer," "I'm only an expert in the voice therapy task, but you are the expert of your experience," "You've got this," or "I think if we try this (task), we might be able to access that area of your range that is giving you trouble—you with me?" are all examples of some of our frequently used meta-therapy dialogues. Surgeons often use the term "in my hands" when describing their successes in surgery. Perhaps as voice clinicians, we should use the same term when talking to our patients about what we expect the course of therapy to look like: "In my hands, people have experienced . . . "

Building the therapeutic alliance begins the minute you meet the patient. Making eye contact, truly listening to the patient tell their story, avoiding judgment about how or what they feel, and conceding the role of "expert" in favor of developing a clinician-patient partnership are all important pieces in developing the therapeutic alliance. Further, we can connect with a patient by acknowledging that the voice is an integral part of what makes us uniquely human and that a voice disorder can impact our sense of self, evoke feelings of defeat, or contribute to social isolation. Additional guidance on building the therapeutic alliance through a culturally responsive lens to respect the unique identities and life experiences of our patients is available in the ASHA Perspectives Forum: *Culturally Responsive Voice Care*.[24,85-89]

Conclusions

As illustrated throughout this chapter, the decision-making process in voice and upper airway is critical for achieving desired goals. It can take time to refine your clinical decision-making skills. To support this development, the cases throughout Chapters 3 through 9 include a section on decision making to offer a peek into the mind of the master clinicians.

References

1. Verdolini K, Rosen CA, Branski RC. *Classification Manual of Voice Disorders-I*. 2nd ed. Psychology Press; 2012.
2. Kirke DN, Sulica L. The natural history of vocal fold cysts. *Laryngoscope*. 2020;130(9): 2202-2207. doi:10.1002/lary.28377
3. Klein AM, Lehmann M, Hapner ER, Johns MM. Spontaneous resolution of hemorrhagic polyps of the true vocal fold. *J Voice*. 2009;23(1):132-135. doi:10.1016/j.jvoice.2007.07.001
4. Kaneko M, Shiromoto O, Fujiu-Kurachi M, Kishimoto Y, Tateya I, Hirano S. Optimal duration for voice rest after vocal fold surgery: Randomized controlled clinical study. *J Voice*. 2017;31(1):97-103. doi:10.1016/j.jvoice.2016.02.009
5. Branski RC. Perioperative voice recovery: A wound-healing perspective. *Perspect Voice Voice Disord*. 2013;23(2):42-46. doi:10.1044/vvd23.2.42
6. Rousseau B, Gutmann ML, Mau T, et al. Randomized controlled trial of supplemental augmentative and alternative communication versus voice rest alone after phonomicrosurgery. *Otolaryngol Head Neck Surg*. 2015;152(3):494-500. doi:10.1177/0194599814566601
7. Rousseau B, Cohen SM, Zeller AS, Scearce L, Tritter AG, Garrett CG. Compliance and quality of life in patients on prescribed voice rest. *Otolaryngol Head Neck Surg*. 2011; 144(1):104-107. doi:10.1177/0194599810390465
8. Abbott KV, Li NYK, Branski RC, et al. Vocal exercise may attenuate acute vocal fold inflammation. 2013;26(June 2005):1-27. doi:10.1016/j.jvoice.2012.03.008
9. Tanner K, Sauder C, Thibeault SL, Dromey C, Smith ME. Vocal fold bowing in elderly male monozygotic twins: A case study. *J Voice*. 2010;24(4):470-476. doi:10.1016/j.jvoice.2008.10.010
10. Fan RS, Yiu Y, Kulesz PA, et al. Clinical voice outcomes for two voice rest protocols after phonomicrosurgery. *Laryngoscope*. 2024; 134(6):2812-2818. doi:10.1002/lary.31250

11. Hantzakos A, Dikkers FG, Giovanni A, et al. Vocal fold scars: A common classification proposal by the American Laryngological Association and European Laryngological Society. *Eur Arch Otorhinolaryngol.* 2019; 276(8):2289-2292. doi:10.1007/s00405-019-05489-3

12. Woo P, Murry T. Short-term voice improvement after repeated office-based platelet-rich plasma PRP injection in patients with vocal fold scar, sulcus, and atrophy. *J Voice.* 2023;37(4):621-628. doi:10.1016/j.jvoice.2021.02.022

13. van der Woerd B, O'Dell K, Castellanos CX, et al. Safety of platelet-rich plasma subepithelial infusion for vocal fold scar, sulcus, and atrophy. *Laryngoscope.* 2023;133(3):647-653. doi:10.1002/lary.30288

14. Santa Maria C, Shuman EA, Van Der Woerd B, et al. Prospective outcomes after serial platelet-rich plasma (PRP) injection in vocal fold scar and sulcus. *Laryngoscope.* 2024;134:5021-5027. doi:10.1002/lary.31683

15. Rumbach A, Aiken P, Novakovic D. Treatment outcome measures for spasmodic dysphonia: A systematic review. *J Voice.* 2024; 38(2):540.e13-540.e43. doi:10.1016/j.jvoice.2021.10.001

16. Lagos-Villaseca A, Bhatt NK, Abdolhosseini P, et al. Assessment of patients receiving short-interval botulinum toxin chemodenervation treatment for laryngeal dystonia and essential tremor of the vocal tract. *JAMA Otolaryngol Head Neck Surg.* 2023;149(7): 615-620. doi:10.1001/jamaoto.2023.0162

17. Samlan RA, Black MA, Abidov M, Mohler J, Fain M. Frailty syndrome, cognition, and dysphonia in the eldery. *J Voice.* 2020; 34(1):160.e15-160.e23. doi:10.1016/j.jvoice.2018.06.001

18. van Leer E, Connor NP. Patient perceptions of voice therapy adherence. *J Voice.* 2010; 24(4):458-469. doi:10.1016/j.jvoice.2008.12.009

19. Tellis C. New concepts in motor learning and training related to voice rehabilitation. *Perspect ASHA Spec Interest Groups.* 2018;3(3):56-67. doi:10.1044/persp3.sig3.56

20. Vinney LA, Tripp R, Shelly S, Gillespie A. Indexing cognitive resource usage for acquisition of initial voice therapy targets. *Am J Speech Lang Pathol.* 2023;32(2):717-732. doi:10.1044/2022_AJSLP-22-00197

21. van Leer E, Hapner ER, Connor NP. Transtheoretical model of health behavior change applied to voice therapy. *J Voice.* 2008;22(6):688-698. doi:10.1016/j.jvoice.2007.01.011

22. Portone C, Johns MM, Hapner ER. A review of patient adherence to the recommendation for voice therapy. *J Voice.* 2008;22(2):192-196. doi:10.1016/j.jvoice.2006.09.009

23. Hapner ER. The ruler exercise. In: Behrman A, Haskell J, eds. *Exercises for Voice Therapy.* 3rd ed. Plural Publishing; 2020:27-29.

24. Castro ME, Enclade H, Biel M. Self-determination theory applications in culturally responsive voice therapy. *Perspect ASHA Spec Interest Groups.* 2024;9(5):1-7. doi:10.1044/2023_persp-23-00168

25. Sackett DL, Rosenberg W, Gray J, Haynes RB, Richardson WS. Evidence based medicine: What it is and what it isn't. *British Medical Journal.* 1996;312:71-72.

26. *ASHA evidence maps.* American Speech-Language-Hearing Association (ASHA). https://apps.asha.org/EvidenceMaps/

27. *Medicare coverage of speech-language pathologists and audiologists.* American Speech-Language-Hearing Association. https://www.asha.org/practice/reimbursement/medicare/

28. Desjardins M, Apfelbach C, Rubino M, Abbott KV. Integrative review and framework of suggested mechanisms in primary muscle tension dysphonia. *J Speech Lang Hear Res.* 2022;65(5):1867-1893. doi:10.1044/2022_JSLHR-21-00575

29. Madill C, Chacon A, Kirby E, Novakovic D, Nguyen DD. Active ingredients of voice therapy for muscle tension voice disorders: A retrospective data audit. *J Clin Med.* 2021; 10(18):4135. doi:10.3390/jcm10184135

30. Hillman RE, Stepp CE, Van Stan JH, Zañartu M, Mehta DD. An updated theoretical framework for vocal hyperfunction. *Am J Speech Lang Pathol.* 2020;29(4):2254-2260. doi:10.1044/2020_AJSLP-20-00104

31. Rubin AD, Sataloff RT. Vocal fold paresis and paralysis. *Otolaryngol Clin North Am.*

2007;40(5):1109-1131. doi:10.1016/j.otc.2007.05.012

32. Mau T, Husain S, Sulica L. Pathophysiology of iatrogenic and idiopathic vocal fold paralysis may be distinct. *Laryngoscope.* 2020; 130(6):1520-1524. doi:10.1002/lary.28281

33. Mau T, Pan HM, Childs LF. The natural history of recoverable vocal fold paralysis: Implications for kinetics of reinnervation. *Laryngoscope.* 2017;127(11):2585-2590. doi: 10.1002/lary.26734

34. Sulica L. Vocal fold paresis: An evolving clinical concept. *Curr Otorhinolaryngol Rep.* 2013;1(3):158-162.

35. Merati AL, Blumin JH, Johns MM, Simpson CB. Decision making in vocal fold paralysis. *Otolaryngol Head Neck Surg.* 2012;147(S2): P23-P23. doi:10.1177/0194599812449008a50

36. Kharidia KM, Bensoussan Y, Rosen CA, Johns MM, O'Dell K. Variations in practices and preferences of vocal fold injection materials: A national survey. *Laryngoscope.* 2023;133(5):1176-1183. doi:10.1002/lary.30331

37. Francis DO, Williamson K, Hovis K, et al. Effect of injection augmentation on need for framework surgery in unilateral vocal fold paralysis. *Laryngoscope.* 2016;126(1):128-134. doi:10.1002/lary.25431

38. Mantel T, Dresel C, Welte M, et al. Altered sensory system activity and connectivity patterns in adductor spasmodic dysphonia. *Sci Rep.* 2020;10(1):1-9. doi:10.1038/s41598-020-67295-w

39. Jinnah HA, Berardelli A, Comella C, et al. The focal dystonias: Current views and challenges for future research. *Mov Disord.* 2013;28(7):926-943. doi:10.1002/mds.25567

40. *Spasmodic dysphonia.* National Institute on Deafness and Other Communication Disorders. https://www.nidcd.nih.gov/health/spasmodic-dysphonia

41. Simonyan K, Frucht SJ, Blitzer A, Sichani AH, Rumbach AF. A novel therapeutic agent, sodium oxybate, improves dystonic symptoms via reduced network-wide activity. *Sci Rep.* 2018;8(1):1-8. doi:10.1038/s41598-018-34553-x

42. Simonyan K, O'Flynn LC, Hamzehei Sichani A, et al. Efficacy and safety of sodium oxybate in isolated focal laryngeal dystonia: A phase IIb double-blind placebo-controlled crossover randomized clinical trial. *Ann Neurol.* 2024:329-343. doi:10.1002/ana.27121

43. *Essential tremor.* International Essential Tremor Foundation. essentialtremor.org

44. Sulica L, Louis ED. Clinical characteristics of essential voice tremor: A study of 34 cases. *Laryngoscope.* 2010;120(3):516-528. doi:10.1002/lary.20702

45. Patel A, Frucht SJ. Isolated vocal tremor as a focal phenotype of essential tremor: A retrospective case review. *J Clin Mov Disord.* 2015;2(1). doi:10.1186/s40734-015-0016-5

46. Barkmeier-Kraemer JM. Isolated voice tremor: A clinical variant of essential tremor or a distinct clinical phenotype? *Tremor Other Hyperkinet Mov.* 2020;10:1-8. doi:10.7916/tohm.v0.738

47. Newland DP, Novakovic D, Richards A. Voice tremor and botulinum neurotoxin therapy: A contemporary review. *Toxins (Basel).* 2022;14(11):773. doi:10.3390/toxins14110773

48. Justicz N, Hapner ER, Josephs JS, Boone BC, Jinnah HA, Johns MM. Comparative effectiveness of propranolol and botulinum for the treatment of essential voice tremor. *Laryngoscope.* 2016;126(1):113-117. doi:10.1002/lary.25485

49. Ho A, Erickson-Direnzo E, Pendharkar A, Sung C, Halpern C. Deep brain stimulation for vocal tremor: A comprehensive, multidisciplinary methodology. *Neurosurg Focus.* 2015;38(6).

50. Khoury S, Randall D. Treatment of essential vocal tremor: A scoping review of evidence-based therapeutic modalities. *J Voice.* 2024;38(4):922-930. doi: 10.1016/j.jvoice.2021.12.009

51. Barkmeier-Kraemer J, Lato A, Wiley K. Development of a speech treatment program for a client with essential vocal tremor. *Semin Speech Lang.* 2011;32(1):43-57.

52. Ghosh N, Eidson E, Derrick E, Lester-Smith RA. Breathy voice as a compensatory strategy for essential vocal tremor: A single case experiment across participants. *J Voice.* 2023:1-17. doi:10.1016/j.jvoice.2023.10.003

53. Lester-Smith RA, Miller CH, Cherney LR. Behavioral therapy for tremor or dystonia

affecting voice in speakers with hyperkinetic dysarthria: A systematic review. *J Voice.* 2023;37(4):561-573. doi:10.1016/j.jvoice.2021.03.026

54. Masic I. Medical decision making. *Acta Inform Medica.* 2022;30(3):230-235. doi:10.5455/aim.2022.30.230-235

55. Pedrosa GF, Lima FV, Schoenfeld BJ, et al. Partial range of motion training elicits favorable improvements in muscular adaptations when carried out at long muscle lengths. *Eur J Sport Sci.* 2022;22(8):1250-1260. doi:10.1080/17461391.2021.1927199

56. McCauley RJ, Strand E, Frymark T. Evidence-based systematic review: Effects of non-speech oral motor exercises on speech. *Am J Speech Lang Pathol.* 2009;18(November).

57. Titze IR. Voice training and therapy with a semi-occluded vocal tract: Rationale and scientific underpinnings. *Hear Res.* 2006;49(April):448-460.

58. Belsky MA, Shelly S, Rothenberger SD, et al. Phonation Resistance Training Exercises (PhoRTE) with and without Expiratory Muscle Strength Training (EMST) for patients with presbyphonia: A noninferiority randomized clinical trial. *J Voice.* 2023;37(3):398-409. doi:10.1016/j.jvoice.2021.02.015

59. Van Stan JH, Roy N, Awan S, Stemple J, Hillman RE. A taxonomy of voice therapy. *Am J Speech Lang Pathol.* 2015;24:101-125. doi:10.1044/2015_AJSLP-14-0030

60. Hart T, Dijkers MP, Whyte J, et al. A theory-driven system for the specification of rehabilitation treatments. *Arch Phys Med Rehabil.* 2019;100(1):172-180. doi:10.1016/j.apmr.2018.09.109

61. Van Stan JH, Whyte J, Duffy JR, et al. Voice therapy according to the rehabilitation treatment specification system: Expert consensus ingredients and targets. *Am J Speech Lang Pathol.* 2021;30(5):2169-2201. doi:10.1044/2021_AJSLP-21-00076

62. Helou LB, Gartner-Schmidt JL, Hapner ER, Schneider SL, Van Stan JH. Mapping meta-therapy in voice interventions onto the rehabilitation treatment specification system. *Semin Speech Lang.* 2021;42(1):5-18. doi:10.1055/s-0040-1722756

63. Vocabulary.com

64. Thesaurus.com

65. Behlau M, Oliveira G. Vocal hygiene for the voice professional. *Curr Opin Otolaryngol Head Neck Surg.* 2009;17(3):149-154. doi:10.1097/MOO.0b013e32832af105

66. Rodríguez-Parra MJ, Adrián JA, Casado JC. Comparing voice-therapy and vocal-hygiene treatments in dysphonia using a limited multidimensional evaluation protocol. *J Commun Disord.* 2011;44(6):615-630. doi:10.1016/j.jcomdis.2011.07.003

67. Desjardins M, Halstead L, Simpson A, Flume P, Bonilha HS. Respiratory muscle strength training to improve vocal function in patients with presbyphonia. *J Voice.* 2020. doi:10.1016/j.jvoice.2020.06.006

68. American College of Sports Medicine. *ACSM's Guidelines for Exercise Testing and Prescription.* Lippincott Williams & Wilkins; 2013.

69. Roy N. Optimal dose-response relationships in voice therapy. *Int J Speech Lang Pathol.* 2012;14(5):419-423. doi:10.3109/17549507.2012.686119

70. Wenke RJ, Stabler P, Walton C, et al. Is more intensive better? Client and service provider outcomes for intensive versus standard therapy schedules for functional voice disorders. *J Voice.* 2014;28(5):652.e31-652.e43. doi:10.1016/j.jvoice.2014.02.005

71. Patel RR, Bless DM, Thibeault SL. Boot camp: A novel intensive approach to voice therapy. *J Voice.* 2011;25(5):562-569. doi:10.1016/j.jvoice.2010.01.010

72. Desjardins M, Halstead L, Simpson A, Flume P, Bonilha HS. Voice and respiratory characteristics of men and women seeking treatment for presbyphonia. *J Voice.* 2022;36(5):673-684. doi:10.1016/j.jvoice.2020.08.040

73. Gartner-Schmidt J, Lewandowski A, Haxer M, Milstein CF. Voice therapy for the beginning clinician. *Perspect ASHA Spec Interest Groups.* 2017;2(3):93-103. doi:10.1044/persp2.sig3.93

74. Enderby P. How much therapy is enough? The impossible question! *Int J Speech Lang Pathol.* 2012;14(5):432-437. doi:10.3109/17549507.2012.686118

75. Fujiki RB, Thibeault SL. Examining therapy duration in adults with voice disorders. *Am*

J Speech Lang Pathol. 2023;32(4):1665-1678. doi:10.1044/2023_AJSLP-22-00390

76. Fujiki RB, Thibeault SL. Pediatric voice therapy: How many sessions to discharge? *Am J Speech Lang Pathol.* 2022;31(6):2663-2674. doi:10.1044/2022_AJSLP-22-00111

77. Gartner-Schmidt J, Gherson S, Hapner ER, et al. The development of conversation training therapy: A concept paper. *J Voice.* 2016; 30(5):563-573. doi:10.1016/j.jvoice.2015.06.007

78. Hapner E, Portone-Maira C, Johns MM. A study of voice therapy dropout. *J Voice.* 2009;23(3):337-340. doi:10.1016/j.jvoice.2007.10.009

79. Gillespie AI, Gartner-Schmidt J. Voice-specialized speech-language pathologist's criteria for discharge from voice therapy. *J Voice.* 2018;32(3):332-339. doi:10.1016/j.jvoice.2017.05.022

80. Zipoli RP, Kennedy M. Evidence-based practice among speech-language pathologists: Attitudes, utilization, and barriers. *Am J Speech Lang Pathol.* 2005;14(3):208-220. doi:10.1044/1058-0360(2005/021)

81. Hapner E, Gartner-Schmidt J. The it factor: Strategies for developing the therapeutic alliance. 2021. https://www.medbridge.com/educate/courses/the-it-factor-strategies-for-developing-the-therapeutic-alliance-edie-hapner-jackie-gartner-schmidt

82. McGrath S, Schultz KR. Mapping the role of therapeutic alliance in speech and language therapy to the rehabilitation treatment specification system. *Perspect ASHA Spec Interest Groups.* 2024;9(2):481-489. doi:10.1044/2024_persp-23-00241

83. Ryan R, Deci E. Self-determination theory and the facilitation of intrinsic motivation, social development, and well-being. *Am Psychol.* 2000;55(1):68-78. doi:10.1037//0003-066x.55.1.68

84. Iwarsson J. Reflections on clinical expertise and silent know-how in voice therapy. *Logop Phoniatr Vocol.* 2015;40(2):66-71. doi:10.3109/14015439.2014.949302

85. Kapila R. Neuro-affirming practices for voice care. 2024;9(October):1314-1323.

86. Moonsammy SU, Procter T, Goodwin ME, Crumpton P. Proactive strategies for breaking barriers: Advancing justice initiatives in speech-language pathology for diverse populations in voice management and upper airway disorders. *Perspect ASHA Spec Interest Groups.* 2024;9(October):1-11. doi:10.1044/2023_persp-23-00138

87. Morton-Jones ME, Timmons Sund L. Exploring culturally responsive voice care: Mitigating disparities by addressing implicit bias. *Perspect ASHA Spec Interest Groups.* 2023;9(October):1-7. doi:10.1044/2023_persp-23-00137

88. Timmons Sund L, Motron-Jones M, Castro M. Exploring culturally responsive voice care: Introduction. *Perspect ASHA Spec Interest Groups.* 2024;9(October):2024-2026.

89. Vastine W, Butcher L. Doing the inner and outer work: Culturally responsive practices in gender-affirming voice care. *Perspect ASHA Spec Interest Groups.* 2024;9(5):1-13. doi:10.1044/2024_persp-23-00151

3

Phonotrauma

Introduction

Ryan C. Branski

In the 1950s, Timex launched an iconic advertising campaign to demonstrate the durability of their timepieces. Commercials showed Timex watches in the dishwasher, jackhammered, or taped to the rotund bellies of Sumo wrestlers. After every failed attempt to destroy the watches, John Cameron Swayze (one of the most famous voices at the time and the sixth cousin once removed of actor Patrick Swayze) delivered the now-famous slogan, "It takes a licking and keeps on ticking." The same can be said for the vocal folds. The architecture of these small structures allows them to withstand nearly unthinkable stresses and strains associated with phonation, and most of the time, they "keep on ticking." On occasion, however, they don't, resulting in chronic injury and tissue changes. This chapter provides innovative examples of therapeutic approaches for challenging patients with phonotraumatic injury.

The vocal folds are supremely engineered to recover from acute, transient injury—we've all sustained phonotraumatic injury after a sporting event or a prolonged coughing episode and recovered to full voice within a few days. Relatively rarely, however, the threshold of tissue tolerance is surpassed and more permanent tissue changes alter voice production.[1] The development of phonotraumatic lesions of the vocal folds, in most cases, is an adaptive response to tissue stress. For example, the first time shoveling snow in the winter will likely yield a blister. After a couple big storms, that blister will be replaced with a callus—new tissue to better withstand the stresses of shoveling. Interestingly, once spring comes and shoveling is extinguished, the callus is likely to resolve. To extend this analogy to the voice, unfortunately, such new tissue is counterproductive to efficient voice production. This process is beautifully described in the Starmer case involving granuloma formation (Case Study 3.5). Perhaps 6 to 8 months of voice rest could be quite therapeutic for phonotraumatic injury but devastating in numerous other ways.

Historically, wound healing across all tissues was thought to be mediated by immobility to allow for rapid healing. Orthopedic dogma required prolonged immobilization following soft tissue injury; a plaster cast was indicated for a simple ankle inversion strain. Unfortunately, suboptimal functional outcomes were rampant, and rapid tissue mobilization has evolved as the new standard. The corollary to these orthopedic developments is the emergence of science and data to direct voice rest strategies following vocal fold injury, both absolute and relative. Although some efficacy was reported for voice rest, and reduced voice use may remain in the clinical armamentarium, compliance with voice rest is poor[2] and the psychosocial impact of voice rest is profound. Grossly, voice rest is thought to be homologous with tissue immobilization. With regard to the voice, the science behind tissue mobilization is emerging. Mobilization has an anti-inflammatory effect on cells from the vocal folds,[3] and intriguing work by Verdolini Abbott found resonant voice exercises reduced vocal fold inflammation more than voice rest in patients with acute phonotrauma.[4] Although not the original intent, Stemple's Vocal Function Exercises (VFEs), presented in the accompanying case (Case Study 3.6), have emerged as a means to "mobilize" the vocal folds in the context of phonotraumatic injury. As outlined in the case by Collum and Lee, voice therapy can enhance vocal fold tissue health, and the biological complexity of wound healing must be incorporated in contemporary therapeutic approaches (Case Study 3.4).

Beyond biology, the cases in this chapter illustrate diversity regarding motor learning approaches to facilitate efficient phonation as a component of the therapeutic process. Traditionally, therapy included a hierarchical structure, paying homage to the "you have to walk before you run" line of thinking. In addition, antiquated therapy sought to perfect technique in the therapy room with little consideration of or practice in more vocally taxing, real-world environments. Most contemporary therapy approaches attempt to simulate scenarios with the potential to yield inefficient voicing after the acquisition of basic skills and awareness. Verdolini Abbott was a pioneer in her approach to therapy, building upon her unique background incorporating speech pathology and psychology. As outlined in Case Study 3.7 by Orbelo, Li, and Verdolini Abbott, her approach to therapy has been adopted nearly universally with the goal of establishing an optimal laryngeal posture to maximize vocal output while minimizing phonotrauma.[5] Generalization of skills obtained in therapy to more challenging scenarios is both critical to success and incredibly challenging.[6-8] More recently, Gillespie, Gartner-Schmidt, and colleagues introduced a novel approach to therapy that circumvents the traditional hierarchical approach (Case Study 3.1); Conversation Training Therapy (CTT) jumps right to conversational speech in initial sessions.[9] Data from their group are impressive.[10]

Collectively, these cases illustrate the diversity of approaches for patients with phonotraumatic vocal fold injury. Voice therapy is no longer one size fits all; creativity is encouraged and required in the pediatric and performing arts populations, as described by Hersan (Case Study 3.2) and Murphy Estes (Case Study 3.3), respectively. This variety allows for therapists to customize therapy for each patient and move the field toward a more personalized approach to voice rehabilitation. In addition, these cases exhibit the immense skill of clinicians treating patients with voice disorders.

Case Studies

 CASE STUDY 3.1

Conversation Training Therapy (CTT) to Treat an Adult With Benign Midmembranous Lesions

Jackie L. Gartner-Schmidt and Amanda I. Gillespie

Voice Evaluation

GZ underwent a comprehensive evaluation by a voice-specialized speech-language pathologist (SLP). The voice evaluation included a case history as well as auditory-perceptual, acoustic, and aerodynamic testing and a standardized stimulability assessment for voice therapy success.

Case History

Patient GZ, a 32-year-old cisgender female worship leader and gospel singer, was referred for voice therapy by an interdisciplinary team consisting of a fellowship-trained laryngologist and a voice-specialized SLP. GZ complained of a gradual onset of dysphonia, low pitch, throat tightness, and vocal fatigue in her speaking voice, as well as difficulty with high-pitched soft sung sounds in her singing voice. These symptoms have been worsening over the past 2 months, precipitated by an upper respiratory infection. GZ reported speaking and singing through her sickness. Her occupational voice demands were many, as she led worship service for 4 hours every Sunday and held rehearsal once a week. GZ was also recording a demo for her solo career as a gospel artist and was embarking on a short tour (12 performances) around the neighboring states in the next 3 months. She was anxious to be helped quickly. GZ also disclosed that she was diagnosed with "nodules" 10 years ago when she was in college and went through voice therapy but stopped going after the ninth session because "it took too long"; she could not remember what she did in therapy, but her voice got better. GZ had 3 singing teachers over her 10 years of vocal training. She was a mezzo-soprano. GZ noted that most of her symptoms were in her speaking voice versus her singing voice, and stated, "I'm much harder on my speaking voice than my singing voice." She was quick to point out that she sang "soulful" gospel, which was safe for her voice, versus "yelling gospel." Her past medical history was significant for seasonal allergies, which were well treated with weekly allergy shots. She was a single mother with an 8-year-old son.

Auditory-Perceptual Evaluation

GZ's voice was assessed using a visual analog scale via the Consensus Auditory-Perceptual Evaluation of Voice (CAPE-V) parameters.[11] The task involved reading aloud the 6 sentences of the CAPE-V protocol and a sustained /a/ vowel. The SLP rated GZ's voice as 38/100 in overall severity with 0 representing "no dysphonia" and 100 being "severe dysphonia," indicating a dysphonia of moderate nature. Perceptually, resonance seemed to be more pharyngeal, or "in the throat," rather than anterior, oral resonance. Respiration seemed within functional limits (WFL), as evidenced by a lack of upper clavicular movement and no report of dyspnea during speaking or other activities of daily living. However, the patient was noted to "breath hold," and there was frequent sighing during connected speech. Other perceptual features included decreased pitch variance (ie, inflection), and vocal fry, especially at the end of phrases. The SLP also asked GZ to glide upwards in pitch softly on the /u/ vowel, feeling airflow on her lips and finger (positioned in front of her lips). GZ was instructed to be as quiet as possible but still phonate. GZ's voice "cracked" around approximately G4 (ie, the G above middle C on a keyboard). Often this brief task can "uncover" midmembranous edema or lesions corroborated by laryngeal videostroboscopy.

Acoustic Analysis

For acoustic analyses, like the auditory-perceptual evaluation, GZ read the 6 sentences of the CAPE-V protocol and sustained the /a/ vowel with a headset microphone (Shure-Beta 54) placed at a 45-degree angle from the mouth. Acoustic measures of cepstral peak prominence (CPP), CPP fundamental frequency (CPP F0) measured in Hz, CPP F0 standard deviation (SD), and cepstral-spectral index of dysphonia (CSID) were taken from the all-voiced sentence "We were away a year ago" using the Analysis of Dysphonia in Speech and Voice (ADSV) program from the Computerized Speech Lab (CSL) (Pentax Medical, Montvale, NJ).[12] Results of the measures are found in Table 3–1.

Aerodynamic Measures

Next, phonatory aerodynamic measurements were obtained by having GZ read the first 4 sentences of the Rainbow Passage using a comfortable pitch and loudness with the Pentax Phonatory Aerodynamic System (model 6600, Pentax Medical, Montvale, NJ).[13,14] Measures and norms are represented in Table 3–2.

Stimulability Testing

Stimulability testing was performed to guide therapeutic decision making and to determine GZ's ability to make phonatory changes in response to a therapeutic prompt.[15] After the first reading of the Rainbow Passage, the SLP instructed GZ to read the sentences again using

"clear speech." Specifically, the SLP asked GZ to "use crisp, clear consonants" and "precise articulation," being sure to also vary the pitch inflection when she read "like you are reading or telling an interesting story." The use of "clear speech" as part of a stimulability assessment is associated with immediate improvement in acoustic and aerodynamic voice outcomes in some patients with voice disorders.[16] Results for both the initial and subsequent "clear speech" productions are found in Table 3–2. Post stimulability trial, the measures were within the normative range for adult phonatory aerodynamics in connected speech.[13]

When GZ was asked if she heard or felt a difference between the 2 different times she read the sentences, she agreed that her voice sounded better and she felt less throat tightness the "second time." GZ then went through a resonant voice and flow phonation stimula-

Table 3–1. ADSV: Cepstral Peak Prominence (CPP), Cepstral Peak Prominence Fundamental Frequency (CPP F0), Cepstral Peak Prominence Fundamental Frequency Standard Deviation (CPP F0 SD), Cepstral-Spectral Index of Dysphonia (CSID)

ADSV Measures	GZ's Scores	Cisgender Female Norms	SD
CPP (dB)	6.00	7.66	0.95
CPP F0 (Hz)	201	200.42	16.49
CPP F0 SD	38	32.66	10.54
CSID	36	6.44	7.94

Table 3–2. Phonatory Aerodynamics in Connected Speech Pretreatment

	Number of Breaths	Passage Duration (seconds)	Mean Pitch (F0) in Hz	Mean Phonatory Airflow in mL/s
Original	3	28	167	92
Stimulability Trial of Clear Speech	6	32	201	180

bility trial in sustained and connected speech stimuli and again reported an improvement in the feel (vibrotactile/kinesthetic awareness) and sound of her voice. Based on the results of the stimulability testing, the SLP counseled GZ that she thought her voice could be improved with voice therapy. She proceeded to give the patient a vocal wellness handout to read before the first voice therapy session and told the patient she would field any questions and individualize a vocal hygiene program for her.

Patient Self-Assessment

In addition to the acoustics, aerodynamics, and stimulability assessment, GZ was also given 4 Patient-Reported Outcome Measures (PROMs). Table 3–3 depicts the scores on the Voice Handicap Index–10 (VHI-10),[17] Dyspnea Index (DI),[18] and Singing Voice Handicap Index–10 (SVHI-10).[19] GZ was also asked to rate vocal effort on a 0 (no vocal effort to produce voice) to 10 (extreme vocal effort to produce voice) scale. GZ reported a 3/10 as it related to singing but a 6/10 as it related to speaking. GZ's self-perception of not having a problem with her singing voice was corroborated by her perceptual reports.

Laryngeal Imaging

Following the SLP assessment, GZ underwent a rigid stroboscopic laryngeal examination with the laryngologist. The exam revealed very small bilateral midmembranous vocal

Table 3–3. Patient-Reported Outcome Measures

VHI-10	*17/40
DI	6/40
CSI	9/40
SVHI-10	25/40

*Indicates a score associated with a voice problem (>11).

fold lesions, appearing to be subepithelial in nature with a good mucosal wave. Specifically, symmetry, amplitude, periodicity, and mucosal wave were all subjectively judged by the laryngologist and SLP to be normal; only closure at high pitch was noted to have a "mild" hourglass closure pattern.

Impressions

GZ's severity of dysphonia was rated moderate secondary to auditory-perceptual, acoustic, and aerodynamic assessment, and her VHI-10 score of 17/40.[17,20] Her prognosis for recovery with behavioral voice therapy was determined to be good secondary to a positive response to stimulability testing, especially her feeling a difference between her presenting dysphonic voice and her voice production in response to stimulability trials,[21] history of some improvement with voice therapy, and her upper respiratory illness (URI)-inciting event having abated. The expected frequency, duration, and goals were as follows: The SLP planned to initiate CTT, which GZ was expected to complete in 2 to 4 sessions (based on results from Gillespie et al that significant gains in all outcomes [PROMs, acoustic, aerodynamic, and auditory-perceptual] were seen following 2 sessions of CTT compared with 4 to 8 sessions of traditional therapy).[10] The duration of each session was set at approximately 45 minutes.

Decision Making

The SLP chose to pursue treatment with CTT. This choice was made based on GZ's positive response to stimulability testing in connected speech, her high occupational voice demands, and the time limitations she had for rehabilitation. The SLP wanted to provide GZ with voice techniques she could immediately use in her everyday conversational speech. CTT exclusively relies on patient-driven conversation rather than the traditional hierarchy of skill building from least (eg, phonemes, words) to most complex (eg, phrases, conversation). CTT was developed based on motor learning theories, which encourage learning through practice in variable, real-life contexts. A full description of each of the 6 components of CTT (clear speech, negative practice, auditory/kinesthetic awareness, prosody, embedded basic training gestures, intensity) and their motor learning scientific rationale is provided in publications regarding the conceptual development of this treatment approach.[9]

Plan of Care

The long-term goal of therapy was for GZ to maximize vocal effectiveness relative to her existing laryngeal disorder and to return to vocal activities of daily living (eg, functional voice communication), especially for her occupational voice demands. Initial short-term goals were as follows but expected to be altered based on session-to-session gains:

1. The patient will perform clear speech in conversational speech at 80% accuracy as assessed by the clinician's auditory perception and patient corroborating vibrotactile sensations.
2. The patient will perform negative practice in conversational speech at 80% accuracy as assessed by the clinician's auditory perception of the "new" and "old" voice and speech production of clear speech, prosody, pauses, projection, and embedded Basic Training Gestures (eBTGs), corroborated by the patient's differentiating the sound and feel between the 2 respective voice productions.
3. The patient will label different voice productions as assessed by names chosen and relevant to the patient, and corresponding analogies/metaphors.

Intervention

The first voice therapy session began with a follow-up to the Vocal Wellness reading material that was given to GZ at the initial voice evaluation. The duration of the personalized indirect voice therapy component was approximately 15 minutes.

GZ was seen for a total of 3 sessions. In the first session, she was prompted to begin a conversation of her choice, using "clear speech with articulatory precision," and to vary her pitch inflection as she had done in the initial voice evaluation. At first, GZ was confused about whether she was "doing it right," but the SLP assured her not to be thinking about "right or wrong" but rather to increase her awareness of the sound and feel of her voice and speech as she attempted the requested changes. The SLP told her to "pretend you have a consonant salad in your mouth." That analogy perplexed GZ, so the SLP took out a piece of paper and drew a simple sagittal view of the head and neck (Figure 3–1) and told her: "We are going to play a game. It's called Fffffffeel the Sssssssoundzzzzzz of Sssssspeech."

The SLP purposely drew out the consonants when she said the sentence. Using Figure 3–1, the SLP asked GZ to hold a /z/ and go up and down in pitch and concentrate on where she felt the /z/ sound. Then, she

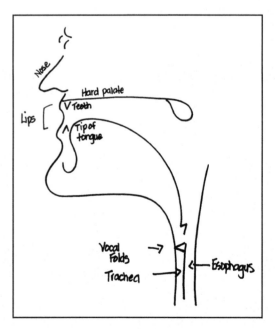

FIGURE 3–1. Simple sagittal-view hand drawing of the head and neck.

gave GZ a highlighter and told her to mark on the figure where she felt the sound. (See Video 1 Mapping Speech Sound Sensations by Gartner-Schmidt.) GZ colored the tip of the tongue of the figure. Next, the SLP asked her to repeat one of the sentences she had said in her prompted speech moments before, "I went to my mom's house," embedding the BTG in connected speech. The BTG is a strategy introduced by Verdolini Abbott in Lessac-Madsen Resonant Voice Therapy (LMRVT) wherein a patient sustains a phoneme (often a nasal consonant) in a word or short phrase to focus on the articulatory sensations (see Case Study 3.7 by Orbelo, Li, and Verdolini Abbott: Lessac-Madsen Resonant Voice Therapy to Treat an Adult With Vocal Fold Nodules). In CTT, the BTG is embedded into the patient's extemporaneous speech and can occur on any sustainable consonant. Again, she was asked if she continued to feel the energy or sensation of the /w/ or the /m/ in her mouth or anterior face. GZ took a different-colored highlighter for various sounds as she felt them and colored the area on the figure (Figure 3–2). After each exploration of the sensation of the consonants, the SLP had GZ repeat the sentence she had generated with an increased focus on the feel of the consonants. This process took less than 10 minutes, and she was now aware of each consonant having a distinct oral-facial vibrotactile sensation. The SLP and GZ immediately engaged in more conversation for a couple of minutes, with GZ concentrating on feeling the consonants in the front of her mouth when she spoke.

Next, the SLP asked GZ to talk, highlighting the complaints that she listed in the initial voice evaluation; namely, she prompted her to speak in a low-pitched and dysphonic voice and to feel throat tightness. The SLP and GZ continued talking about the initial patient narrative, which was about visiting her mom. The SLP abruptly stopped the conversation and asked GZ to immediately switch back to the "clear speech and increased pitch inflection" style of talking. Here the SLP was covertly

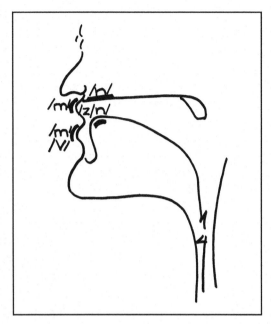

FIGURE 3–2. GZ's sensory reference for 4 phonemes.

introducing negative practice (discriminatory practice) in conversational speech. (See Video 2 Clear Speech and Negative Practice by Gillespie.)

When asked, GZ stated she could feel and hear a difference in the 2 voices and preferred the "new" voice. GZ left the therapy session feeling confident about using her "new" voice, even though, as she reported, "I have no clue what I am doing but I can feel a difference!" The SLP assured GZ that her impression was perfectly fine and vibrotactile awareness was the goal, not biomechanical knowledge of what she was doing with her voice production.

It was recommended that she practice at least 7 times a day using her "new" voice for 1 minute and then switching immediately to her "old" voice for approximately 30 seconds and finally returning to the "new" voice to train her awareness of the differences in sound and feel between the 2 conversational voices. This training protocol also aimed to establish a sense of control for the patient concerning her differing voice productions versus continuing to be a "victim" of her voice.

The next 2 voice therapy sessions focused on differentiating projection using the "old" and "new" voice in conversation. GZ was asked to increase and decrease the sensation of the anterior energy of the consonants while talking and become aware of the resulting dynamic changes in loudness. This increased consonant energy served as a sensory target when GZ wanted to project her voice. She was also taught to decrease the rate of speech so that the vowels could "carry the loudness" much like in singing. The ends of words and phrases were also recommended to have crisp consonants, as this technique can allow for linguistically appropriate pauses for breath replenishment. GZ was also asked to become aware of dropping her pitch and airflow at the ends of linguistic strings and not to talk in the "pitch ditch" (eg, vocal fry).

To make these different voice productions more personal and easier to remember than "old" versus "new," GZ was asked to label them, which is a tenet of meta-therapy.[22] GZ referred to her old voice as "the Redrum voice" from Stephen King's novel and movie *The Shining*, and her new voice as "free voice." Naming 2 different voice productions ostensibly creates a (sensory) metaphor for remembering the auditory/kinesthetic sensations of the "new" voice production. During the last 2 sessions, GZ was asked to bring "scripts" that she used for her worship so the connected speech therapy stimuli would be even more ecologically valid to the patient's occupational conversational voice.

GZ returned to the follow-up clinic 2 months later. This time frame was intentional to examine whether GZ had retained the tenets of CTT in her occupational and avocational voice demands. At follow-up, GZ repeated the same voice laboratory measurements: auditory-perceptual judgment of overall severity of voice, acoustics, aerodynamics, and patient-reported outcomes questionnaires. Her self-assessment scores all improved, as did her acoustic and aerodynamic measures (Table 3–4).

> Here, Gartner-Schmidt and Gillespie demonstrate the value of following up with the patient after a period of time in which they have returned to typical voice use. Patients are often lost to follow-up after voice therapy, and we do not always know the long-term outcomes. Perhaps periodic monitoring or long-term follow-up could better elucidate the sustainable benefits of voice therapy.

Table 3–4. Patient-Reported Outcomes and Auditory-Perceptual, Acoustic, and Aerodynamic Measures Pre- and Post-Voice Therapy

Patient-Reported Outcomes	Pre-CTT	Post-CTT
VHI-10	*17/40	7/40
DI	6/40	NA
CSI	9/40	NA
SVHI-10	25/40	16/40
Auditory-Perceptual (CAPE-V overall severity)	41/100	24/100
Acoustics in Speech		
CPP (dB)	6.00	8.02
CPP F0 (Hz)	201	226
CPP F0 SD	38	42
CSID	36	21
Aerodynamics in Speech		
Number of breaths	6	6
Passage duration (s)	32	36
Mean pitch (Hz)	201	232
Mean phonatory airflow (mL/s)	180	230

*indicates a score associated with a voice problem (>11)

Laryngeal Imaging

Her laryngeal videostroboscopy revealed a perceptual reduction in size of the vocal fold lesions and an increase in mucosal wave consistent with improvement in function but not full reduction of the lesions. At high pitches, the hourglass closure was gone.

Summary and Conclusion

Because CTT focuses on voice awareness and production in conversational speech (in the first session and throughout), the number of voice therapy sessions required for CTT is often lower than with traditional therapies. In addition, the functional specificity of CTT (ie, conversation) seemed important to GZ based on her remarks about her prior voice therapy. GZ felt confident about using her "free voice" and "getting her voice production back" if she reverted to her "Redrum voice" based on her ability to feel and hear the difference between the 2 voice productions in connected speech.

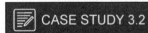

CASE STUDY 3.2

Treating a Child With Dysphonia Using Concepts From "Adventures in Voice"

Rita Hersan

Voice Evaluation

Case History

Chief Complaint. Gradual onset of dysphonia described as "hoarseness" and periods of soreness in the neck, which was aggravated after extensive voice use during summer camp activities.

History of Voice Complaint. MJ, a 7-year-old boy, is accompanied by his parents and referred to the SLP by a laryngologist. The parents report a gradual change in voice quality over the preceding 9 months. Initially, the voice problem was considered transient and did not seem to bother the child or impact communication in daily activities. MJ's parents noticed frequent periods of "hoarseness," which they considered normal until the voice quality worsened and persisted after attending a summer camp. MJ's parents decided to pursue a voice evaluation once he expressed frustration, saying his voice "was not working right." The parents described MJ as healthy with a normal developmental history. He had tympanostomy tubes placed when he was 3 years old, and a recent hearing test was within normal limits. His medical history revealed no evidence of allergies or acid reflux symptoms.

Voice Use. MJ is the oldest of 3 children; his younger brothers are 5 and 3 years old. His parents describe him as a socially and academically well-adjusted second-grade student who shows special interest in soccer and recently joined the school choir. Both parents are professional classical musicians. The family environment is characterized as moderately noisy because MJ's mother teaches piano lessons at home. The parents report that MJ strains his voice frequently during soccer practice and occasionally imitates different character voices when playing with toy figures or video games.

Laryngeal Imaging

Laryngeal videostroboscopy was performed transnasally with a flexible distal chip laryngoscope. The exam revealed bilateral symmetric midmembranous vocal fold lesions, appearing to be subepithelial in nature, with normal mucosal wave and slightly reduced amplitude of vibration bilaterally. Glottal closure was marked by an hourglass configuration.

Quality-of-Life Impairment

The parental proxy Pediatric Voice Handicap Index (pVHI)[23] was administered to quantify the effects of the voice problem, with a score of 45/92 indicating a moderate impact on the child's life. Additionally, MJ was asked to answer the following questions for self-assessment of his voice problem:

1. "How much does your voice problem bother you? Does it bother you a little bit (mildly), quite a bit (moderately), or a lot (severely)?" MJ answered, "Sometimes it bothers me a lot!"
2. "How is your voice today?" The voice therapist provided a chart representing 10 steps. Step 1 represented the worst voice and step 10 represented the best voice. MJ pointed to step 5.

Auditory-Perceptual Assessment

Auditory-perceptual evaluation was administered using the CAPE-V.[11] The child's overall CAPE-V score was 48/100, which indicates a moderately deviant voice. Aberrant perceptual voice features included: moderate roughness (45/100), mild breathiness (20/100), mild to moderate strain (30/100), mild to moderate low pitch (28/100), and mild increased loudness (20/100).

Acoustic and Aerodynamic Assessment

Acoustic data were acquired utilizing the Multi-Dimensional Voice Program (MDVP) from CSL (Pentax Medical, Montvale, NJ) with a headset microphone placed at a 45-degree angle at 4 inches from the mouth.

Acoustic measures revealed a mean fundamental frequency of 238 Hz on the Rainbow Passage and 226 Hz taken on sustained vowel /a/ at comfortable loudness. A mean fundamental frequency of 260 Hz was expected for the child's age on sustained /a/ at comfortable loudness. Frequency range varied from 200 to 295 Hz on sustained /a/; a range of 220 to 310 Hz was expected for his age.[24] Mean intensity was 68 dB SPL measured during connected speech (Rainbow Passage) and the dynamic intensity range was 65 dB to 86 dB SPL on sustained /a/. Intensity measures were within normal range.[25]

Aerodynamic measures were obtained on repeated syllable trains of /pa/ at comfortable pitch and loudness using the Phonatory Aerodynamic System (PAS). Results showed mean airflow of 250 mL/sec at comfortable pitch and loudness and estimated subglottal pressure at 8.5 cmH$_2$O, which was expected for his age.[26,27]

Stimulability

MJ was stimulable for voice improvement utilizing the following strategies: (1) producing voiceless fricatives and releasing airflow, (2) transitioning from voiceless to voiced fricatives, and (3) repeating words initiated with /m/, /n/, /v, and /z/ and prolonging the consonants while focusing on anterior sensation of vibration on lips or tongue. MJ felt a "tickle" on his lips and a "buzz" in his voice. The voice therapist and the child heard a consistent and clearer voice quality during stimulability tasks.

Impressions

MJ interacted attentively and showed interest during the voice evaluation and stimulability tasks. He seemed motivated to explore his voice symptoms and go on a "voice journey." His parents were supportive and confirmed their availability to initiate voice therapy. All these factors contributed to a good prognosis for the therapy outcome.

Plan of Care

The SLP recommended that MJ attend a total of eight 45-minute voice therapy sessions over a 10-week period. The initial 6 sessions were scheduled once a week and were recommended to be conducted in person. The last 2 sessions were spaced out every 2 weeks and could be delivered via teletherapy. The parents opted for in-person sessions.

The SLP introduced the concepts of *Adventures in Voice* and explained that the program was developed to help children use their voices strongly, when needed, while avoiding damage and promoting healing to existent vocal injury.[28,29]

The long-term therapy goal for MJ was to maximize his vocal output relative to the existing laryngeal disorder. It was expected that he would be able to acquire a healthy vocal pattern, produce clearer and stronger voice with minimal vocal fold impact stress, and integrate target vocal behaviors in a variety of contexts, including background noise and emotional situations. The voice therapist clarified that a healthy vocal pattern involved barely ad-/abducted vocal folds, perceptually corresponding to resonant voice or "easy voice" associated with perceptible anterior oral vibrations.[5]

The short-term goals included:

1. Provide education about voice production and work on perception and production of easy anterior vibrations versus no vibrations
2. Increase perception and production of resonant voice or "easy voice" associated with perceptible anterior oral vibrations
3. Identify situations with an emotional content and describe their possible effect on voice
4. Perceive and produce vocal loudness variations focusing on strong anterior vibrations.
5. Vary vocal loudness according to the circumstances.

Decision Making: Why use the concepts from Adventures in Voice?

Children often use their voices extensively and vigorously, placing them at risk for phonotrauma. Noisy playgrounds, sports events, and outdoor activities are typical environments sought by this population, which consequently promote yelling, cheering, and loud talking. These are common vocal behaviors in children and should not be considered aberrant. For this reason, the traditional therapy approach for children, which focuses on voice conservation by encouraging them to reduce or eliminate phonotraumatic behaviors, historically referred to as vocal "abuse" and "misuse," seems pragmatically hopeless from the outset. It usually provides dysphonic children with long lists of "do"s and "don't"s, lacking a cohesive framework and ultimately poten-

tially promoting fear of talking, singing, and even laughing. *Adventures in Voice* promotes targeting and tailoring individualized vocal care activities, which are more likely to benefit the child, as compared with generic programs that may be overwhelming and irrelevant to the patient.[30]

> The reader is encouraged to read the above section again given the importance of the concepts described. Successful voice therapy embraces principles of self-efficacy and building the therapeutic alliance. Here, Rita Hersan beautifully highlights these principles.

Intervention

Short-Term Therapy Goal #1

Goal #1. Provide education about voice production and work on perception and production of easy anterior vibrations versus no vibrations. *"Are you ready for this adventure with your voice?"*

The child heard a simple story about how "hurt voices and healing voices" may happen to children and adults because we all use our voices frequently and not always in the best conditions.[8] He learned about facts that can cause hurt voices, such as not drinking enough water, talking loudly with background noise, clearing the throat often, yelling and screaming, and talking a lot while feeling sick. When asked about what he thought may have contributed to his "hurting" voice, MJ responded, "Maybe I yelled a lot at the soccer games and didn't drink much water!"

The program *Adventures in Voice* for this particular child was called "A Journey to Discover My Easy Voice." For each therapy session, MJ was asked to self-assess his voice using the same representation of steps that was used in the initial evaluation. Most of the activities were planned using the child's own ideas. He prepared a map of the journey, and the voice therapist, also known as the "Journey Guide," proposed a visit to different "towns." MJ received a bottle of water, a backpack, a journey diary, and a passport before starting his journey. He was told that he could help his voice by taking sips of water and eating watery fruits to increase vocal fold hydration. He was asked to press and rub one hand against the other and describe the feel. Then, he was asked to clap forcefully for a few seconds and look at his hands. He noticed that the friction while rubbing and the force while clapping were causing redness on his hands. These demonstrations were appropriate for MJ to understand the negative impact of throat clearing, screaming, and yelling on the vocal folds. MJ received a stamp on his passport for following the directions well.

Taking into account MJ's recent interest in music and singing, the Journey Guide suggested that the first stop would be at "Wind Town" and all the visitors were requested to produce special sounds. Pictures of some wind instruments in an orchestra were shown, and the target sounds /v/, /z/, and /ʒ/ introduced. To incorporate the activity into something meaningful, MJ selected cards with written words and pictures from a small backpack. The Journey Guide produced target sounds with exaggerated vibration on words, such as: zebra, viola, measure, very, zero, television, voice, zoo, treasure. MJ heard the difference when the Journey Guide alternated voice with vibrations and voice without vibrations on words beginning with /f/, /s/, and /ʃ/, such as: sea, fifth, shop, fat, ship, soup, shoe, feet, shelf, soap, face. The Journey Guide asked if the child would like to practice "vibration sounds" while playing a game: each player got 3 points if a word with /v/, /z/, or /ʒ/ was pulled out from the backpack and produced with a tickle, and only 1 point for a word with /f/, /s/, or /ʃ/ and no tickle. Together, MJ and the Journey Guide prepared a home package called "Tracking My Voice." They used a chart and added

personalized vocal care and vocal activities to be practiced at home.

Short-Term Therapy Goal #2

Goal #2. Increase perception and production of resonant voice or "easy voice" associated with perceptible anterior oral vibrations. *"Our voice journey continues."*

The Journey Guide pretended to play string instruments while producing easy anterior vibrations on /m/, /n/, and /ŋ/, and immediately MJ guessed that he was going to visit "String Town" on the second voice therapy session. He was asked to cover his mouth and nose to feel the vibrations on the palm of his hands. Once he was able to feel the buzzing, he was asked to use contrastive drills, keeping his lips very tight while producing /m/ or the tongue very pressed while producing /n/. MJ recognized the difference between easy vibration and no vibration. He was told that in "String Town" everyone enjoyed humming, so they were known as "Humming People." Humming was helpful because prolonging sounds caused stronger sensations of a tickle inside the mouth, around the lips, or behind the teeth. MJ and the Journey Guide played a game filling in blanks in sentences using words beginning with /m/ and /n/, while "humming" or chanting the words. Examples: Many men on the . . . (moon), My nanny . . . (made) lemonade, String Land is . . . (magical), My Mom is a . . . (musician), I love lemon . . . (muffins), Manny and Lenny are . . . (nice), Mona made me . . . (mad), No one found the . . . (money), Noah is . . . (mowing) the lawn, May I know your . . . (name)?

Once MJ felt stronger anterior vibrations while chanting the words, he was asked to prolong the target sounds just a bit, and this time, combine target sounds from Wind and String Town while playing bingo: van, music, dozen, vision, news, visit, museum, nose, violin, television, navy, eleven, venture, zombie. To transition from structured activity to natural voice production, the child, his mother, and the Journey Guide had to answer 10 questions each, just using "mhmm" for "yes" or "nnno," gliding the voice and focusing on easy anterior vibrations.

MJ heard a story about "Phone," a telephone that enjoyed long conversations, until the day when nobody was at home and "Phone" felt exhausted after hours of constant ringing. The story reinforced the idea that "Phone" recovered its clear ringing sound after some rest and care. MJ prepared his version of the story using the "Little Story Creator" iPad app, and he repeated tongue trills to imitate "Phone's" clear ringing sound.

Short-Term Therapy Goal #3

Goal #3. Identify situations with an emotional content and describe their possible effect on voice. *"Where are we going now?"*

The third voice therapy session was a visit to "Brass Town" and the target sounds /l/ and /r/ were introduced, with emphasis on pitch glides and anterior vibrations in the mouth. MJ and the Journey Guide prepared a road template using curves, ups, and downs through the mountain scene. MJ was asked to create a story using suggested pictures and words with target sounds: **r**ed, ca**r**, **r**ock, **r**ain, **r**ainbow, pa**r**rot, ye**ll**ow, ti**r**e, **r**un, long **r**iver, **l**izard, **r**oll-ing, **L**ori, **R**osie, **L**arry, **L**iz, **R**yan. He called it "The Road to Brass Town." MJ learned about "voice release" using strategies such as sighing, lip trills, stretches, and yawning associated with body movement and embedded in different emotional situations related to the story. Examples of an emotional situation: The car ran out of gas and the Journey Guide felt upset; she said "arr" with tight /r/ and then she "released" her voice, saying "ahh" on a glid-ing sigh. Then, the car got a flat tire, and MJ expressed frustration with a tight "uhh" and then he released his voice with lip trill glides and a shoulder shrug. Feeling exhausted by driving, MJ and the Journey Guide stretched their arms and yawned widely!

Short-Term Therapy Goal #4

Goal #4. Perceive and produce vocal loudness variations focusing on strong anterior vibrations. *"When is loud too loud?"*

Another series of target sounds, /b/, /d/, and /g/, was introduced for the specific work on loudness variation associated with precise articulation. The fourth voice therapy session was the visit to "Percussion Town." Different sizes of fake pebbles made of cardboard were used to build a trail on the floor and help the patient to engage in functional use of loudness variation. MJ was shown how to vary the vocal loudness while stepping on the pebbles: the bigger the pebble, the louder the voice. Syllable trains with target sounds were included in a variety of rhythmic patterns, such as: BOM-BOM bombombom; dan DAN danDANdan, gogoGOgogoGOgogo.

MJ read a story about Zane, a boy who yelled frequently at soccer games until he finally realized that it was not his loud voice that helped him to score a goal, but rather his strong legs. Yelling was just causing confusion among the other players and affecting Zane's voice to the point that he had almost no voice after soccer games. Loud background noise with headphones was played during the read-ing activity. MJ's voice was recorded and played back after his reading. MJ and his mother were impressed by the effect of background noise on voice loudness. Using the "Little Story Creator" iPad app, MJ wrote his version of Zane's story, drawing and adding some voice recordings.

Short-Term Therapy Goal #5

Goal #5. Vary vocal loudness according to the circumstances. *"Let's invite a friend to our voice journey."*

It was arranged with the child's mother that MJ could invite a friend to participate in his voice journey. This strategy was particu-larly important to engage MJ in activities that were more representative of his habitual behav-ior. MJ showed the journey map to his friend, including all the towns he had visited and the most special characteristics of each town. MJ felt excited to share with his friend what he had done on the journey to discover his easy voice! To work on loud and safe voices, MJ and his friend used a sound level meter to monitor the loudness of their voices while playing a video game. To address loudness variation in different situations, the Journey Guide suggested a role-play activity:

1. MJ went to the library and needed to ask for a book using his soft voice.
2. The rocket was about to launch, and MJ's friend had to count "5, 4, 3, 2, 1" while projecting his voice.
3. Dad was taking a nap, and MJ wanted to ask Mom to play outside, so he used a softer voice.
4. The soccer coach was teaching the team how to dribble and used a strong voice.
5. MJ's friend wanted to watch TV, so he asked his mother in a normal loudness.
6. Mom was asking her kids to come for dinner, so she projected her voice.

The last 2 therapy sessions were less structured and reviewed all concepts of healthy voice use through stories and games. They focused on applying target sounds to spontaneous conversation and challenging the child to recognize risky situations.

Therapy Outcomes

Auditory-Perceptual Evaluation

The overall severity of voice quality that was considered moderately deviant (48/100) at the initial evaluation indicated a marked improvement (15/100) at 1 month post therapy reassessment. Perceptually, his voice showed no evidence of breathiness or strain and only mild intermittent roughness. The pitch and loudness of his voice were considered normal.

Laryngeal Imaging

Videolaryngostroboscopy revealed mild edema of true vocal folds with considerable reduction of bilateral subepithelial lesions, normal mucosal wave, normal amplitude of vibration, and a small posterior glottic gap.

Acoustic Analysis

The acoustic measures revealed a speaking fundamental frequency of 250 Hz in connected speech and 246 Hz on sustained /a/. These measures showed a significant improvement, since a mean fundamental frequency of 260 Hz was expected for the child's age in connected speech. Frequency range revealed a slight improvement, from 200 to 295 Hz at initial evaluation to 210 to 310 Hz. The mean intensity did not show much difference. It was 68 dB SPL at the initial evaluation and 69 dB SPL in connected speech (Rainbow Passage) post therapy. However, the dynamic range indicated a widening from 65 to 86 dB SPL at the initial evaluation to 62 to 90 dB SPL post treatment, which is within a normal range.

Aerodynamic Measures

Aerodynamic measures based on 5-syllable trains of /pa/ showed mean airflow of 160 mL/sec and estimated subglottal pressure of 7.5 cmH$_2$O. Both measures were considered normal for his age.

Patient Self-Assessment

The pVHI score was 12/92 at the 1-month post-therapy follow-up visit. The total score of the pVHI showed a significant improvement, especially on the physical and emotional subscales. MJ reported that the sound of his voice was not bothering him anymore and he described needing no effort to produce his voice.

Summary

Some voice therapists may argue that children, who are not aware of the voice problem, consequently have no motivation to engage in a therapeutic program such as *Adventures in Voice*. In fact, in challenge situations, motivation is also addressed by keeping the child actively involved as co-creator of the tasks in all phases of the program. Moreover, the attention required to learn a new motor task is continually encouraged by requiring the child's participation. Children require frequent and tangible evidence of progress across time. Visual charts assume great importance in analyzing the child's progress. The notion of getting better was translated by going higher in numbers using a chart representing steps from 1 to 10. This idea was very beneficial for motivation, helping the child to quantify his progress and to understand the long-term goals. MJ perceived a significant improvement after the third and fourth sessions, jumping from step 5 of his self-evaluation of voice to step 7 using the chart. Then he went back one point in session 5, most likely because he had a cold. He plateaued on step 7 for 2 consecutive sessions and finished on step 9 at the last session. He expressed great satisfaction with his progress.

Home practice should be part of real life, not time out from it. In this particular case, the family participation was remarkable, but even with their incredible support, the voice therapist was attentive to not overload the parents with too many tasks. Based on the progress noted in each therapy session, only 1 or 2 voice activities were selected each week for the home program, besides the vocal care recommendations. The use of recordings on the mother's cell phone and on the iPad during the therapy sessions, the journey diary containing a summary of all the activities worked in therapy, and the "Tracking My Voice" chart assisted the patient and his parents in adhering to the therapy process. The voice therapist reviewed the chart at the beginning of each therapy session. She suggested specific times for home practice according to the family availability.

> With both children and adults, making home practice a natural part of daily activities is critical. This reduces the burden of finding time to practice, which can be a barrier to behavior change. Weaving practice into daily life can support more sustainable voice changes and better outcomes overall.

Informational feedback was present throughout the therapy process to reflect how well the patient was doing with great emphasis on positive reinforcement. In addition, motivational feedback was applied in the form of extrinsic rewards (stickers on passport) every time the patient "journeyed" well during a therapy session and completed the daily assignments of the home program.

CASE STUDY 3.3

Multimodality Voice Therapy to Treat an Adult Female Opera Singer With a Vocal Fold Pseudocyst

Christine Murphy Estes

Voice Evaluation

Case History

Chief Complaint. Loss of singing range, increased vocal effort, vocal fatigue, "husky" quality in speaking voice

History of Voice Complaint. Patient B, a 48-year-old cisgender female operatic lyric soprano and voice teacher, sought evaluation for 4 months of voice symptoms. Onset coincided with a period of particularly heavy voice use while sick with a URI. She initially noticed a "flutter" in her high range. Symptoms progressively worsened, leading to inconsistency singing softly above G5, increased vocal effort, and vocal fatigue. Voice rest provided relief, but symptoms returned when she resumed singing. She later noticed a "husky" quality

62 Voice Therapy: Clinical Case Studies

to her speaking voice. She denied odynophonia, dysphagia, odynophagia, or dyspnea, but endorsed throat clearing. Past laryngeal examinations (>5 years) were unremarkable beyond edema from illness or allergies. Remarkable medical history included seasonal allergies and sinus infections. Medications included over-the-counter treatments for rare heartburn, and fluticasone and loratadine as needed for allergies.

Patient B began classical voice training at age 14 and earned bachelor's and master's degrees in vocal performance. She reported a history of "pushing" for fullness and straining in her high singing range. After graduation she worked with a voice teacher for a short time, but still experienced habitual "pushing and muscling." Her last voice lesson was 8 years ago, and she relied on past recordings as warm-ups, which she admitted to completing inconsistently.

Patient Self-Assessment
- OMNI Vocal Effort Scale[31]: 4/10 with speech, 7-8/10 with singing
- Voice Handicap Index–10 (VHI-10)[17]: 13/40 (threshold = 11)[20]
- Singing Voice Handicap Index–10 (SVHI-10)[19]: 28/40
- Reflux Symptom Index (RSI)[34]: 7/45

Voice Use/Vocal Demands
- Led soprano section of church choir (1 rehearsal and 1-2 services per week)
- Soloist for church services, such as funerals and weddings (0-2 per week, with amplification)
- Taught voice students (9-12 per week ranging in age from 13 to 64, in person and virtually)
- Upcoming contracts: soprano soloist for Mozart's *Requiem* in 2 months, summer festival as The Marschallin in *Der Rosenkavalier* in 4 months
- Inconsistent with vocal warm-ups when not in a performance contract, no cool-

down regimen (warm-ups included lip trills on 9-note scales and /ma-i/ on ascending/descending arpeggios)
- "Social and talkative" with mild difficulty speaking in noisy settings

Vocal Hygiene
- Drank 48 to 80 oz water and 8 to 16 oz caffeinated beverages daily, rarely drank seltzer, 1 to 3 EtOH weekly
- Inconsistently used humidifier due to difficulty with maintenance
- Tendency to eat late, occasional reflux symptoms (eg, heartburn)
- Nasal saline irrigation for allergies

> Throughout this text, in the research literature, and in clinical practice, a variety of terms have been suggested to describe healthy vocal behaviors, including vocal hygiene, vocal health, and vocal health and wellness. While terminology may differ, the general concepts are consistent.

Acoustic and Aerodynamic Assessment
Results are detailed in Tables 3–5 and 3–6. Assessment protocols and normative data are based on references.[33-37]

Interpretation and Stimulability Trials
Acoustic Analysis. Within normal limits (WNL) (low end) speaking pitch in speech, inconsistent with mean F0 on sustained /a/ (above norm). Pitch range reduced from reported baseline. CPP and intensity WNL.

Aerodynamic Analysis. Maximum phonation time (MPT) was WNL, but with moderate muscle tension (base of tongue, sternocleidomastoid muscle).

Stimulability with voiced fricative /z/ preceding /a/ reduced tension and the patient endorsed decreased vocal effort. Sensation was extended into "Zip up the zipper" and "Zoom" with cueing to notice a sensation of anterior-focused resonance with and without

3. Phonotrauma 63

Table 3–5. Acoustic Analysis (Pentax Medical Computerized Speech Lab)

Measure	Result	Analysis	F0 Mean (SD)
Sustained /a/ 3-5 Seconds			
Mean F0 (Hz)	241.92 (B3)	Above norm	211.47/range 191.28-235.07
Cepstral Peak Prominence (CPP) (dB)	10.51	WNL	10.894 (1.751)
All-Voiced Sentence			
Speaking sF0 (Hz)	168.51 (E3)	WNL	177.34/range 165-201.66
CPP (dB)	8.372	WNL	7.898 (0.721)
Ascending/Descending /a/			
Semitone Pitch Range (Hz)	163.75 (E3) to 1029.17 (C6)	WNL, but reduced from baseline	For reference only
Softest and Projected Sustained /a/			
Min Intensity (dB SPL)	45.62	Within range	Range 41-53
Max Intensity (dB SPL)	79.35	For reference only	No norms available

the face mask from the PAS. Patient B was able to feel and hear favorable changes, confirming good kinesthetic and auditory awareness for purposes of engaging in voice therapy if recommended.

Auditory-Perceptual Analysis
The CAPE-V[11] was completed. Results are documented in Table 3–7.

Manual Palpation
Results of manual palpation are documented in Table 3–8.

Patient B exhibited rigid physical alignment with elevated shoulders (right higher than left) and locked knees, resulting in restricted thoracic movement during inhalation. Additionally, she demonstrated a tendency to vacillate between insufficient airflow and overbreathing for singing.

Initial Impressions
Based on symptoms of vocal fatigue, breathiness, and decreased range, supported by instrumental vocal function assessment, the SLP suspected edema or a phonotraumatic lesion. As symptom onset followed a URI, there was also a possibility of post-viral paresis.

Laryngeal Imaging
A rigid laryngeal videostroboscopic examination was completed. A semitransparent superficial lesion was seen on the right vocal fold vibratory margin, and an inspiratory phonatory maneuver revealed a broad base. Hourglass glottic closure was observed at modal register, more pronounced in her upper register, causing difficulty with sustained high-pitched phonation. An ascending pitch glide revealed a pronounced break at E5 to G5, with moderate circumferential hyperfunction and

Table 3–6. Aerodynamic Analysis (Pentax Medical Phonatory Aerodynamic System)

Measure	Result	Analysis	Mean (SD) Normative Values for Females Aged 40-59
Maximum Sustained /a/			
Maximum Phonation Time (sec)	24	WNL	21.24 (5.79)
Mean Airflow (L/sec)	0.07	WNL	0.14 (0.08)
Comfortable Sustained /a/			
Mean Airflow (L/sec)	0.08	WNL	0.15 (0.07)
All-Voiced Sentence			
Mean Airflow (L/sec)	0.210	N/A	For reference only
Voicing Efficiency on /pipipipipi/ at Comfortable Loudness			
Mean Peak Air Pressure (cmH$_2$O)	4.29	WNL	5.76 (1.51)
Mean Airflow During Voicing (L/sec)	0.21	Exceeds norm	0.13 (0.06)
Mean Pitch (Hz)	198.48	WNL	183.58 (21.74)
Mean SPL During Voicing (dB)	79.35	WNL	75.68 (4.24)
Voicing Efficiency on /pipipipipi/ at Softest Intensity			
Mean Peak Air Pressure/PTP (cmH$_2$O)	5.59	Exceeds norm	4.22 (1.02)
Mean Airflow During Voicing (L/sec)	0.16	N/A	No norms available
Mean Pitch (Hz)	199.08	N/A	No norms available
Mean SPL During Voicing (dB)	73.14	N/A	No norms available
Voicing Efficiency on /pipipipipi/ at Projected Loudness			
Mean Peak Air Pressure (cmH$_2$O)	9.35	N/A	No norms available
Mean Airflow During Voicing (L/sec)	0.19	N/A	No norms available
Mean Pitch (Hz)	203.03	N/A	No norms available
Mean SPL During Voicing (dB)	82.33	N/A	No norms available

tongue tension with retraction, despite the tongue being held for purposes of performing the rigid exam. Sustained /i/ at various pitches, ascending /i/, and production of /hi hi hi hi hi/ revealed no motion abnormalities suggestive of paresis. Patient B was diagnosed with a right vocal fold pseudocyst with moderate compensatory hyperfunction.

As an important point of clarification, pseudocysts have a translucent, blisterlike

Table 3–7. Auditory-Perceptual Analysis

CAPE-V Parameter	Severity (Inconsistent/Consistent)
Overall	26/100; moderate dysphonia
Roughness	17/100 (I)
Breathiness	18/100 (C)
Strain	28/100 (I)
Pitch	22/100 (I) decreased
Loudness	18/100 (I) decreased at E5 to G5
Resonance	Fluctuates between posterior/anterior
Other	Vocal fry (I), hard glottal attack (I)

Table 3–8. Laryngeal Palpation

Region	Tension	Pain (0-5)
Scalenes	Mild	1
SCMs	Mild	2
Cricothyroid	Mild	0
Tongue base	Moderate	1
Suprahyoids	Mild	0
Thyrohyoid	Mild	1
Hyoid	Elevated	0
Jaw	None	0

appearance, with semisolid material beneath a thinned epithelium without a capsule.[38,39] Several names are used to describe them, such as translucent polyp, paresis podule, localized Reinke's edema, unilateral nodule and polypoid degeneration.[40] They may be associated with glottic insufficiency from paresis or a posterior glottic gap, a common normal variant in the female larynx.[39-41] Because they may arise from underlying anatomical factors that do not change with surgery, they have a relatively high recurrence rate,[39-41] which should be considered when making treatment recommendations.

Decision Making

The first line of recommended treatment was voice therapy with the goal of optimizing vocal function. The SLP discussed realistic expectations, explaining that treatment may improve the pliability of the pseudocyst and potentially reduce its size, but complete resolution of the lesion was unlikely. The laryngologist explained the role of surgical intervention if Patient B was unable to achieve satisfactory and consistent vocal function through behavioral means.

Plan of Care

The expected trajectory included 6 sessions of voice therapy over 8 to 12 weeks, initially scheduled weekly, with a gradual increase in the spacing between sessions to foster independence. Additionally, the SLP counseled the patient on the importance of establishing a relationship with a voice teacher to address technical concerns and, per request, provided recommendations for classical voice teachers with understanding of phonotraumatic injury. It was recommended that Patient B contact a teacher early in the treatment process to facilitate an easy transition to habilitation.

Long-Term Goals. Patient B will:

- Implement vocal hygiene routines to maintain vocal health and improve the vocal pathology
- Adapt voice use to optimize function and prevent strain while maintaining vocal demands
- Achieve improved speaking voice behaviors in the presence of the vocal pathology
- Achieve improved singing voice function with eventual transfer to a voice teacher

Short-Term Goals. Patient B will:

- Integrate vocal hygiene and pacing strategies (maintain adequate hydration, decrease late-night eating, substitute throat clearing with nonphonotraumatic behaviors, and monitor voice use in various contexts)
- Incorporate individualized rehabilitative interventions to enhance vocal tract inertance, promote optimal vocal fold vibration, reduce vocal effort to 1/10, and optimize voice quality in the presence of the pathology. Interventions will incorporate respiratory-phonatory coordination, semi-occluded vocal tract (SOVT) therapy, and resonant voice therapy (RVT).
- Demonstrate increased ease and stamina in CTT and in the context of a mock voice lesson delivered in person and virtually
- Demonstrate increased ease and efficiency in the singing voice through performance of vocalises and repertoire selections from upcoming scheduled performances.

Patient B was encouraged to record sessions to ensure accurate self-practice. It was typically recommended to practice specific interventions 5 times per week, with frequent "resets" to promote and maintain target behaviors. She was encouraged to incorporate these behaviors into daily activities such as conversations, telephone calls, and teaching.

Intervention

Session #1, Week 1

Patient B used a voice journal provided by the SLP (Table 3–9), which helped her identify patterns contributing to vocal fatigue.

With increased hydration and avoiding late-night eating, she felt less mucus in the morning. When needed, she sipped water instead of throat clearing. Vocal effort ranged from 2/10 to 7/10.

Observations. Moderate dysphonia (raspy quality, intermittent vocal fry), rigid posture with elevated shoulders and locked knees, overbreathing and withholding breath during vocalises

Interventions:

- **Respiratory-Phonatory Coordination.** Patient B performed a physical roll-down exercise, reaching maximum forward flexion (Figure 3–3; See Video 3 Physical Roll-down Stretch by Murphy Estes). The SLP addressed patterns of overbreathing and breath holding by using the term "breath buoyancy" to promote a more relaxed and flowing pattern while cueing Patient B to observe gentle abdominal engagement and low back expansion. Patient B produced "hum-ahh" with easy onset, noticing anterior-focused resonance. She slowly rolled to an upright position, with cueing to maintain grounded thighs, soft knees, relaxed shoulders, and a gentle lift from the top back of the head. She again

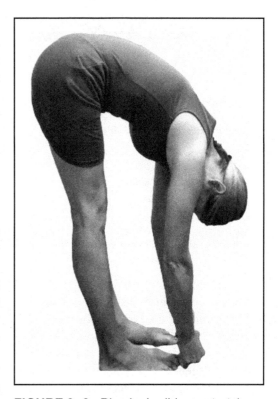

FIGURE 3–3. Physical rolldown stretch.

Table 3–9. Vocal Pacing Journal

	Sunday	Monday	Tuesday
VOCAL HYGIENE			
Sleep Quality			
Hydration			
Health Notes			
Allergy Symptoms			
Reflux Triggers			
Medications			
VOICE USE			
Normal Speaking			
Loud Speaking			
General Vocalizing			
Singing			
STRATEGIES			
Vocal Naps			
Raspberries			
Resonance Strategies			
Conversational Practice			
Other			
HOW DID YOUR VOICE FEEL/SOUND TODAY?			
Voice Quality			
	worst best	worst best	worst best
Vocal Effort			
	least most	least most	least most
Details			
Goals for Tomorrow			

produced "hum-ahh" and experienced a sensation of increased oral resonance with repetition.
- **SOVT.** Instead of lip trills, Patient B practiced "raspberries" (labio-lingual trills), starting unvoiced and gradually adding phonation. (See Video 4 Labio-Lingual Trills [Raspberries] by Murphy Estes.) This maintained the benefits of SOVT while reducing base of tongue engagement. Patient B practiced descending 5-1 patterns (range: G3 to D5) (Figure 3–4) and 1-3-5-4-3-2-1 patterns (range: Eb5 to Bb5) (Figure 3–5). Cueing to "breathe with the high note in mind" helped reduce excessive weight on the lower starting pitch, allowing for smoother register transitions. Physical movements, such as swaying and arm stretches, were incorporated to promote airflow connection and to decrease breath holding and other hyperfunctional behaviors. Movements were gradually faded while maintaining the achieved benefits.
- **CTT.** Patient and SLP had a 10-minute conversation, focusing on maintaining target sensations, using phonemes /m/, /n/, /v/, and /z/ as reset cues. She endorsed decreased vocal effort (3/10). There was limited generalization to spontaneous speech, but she noticed reduced throat clearing with target behaviors (named "Smooth Voice") and increased throat clearing with habitual behaviors (named "Husky Voice"). The SLP helped the patient recognize the correlation between increased strain/effort and an increased urge to clear the throat.

Session #2, Week 2

B began using a handheld nebulizer with isotonic saline. She maintained good hydration, avoided late-night eating, and completed the home exercise program (HEP) daily. She found it challenging but beneficial to try to maintain target speaking voice behaviors. Vocal effort ranged from 2/10 to 5/10.

Observations. Decreased vocal fry, more optimal speaking pitch, mildly increased breathiness suggesting reduced compensatory hyperfunction, improved physical alignment with decreased breath holding

Interventions:

- The patient practiced the respiratory-phonatory coordination exercise described above.
- **SOVT.** The patient performed the raspberry exercise with increased agility on ascending/descending arpeggios within range of G3 to B5 (Figure 3–6).
- The SLP used CTT tenets while discussing the patient's weekly voice journal, with added cueing for "clear speech."

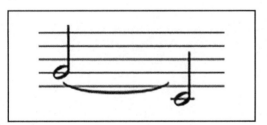

FIGURE 3–4. Descending 5-1 pitch pattern.

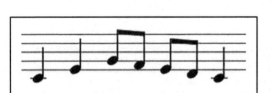

FIGURE 3–5. Ascending-descending 1-3-5-4-3-2-1 pitch pattern.

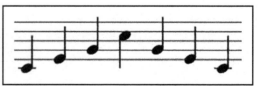

FIGURE 3–6. Ascending-descending arpeggios.

3. Phonotrauma 69

- **Manual Therapy.** The SLP addressed mild but persistent tension in the thyrohyoid space with manual therapy, applying gentle and sustained pressure while stretching in a downward direction. At times, gentle side-to-side motions were incorporated to further promote release and encourage a neutral laryngeal position. Patient B was taught self-care massage techniques, which she demonstrated during the session to ensure safe and accurate home practice.
- **RVT.** Patient practiced 9-note scales from G3 to F5 on /m/ with gentle chewing, transitioning to /mi-a/ on ascent to C6. She maintained a forward, relaxed tongue position for the /a/ vowel. Cueing to "filter /a/ through the /i/ space" helped her achieve a sensation of pharyngeal space without false vocal fold constriction or tongue base retraction. This made her recognize a pattern of trying to "make space," which contributed to her muscle tension when singing.
- A second round of CTT was conducted, this time with background noise ("Busy Restaurant" video played from the SLP's computer). Patient B maintained target resonant sensation while speaking with gradually increased projection. "Mhm" was cued to support target sensations.

Session #3, Week 3

Session #3 was conducted via telehealth to promote generalization and transfer of skills. Patient B reported more consistent access to her higher singing range and decreased vocal effort, with ratings ranging from 1/10 to 4/10. She sang at a wedding and a funeral with minimal concern.

Observations. Decreased breathiness, rare vocal fry, elevated loudness over telehealth

Interventions:

- **CTT.** Patient B was cued to reduce her loudness while maintaining anterior-resonant sensation, with nasal continuants and voiced fricatives to facilitate. Laptop volume was lowered to avoid hearing the SLP at an unnecessarily high volume, causing reflexive elevated loudness. The patient's headset microphone served as a visual cue to maintain normal conversational loudness.
- **SOVT/RVT.** Patient B achieved ease and agility in raspberry ascending/descending scales to C#6. She followed these with descending 8-1 lip trills extending to /mi me ma/ while maintaining target sensations and avoiding excessive tongue base retraction on /a/.
- During a mock virtual voice lesson, the SLP took the role of the student. It was noted that Patient B dedicated more time than necessary demonstrating problematic technical issues for the student. This observation was significant for the patient, as it made her aware that such demonstrations led to unnecessary vocal fatigue. With this newfound knowledge, Patient B focused on allowing the student to experience her own kinesthetic changes through negative practice, which in turn reduced Patient B's vocal dose and vocal effort.

Session #4, Week 5

Session #4 resumed in-person sessions. Patient B successfully implemented therapy goals and had no difficulty with her choral or solo church repertoire during the week. She also contacted a voice teacher and had an encouraging first lesson. She signed a release form to allow the SLP to communicate with the teacher.

Observations. Very mild intermittent breathiness

Interventions:

- Patient B independently demonstrated her current regimen of rehabilitative voice exercises (alignment, respiratory-phonatory coordination, SOVT, RVT). At times she was cued to feel coordinated onset, as opposed to breath holding prior

70 Voice Therapy: Clinical Case Studies

to onset. Brief instances of tongue tension were relieved with tongue stretches. In general, Patient B demonstrated mostly independent mastery of therapy goals with minimal cueing from the SLP.

■ Patient B conducted a mock in-person voice lesson while implementing target behaviors. The SLP suggested speaking more slowly and providing concise explanation, which would simultaneously reduce the patient's vocal demand and give students more opportunity to process information.

Session #5, Week 7

The patient's voice teacher was invited to attend session #5. Patient B continued to find her current regimen helpful. She no longer needed to use the voice journal, nor did she experience vocal fatigue. Vocal effort was 1-2/10.

Observations. Perceptually "normal" speaking voice with WNL habitual pitch and prosody

Interventions:

■ Patient B, the SLP, and the voice teacher discussed her progress and future goals. They reviewed the initial videostrobsocopic examination and discussed the chronic nature of pseudocysts, including exacerbating and relieving factors.

■ Patient B demonstrated her current regimen of rehabilitative exercises. The SLP addressed a newly observed pattern of B turning her head to the right at and above F5, and the patient instead vocalized with her head turned to the left with gradual return to center. Patient B sang portions of Mozart's *Requiem* in anticipation of her upcoming performance with the goal of feeling consistent airflow and movement through long, sustained phrases and avoiding tongue base retraction. The voice teacher was invited to address technical concerns as part of team treatment.

Outcome Measures and Repeat Videostroboscopic Examination

Patient B's VHI-10 score improved to 6/40, and SVHI-10 score improved to 12/40. As expected, the pseudocyst remained and was unchanged in size, but it had increased pliability. Patient B produced pianissimo /i/ glides in her high range without breaks in her upper passaggio. Overall, there was decreased hyperfunction. The voice team reiterated that the measure of treatment success was improved vocal function. Surgical intervention was not advised at that time.

> An important concept is highlighted above. Though the patient's lesion was still present after therapy, the voice care team did not recommend surgery since the patient's voice was able to function at a high level and meet her needs. In this situation, surgery may not make the voice any better. Benign lesions do not need to be removed if their impact on vocal function is negligible after voice therapy.

Session #6, Week 11

Patient B returned after performing Mozart's *Requiem*. She used her voice journal regularly during rehearsals. She was satisfied with her performance and pleased to socialize with industry sponsors at a postconcert event with only mild vocal fatigue, resolved by the next day. This served as a reminder to be mindful of her vocal behaviors and maintain a consistent regimen.

Observations. "Normal" speaking voice quality

Interventions: Patient B independently demonstrated her vocal regimen and engaged with the SLP in 25 minutes of CTT with and without background noise. She sang portions of "Die Zeit, die ist ein sonderbar Ding" from *Der Rosenkavalier* with mild habitual muscle tension, reduced when vocalizing on a syllable

/zi/. The SLP counseled the patient that technical issues would be best addressed by the voice teacher. The patient stated that she had achieved or even exceeded her prior baseline and agreed that it was appropriate to transition to singing voice habilitation.

Discharge

Patient B was discharged from voice therapy, based on (1) improved vocal function in the presence of the pseudocyst; (2) increased self-awareness of vocal hygiene and vocal pacing; (3) demonstrated ability to maintain target behaviors in conversational speech, a mock voice lesson, vocalises, and repertoire; and (4) successful transfer to a voice teacher for continued singing voice habilitation. She was encouraged to return to the voice clinic should she experience an acute voice change, a decline in function beyond 2 weeks, new vocal symptoms, or as needed for surveillance.

Summary

This case study aligns with clinical observations of many performers with pseudocysts, demonstrating that they often achieve restored vocal function after voice therapy. Surgical intervention may be an option if vocal function remains impaired or inconsistent. It is important to provide outreach to the performing arts community to educate on treatment options and dispel stigmas about voice injury.

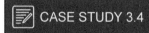

CASE STUDY 3.4

Perioperative Therapeutic Care for an Adult With a Vocal Fold Cyst

Austin Collum and Megan Lee

Voice Evaluation

Chief Complaint. Vocal deterioration, reduced volume, dysphonia

Patient KZ was referred for a team-based voice evaluation by a local otolaryngologist. The patient was diagnosed with dysphonia and a recurrent right true vocal fold lesion.

History of Voice Complaint. Patient KZ is a 75-year-old cisgender woman with gradual and intermittent onset of voice problems starting about 5 years ago. The patient reported that dysphonia improved after a previous surgery 1 year prior but noted her symptoms recurred within several months. Current voice symptoms include reduced volume, deterioration with use, increased effort and strain, difficulty being heard on the phone and in background noise, and the need to repeat herself frequently. The patient reportedly underwent vocal fold surgery to address a vocal fold cyst with 3 sessions of postoperative voice therapy at an outside ENT clinic. The patient reported a comorbidity of arthritis and takes progesterone for hormone replacement therapy.

Voice Use. KZ denied significant voice use, as she is retired. However, she noted dysphonia has impacted her ability to participate in social settings with family and friends. She previously taught classes at her local church on Sundays but had to discontinue due to ongoing voice issues.

Laryngeal Videostroboscopy

Videolaryngostroboscopy was performed transnasally with a flexible distal chip scope.

Salient Examination Findings. The exam found irregular free edge contour of the right true vocal fold due to a subepithelial space-occupying cyst (physician confirmed) and convex free edge contour of the left vocal fold due to a small reactive contralateral lesion. These structural findings resulted in an anterior glottic gap, mild sphincteric supraglottic compression, open phase dominance, intermittent phase asymmetry, and intermittent strobe tracking (periodicity). Mucosal wave and amplitude were within normal limits bilaterally.

Voice Therapy: Clinical Case Studies

Quality-of-Life Impairment

KZ rated the impact of her voice disorder on quality of life using the VHI,[42] with the following results:

Voice Handicap Index: 54/120 (moderate)

Seriousness of voice problem overall: Moderate

Seriousness of voice problem today: Moderate

Voice percentage of normal: 50%

Auditory-Perceptual Assessment

The GRBAS scale was administered to qualify dysphonia severity, with the following ratings: Grade: 2; Roughness: 1; Breathiness: 2; Asthenia: 1; Strain: 2, where 0 indicates "within normal limits," 1 indicates "mild," 2 indicates "moderate," and 3 indicates "severe." The patient's overall dysphonia severity was rated as "moderate," with the most aberrant features identified as breathiness and strain. Roughness and asthenia were rated as "mild." The patient's speaking voice was additionally perceived to be consistently too quiet with pitch instabil-

ity, back-focused resonance, inadequate breath support, and concomitant, frequent throat clearing. Her maximum phonation time was 9.3 seconds, below the expected 18.9 seconds (SD: 7.3 seconds) for her age and sex.[45]

Manual Palpation Assessment

Palpation of the extralaryngeal region was conducted to assess paralaryngeal muscle tension that may be contributing to symptoms (Table 3–10).

Acoustic and Aerodynamic Assessment

The patient was seated with a head-mounted AKG microphone placed at a 45-degree off axis position and 5 cm from the mouth. The patient was asked to read sentences and the Rainbow Passage from printed materials and then received instructions for sustained phonation tasks. Results are detailed in Table 3–11 and Figure 3–7; normative measures were obtained from Goy et al (2013) and Buckley et al (2023).[43,44]

The patient was seated while placing the face mask over her mouth and nose during sustained vowel production. The same

Table 3–10. Manual Palpation Results

	Tension Severity at Rest	Tension Severity During Phonation	Patient-Reported Pain/Tenderness
Suprahyoid/Base of Tongue	Mild to moderate	Moderate	None
Posterior Suprahyoid Region	Mild	Unchanged	None
Thyrohyoid Space	Mild to moderate	Moderate	None
Lateral Hyoid Movement	Resistance to movement bilaterally	Unchanged	None
Lateral Thyroid Cartilage Movement	Resistance to movement bilaterally	Unchanged	None
Sternocleidomastoids	Mild tension	Unchanged	None

Table 3–11. Pretreatment Acoustic Analysis

Baseline Acoustic Measures	/a/	CAPE-V Sentences	Rainbow Passage	*Normative Measures for Older Cisgender Females*[45,46]
Average Fundamental Frequency	186 Hz	193 Hz	180 Hz	/a/: 211 Hz (SD: 42 Hz) Reading tasks: 174 Hz (SD: 22 Hz)
F0 Standard Deviation		50 Hz	36 Hz	38 Hz (SD: 10 Hz)
Average Vocal Intensity	55.2 dB	53.5 dB	55.4 dB	/a/: 74 dB (SD: 4.2 dB) Reading tasks: 66.4 dB (SD: 4.0 dB)
Smoothed Cepstral Peak Prominence	9.9 dB	5.2 dB	5.9 dB	/a/: 16.17 (SD: 2.56) Rainbow Passage: 9.17 dB (SD: 1.34 dB)
Physiologic Pitch Range	165–466 Hz			>2 octaves (lowest F0×4)
Vocal Intensity Range	40.7–82.2 dB			>30 dB SPL range

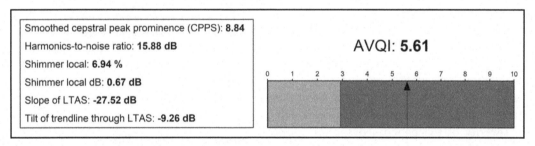

FIGURE 3–7. Pretreatment Acoustic Voice Quality Index as displayed in Praat Phonanium script by Youri Maryn.

task was also performed with placement of a polyethylene tube on the surface of the tongue while repeating /pi:pi:pi:/ at 1.5 syllables per second at comfortable loudness and then at double the loudness. Measures of average airflow and intraoral pressure (inferred measure of lung pressure) were calculated with the Pentax Medical Phonatory Aerodynamic System: Model 6600 and used to determine the average laryngeal resistance during voice production. Results are detailed in Table 3–12 and normative data are from Zraick et al (2012).[36]

Clinical Decision Making

Given that the patient presented with recurrent phonotraumatic lesions, the attending laryngologist and the clinical SLP jointly

Table 3–12. Pretreatment Aerodynamic Analysis

Baseline Aerodynamic Measures	/a/	/i/	/pi/ at Comfortable Volume	/pi/ at Loud Volume	Normative Measures for Cisgender Females 60-89 Years Old
Mean Glottal Airflow	0.12 L/sec	0.12 L/sec	0.19 L/sec	0.35 L/sec	0.11 L/sec (SD: 0.06)
Mean Subglottal Air Pressure			10.77 cmH$_2$O	11.20 cmH$_2$O	7.78 cmH$_2$O (SD: 4.23)
Mean SPL (dB)	61.58 dB	61.42 dB	67.38 dB	71.94 dB	76.93 dB (SD: 7.64)
Mean F0 (Hz)	190 Hz	198 Hz	200 Hz	199 Hz	182.94 Hz (SD: 24.42)

decided to proceed with a combined approach of therapeutic and surgical management. From the surgical perspective, microdirect laryngoscopy with microflap excision and Kenalog injection of the right true vocal fold cyst was recommended. No surgical intervention was recommended for the left true vocal fold reactive lesion. Therapeutic intervention was divided into 2 segments: pre- and postoperative therapy. The long-standing nature of the patient's dysphonia and perceived reduction in severity of the patient's dysphonia during stimulability testing led the clinician to proceed with preoperative therapy. Sessions prior to surgical intervention were utilized to counsel the patient on expectations for postoperative recovery and to begin utilizing RVT techniques to assist with attenuating vocal fold inflammation.[4] In total, 6 sessions of therapy were recommended per the plan of care: 2 sessions preoperatively and 4 sessions postoperatively. The patient's prognosis was judged to be excellent, with no negative prognostic factors indicated.

A microflap excision is a surgical procedure that removes benign vocal fold lesions while preserving surrounding delicate vocal fold tissue. The procedure reduces scarring, improves vocal fold healing, and generally results in improved voice outcomes compared to historically more invasive surgeries such as vocal fold stripping or CO_2 laser.

Therapeutic Intervention

To illustrate appropriate timing of evaluation, intervention, and return to voice use through the perioperative period, a detailed outline is included in Table 3–13, followed by discussion of goals and the patient's completion of voice therapy.

Long-Term Goal #1. The patient will identify factors affecting her laryngeal health and independently implement changes to maintain vocal health throughout the perioperative course of behavioral voice therapy.

3. Phonotrauma   75

Table 3–13. Perioperative Care Timeline

Timing	Appointment	Therapeutic Intervention and Recommendations
Preoperative Intervention		
	Initial Evaluation	
	Session 1	Introduction of throat clear alternative strategies, rescue breathing, voice rest recommendations for postoperative voice use, and SOVTEs
	Session 2	Review of respiratory retraining strategies, monitoring of throat clear alternatives, review of SOVTEs, brief introduction of resonant voice facilitator /m/
Surgical Intervention		
Postoperative Intervention		
Days 1-3	**Complete Voice Rest**	Complete voice rest includes no talking, yelling, whispering, whistling, humming, laughing, coughing, throat clearing, and heavy lifting during this first week
Days 4-6	**Modified Voice Use**	Resume 5 minutes per hour of voice use, completing SOVTEs in 1- to 2-minute practice sessions.
Day 7	**Reevaluation**	Repeat laryngeal videostroboscopy exam completed. Continuation of modified voice rest of 5 minutes per hour including SOVTEs for approximately 2-3 minutes per hour and speaking for no more than 1-2 minutes per hour.
Day 14	**Session 3**	Review of throat clear alternative strategies, review of SOVTEs, reintroduction of resonant voice facilitator /m/. Increase modified voice use to 10 minutes per hour divided into 2-3 minutes of SOVTEs, 2-3 minutes of Resonant Voice Therapy exercises, and 2-3 minutes of speaking.
Day 21	**Session 4**	Review of respiratory retraining strategies for cough suppression, resonant voice /m/ facilitator combined with tongue-out speech at phoneme, word, and short phrase level. Increase modified voice use to 10-15 minutes per hour, 4-6 minutes of therapeutic exercises every hour/every other hour, and remaining time speaking.
Day 28	**Session 5**	Continuation of Resonant Voice Therapy to short phrase, sentence, and functional phrase level. Increase modified voice use to 15-20 minutes per hour with 2-3 minutes per hour of therapeutic exercises and remaining time speaking.

continues

76 Voice Therapy: Clinical Case Studies

Table 3–13. *continued*

Timing	Appointment	Therapeutic Intervention and Recommendations
Day 35	**Session 6**	Completion of Resonant Voice Therapy, use of negative practice to reinforce optimal resonance. Increase to full voice use, completing exercises 3-5 times daily, avoiding background noise, overuse, and monitoring for fatigue or return of symptoms.
Day 42	**Final Evaluation**	Clearance for full voice use and discontinuation of restrictions.

Long-Term Goal #2. The patient will implement evidence-based behavioral voice strategies across the hierarchy of speech to assist with reducing severity of dysphonia and to improve voice use throughout all activities of daily living.

Short-Term Goal #1. The patient will report adherence to recommendations for management of vocal load/voice rest weekly across the course of perioperative therapy.

Preoperative therapy primarily utilized indirect voice interventions focused on counseling the patient on expectations of wound healing of the vocal folds post phonosurgery. The patient underwent 3 days of complete voice rest immediately following completion of surgery.[45] Nonverbal means of communication, such as text-to-speech apps, dry erase boards, and prerecorded voice memos, were discussed preoperatively to ease the burden of complete voice rest. The patient opted to prerecord bedtime stories for her grandchildren to allow her to participate in her activities of daily living without sacrificing the need for voice rest. Direct interventions, including RVT and SOVT exercises, were also trained preoperatively. For days 4 to 6 postoperative, voice use was reintroduced at 5 minutes per hour using identified therapeutic techniques. Specifics regarding these interventions will be discussed in detail in short-term goal #3.

> Postoperative voice rest and return to voicing protocols vary across practices, as does timing of follow-up laryngeal videostroboscopy. Commonly, a period of 3 to 7 days is recommended for complete voice rest followed by a gradual return to voicing, as is detailed in this case. Research on voice rest continues to actively shape clinical practice in this area.

On the seventh day of postoperative healing, the patient was seen for repeat laryngeal imaging to determine if advancing voice use was feasible. A normal degree of erythema with expected reduced vibratory capabilities of the right true vocal fold was observed. These results were reviewed with the patient's laryngologist, and a joint decision was made for the patient to proceed with increasing voice use according to the protocol. The protocol was initiated beginning at a rate of 5 minutes of voice use per hour. As this is challenging to monitor, the patient was encouraged to utilize a stopwatch as needed to monitor her vocal load. The patient was also encouraged to utilize her voice in 1- to 3-minute increments to avoid prolonged vocal dose. The patient was encouraged to keep track of her vocal fatigue and rest for longer periods of time should fatigue present itself. Voice use was increased weekly under direct supervision of the clinician. The patient increased her voice use by 5 minutes each week. Five weeks after phonosurgery, the patient was cleared to resume full voice use while continuing to monitor for vocal fatigue and utilizing her voice exercise routine, as described in short-term goal #3, 3 to 5 times daily.

Short-Term Goal #2. The patient will consistently and independently employ breathing techniques, laryngeal control exercises, and laryngeal desensitization techniques to eliminate phonotraumatic behaviors and to reduce the frequency, duration, and severity of irritation sustained due to coughing and/or throat clearing.

During the patient's initial evaluation, a consistent pattern of throat clearing and intermittent coughing was observed. The phonotraumatic nature of chronic coughing and throat clearing was identified as a risk factor for preventing optimal wound healing post phonosurgery. Behavioral cough/throat clearing suppression strategies were introduced during the patient's preoperative course of therapy.

Stemple's throat clearing substitutes, outlined in *Clinical Voice Pathology*[46] and Case Study 3.6, were discussed in full. Suppression strategies included an effortful swallow, multiple sips of water, sniff-swallow technique, and a hum-swallow technique. These strategies are to be utilized immediately when sensing any form of laryngeal irritation to replace the phonotraumatic behavior of throat clearing. Respiratory retraining strategies,[47] such as pursed lip breathing or 3 sniffs paired with pursed lip exhalation, were also introduced to avoid physiologic respiratory and laryngeal behaviors that precipitate chronic cough and throat clearing. The patient was instructed to use these breathing exercises in a cyclical fashion until the urge to cough subsided or lessened significantly. This goal was readdressed weekly during the postoperative phase of treatment to continue to reduce phonotraumatic events. (See Video 19 Throat Clearing Reduction Strategies by Zughni.)

Short-Term Goal #3. The patient will consistently produce anterior resonance during voicing tasks at the phoneme, syllable, word, phrase, sentence, paragraph, and spontaneous speech levels without direct models and with minimal cueing through the use of varying direct voice interventions.

Stimulability testing was completed at the patient's initial evaluation. Improved voice quality was perceived by the patient and the clinician when utilizing targeted productions of /m/ with and without her tongue protruded and targeted productions of /wu/ with and without straw phonation. Somatosensory cues regarding anterior resonance versus back-focused resonance were especially helpful per the patient's feedback. The patient opted to proceed with /m/ exercises, as she noted more somatosensory feedback with this exercise. Carryover to conversation was completed through the use of a hierarchical approach. This basic training gesture of humming was then shaped to phonemes, words, phrases, and sentences. Negative practice and tongue-out speech were utilized concomitantly as needed to assist with entrainment of the target motor pattern. The patient was informed to practice these exercises at least 3 times daily prior to her surgery. Once initial voice rest was completed, the patient was encouraged to complete these exercises in an abbreviated format approximately once every other hour to optimize anterior resonance for speech and to attenuate vocal fold inflammation.

Posttreatment Outcomes

Laryngeal Imaging. Six weeks after surgical intervention, laryngeal videostroboscopy was performed transorally with a 70-degree rigid endoscope. The leading edge of the right true vocal fold was smooth and straight without mass or lesion. Amplitude and mucosal wave were rated as within normal limits. The leading edge of the left true vocal fold was judged to be convex in nature with continued reactive

Voice Therapy: Clinical Case Studies

lesion. Amplitude and mucosal wave of the left true vocal fold were rated as within functional limits. Vocal fold closure was now rated as complete. Given the mass differential, slight phase asymmetry was consistent throughout phonatory tasks. Continued mild medial compression of the supraglottis occurred throughout phonatory tasks in modal and falsetto registers. All other stroboscopic parameters were rated within functional limits.

Patient-Reported Outcome Measures (PROMs). The VHI was recorded to determine the impact of the patient's dysphonia on her quality of life. Following completion of postoperative voice therapy, the patient scored a 7 out of 120. This is a significant improvement when compared to her baseline measurement of 54 out of 120. Subjectively, the patient rated her voice as approximately 90% of normal (0 = abnormal; 100 = normal). Her perceived talkativeness changed from a 4 out of 10 to an 8 out of 10.

Acoustic and Aerodynamic Assessment. Results of the posttreatment assessment are detailed in Table 3–14 and Figure 3–8. Aerodynamic measures were not taken following completion of postoperative therapy.

Discussion

This case highlights the delicate balance of surgical and therapeutic voice care needed for all patients undergoing phonosurgery. This case also serves as an example of the necessity of pre- and postoperative behavioral voice therapy. In prior courses of surgical intervention, this patient had recurrence of her lesion due to a lack of consistent perioperative therapeutic management. Adherence to evidence-based recommendations regarding postoperative voice rest and maintenance of laryngeal hygiene throughout her course of treatment were imperative to reduce risk of recurrence of her vocal fold lesion. Addition-

Table 3–14. Posttreatment Acoustic Analysis

Post-Acoustic Measures	/a/	CAPE-V Sentences	Rainbow Passage	Normative Measures for Older Cisgender Females
Average Fundamental Frequency	186 Hz	171 Hz	170 Hz	/a/: 211 Hz (SD: 42 Hz) Reading tasks: 174 Hz (SD: 22 Hz)
F0 Standard Deviation		32 Hz	25 Hz	38 Hz (SD: 10 Hz)
Average Vocal Intensity	54.8 dB	48.3 dB	53.3 dB	/a/: 74 dB (SD: 4.2 dB) Reading tasks: 66.4 dB (SD:4.0 dB)
Smoothed Cepstral Peak Prominence	10.7 dB	7.2 dB	8.5 dB	/a/: 16.17 (SD: 2.56); Rainbow Passage: 9.17 dB (SD: 1.34 dB)
Physiologic Pitch Range	148-348 Hz			>2 octaves (lowest F0×4)
Vocal Intensity Range	40.7-79.4 dB			>30 dB SPL range

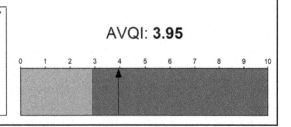

FIGURE 3–8. Posttreatment Acoustic Voice Quality Index as displayed in Praat Phonanium script by Youri Maryn.

ally, early entrainment of anterior resonance was provided prior to surgical intervention to optimize vocal fold wound healing. This likely helped the patient maintain optimal voicing patterns upon her return to modified voice use. At the patient's 1-year follow-up, all subjective and objective voice outcome measures remained stable. This demonstrates that perioperative care proved beneficial for this patient, ensuring a lack of recurrence across the span of a year post phonosurgery through the continued generalization of vocal hygiene and optimal voicing patterns.

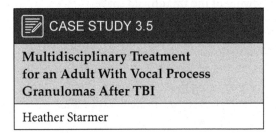

CASE STUDY 3.5

Multidisciplinary Treatment for an Adult With Vocal Process Granulomas After TBI

Heather Starmer

Voice Evaluation

Case History

Chief Complaints. Dysphonia, chronic throat clearing, and throat pain.

I had the pleasure of seeing this patient in conjunction with the laryngologist for a comprehensive voice and upper airway evaluation. The laryngologist diagnosed the patient with vocal process granulomas.

History of the Voice Complaint. Patient RC is a 36-year-old cisgender male referred for an outpatient voice evaluation following prolonged hospitalization. He sustained a closed head injury after falling from a ladder 3 months prior to referral. During his hospitalization, a craniotomy was performed for decompressive purposes. He required prolonged orotracheal intubation due to difficulty weaning from the ventilator and underwent tracheotomy 16 days following intubation. Speaking valve intervention was implemented during his hospital stay and the patient reportedly had a rough, coarse vocal quality from initiation of voicing. Voice worsened over the month following decannulation and the patient was able to discern a greater sense of vocal strain/effort, which has remained unchanged since that time. Disinhibition, impulsivity, and tangential speech were observed following the injury and the patient underwent intensive cognitive rehabilitation in both inpatient and outpatient settings prior to reporting to the voice clinic. He has not yet returned to work and voice use is limited to conversation in the home at this time. He denies any history of vocal difficulties prior to his injury.

Medical History. Pertinent medical history for this patient includes significant alcohol abuse, severe seasonal allergies, and gastroesophageal reflux disease (GERD). He is not currently taking any medications for his allergies or GERD.

Social History. The patient does not smoke. Alcohol intake has been minimal since the injury despite a history of heavy use prior. He consumes 3 to 4 cups of coffee per day and 2 to 3 caffeinated sodas. Water intake is estimated to be 8 to 16 ounces per day. He is

80 Voice Therapy: Clinical Case Studies

married with a 4-year-old son. He previously worked in construction, but has been on disability following his injury.

Laryngeal Imaging

Videostroboscopic evaluation was performed using a flexible, distal chip endoscope. There was normal mobility of the true vocal folds bilaterally. Large, bilateral lesions were observed on the vocal processes, left greater than right. The vibratory portion of the vocal folds was smooth and straight bilaterally. There was mild erythema of the striking edges of the vocal folds bilaterally. Full glottic closure was accomplished despite the presence of vocal process granulomas. Slight edema of the vocal folds was observed, greater on the left than right, leading to mild reduction of amplitude and mucosal wave. Closed-phase vibration predominated. He had moderate anterior-posterior and lateral supraglottic compression.

> Vocal process granulomas can be post-intubation related. The complaint of pain, often accompanied by pointing to the location of the thyrohyoid space, is a clue to the possibility of a granuloma. The results of laryngeal imaging demonstrated lesions on the vocal processes, the location of a great majority of postintubation granulomas. This lesion type has been described as exuberant healing tissue at the site of a chronic irritation, as can be assumed from an endotracheal tube. It is benign in nature.

Vocal Effort, Fatigue, and Pain

The OMNI Vocal Effort Scale (OMNI-VES)[31] was completed. The patient rated vocal effort on a 0 to 10 where 0 = "extremely easy" and 10 = "extremely hard" to produce voice. The patient reported vocal effort of 7/10.

Quality-of-Life Impairment

The VHI[42] and Reflux Symptom Index (RSI)[32] were administered. On the VHI, the patient scored 20/40 points on the functional subscale, 10/40 points on the physical subscale, and 6/40 points on the emotional subscale, yielding a total score of 36/120, indicating mild self-perceived voice handicap. On the RSI, he scored a total of 22 points, indicating some concern for potential reflux contributions (scores >13 are considered clinically significant).

Auditory-Perceptual Evaluation

The patient presented with a mild-moderate dysphonia characterized by a pressed, strained quality with a rough component. The CAPE-V[11] was administered with an overall severity score of 26, indicating mild-moderate dysphonia. While pitch levels and variability were appropriate for conversation, he habitually spoke louder than appropriate for a clinical setting. He cleared his throat habitually throughout the session and did not appear to have awareness of this occurring. Impulsivity and tangential speech were noted throughout the evaluation.

Manual Palpation Assessment

There was mild muscular tension and tenderness in the thyrohyoid region with mild narrowing of the thyrohyoid space.

Acoustic and Aerodynamic Assessment

Acoustic analysis was performed using the MDVP and aerodynamic analysis was performed using the PAS (Pentax Medical, Montvale, NJ). Results are detailed in Tables 3–15 and 3–16 with normative data according to Zraick et al (2012).[36]

Stimulability

Despite impulsivity, the patient was able to follow directions during stimulability testing. Best voice was noted during production of a gentle, resonant hum.

Impressions

Patient RC presents with a mild-moderate dysphonia related to laryngeal granulomas and reactive laryngeal tension. Contributing factors include poor laryngeal hygiene

Table 3–15. Pretreatment Acoustic Analysis

Acoustic Measures	Sustained Vowel	Norms	X Indicates Abnormal
Mean F0 (Hz)	137	128	
Jitter (%) at Modal Pitch	1.6	≤1.04	X
Shimmer (dB) at Modal Pitch	0.08	0.35	
Noise: Harmonics Ratio (%)	0.32	0.19	X
Pitch Range	111-431 (23 semitones)	24	

Table 3–16. Pretreatment Aerodynamic Analysis

Aerodynamic Measures	Results	Norms	X Indicates Abnormal
Maximum Sustained Phonation (seconds)	15	21.29 (SD 5.92)	X
Vital Capacity (L)	3.65	4.14 (SD 1.14)	X
Mean Airflow During Sustained /a/ (mL/sec)	120	170 (SD 90)	
Mean Peak Air Pressure (cmH$_2$O)	9.76	6.65 (SD 1.98)	X
Aerodynamic Resistance	88.76	68.20 (SD 53.08)	

(chronic throat clearing and poor hydration) and unmanaged reflux disease. He is a good candidate for therapy given stimulability for improved voice. Prognosis is guarded due to impulsivity and lack of awareness of throat-clearing behaviors.

Plan of Care

Voice therapy was recommended on a weekly basis. Six sessions were recommended, with potential for additional sessions based upon response to treatment.

Long-Term Goal #1. Patient will eliminate throat-clearing behaviors.

Long-Term Goal #2. Patient will maintain low-effort voicing (OMNI-VES <4) in a variety of communication settings 90% of the time.

Short-Term Goal #1. Patient will consume and log a minimum of 24 ounces of water daily.

Short-Term Goal #2. Patient will correctly identify throat-clearing behavior in the clinical setting 60% of the time without clinician cues.

Short-Term Goal #3. Patient will produce sustained phonation using a resonant hum with OMNI-VES score of 5 or less in 80% of trials with moderate clinician cues.

Decision Making

The plan of care was established collaboratively by the SLP and the laryngologist and included both medical and behavioral interventions based upon existing evidence.[48] Medical management was directed at the patient's vocal process granulomas and reflux. Twice daily proton-pump inhibitors (PPIs) and inhaled steroids were recommended based upon evidence of their benefit in the management of vocal process granulomas.[49] In-person voice therapy was recommended due to evaluation findings of poor vocal hygiene, excessive throat clearing, and vocal strain/muscular tension. The role of voice therapy in the management of patients with vocal process granulomas has been previously established.[48-50] There is level 2A evidence for conservative management of vocal process granulomas including medication and voice therapy.[48] In patients who do not respond to conservative management, other options include Botox® injection into the lateral cricoarytenoid muscles,[51] KTP (potassium titanyl phosphate) laser ablation,[52] and resection.[53]

Intervention: Voice Therapy

Therapeutic approaches selected for this patient included vocal hygiene education with emphasis on improved hydration, behavioral reflux management, and elimination of throat clearing. Additionally, resonant voice was utilized to help reduce vocal strain/tension. Each therapy technique is outlined below with rationale for selection of particular therapy tasks.

Improved Hydration

Short-Term Goal #1. Patient will consume and log a minimum of 24 ounces of water daily. The patient was educated regarding the importance of hydration for laryngeal function and voicing. The concept of phonation threshold pressure was described as the amount of air pressure required to initiate vocal fold vibration. The clinician and patient discussed that poorly hydrated vocal folds require more air pressure to initiate vibration and therefore may lead to greater vocal strain and fatigue.[54] They discussed that both systemic and direct hydration may have an impact on vocal fold vibration. In respect to systemic hydration, RC had a significant imbalance between hydrating and dehydrating agents. It was discussed that caffeine and alcohol are drying agents and that he needed to balance drying agent intake with increased water intake. They discussed that optimizing hydration would reduce the amount of effort required to produce voice and reduce the sensation of the need to clear his throat. He was advised to increase his water intake to at least six to eight 8-ounce servings of water per day. The clinician discussed strategies to help RC achieve this goal, such as filling a premeasured container in the morning and setting subgoals for water intake throughout the day. Together, they determined that RC would drink at least 16 ounces in the morning before lunchtime, 8 ounces with lunch, 16 ounces in the afternoon before dinner, and 8 ounces with dinner. RC installed a water tracker mobile application on his cell phone to increase his awareness of and adherence to this recommendation.

Elimination of Throat-Clearing Behaviors

Short-Term Goal #2. Patient will correctly identify throat-clearing behavior in the clinical setting 60% of the time without clinician cues. RC had poor awareness of his habitual throat-clearing behavior. The clinician and patient discussed that throat clearing can be traumatic to the tissues of the larynx and discussed the relationship between throat clearing, vocal process granulomas, and vocal fold edema/erythema, which was viewed on the videostroboscopic evaluation. The patient was educated regarding the cyclical nature of throat clearing. He was told that each throat clear caused irritation of the laryngeal mucosa, which would lead to inflammation and a sense of fullness, resulting in the perceived need to clear the throat again.

Once RC was able to demonstrate understanding of this relationship, efforts shifted to increasing awareness of the throat-clearing behavior. This was accomplished through clinician feedback of raising the hand whenever a throat clear occurred. Further, the patient listened to a sample of a 5-minute conversation with the clinician, raising his hand whenever the throat clearing behavior occurred. Once the patient demonstrated greater awareness of throat clearing, alternative behaviors were suggested to be used at times when he felt the urge to clear his throat. The alternative behaviors discussed were an effortful swallow and a silent cough. Both strategies are gentler on the vocal folds and will result in clearance of accumulated mucus. RC was counseled that improved hydration would help thin the mucus and reduce the perceived need to clear the throat. RC asked his wife to help with improving his awareness of throat clearing at home. She was asked to simply raise her hand whenever she observed RC clearing his throat as a reminder to use his alternate behaviors. During clinical visits, both RC and the clinician completed throat-clearing logs and compared the frequency of throat clearing at the end of each visit. Whenever the patient caught himself clearing his throat during the session, he was asked to implement one of the alternative behaviors.

Reduction in Vocal Strain

Short-Term Goal #3. Patient will produce sustained phonation using a resonant hum with OMNI-VES score of 5 or less in 80% of trials with moderate clinician cues. The anatomy and physiology of voice production was reviewed using the patient's own videostroboscopy to demonstrate the increased strain evidenced by closed-phase vibration and false vocal fold compression. The clinician discussed how the aerodynamic findings of elevated peak air pressure and aerodynamic resistance related to the endoscopic findings. RC was educated that the primary goal for all vocal exercises was to reduce the effort and strain and to adopt a gentler voicing pattern.

Several therapeutic strategies were attempted to assess their ability to reduce strain and tension. A resonant voice approach appeared to be of greatest benefit for this patient and was the primary target for treatment. RC was guided to relax the jaw, lips, and throat to create a "cavernlike" feeling in the oral cavity (like holding a hard-boiled egg in the mouth). He was then asked to yawn and feel the retraction and openness of the throat. Once able to consistently assume this relaxed posture, he was asked to sigh out a relaxed and resonant hum. He was cued to focus the sound of the voice forward and upward toward the nasal cavity to minimize strain and tension in the throat. Often, he produced hard onsets at the initiation of the hum and was therefore instructed to allow a small escape of air prior to voice onset. This resulted in more gentle voice onsets. The clinician discussed the importance of self-awareness and kinesthetic feedback, particularly for home practice. RC was informed that he needed to be able to judge for himself whether he was using too much effort/strain, since the clinician would not be with him when he used his voice outside of the clinic. Throughout the sessions, he was asked to comment on the physical effort/strain level as well as his mental effort during tasks.

Once the patient was able to consistently replicate resonant voice and easy onset, he was taken through a hierarchy where he advanced to gentle pitch glides up and down the scale using the relaxed jaw posture resonant hum. Once he was able to maintain an open resonant voice for humming and pitch glides, consonant-vowel (CV) syllables were introduced (eg, "me, me, me," "my, my, my," "ma, ma, ma," "mow, mow, mow," "moo, moo, moo"), avoiding any strain or tension, particularly as he varied vowel sounds. He then progressed to single words, starting with nasal continuants with a gradual increase in syllable count and complexity. He was asked initially to extend the nasal /m/ sound and then

84 Voice Therapy: Clinical Case Studies

to gradually blend the sounds together for more natural speech. During the second session, he was asked to complete a negative practice task where he alternated between resonant voice and the old, pressed voice. He was able to perform this task and identified the difference in sensation between the two. He reported that the resonant voice was more comfortable and noted that when he was using relaxed, resonant voice he did not feel the need to clear his voice as frequently. He rated his vocal effort as a 5 during this session using the OMNI-VES.

By the third therapy session, focus moved to generalization of the vocal technique into more functional contexts. RC was presented with a list of phrases and sentences heavily weighted with nasal consonants (eg, "more and more," "maybe Monday"). Initially, he was asked to chant these stimuli, but then gradually increased the naturalness while maintaining forward focus. Once he was able to perform sentences with consistent accuracy, he was provided with unconstrained reading passages and asked to maintain his relaxed-throat resonant voice. This task proved to be slightly more difficult for RC, and he was prompted to use a gentle hum as a "reset button" when tension/strain was observed. He demonstrated surprisingly good self-awareness despite his persisting cognitive issues and was able to self-correct performance with good accuracy after 2 sessions working on unconstrained passages. At the same time, he began work on short conversational tasks to assist with generalization. At home, RC was asked to participate in 5-minute conversations, 3 times per day, while focusing on his vocal technique. His wife was asked to help monitor his techniques and provide him with supportive feedback. These same conversational tasks were targeted during the therapy sessions. Once RC was able to consistently demonstrate resonant voice in all contexts with his wife and the clinician, he was asked to focus on techniques in a variety of settings and with varied interlocutors. By his sixth session, he realized that he was often using his techniques with minimal mental effort and was able to repair the times he noted strain. At that point, he was weaned to home practice and returned 1 month later for reevaluation.

> The reader may notice that this patient benefited from a more structured voice therapy program compared to preceding cases in this chapter. At times, a more structured approach can be necessary depending on various patient factors. In this case, the patient was impacted by cognitive impairments including impulsivity and reduced insight after a closed head injury, warranting a higher level of structure and clinician support to meet his voice goals.

Therapy Outcomes

RC responded very well to voice therapy despite his preexisting head injury. He adjusted his hydration according to recommendations by his second session. He was less enthusiastic, however, about dietary changes for reflux and though he became more moderate in his food intake, he continued eating spicy foods frequently. Elimination of throat-clearing behaviors was the most difficult aspect of treatment for RC He needed a significant amount of clinician and spousal feedback, but approximately 1 month following initiation of treatment had eliminated throat clearing most of the time. He was able to adopt the target resonant voice and extend it to functional contexts by his fifth or sixth therapy session. He no longer felt he was straining to produce a voice.

Auditory-Perceptual Evaluation. Reevaluation revealed improvement across domains. At the 1-month posttreatment visit, his voice was clear and resonant with only mild, intermittent roughness appreciated. The strained/pressed aspect of voice had fully resolved. CAPE-V severity rating improved from 26 to 12.

Laryngeal Imaging. Videostroboscopic evaluation revealed near-full resolution of the vocal process granulomas, with the posttreatment lesions being ~20% of the size of the original lesions. Vocal fold edema and erythema were resolved, and he had full glottic closure and normal amplitude and mucosal waves. He had balanced and periodic vibration with no significant supraglottic hyperfunction.

Acoustic and Aerodynamic Assessment. Acoustic measures of pitch perturbation and pitch range were more normalized. In regard to aerodynamics, he had improved maximum sustained phonation, nearly normal mean peak air pressure, and marked improvement in aerodynamic resistance.

Quality-of-Life Impairment. On the posttreatment VHI, the patient scored 10/40 points on the functional subscale, 5/40 points on the physical subscale, and 2/40 points on the emotional subscale, yielding a total score of 17/120, which indicated minimal self-perceived voice handicap and a clinically significant improvement from his baseline of 36/120.

Summary

Multidisciplinary intervention for vocal process granulomas optimally includes identification of precipitating factors associated with development and persistence of the lesions. In RC's case, endotracheal intubation was likely the primary factor associated with development of granulomas; however, untreated reflux disease, poor hydration, and chronic throat clearing contributed to their persistence. Secondary muscle tension dysphonia developed due to chronic laryngeal irritation. Medical management of inflammation and reflux, combined with lifestyle modifications and voice therapy, significantly improved his laryngeal exam, voice quality, acoustic/aerodynamic measures, and patient-perceived voice-related quality of life.

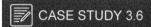

CASE STUDY 3.6

Vocal Function Exercises to Treat an Adult With Undifferentiated Phonotrauma

Joseph C. Stemple

Voice Evaluation

Case History

Patient F, a 26-year-old cisgender female second-grade teacher, was referred by a laryngologist to the voice center for a comprehensive voice evaluation following a diagnosis of large bilateral vocal fold nodules and a left vocal process ulcer. Patient F first became symptomatic in the fall of her first year of teaching and by October of that year, she became dysphonic. When the dysphonia persisted, she sought the opinion of a laryngologist, whose examination revealed mild bilateral vocal fold edema. The physician instructed her to reduce caffeine intake and increase intake of water and briefly counseled her regarding vocal hygiene. The patient followed these instructions, and her voice quality improved.

Between fall and late winter, the patient again experienced intermittent dysphonia. She thought the mild "hoarseness" was fairly normal considering her level of voice use in the school setting. In late February, however, she became moderately dysphonic during a URI but continued to work a normal schedule during her illness. She began to notice not only dysphonic voice changes but also voice fatigue and a burning sensation on the left side of her throat. When the URI resolved and her voice symptoms persisted, she again sought the opinion of the laryngologist.

On seeing the vocal nodules and the ulcerated tissue located on the vocal process of the left arytenoid cartilage, the laryngologist prescribed reflux medication (PPI) and referred the patient for a voice evaluation and therapy. The PPI was prescribed as a precaution because of the implications of acid reflux on the development of contact ulcers and granulomas.

The information gathered during the voice evaluation confirmed the nature of the voice trauma that had significantly increased the patient's symptoms in February. Patient F had indeed experienced a mild dysphonia since school began that fall. She reported that her voice quality typically was better on Monday and much worse by Friday but that she always had some level of dysphonia. Daily, she was more symptomatic during the early morning. The dysphonia would clear somewhat by midmorning and worsen again by afternoon.

With the onset of the respiratory infection, Patient F began coughing and throat clearing. By the time of the voice evaluation, the coughing had decreased, but chronic throat clearing was noted. Her voice use was typical for a second-grade teacher. Students of this age require much instruction, and non-speech times in the classroom were reported to be minimal. In addition, the patient was assigned playground and school bus duty, which required occasional shouting and raising the voice above noise to be heard.

There was no evidence of phonotraumatic behaviors outside of the work environment. She was married and had a 2-year-old daughter. She denied any direct vocal trauma or environmental contributions, such as inhaled dust, fumes, chemicals, or paints. She reported that her voice improved on weekends and always returned to "normal" during the summer months. The remaining social history was unremarkable as related to this problem.

Medical History. The patient's medical history also was unremarkable. She was free of any chronic illnesses or disorders and took only the PPI, although she was not symptomatic with "heartburn." She was a nonsmoker, living and working in a nonsmoking environment. Her liquid intake was not adequate. She drank 2 cans of caffeinated soda and 2 glasses

of iced tea per day. Patient F reported that she "loved" teaching and felt "great" daily.

Auditory-Perceptual Evaluation

The CAPE-V[11] yielded a score of 38/100, indicating a moderate dysphonia. The voice was breathy and rough.

Laryngeal Imaging

Transoral laryngeal videostroboscopic examination revealed large bilateral vocal fold nodules, larger on the right than on the left; bilateral edema and erythema; and an apparent resolving left contact ulcer. The nodules caused glottic closure to demonstrate an hourglass configuration with a slight bilateral ventricular fold compression. Both the amplitude of vibration and the mucosal waves were severely decreased bilaterally. The open phase of the vibratory cycle was dominant, whereas the symmetry of vibration generally was irregular. In other words, she presented with significant tissue changes that would present a challenge to functional voice therapy.

Acoustic and Aerodynamic Assessment

Salient acoustic measures demonstrated a limited frequency range of 147 to 562 Hz; fundamental frequency remained appropriate at 211 Hz; jitter measures were within normal limits while shimmer measures were high at 0.46 dB. Aerodynamic measures yielded significantly high airflow rates for high pitches, averaging 305 mL/H_2O. Comfortable and low pitches were borderline high at 180 and 189 mL/H_2O, respectively. The patient was required to push more air through her vocal system to support the vibration because of increased vocal fold mass and the hourglass glottal closure. Her subsequent phonation times at all pitch levels were only 11 seconds or less.

Quality of Life

Patient F completed the Voice-Related Quality of Life (V-RQOL)[55] assessment to document the effect the voice disorder was having on her life. Results demonstrated a moderate life impact.

Impressions

This patient presented with persistent dysphonia secondary to bilateral vocal nodules as a result of phonotraumatic behaviors while teaching, inadequate hydration, and persistent throat clearing.

Plan of Care

After the voice evaluation, the following treatment plan was proposed:

- Temporary reassignment from playground and school bus duties
- Site visit to determine environment and teaching style
- Elimination of phonotraumatic throat clearing
- Oral hydration program
- Vocal function exercises designed to rebalance respiration, phonation, and resonance.

Intervention

Temporary Reassignment

To immediately eliminate the potential for the most obvious vocal traumas, the patient was guided to request to be assigned to other duties away from the playground and school buses where voice would not be a factor and she would not be required to raise her vocal loudness.

Site Visit

Site visits are time consuming and not always practical, but the value of seeing the patient in the implicated environment cannot be overemphasized. Other useful options include remote observations or video and audio recordings of the patient in the speaking environment.

Patient F's school was convenient to the voice center, so a 1-hour site visit was arranged. Observations made during the visit included:

- Large room
- Unusually high (16-18 feet) acoustical tile ceilings
- Sound was lost in space
- Only 24 students spread throughout the large room at different "stations"
- All sounds (scooting chairs, dropped books, and so forth) were magnified by glass and plastic
- Speech was hard to discriminate.

It was obvious that Patient F indeed "loved" her work. She was enthusiastic and had complete control of the classroom. Observations made regarding her teaching style included:

- Vocally enthusiastic, but does not shout
- Room requires that she speak loudly and precisely, not to be heard but to be understood
- Spends a good deal of time "directing" children when not actually teaching
- Uses high pitch, limited inflection, and back focus; constantly strains voice.

An audio recording was made during the visit that was reviewed later in therapy.

The opportunity to visit the patient's classroom led to several suggestions:

- Decrease the physical space by rearranging seating and using approximately two-thirds of the classroom. With a class size of only 24 students, this was easy to accomplish. The patient herself suggested an additional change. She physically decreased the room size by using large, free-standing display boards (which were normally in school storage) as temporary walls.
- Soften the acoustics of the room by using the window blinds, pulled halfway down. Use fabric in a work display area by hanging a sheet on the wall to display student papers, pictures, tests, and similar exhibits.

The large display boards also functioned well as an acoustic barrier.

■ Build into the schedule a vocal "time out" for both the teacher and the students. Learn to respect and appreciate the silent time as a chance to rest the voice and as a reminder to talk only as loudly as necessary in the newly configured classroom.

■ Develop a sign system for common instructions and requests. It was noted during the site visit that the patient was constantly correcting and directing students' actions while instructing. When this was brought to her attention, she decided to implement an interesting sign-symbol system that would preclude voice commands. She listed the names of the students on a large magnetic board in the corner of the classroom. Signs were then made with picture symbols depicting the most common corrections and directions that she made. They included symbols representing directions such as: be quiet, don't tilt your chair, slow down, stop talking, talk softer, and pay attention. These symbol pictures were attached to magnets. When the need arose, the patient would place the symbol next to the name of the offending child, all the while continuing her teaching. A list of consequences for receiving more than one symbol correction was established by the teacher and well understood by the children.

> Stemple highlights the immense value of a site visit to observe ecologically valid voice use. Voice use in daily life can differ dramatically compared to the environment of the voice therapy room. While many clinicians may not have the time or flexibility to personally make a site visit, telehealth services can be pragmatically used to similar effect.

Elimination of Habitual Throat Clearing

The previous suggestions immediately decreased the daily vocal fatigue but did not eliminate the dysphonia. The therapy plan introduced a behavior modification approach for eliminating the phonotraumatic behavior of throat clearing. Until the therapist brought it to her attention, the patient was not aware of the frequency of her throat clearing. Throat clearing may be traumatic to the tissue lining of the vocal folds and arytenoid cartilages. Once she became aware of it, the patient was surprised by the number of times she cleared her throat during the session. To modify this behavior, she was told the following:

Throat clearing is one of the most traumatizing things you can do to your vocal folds. When you clear your throat like this [demonstrate], you create an extreme amount of movement of your vocal folds, causing them to slam and rub together [demonstrate using your hands]. You should understand that it is not unusual to have developed this habit. Many patients we see with this type of voice problem also have this habit. Sometimes people do not even know that they are doing it, but often they say that they feel something in their throat, such as a lump sensation or mucus. The majority of the time, however, when you clear your throat, there is nothing there. Often, patients only feel a sensation of thickness from chronic vocal strain. The only thing you have accomplished when throat clearing is to create more vocal fold trauma.

We have demonstrated to you with the audio recording from your class that, most of the time, you clear your throat right before you begin to speak. We call that a preparatory throat clear. Also, you are clearing many more times than you realized. This is a sign that throat clearing is a habit. As with all habits, it is difficult to break. We are, therefore, going to try to make it easier by giving you a substitute habit that (1) will take the place of throat clearing, (2) will accomplish the same thing as throat clearing, and (3) is not vocally traumatic. This substitute habit is a hard, forceful swallow.

If you do, in fact, occasionally have increased amount of mucus on your vocal folds, a forceful swallow will accomplish the same thing as throat clearing, minus the trauma. The only difference is that throat clearing feels good. It psychologically gives you more relief than the forceful swallow, even though it physically accomplishes no more. It is your goal to overcome the psychological dependence. Understand that this habit is harmful and that it must be broken.

To break this habit, you need to tell everyone in your family and any friends who are often around you (and whom you feel comfortable telling) that you're not permitted to clear your throat anymore. When these "helpers" hear you clear your throat, and they will, they are to immediately point it out. You may even consider using your students as helpers. Your task, then, is to swallow forcefully. Obviously, it will not be necessary to swallow because you just cleared your throat, but this is your first step in substituting the hard swallow for the throat clearing.

After your family, friends, or students have pointed out your throat clearing to you several times, your level of awareness will rise and you will begin to "catch" yourself. You will clear your throat and almost immediately think, "Oops! I am not supposed to do that." Your response again should be to swallow forcefully.

When you have caught yourself clearing your throat several times, you begin to halt yourself just prior to clearing. Once again, you will substitute the hard swallow, but this time the throat clearing was stopped. By the time you have reached this point, you will be close to breaking the habit totally. The final goal will be met when you realize that you are swallowing many fewer times than the number of times you previously were clearing your throat.

I want you to work hard on this problem. I think you will be surprised just how quickly you are able to break this habit. As a matter of fact, the majority of our patients have significantly reduced the habit within 1 to 2 weeks. Most patients, however, cannot do it alone. So please, find other people to help you by having them point out when you are doing it. Any questions?

Following this explanation, the patients typically will clear their throats more times during the session. The speech pathologist immediately points this out, and the patient initiates a forceful swallow substitution while in the therapy session. Often, patients make great gains in habit modification during this initial session. Patient F received help from her husband, mother, and a friend and was able to eliminate the habit of throat clearing within 2 weeks.

Oral Hydration Program

The vocal folds must be well lubricated to decrease the heat and friction of vibration. Thin, slippery mucus secreted onto the vocal folds serves the same purpose as oil serves to the engine of a car. It was explained to Patient F that what she swallows does not touch her vocal folds but is diverted around them. Therefore, the amount and type of liquid intake will either permit or inhibit the normal mucus flow to the vocal folds. Caffeine, alcohol, and many medications are drying agents. Many times, when patients feel as if they have too much mucus on the vocal folds, they actually have increased mucus viscosity, which is thicker and stickier than is desirable.

This patient's liquid intake was minimal and caffeinated. She therefore was placed on a hydration program that required a minimum intake of six 8-ounce glasses of water or fruit juice per day. In addition, she was asked to decrease her caffeine intake but was not required to eliminate caffeine from her diet.

Vocal Function Exercises. An important part of this patient's voice therapy program was the use of VFEs. These exercises, first described by Barnes[56] and modified by Stemple,[57] strive to balance the subsystems of voice production. The exercise program has proven successful in improving and enhancing the vocal function of speakers with normal voices, singing voices, and disordered voices.[58]

The program is as follows: Describe the voice problem to the patient, using illustrations as needed or the patient's own stroboscopic evaluation video. Then, teach the patient a series of 4 exercises to be done at home, twice each, 2 times per day, preferably morning and evening. (See Video 5 Vocal Function Exercises by Stemple.) These exercises include:

1. Sustain the /i/ vowel for as long as possible on the musical note F above middle C for all higher-pitched voices and children prior to puberty and F below middle C for lower-pitched voices. (Notes may be modified up or down to fit the needs of the patient. Seldom are they modified by more than 2 notes in either direction.)
   Goal. Based on airflow volume. In our clinic, the goal is based on reaching 80 to 100 mL/sec of airflow. If the flow volume is equal to 4000 mL, then the goal is 40 to 50 seconds. When airflow measures are not available, the goal is equal to the length of time the patient can maximally sustain a soft /s/. Placement of the tone should be in an extreme forward focus that is almost, but not quite, nasal. All exercises are produced as softly as possible, but not breathy. The voice must be "engaged." This is considered a warm-up exercise.
2. Glide from your lowest note to your highest note on the word "knoll."
   Goal. No voice breaks. The glide requires the use of all laryngeal muscles. It stretches the vocal folds and encourages a systematic, slow engagement of the cricothyroid muscles. The word "knoll" encourages a forward placement of the tone as well as an expanded, open pharynx. The patient's lips are to be rounded and a sympathetic vibration should be felt on the lips. (May also use a lip trill, tongue trill, or the word "whoop.") Voice breaks typically will occur in the transitions between low and high registers. When breaks occur, the patient is encouraged to continue the glide without hesitation. When the voice breaks at the top of the current range and the patient typically has more range, the glide may be continued without voice as the folds will continue to stretch. Glides improve muscular control and flexibility. This is considered a stretching exercise.
3. Glide from a comfortable high note to your lowest note on the word "knoll."
   Goal. No voice breaks. The patient is instructed to feel a half-yawn in the throat throughout this exercise. By keeping the pharynx open and focusing the sympathetic vibration at the lips, the downward glide encourages a slow, systematic engagement of the thyroarytenoid muscles without the presence of a back-focused growl. In fact, no growl is permitted. (May also use a lip trill, tongue trill, or the word "boom.") This is considered a contracting exercise.
4. Sustain the musical notes C, D, E, F, and G for as long as possible on the word "knoll" minus the "kn." (Middle C for higher voices and an octave below middle C for lower voices.)
   Goal. Remains the same as for exercise 1. The "oll" is once again produced with an open pharynx and constricted, sympathetically vibrating lips. The shape of the pharynx to the lips is likened to an inverted megaphone. The fourth exercise may be tailored to the patient's present vocal ability. Although the basic range starting at middle C, or an octave lower for mature male patients, is appropriate for most voices, the exercises may be customized up or down to fit the current vocal condition or a particular voice type. Seldom, however, are the exercises shifted more than 2 notes in either direc-

tion. This is considered a low-impact adductory power exercise.

Quality of the tone is also monitored for voice breaks, wavering, and breathiness. Quality improves as times increase and pathologies begin to resolve.

All exercises are done as softly as possible, but engaged. It is much more difficult to produce soft tones; therefore, the vocal subsystems will receive a better "workout" than if louder tones were produced. Extreme care is taken to teach the production of a forward tone that lacks tension. In addition, attention is paid to the glottal onset of the tone. The patient is asked to breathe in deeply while paying attention to training abdominal breathing, posturing the vowel momentarily, and then initiating the exercise gesture without a forceful glottal attack or an aspirate breathy attack.

It is explained to the patient that maximum phonation times increase as the efficiency of the vocal fold vibration improves. Times do not increase because of improved "lung capacity." Indeed, even aerobic exercise does not improve lung capacity but rather the efficiency of oxygen exchange with the circulatory system, thus giving the sense of more air.

The patient is provided with a cell phone video or audio recording of the clinician demonstrating the exercises, which is used to guide the home exercise sessions. We have found that patients who complain of "tone deafness" often can be taught to approximate the correct notes with practice and guidance from the speech pathologist.

Finally, the patient is given a chart on which to mark sustained times, which is a means of plotting progress (Table 3–17). Progress is monitored over time, and because of

Table 3–17. Vocal Function Exercises Practice Chart for Exercises #1 and #4

		MON	TUE	WED	THU	FRI	SAT	SUN
	Date							
AM								
#1	E/F	/	/	/	/	/	/	/
#4	C	/	/	/	/	/	/	/
	D	/	/	/	/	/	/	/
	E	/	/	/	/	/	/	/
	F	/	/	/	/	/	/	/
	G	/	/	/	/	/	/	/
PM								
#1	E/F	/	/	/	/	/	/	/
#4	C	/	/	/	/	/	/	/
	D	/	/	/	/	/	/	/
	E	/	/	/	/	/	/	/
	F	/	/	/	/	/	/	/
	G	/	/	/	/	/	/	/

normal daily variability, patients are encouraged not to compare one day with the next. Rather, weekly comparisons are encouraged. Estimated time of completion for the program is 8 to 10 weeks.

When the patient has reached the predetermined therapy goal and the voice quality and other vocal symptoms are improved, a tapering maintenance program is recommended. Although some professional voice users choose to remain in peak vocal condition using the exercises, many of our patients desire to taper the program. The following systematic taper is recommended:

- Full program 2 times each, 2 times per day
- Full program 2 times each, 1 time per day (morning)
- Full program 1 time each, 1 time per day (morning)
- Exercise 4, 2 times each pitch, 1 time per day (morning)
- Exercise 4, 1 time each pitch, 1 time per day (morning)
- Exercise 4, 1 time each pitch, 3 times per week (morning)
- Exercise 4, 1 time each pitch, 1 time per week (morning)

Each taper should last 1 week. Patients should maintain 85% of their peak time, otherwise they should move up one step in the taper until the 85% criterion is met.

VFEs helped to improve the overall condition of Patient F's vocal folds and to retrain frontal focus. The patient's baseline mean phonation time for sustaining the appropriate notes was 8.5 seconds. This measure improved to a mean of 18 seconds during 6 weeks of therapy.

Results of Initial Therapy

Significant improvement was noted during 6 weeks of therapy for both subjective observations of voice quality and objective measures of vocal function. The patient was experiencing much less vocal fatigue and laryngeal discomfort. Audio recordings made while teaching demonstrated stabilization of new voicing habits and only very occasional throat clearing. She did, however, remain mildly dysphonic, characterized by slight breathiness.

Selected Acoustic and Aerodynamic Measures and Assessment. Objective measures demonstrated a fundamental frequency of 196 Hz (pretreatment 211 Hz) and an expanded frequency range of 165 to 720 Hz (pretreatment 147 to 562 Hz). Jitter and shimmer measures were both within normal limits. Airflow rates for comfortable and low-pitched voices were decreased to 136 and 150 mL/sec, respectively (pretreatment 180 and 189 mL/H_2O, respectively). Airflow rate for high-pitched voice also decreased to 240 mL/sec but was still above the normal limit of 200 mL/sec.

Laryngeal Imaging. Videostroboscopy also demonstrated improvement. The edema and erythema were resolved, and there was no evidence of the contact ulcer. A slight thickness was noted where the left nodule had been. The right nodule was still present but appeared much more cystlike. Glottic closure retained an hourglass shape; however, the glottal gaps were much smaller. The amplitude of vibration was only slightly decreased on the left and moderately decreased on the right. The mucosal wave was normal on the left and moderately decreased around the right lesion. The open phase of the vibratory cycle was slightly dominant, while the symmetry of vibration remained irregular.

The results of the therapy program were discussed with Patient F's physician and Patient F. Given the cystlike nature of the vocal fold lesion, there was not an expectation that the lesion would resolve with voice therapy alone. However, Patient F was happy with the voice outcome and decided that she did not want surgery. She reported understanding that, should she experience future voice concerns, surgery may be needed to address the lesion to achieve further voice improvement.

CASE STUDY 3.7

Lessac-Madsen Resonant Voice Therapy to Treat an Adult With Vocal Fold Nodules

Diana Marie Orbelo, Nicole Y. K. Li-Jessen, and Katherine Verdolini Abbott

Voice Evaluation

Case History

Patient K, a 21-year-old cisgender female college student and avid singer, was referred to voice therapy by laryngology with bilateral vocal fold nodules. She presented with a 9-month history of worsening voice fatigue following school-related performances and a precipitating upper respiratory tract infection. She described instability in her upper singing range, throat discomfort, and hoarseness when speaking. Other medical concerns were denied.

Pre- and Posttherapy Measures

Pre- and posttherapy voice evaluations included an auditory-perceptual voice evaluation using the CAPE-V,[11] instrumental assessment with videostrobolaryngoscopy, and patient self-assessments using the Voice Symptom Scale (VoiSS)[59] and the SVHI.[60] All results are presented in Figures 3–9 through 3–12.

Decision Making

History and observations suggested the most obvious contributor to K's physical pathology and dysphonia was voice use patterns, which by clinical observation included both adducted and nonadducted hyperfunction. The biomechanical result of adductory hyperfunction, which K often used during singing, would be large inter-vocal-fold impact stresses that increase susceptibility to nodules and attendant voice changes.[61] In contrast, the nonadducted hyperfunction, which can also constitute vocal dysfunction and even episodic voice loss,[62] characterized K's speaking voice,

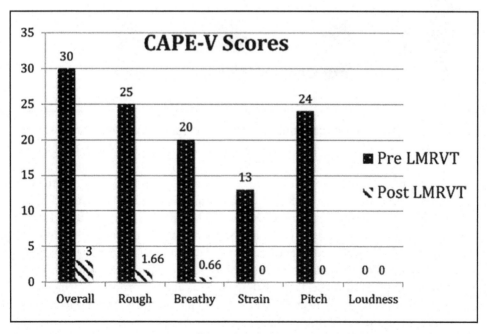

FIGURE 3–9. Pre- and posttreatment Consensus Auditory-Perceptual Evaluation of Voice (CAPE-V) scores.

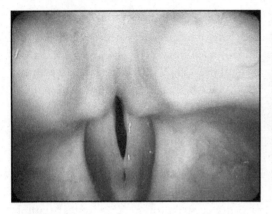 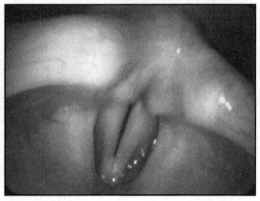

FIGURE 3–10. Pre- and posttreatment laryngeal imaging.

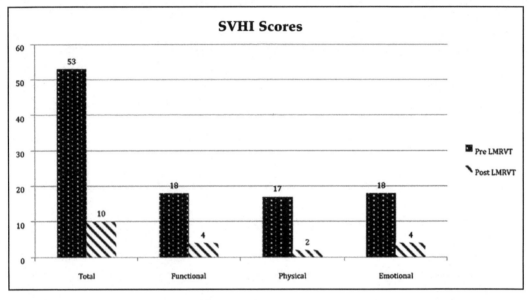

FIGURE 3–11. Pre- and posttreatment Singing Voice Handicap Index (SVHI) scores.

along with a chronic "throaty resonance" and vocal fry. A second potential factor of K's dysphonia was relative dehydration evidenced by her frequent throat clearing in reaction to a "feeling of mucus" and acknowledgment that she drank little water. The literature indicates that dehydration may predispose laryngeal tissue to injury or slow recovery from injury, while also increasing the subglottic pressure required for phonation, especially for high pitches.[63]

Considering the clinical picture, Lessac-Madsen Resonant Voice Therapy (LMRVT)[64,65] was selected as the therapy tool. LMRVT has origins in a convergence of performing arts traditions and basic science in biomechanics, biology, and perceptual-motor learning. The program also incorporates principles in the clinical literature on factors affecting patients' adherence with health care recommendations. LMRVT is an integrated program that differs from traditional models of voice con-

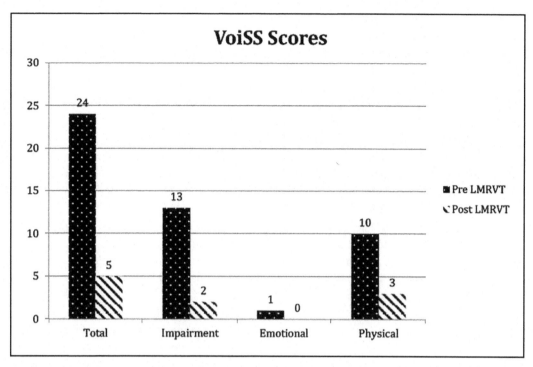

FIGURE 3–12. Pre- and posttreatment Voice Symptom Scale (VoiSS) scores.

servation. Many people with voice problems use their voices often and even loudly due to occupational or other life circumstances, and sometimes due to a personality component. A basic premise in LMRVT is that our job, as clinicians, is not to encourage people with voice problems to adopt a quiescent lifestyle in the interest of vocal health but rather to figure out how people can accomplish their vocal tasks effectively and safely without incurring injury. Emerging biomechanical and biological data suggest that voice produced with a barely ad-/abducted vocal fold configuration, often corresponding to the perceptual phenomenon called "resonant voice," can help many people with voice problems achieve this goal regardless of the origin of their pathology. In fact, data suggest that "resonant voice" (RV) may not only help prevent aggravating pathology that may be cumulative in an individual with voice problems but may also help repair acute phonotrauma.

Treatment Goals

In-person treatment was based on a standard LMRVT program, which is intended as a general platform for treatment that clinicians and patients should vary depending on the situation. For K, and as typical for LMRVT, 3 levels of treatment goals were established: (1) functional, (2) medical, and (3) behavioral.

Goal #1. Functional. For benign conditions affecting voice, such as nodules, functional goals are considered the ultimate target of treatment and are determined by the patient. K's functional goal was to have a fully functional speaking and singing voice without dysphonia or voice breaks, and to reestablish pain-free and effort-free phonation without constant vigilance.

Goal #2. Medical. The medical goal, implied by the referral to voice therapy, was to reduce or resolve vocal fold nodules.

Goal #3. Behavioral. Behavioral/biomechanical goals, established by the SLP, were divided into 2 subtypes, as typical for most voice therapy, including (1) goals pertinent to the viscoelastic properties of the tissue, targeted using "indirect methods" ("vocal hygiene"), and (2) goals that address phonation modality itself ("direct methods"). Behavioral and biomechanical goals are the only ones specifically addressed in voice therapy in LMRVT under the assumption that, if these goals are appropriately established and achieved, functional and medical goals will be attained as a result. For K, biomechanical goals were to increase both systemic and surface hydration (indirect treatment) and to establish a voice-production pattern associated with barely ad-/abducted vocal folds for most phonation in speech and singing (direct goal).

Intervention

LMRVT is typically delivered in 6 to 8 sessions over 4 to 8 weeks. However, given constraints in K's schedule, a more intensive approach was taken and the entire LMRVT course was completed in 4 weeks. Beyond voice therapy, K received no other treatments or training during the active therapy period, either medical or vocal (as with singing training). The overarching therapeutic framework—for K and for LMRVT in general—identifies 3 critical factors that are both "necessary" and "sufficient" to address in physical training of any type. Those factors are (1) the "what," (2) the "how," and (3) the "if" of training. The "what" refers to behaviors and biomechanical targets that are addressed in training. "What" are behavioral and biomechanical goals (eg, drink more water and use a barely adducted vocal fold configuration during phonation, respectively) across therapy. The "how" of voice therapy refers to the approach to training, independent of the biomechanical target. That is, "how" will patients acquire the behaviors and biomechanical targets we identify for them? The "if" of voice therapy refers to patient adher-

ence—"if" the patient will do what we might suggest, especially outside the clinic. Summary details regarding these parameters are as follows.

The "What" of Training

The "what" piece of LMRVT therapy is subdivided into 2 parts: voice care education ("hygiene") and voice training. One emphasis in LMRVT is that voice care education should limit the number of parameters we suggest patients address rather than creating a large list of "do"s and "don't"s, which can be overwhelming and generally lack specificity for a given patient. We consider the "short list" of key domains to address in hygiene as (1) systemic and surface hydration; (2) exogenous inflammation control, environmental pollutants, illness allergens, medications, smoke, and so on; and (3) patent phonotraumatic behaviors such as uncontrolled, unskilled screaming. The key in Patient K's program, and in LMRVT in general, was the identification of only those hygiene parameters relevant to the patient in question, based on case history and observations. Targeted hygiene programs have been found to improve patient adherence[4,68] compared to one-size-fits-all programs.[11] Slimmed down, targeted hygiene interventions may be sufficient to help prevent the onset of new voice problems in at-risk populations (eg, teachers), although such interventions may be insufficient as a single treatment modality in cases of existing pathology.[66,67]

Regarding actual voice training, in LMRVT for this patient and others, most sessions initiate with exercises to stretch extrinsic and intrinsic structures involved in phonation. This approach is based on the notion that skilled perceptual-motor behavior in most domains fundamentally involves inhibition of musculature irrelevant to a task, with concomitant activation of relevant musculature. Support for this approach is found in the developmental motor learning literature pointing to selective activation as a hallmark of skilled performance.[68] Accordingly, all therapy sessions for Patient K initiated with a series of stretches targeting the thorax, cervical region, face, oral structures, oropharynx, and vocal folds to minimize activation of musculature in the phonatory substrate.[65] Selective activation exercises followed. Conceptually, the selective activation piece of therapy may proceed according to any one of several specific therapy interventions, including VFEs and Flow Phonation, described elsewhere in this text and in the literature (see Case Study 3.6 by Stemple: Vocal Function Exercises to Treat an Adult With Undifferentiated Phonotrauma and Case Study 4.3 by Gartner-Schmidt: Flow Phonation to Treat a Teenager With Primary Muscle Tension Aphonia).[64,65]

Table 3–18 describes the specific contents of K's therapy, which arose from the general framework described. Additional information about the contents of current LMRVT can be obtained through Plural Publishing,[64,65] coupled with hands-on training in seminar and webinar formats. Here, discussion is limited to general "philosophical" comments around LMRVT and to newer findings and speculations pertinent to LMRVT for this patient and others.

As already implied, in LMRVT the target voice-production modality is defined both productively and perceptually. Productively, the target involves voicing with barely adducted or slightly abducted vocal folds. This configuration, and specifically a configuration involving an approximately 0- to 1.0-mm separation between the vocal processes at phonation onset, appears to generate an optimized ratio of voice output intensity versus vocal fold impact intensity under constant subglottic pressure (Ps) and fundamental frequency (F0) conditions.[5] Not incidentally, this same general vocal fold configuration requires relatively limited subglottal pressure to initiate and maintain vocal fold oscillation, and thus should be physiologically "easy." Perceptually,

one correlate of this laryngeal setup—when trained using a semi-occluded vocal tract, as occurs with LMRVT—is RV, which involves vibratory sensations in the anterior oral cavity in the context of "easy" phonation.[69,70]

Advantages of RV in voice therapy may be linked to its likely connection to a biomechanical setup that favors strong voice production (when needed) while protecting from laryngeal injury.[5] Preliminary data from biological studies indicate that this voicing approach can have therapeutic properties. For instance, RV exercises may help to attenuate acute vocal fold inflammation even more than voice rest in some cases.[4]

The "How" of Voice Therapy

LMRVT is similar in emphasis to traditional "forward focus" approaches. The laryngeal goal is essentially identical to the goal implicitly targeted in VFEs.[57] One of the features of LMRVT that distinguishes it from "resonant voice" or "forward focus" training approaches in general lies with its systematic incorporation of well-vetted principles of perceptual motor learning documented in peer-reviewed literature.[71] In brief, clinicians are asked to avoid instructions about how a person should attempt to achieve a target voice pattern biomechanically. Instead, the training focuses on biomechanical outcomes such as sound and feel of the voice. ("Does your voice sound clear? Does your voice feel easy?") Perception and an experiential approach rather than biomechanical instructions are emphasized. Also, "laws of practice" are used to structure exercises, including "laws" indicating that augmented feedback should be minimized and provided terminally during training (eg, after a vocalization) rather than concurrent with production. Random practice is emphasized, as are "whole" as opposed to "part" practice and variable practice of the target RV in numerous phonetic, acoustic, and emotional contexts (for details, see Schmidt et al, 2018[72]).

Table 3–18. Description of Each Therapy Session (RV = Resonant Voice; BTG = Basic Training Gesture)

Session	Status at Start of Session	Therapy Provided During Session	Patient's Performance Within Session	Home Tasks and Exercises	Time to Next Session
Initial Evaluation	Intermittent dysphonia, throat pain, and pitch instability	• *Hygiene:* hydration instructions provided • *Voice training:* stretches; RV BTG exercises (RV explorations in single consonants); words	• *Hygiene:* instructions understood • Produced RV well at 85% for nasal consonants	• 2-3 qt water daily, steam inhalations, 5-min BID • Stretches; RV foundation BTG exercises and RV chants, 10-min BID, frequent mini-practices	4 days
Therapy #1	Voice unchanged	• *Voice training:* stretches; RV BTG exercises; words/sentences with multiple phonemic contexts	• Produced RV relatively well to sentence level without models; hyperfunction decreased particularly when models stimulated increased air flow	• Continue hygiene • Stretches; RV BTG words/sentences 10-min BID, frequent mini-practices	18 days (patient was extremely busy with upcoming show)
Therapy #2	Voice unchanged	• *Voice training:* stretches; RV BTG words/sentences; worked on singing techniques for upcoming performance	• Produced RV well to sentence level with models; patient was focused on singing issues	• Continue hygiene • Stretches; RV BTG words/sentences including loudness variations, 10-min BID, frequent mini-practices	9 days

Table 3–18. *continued*

Session	Status at Start of Session	Therapy Provided During Session	Patient's Performance Within Session	Home Tasks and Exercises	Time to Next Session
Therapy #3	Singing voice feeling better, less pain with singing	• *Voice training:* stretches; RV BTG words/sentences; worked on singing techniques for upcoming performance	• Produced relatively good RV without hyperfunction to phrase level; singing was consistently on pitch without breaks	• Continue hygiene • Stretches; RV BTG words/sentences including loudness variations, 10-min BID, frequent mini-practices	2 months (left for summer vacation, reported doing exercises 1x per day "most days")
Therapy #4	Voice less frequently hoarse, still experiencing some pain with long periods of speaking	• *Voice training:* reviewed hygiene, stretches, RV core, chant, vocal communicators, mini-practice with practice to carry over into conversation. Use of real-time visual of pitch and roughness focusing on ends of phrases. Introduced loudness work.	• Produced RV with intermittent mild hyperfunction to 85% with prompts and models (session materials recorded on smartphone for patient use)	• Continue hygiene • Stretches; RV BTG words/sentences, including loudness variations on vowels, 10-min BID, frequent mini-practices, use of vocal communicator	3 days
Therapy #5	Voice generally feeling "good" and noticing speaking patterns on phone, in loud environments, and when physically tired	• *Voice training:* stretches; RV BTG adding phonemic complexity, variable loudness work, conversation	• Produced completely hyperfunction-free voice on 50%-60% of conversational trials and good approximations on remainder of trials, with some models	• Continue hygiene • Same as last session, but adding loudness work and mindfulness about speaking pattern during everyday conversation	4 days

continues

Table 3–18. *continued*

Session	Status at Start of Session	Therapy Provided During Session	Patient's Performance Within Session	Home Tasks and Exercises	Time to Next Session
Therapy #6	Voice "very good most of the time" but still falling into hyperfunctional habits during long social conversations. No pain with speaking.	• *Voice training:* stretches; review and warm-up using RV BTG, core, and chants. Work on phrase and conversational-level exercises in quiet environment with model challenges.	• By end of session, patient produced hyperfunction-free voice on about 75% of trials during structured conversation, with minimal cues	• Continue hygiene • Continue exercises • Continue mini and mindful practices throughout the day	2 days
Therapy #7	Voice "feeling very good"; patient confident that she can continue with techniques as she returns to school	• *Voice training:* stretches; review and warm-up using RV BTG, core, and chants. Work on phrase and conversational-level exercises in challenging environments outside the therapy room, including places where loud and soft voice is required.	• Throughout session, patient was able to produce RV approximately 90% of the time in challenging environments with minimal modeling and cues	• Continue hygiene • Continue exercises as previously added • Start work with a local singing teacher	7 months to reevaluation

The "If" of Training

Full discussion of factors thought to influence patient adherence or compliance is beyond the scope of the present venue (for review, see Titze and Verdolini[71]). Briefly, key factors include the concept of self-efficacy for voice (does a patient believe they can perform exercises?) and readiness for voice change (is a patient ready to make changes, as discussed in motivational interviewing techniques?)[73,74] In addition, the clinician must be engaged, attentive, empathetic, and mindful throughout the interaction. These principles are folded into standard LMRVT.

Treatment Outcome and Recommendations

Patient K underwent reevaluation of baseline measures 7 months following therapy termination. K felt she had met her functional goal and was now speaking normally without discomfort during most speech. She no longer experienced fatigue during social or occupational conversation, and she was able to sing more consistently and without discomfort or voice breaks.

Auditory-perceptual findings, laryngeal imaging, and patient self-assessment agreed. CAPE-V results indicated that K's voice was perceived as normal, implying that biomechanical goals had been achieved (see Figure 3–9). Laryngeal imaging showed the resolution from hourglass-shape glottis to normal vocal fold edges, suggesting that medical goals were also achieved (see Figure 3–10). Likewise, laryngeal videostroboscopy revealed complete glottic closure consistent with barely ad-/abducted vocal folds, normal amplitude of vocal fold vibration, and normal mucosal wave bilaterally at discharge, compared with reduced amplitude of vibration and reduced mucosal wave bilaterally at baseline. K reported meeting her functional goals for pain-free, clear speaking and singing without constant self-monitoring and was observed by the treating clinician to produce resonant voice at least 90% of the time. Self-assessment tools completed by K corroborated observed improvements (see Figures 3–11 and 3–12). Based on medical and biomechanical findings at treatment termination, it was recommended that K continued using stretches and resonant voice exercises at least 3 to 4 times weekly, prophylactically, and that she work with a local singing voice teacher.

References

1. Branski RC, Verdolini K, Sandulache V, Rosen CA, Hebda PA. Vocal fold wound healing: A review for clinicians. *J Voice.* 2006;20(3):432-442. doi:10.1016/j.jvoice.2005.08.005
2. Rousseau B, Cohen SM, Zeller AS, Scearce L, Tritter AG, Garrett CG. Compliance and quality of life in patients on prescribed voice rest. *Otolaryngol Head Neck Surg.* 2011;144(1):104-107. doi:10.1177/0194599810390465
3. Branski R, Perera P, Verdolini K, Rosen C, Hebda P, Agarwal S. Dynamic biomechanical strain inhibits IL-1β–induced inflammation in vocal fold fibroblasts. *J Voice.* 2016;21(6):651-660. doi:10.1016/j.jvoice.2006.06.005
4. Abbott KV, Li NYK, Branski RC, et al. Vocal exercise may attenuate acute vocal fold inflammation. 2013;26(6):814.e1-814.e13. doi:10.1016/j.jvoice.2012.03.008
5. Berry DA, Verdolini K, Montequin DW, Hess MM, Chan RW, Titze IR. A quantitative output-cost ratio in voice production. *J Speech Lang Hear Res.* 2001;44(1):29-37. doi:10.1044/1092-4388(2001/003)
6. Ziegler A, Dastolfo C, Hersan R, Rosen CA, Gartner-Schmidt J. Perceptions of voice therapy from patients diagnosed with primary muscle tension dysphonia and benign mid-membranous vocal fold lesions. *J Voice.* 2014;28(6):742-752. doi:10.1016/j.jvoice.2014.02.007
7. Iwarsson J. Facilitating behavioral learning and habit change in voice therapy—Theoretic premises and practical strategies. *Logop Phoniatr Vocol.* 2015;40(4):179-186. doi:10.3109/14015439.2014.936498

8. Van Stan J, Mehta D, Petit R, et al. Integration of motor learning principles into real-time ambulatory voice biofeedback and example implementation via a clinical case study with vocal fold nodules. *Am J Speech Lang Pathol.* 2017;26(1):1-10. doi:10.1044/2016_AJSLP-15-0187

9. Gartner-Schmidt J, Gherson S, Hapner ER, et al. The development of conversation training therapy: A concept paper. *J Voice.* 2016;30(5):563-573. doi:10.1016/j.jvoice.2015.06.007

10. Gillespie AI, Yabes J, Rosen CA, Gartner-Schmidt JL. Efficacy of conversation training therapy for patients with benign vocal fold lesions and muscle tension dysphonia compared to historical matched control patients. *J Speech Lang Hear Res.* 2019;62(11):4062-4079. doi:10.1044/2019_JSLHR-S-19-0136

11. Kempster GB, Gerratt BR, Abbott KV, Barkmeier-Kraemer J, Hillman RE. Consensus auditory-perceptual evaluation of voice: Development of a standardized clinical protocol. *Am J Speech Lang Pathol.* 2009;18(2):124-132. doi:10.1044/1058-0360(2008/08-0017)

12. Gillespie AI, Dastolfo C, Magid N, Gartner-Schmidt J. Acoustic analysis of four common voice diagnoses: Moving toward disorder-specific assessment. *J Voice.* 2014;28(5):582-588. doi:10.1016/j.jvoice.2014.02.002

13. Lewandowski A, Gillespie AI, Kridgen S, Jeong K, Yu L, Gartner-Schmidt J. Adult normative data for phonatory aerodynamics in connected speech. *Laryngoscope.* 2018;128(4):909-914. doi:10.1002/lary.26922

14. Dastolfo C, Gartner-Schmidt J, Yu L, Carnes O, Gillespie AI. Aerodynamic outcomes of four common voice disorders: Moving toward disorder-specific assessment. *J Voice.* 2016;30(3):301-307. doi:10.1016/j.jvoice.2015.03.017

15. Powell TW, Miccio AW. Stimulability: A useful clinical tool. *J Commun Disord.* 1996;29(4):237-253. doi:10.1016/0021-9924(96)00012-3

16. Gillespie AI, Gartner-Schmidt J. Immediate effect of stimulability assessment on acoustic, aerodynamic, and patient-perceptual measures of voice. *J Voice.* 2016;30(4):507.e9-507.e14. doi:10.1016/j.jvoice.2015.06.004

17. Rosen CA, Lee AS, Osborne J, Zullo T, Murry T. Development and validation of the voice Handicap Index-10. *Laryngoscope.* 2004;114(9 I):1549-1556. doi:10.1097/00005537-200409000-00009

18. Gartner-Schmidt JL, Shembel AC, Zullo TG, Rosen CA. Development and validation of the Dyspnea Index (DI): A severity index for upper airway-related dyspnea. *J Voice.* 2014;28(6):775-782. doi:10.1016/j.jvoice.2013.12.017

19. Cohen SM, Statham M, Rosen CA, Zullo T. Development and validation of the singing Voice Handicap-10. *Laryngoscope.* 2009;119(9):1864-1869. doi:10.1002/lary.20580

20. Arffa RE, Krishna P, Gartner-Schmidt J, Rosen CA. Normative values for the voice Handicap Index-10. *J Voice.* 2012;26(4):462-465. doi:10.1016/j.jvoice.2011.04.006

21. Shelly S, Rothenberger SD, Gartner-Schmidt J, Gillespie AI. Assessing candidacy for conversation training therapy: The role of patient perception. *J Voice.* Published online March 10, 2023. doi:10.1016/j.jvoice.2023.02.008

22. Helou LB, Gartner-Schmidt JL, Hapner ER, Schneider SL, Van Stan JH. Mapping meta-therapy in voice interventions onto the rehabilitation treatment specification system. *Semin Speech Lang.* 2021;42(1):5-18. doi:10.1055/s-0040-1722756

23. Zur KB, Cotton S, Kelchner L, Baker S, Weinrich B, Lee L. Pediatric Voice Handicap Index (pVHI): A new tool for evaluating pediatric dysphonia. *Int J Pediatr Otorhinolaryngol.* 2007;71(1):77-82. doi:10.1016/j.ijporl.2006.09.004

24. Wilson D. *Voice Problems of Children.* Williams and Wilkins; 1987.

25. Glaze L, Bless D, Susser R. Acoustic analysis of vowel and loudness differences in children's voice. *J Voice.* 1990;4(1):37-44.

26. Weinrich B, Salz B, Hughes M. Aerodynamic measurements: Normative data for children ages 6:0 to 10:11 years. *J Voice.* 2005;19(3):326-339. doi:10.1016/j.jvoice.2004.07.009

27. Weinrich B, Brehm SB, Knudsen C, McBride S, Hughes M. Pediatric normative data for the KayPentax phonatory aerodynamic system model 6600. *J Voice.* 2013;27(1):46-56. doi:10.1016/j.jvoice.2012.09.001

28. Verdolini Abbott K, Hersan R, Hammer D, Reed J. *Adventures in Voice: Clinician Manual*. Multivoice Dimensions; 2012.

29. Verdolini Abbott K, Hersan R, Hammer D, Reed J. *Adventures in Voice: Patient Materials*. Multivoice Dimensions; 2012.

30. Verdolini Abbott K, Hersan R, Kessler L. Voice therapy for children. In: Hartnick C, Boseley M, eds. *Clinical Management of Children's Voice Disorders*. Plural Publishing; 2010:111-134.

31. Shoffel-Havakuk H, Marks KL, Morton M, Johns MM III, Hapner ER. Validation of the OMNI vocal effort scale in the treatment of adductor spasmodic dysphonia. *Laryngoscope*. Published online October 12, 2018. doi:10.1002/lary.27430

32. Belafsky PC, Postma GN, Koufman JA. Validity and reliability of the Reflux Symptom Index (RSI). *J Voice*. 2002;16(2):274-277. doi:10.1016/S0892-1997(02)00097-8

33. Patel RR, Awan SN, Barkmeier-Kraemer J, et al. Recommended protocols for instrumental assessment of voice: ASHA expert panel to develop a protocol for instrumental assessment of vocal function. *Am J Speech Lang Pathol*. 2018:1-19.

34. Kent SAK, Fletcher TL, Morgan A, Morton M, Hall RJ, Sandage MJ. Updated Acoustic normative data through the lifespan: A scoping review. *J Voice*. Published online March 18, 2023. doi:10.1016/j.jvoice.2023.02.011

35. Šrámková H, Granqvist S, Herbst CT, Švec JG. The softest sound levels of the human voice in normal subjects. *J Acoust Soc Am*. 2015;137(1):407-418. doi:10.1121/1.4904538

36. Zraick RI, Smith-Olinde L, Shotts LL. Adult normative data for the KayPentax phonatory aerodynamic system model 6600. *J Voice*. 2012;26(2):164-176. doi:10.1016/j.jvoice.2011.01.006

37. KayPentax. *Phonatory Aerodynamic System (PAS) 6600 Instruction Manual*. 2010.

38. Bouchayer M, Cornut G, Witzig E, Loire R, Roch J, Bastian R. Epidermoid cysts, sulci, and mucosal bridges of the true vocal cord: A report of 157 cases. *Laryngoscope*. 1985; 95:1087-1094.

39. Rosen CA, Gartner-Schmidt J, Hathaway B, et al. A nomenclature paradigm for benign midmembranous vocal fold lesions. *Laryngoscope*. 2012;122(6):1335-1341. doi:10.1002/lary.22421

40. Estes C, Sulica L. Vocal fold pseudocyst: Results of 46 cases undergoing a uniform treatment algorithm. *Laryngoscope*. 2014; 124(5):1180-1186. doi:10.1002/lary.24451

41. Estes C, Sulica L. Vocal fold pseudocyst: A prospective study of surgical outcomes. *Laryngoscope*. 2015;125(4):913-918. doi:10.1002/lary.25006

42. Jacobson BH, Johnson A, Grywalski C, et al. The Voice Handicap Index (VHI): Development and validation. *Am J Speech Lang Pathol*. 1997;6(3):66-69. doi:10.1044/1058-0360.0603.66

43. Goy H, Fernandes DN, Pichora-Fuller MK, Van Lieshout P. Normative voice data for younger and older adults. *J Voice*. 2013; 27(5):545-555. doi:10.1016/j.jvoice.2013.03.002

44. Buckley DP, Abur D, Stepp CE. Normative values of cepstral peak prominence measures in typical speakers by sex, speech stimuli, and software type across the life span. *Am J Speech Lang Pathol*. 2023;32(4):1565-1577. doi:10.1044/2023_AJSLP-22-00264

45. Kaneko M, Shiromoto O, Fujiu-Kurachi M, Kishimoto Y, Tateya I, Hirano S. Optimal duration for voice rest after vocal fold surgery: Randomized controlled clinical study. *J Voice*. 2017;31(1):97-103. doi:10.1016/j.jvoice.2016.02.009

46. Stemple J, Roy N, Klaben B. *Clinical Voice Pathology: Theory and Management*. 6th ed. Plural Publishing; 2018.

47. Vertigan AE, Theodoros DG, Gibson PG, Winkworth AL. Efficacy of speech pathology management for chronic cough: A randomised placebo controlled trial of treatment efficacy. *Thorax*. 2006;61(12):1065-1069. doi:10.1136/thx.2006.064337

48. Karkos PD, George M, Van Der Veen J, et al. Vocal process granulomas: A systematic review of treatment. *Ann Otol Rhinol Laryngol*. 2014;123(5):314-320. doi:10.1177/0003489414525921

49. Hillel AT, Lin LM, Samlan R, Starmer H, Leahy K, Flint PW. Inhaled triamcinolone with proton pump inhibitor for treatment of

vocal process granulomas: A series of 67 granulomas. *Ann Otol Rhinol Laryngol.* 2010;119(5):325-330. doi:10.1177/0003489 41011900509

50. Leonard R, Kendall K. Effects of voice therapy on vocal process granuloma: A phonoscopic approach. *Am J Otolaryngol Head Neck Med Surg.* 2005;26(2):101-107. doi:10 .1016/j.amjoto.2004.08.010

51. Gandhi S, Ganesuni D, Shenoy SS, Bhatta S, Ghanpur AD. Arytenoid granuloma: A single-institution experience of management of 62 cases. *J Laryngol Otol.* 2023;137(2):186-191. doi:10.1017/S0022215121003662

52. Dominguez LM, Brown RJ, Simpson CB. Treatment outcomes of in-office KTP ablation of vocal fold granulomas. *Ann Otol Rhinol Laryngol.* 2017;126(12):829-834. doi:10 .1177/0003489417738790

53. Ma L, Xiao Y, Ye J, Yang Q, Wang J. Analysis of therapeutic methods for treating vocal process granulomas. *Acta Otolaryngol.* 2015; 135(3):277-282. doi:10.3109/00016489.2014 .986756

54. Alves M, Kruger E, Pillay B, van Lierde K, van der Linde J. The effect of hydration on voice quality in adults: A systematic review. *J Voice.* Published online November 6, 2017. doi:10.1016/j.jvoice.2017.10.001

55. Hogikyan ND, Sethuraman G. Validation of an instrument to measure voice-related quality of life (V-RQOL). *J Voice.* 1999;13(4):557-569. doi:10.1016/S0892-1997(99)80010-1

56. Barnes J. Voice therapy: Briess exercises. In: *Meeting of the Southwestern Ohio Speech and Hearing Association;* Cincinnati, OH; 1977.

57. Stemple JC, Lee L, D'Amico B, Pickup B. Efficacy of Vocal Function Exercises as a method of improving voice production. *J Voice.* 1994;8(3):271-278. doi:10.1016/S0892-1997 (05)80299-1

58. Angadi V, Croake D, Stemple J. Effects of Vocal Function Exercises: A systematic review. *J Voice.* 2019;33(1):124.e13-124.e34. doi:10.1016/j.jvoice.2017.08.031

59. Deary IJ, Wilson JA, Carding PN, MacKenzie K. VoiSS: A patient-derived voice symptom scale. *J Psychosom Res.* 2003;54(5):483-489. doi:10.1016/S0022-3999(02)00469-5

60. Cohen SM, Jacobson BH, Garrett CG, et al. Creation and validation of the singing voice handicap index. *Ann Otol Rhinol Laryngol.* 2007;116(6):402-406. doi:10.1177/00034894 0711600602

61. Jiang JJ, Titze IR. Measurement of vocal fold intraglottal pressure and impact stress. *J Voice.* 1994;8(2):132-144. doi:10.1016/S08 92-1997(05)80305-4

62. Hillman RE, Holmberg EVAB, Perkell JS. Objective assessment of vocal hyperfunction: Experimental framework and initial results. 1989;32(June):373-392.

63. Tanner K, Roy N, Merrill RM, et al. Nebulized isotonic saline versus water following a laryngeal desiccation challenge in classically trained sopranos. *J Speech Lang Hear Res.* 2010;53(6):1555. doi:10.1044/1092-4388(20 10/09-0249)

64. Verdolini Abbott K. *Lessac-Madsen Resonant Voice Therapy Patient Manual.* Plural Publishing; 2008.

65. Verdolini Abbott K. *Lessac-Madsen Resonant Voice Therapy Clinician Manual.* Plural Publishing, Inc.; 2008.

66. Nanjundeswaran C, Li NYK, Chan KMK, Wong RKS, Yiu EML, Verdolini Abbott K. Preliminary data on prevention and treatment of voice problems in student teachers. *J Voice.* 2012;26(6):816.e1-816.e12. doi:10 .1016/j.jvoice.2012.04.008

67. Roy N, Gray SD, Simon M, Dove H, Corbin-Lewis K, Stemple JC. An evaluation of the effects of two treatment approaches for teachers with voice disorders: A prospective randomized clinical trial. *J Speech Lang Hear Res.* 2001;44(2):286-296. doi:10.1044/1092-4388(2001/023)

68. Lee T, Swinnen S. Three legacies of Bryan and Harter: Automaticity, variability and change in skilled performance. In Starkes JL, Allard F, eds: *Advances in Psychology.* Elsevier; 1993:295-315.

69. Peterson KL, Verdolini-Marston K, Barkmeier JM, Hoffman HT. Comparison of aerodynamic and electroglottographic parameters in evaluating clinically relevant voicing patterns. *Ann Otol Rhinol Laryngol.* 1994;103(5): 335-346. doi:10.1177/000348949410300501

70. Verdolini K, Druker DG, Palmer PM, Samawi H. Laryngeal adduction in resonant voice. *J Voice*. 1998;12(3):315-327. doi:10.1016/S0892-1997(98)80021-0

71. Titze I, Verdolini K. *The Science and Practice of Voice Habilitation*. National Center for Voice and Speech. 2012

72. Schmidt R, Lee T, Winstein C, Wulf G, Zelaznik H. *Motor Control and Learning: A Behavioral Emphasis*. Human Kinetics; 2018.

73. Rollnick S, Miller W, Butler C, Aloia M. *Motivational Interviewing in Health Care: Helping Patients Change Behavior*. Guilford Press; 2008.

74. Behrman A. Facilitating behavioral change in voice therapy: The relevance of motivational interviewing. *Am J Speech Lang Pathol*. 2006;15(3):215-225. doi:10.1044/1058-0360 (2006/020)

4

Muscle Tension Dysphonia

Nelson Roy

Introduction

Poorly regulated activity of the perilaryngeal muscles affects phonatory function and contributes to a heterogeneous class of disorders known as hyperfunctional or musculoskeletal tension voice disorders.[1] Several characterizations of laryngeal hyperfunction exist, but a recurrent feature in almost all descriptions includes excessive, imbalanced, or dysregulated laryngeal musculoskeletal activity, force, or tension during voice production. Over the past 2 decades, muscle tension dysphonia (MTD) has become the preferred diagnostic label for such hyperfunctional syndromes,[2,3] with some clinicians preferring the term "primary MTD" (pMTD), to refer to a voice disturbance that exists in the absence of obvious structural or neurological pathology.[4] "Primary" emphasizes the principal role of dysregulated muscle activity as the proximal cause of the dysphonia and distinguishes it from "secondary" MTD, wherein the hyperfunctional muscle activity is interpreted to either coexist with or compensate for some underlying

mucosal disease, glottic insufficiency, and/or involuntary movements observed in laryngeal dystonia.[4–7] Braden describes secondary MTD in a child with recurrent respiratory papillomatosis in Case 4.6.

In primary MTD, the origin of this abnormal muscle activity is not fully elucidated, but it has been attributed to a variety of potentially overlapping sources, including: (1) psychological and/or personality factors that tend to induce elevated perilaryngeal tension and/or muscular laryngeal inhibition,[8–12] (2) technical misuses of the vocal mechanism in the context of extraordinary voice demands,[13–16] (3) learned adaptations following upper respiratory tract infection,[17] (4) increased pharyngolaryngeal tone as a result of persistent laryngopharyngeal reflux,[18] and/or (5) possible sensorimotor deficits.[19] Despite considerable uncertainty surrounding factors that predispose, precipitate, or perpetuate pMTD (and whether pMTD is one disorder or many),[1] these heterogeneous tension-based disorders often represent the most perceptually abnormal voices encountered clinically.[8]

For example, Gartner-Schmidt describes a case of a teenager who presents with near-complete aphonia in Case 4.3. Furthermore, most clinicians agree that recognizing the untoward effects of abnormal musculoskeletal tension is an important component of the diagnostic process and that restoring normal laryngeal muscle activity (ie, muscular balance) is an essential part of successful voice therapy.

Muscle tension voice disorders often leave the impression that the speaker is expending considerable physical effort to produce voice, and there is a decidedly laryngeal/perilaryngeal focus to this effort.[18,20,21] Perilaryngeal tension typically refers to tension primarily in the extrinsic and intrinsic laryngeal muscles, but this tension may also extend to include the pharyngeal constrictor muscles and the deep muscles of the neck. The putative effect of such excess tension is foreshortening and stiffening of muscles, which interferes directly or indirectly with normal voice production.[20] Because excess perilaryngeal tension tends to restrict vocal flexibility, most patients are described as pitch and loudness "locked," often displaying a markedly reduced dynamic range in both speaking and singing. Case 4.2 by Milstein and Adessa and Case 4.1 by Roy highlight direct targeting of perilaryngeal tension in voice therapy with manual techniques. Vocal fatigue and discomfort are frequent concomitants,[13,20] as is evident in Case 4.4 by Nanjundeswaran. Voice quality symptoms can vary in severity and type, ranging from severely pressed to extreme breathiness with myriad combinations depending on the muscle groups involved.[18] Patients present with several dysphonia types, including hoarseness, pressed voice, glottal fry, breathiness, high-pitched falsetto, and diplophonia, as well as voice and pitch breaks that vary in consistency and severity.[1,22] In Case 4.5, Fry describes a case of mutational falsetto, or puberphonia, in which the patient is "locked" at a higher pitch. Although the term "muscle tension" typically implies *sustained* overactivation of laryngeal and extralaryngeal muscles (both at rest and during phonation), in some cases of pMTD (1) signs of aberrant laryngeal or extralaryngeal muscle activity may be intermittent and phasic (ie, present during phonation only) and/or (2) specific laryngeal muscles may actually be underactivated or work at cross-purposes with others, thereby compromising normal synergy during phonation. In clinical circles, this loss of synergy in muscle activation or force is generically referred to as "muscle imbalance" or "muscle misuse." Thus, in the absence of mucosal, structural, or neurological pathology, these myriad voice effects can only be explained based on the potential deleterious effects of both sustained and phasic abnormal muscle contraction patterns on laryngeal and extralaryngeal structures. That is, the disordered voice in pMTD reflects the cumulative effects of sustained and/or variable abnormal muscle activity affecting both the source and the filter (ie, the entire vocal tract).

In cases where excess perilaryngeal tension has persisted for some time, additional features may be present. Patients commonly report a dull to severe ache and tightness of the anterior neck, larynx, and shoulder regions that intensify with extended voice use.[18,20,21] According to Morrison, the inferior bellies of the omohyoid muscles where they cross the supraclavicular fossae are often tense and prominent during speech. General body posture may be rigid with the jaw jutting forward.[23] Jaw, tongue, and respiratory movements can be restricted, reflecting the held nature of the voice and articulatory system.[18,24] Boone and McFarlane observed, "We see too many people with vocal hyperfunction who appear to speak through clenched teeth, with very little mandibular or labial movement."[25(p177)] Similarly, Sapir recognized the complex effects of laryngeal tension on both voice and articulation.[26] He noted "articulatory movements may induce or exacerbate, via mechanical or neural coupling, the phonatory abnormalities."[26(p49)] Although pMTD is properly regarded as a "voice" disorder, excess activity of the perilaryngeal muscles could also constrain articulatory movements and vocal tract dynamics by virtue of the mechanical linkage of the articulators to the hyolaryngeal complex, central nervous system influences (eg, heightened muscle tension in the jaw muscles), orolaryngeal sensorimotor interactions, or a combination of these.[26-29] Recent research suggests that successful treatment of pMTD appears to positively affect vocal tract dynamics, with acoustic evidence of vowel space expansion to suggest improved articulatory movements after treatment.[27,30] In Case 4.7, Kang Rosow describes muscle tension dysphagia, wherein abnormal laryngeal and perilaryngeal muscle tension negatively impacts swallow function.

Dysregulated laryngeal and perilaryngeal muscle tension can often be observed laryngoscopically. In this regard, a variety of glottic and supraglottic contraction patterns have been associated with pMTD, and several classification systems have been offered to describe these laryngoscopic features.[2,17,18] Often-cited laryngeal manifestations of dysregulated laryngeal muscle tension include tight mediolateral glottic and/or supraglottic contraction, anteroposterior glottic and/or supraglottic compression, incomplete glottic closure, posterior glottic gap, and bowing of the vocal folds.[2,31] It should be noted, however, that researchers have recently challenged the existence of specific laryngoscopic clusters/features believed to uniquely and reliably distinguish pMTD from nondysphonic speakers and other voice disorder types including laryngeal dystonia (aka spasmodic dysphonia).[32-35] According to these investigators, many of the laryngoscopic patterns used to classify pMTD, such as supraglottic mediolateral and/or anterior-posterior compression, are frequently observed in individuals with normal voices and subtypes of laryngeal dystonia, and thus clinicians often fail to distinguish such individuals from patients with pMTD. Given the likely involvement of a variety of intrinsic and extrinsic laryngeal muscles—in diverse states of relaxation and contraction—myriad laryngeal configurations may be present in pMTD. So, although no single laryngoscopic pattern should be uniquely and definitively identified with musculoskeletal tension voice disorders, observing certain glottic and supraglottic contraction patterns should raise the suspicion of a tension-based voice disorder but not confirm it.

Despite some controversy surrounding causal mechanisms and nosological imprecision,[36] the clinical voice literature is replete with evidence that symptomatic and/or physiologic voice therapy for hyperfunctional voice disorders such as pMTD often results in rapid and dramatic voice improvement. Because there are few studies directly comparing the effectiveness of specific therapy techniques, not much is known as to whether one therapy approach for primary or secondary MTD is superior to another. In the following section, numerous case examples illustrate the various approaches used to manage MTD.

Case Studies

 CASE STUDY 4.1

Manual Circumlaryngeal Techniques to Treat an Adult With Primary Muscle Tension Dysphonia

Nelson Roy

Voice Evaluation

Case History

History of Voice Complaint. Patient XX, a 55-year-old paralegal, reported a 6-month history of chronic mild to moderate dysphonia with sporadic acute exacerbations. These acute episodes, which bordered on aphonia, persisted for less than a week and resolved gradually. The patient indicated that she seemed to be progressively "losing the full force of her voice." She reported a persistent ache and tightness of the anterior neck, larynx, and shoulder regions. She also noticed episodic neck swellings that she labeled as "swollen glands." These "lumps" would worsen according to her amount of voice use and the degree of perceived laryngeal tension, fatigue, and effort. She added that the swellings coincided with the acute dysphonic exacerbations and that their appearance was not accompanied or preceded by symptoms of an upper respiratory infection (URI). The patient reported no change in health status and occupational or social voice use preceding the onset of vocal symptoms.

Medical History. The patient's recent medical history included treatment for asthma, allergies, hypertension, depression, tension headaches, gastroesophageal reflux disease (GERD), and temporomandibular joint dysfunction. Her current medications included Altace (antihypertensive), Prozac (antidepressant), cimetidine (antacid), and Premarin (estrogen replacement). She had received psychological treatment for clinical depression 4 years prior, but she was not consulting a mental health professional currently.

Psychosocial Interview. The clinician conducted a brief psychosocial interview and Patient XX reported numerous work-related stresses. She indicated that, just prior to the onset of her voice difficulties, her "workload at the law firm had become horrendous and had doubled following a company takeover." Patient XX explained, "I found every single day stressful at work, and that's when some of this started . . . Every day I went into work to put out the fires, rather than doing something fresh—it was constant pressure." She admitted feeling overwhelmed and exhausted. Patient XX indicated that 2 months earlier, she had missed work for 1 week with "chronic fatigue" accompanied by complete voice loss. Although she was frustrated by the increased workload and the limited support offered by her superiors, she had not expressed this dissatisfaction to her manager and was reluctant to do so. Her employer had hired additional office help recently, but she was solely responsible for training that individual. Consequently, she was forced to neglect some of her own duties in the process, only adding to the burden. In addition to the work-related stresses, the patient admitted to a long-standing communication breakdown with her only daughter. She had not communicated with her daughter over the past several years. Despite probing by the clinician, Patient XX denied knowing the precise cause of the communication breakdown, but she confessed to thinking about the unresolved conflict on a daily basis.

Auditory-Perceptual Assessment

Perceptually, Patient XX's connected speech was characterized by a mildly pressed, tight vocal quality, which worsened over the course of the assessment period. By the end of the psychosocial interview, Patient XX was in glottal fry 80% of the time. Repeated readings of a standard passage produced further deterioration in voice. Sustained vowel production was somewhat superior in quality when compared with connected speech. She displayed reduced pitch range and experienced noticeable phonatory disintegration early during upward pitch glides. She seemed to be functioning toward the bottom of her phonatory frequency range. GRBAS ratings for connected speech were as follows: Grade = 1, Roughness = 1, Breathiness = 0, Asthenia = 0, Strain = 1, which were consistent with a generally mild dysphonia.

Laryngeal Imaging

Videolaryngostroboscopy conducted with a 70-degree rigid endoscope revealed no evidence of structural or neurological pathology. Both vocal folds moved symmetrically and were free of mucosal disease. Mild mediolateral supraglottic compression was noted. Vocal fold vibratory characteristics, including mucosal wave and amplitude of vibration, were essentially within normal limits; however, the closed phase dominated the vibratory cycle.

> Episodic "swelling" in the neck is not an uncommon symptom reported by patients with pMTD. Concerns of swelling should always be evaluated by the physician.
> In most cases of MTD, if the swelling is transient and is not associated with illness or allergies, the "swelling" may be a focal area of muscle tension.

Focal Laryngeal Palpation

At rest, musculoskeletal tension was appraised manually by palpation of the laryngeal area to assess the degree, nature, and location of focal tenderness, muscle tautness, muscle nodularity (ie, well-circumscribed "knots" within the belly of a muscle), or pain. Care was taken to avoid sustained carotid artery compression during these maneuvers. With the occiput gently supported in a neutral position, pressure was directed: (1) over the major horns of the hyoid bone, (2) over the superior cornu of the thyroid cartilage, (3) within the thyrohyoid space, (4) within the suprahyoid region, and (5) along the anterior border of the sternocleidomastoid muscle. During palpation, the degree of compression applied was roughly equal to the pressure required to cause the thumbnail tip to blanch when pressed against a firm surface. When this amount of pressure was applied, focal sites of tension evoked discomfort and pain. The patient winced, withdrew, and vocalized her discomfort when tender points were specifically identified. These sites of tenderness were over the major horns of the hyoid and the superior cornu of the thyroid cartilage. The patient confirmed that these sites were the location of her episodic laryngeal swellings. The discomfort was more pronounced on the left than on the right and radiated to both ears. This severe tenderness in response to pressure in the laryngeal region, along with extreme muscle tautness, was considered abnormal and highly suggestive of excess laryngeal musculoskeletal tension.

The extent of laryngeal elevation was examined by palpating within the suprahyoid region and the thyrohyoid space from the posterior border of the hyoid bone to the thyroid notch. Noticeable muscle tautness was appreciated in the suprahyoid region. The patient also demonstrated a narrowed thyrohyoid space with the larynx and hyoid suspended high in the neck. This finding was also highly suggestive of excess muscle tension. Attempting to maneuver the larynx from side to side along the horizontal plane tested its mobility. Ample resistance to lateral movement indicated generalized extralaryngeal tension.

Stimulability Testing Using Manual Laryngeal Reposturing Techniques

With the index finger and thumb situated within the thyrohyoid space, gentle downward traction was applied over the superior border of the thyroid lamina while the patient vocalized a sustained "ah" vowel. The voice improvement associated with such laryngeal lowering (reposturing) was immediate and audible to both the patient and the clinician. Such a positive response to laryngeal reposturing and stimulability testing informed the patient's likely potential for normal voice and suggested muscular tension and laryngeal elevation as possible causal mechanisms. (Other manual reposturing techniques, including pressure in a posterior and downward direction within the suprahyoid region and over the anterior body of the hyoid bone, did not noticeably improve voice quality.)

Patient Education

Before proceeding with manual circumlaryngeal therapy (ie, circumlaryngeal massage), the clinician explained the diagnosis of MTD to the patient and educated her regarding the negative effects of excessive musculoskeletal tension on voice and the possibility that such tensions may be responsible, solely or in part, for her voice disorder. In addition, the results of the videolaryngostroboscopic examination were reviewed, emphasizing the absence of vocal fold pathology sufficient to account for the severity and fluctuating nature of her voice symptoms. Once she appeared to understand the relationship between muscle tension dysregulation, stress, and voice, the clinician outlined the manual therapy procedure and explained the positive outlook for recovery. She was warned that the technique may produce some initial discomfort but that with continued kneading of the musculature, the pain would gradually remit. She was also encouraged to attend carefully to any voice improvement and the laryngeal sensation accompanying such improvement.

Impressions

The patient's history and assessment findings suggested pMTD. These findings included (1) no structural or neurological laryngeal pathology observed during laryngeal imaging sufficient to explain the nature and fluctuating course and severity of her voice problems; (2) auditory-perceptual features consistent with a strained, pressed vocal quality; (3) laryngeal pain, tightness, elevation, and muscle tautness observed during laryngeal palpation; and (4) a positive response to voice stimulability testing using manual reposturing maneuvers (specifically downward traction applied over the superior border of the thyroid cartilage).

Plan of Care

Given the diagnosis, the short-term goal was to assess the effects of circumlaryngeal massage on voice production and to provide follow-up instructions/care as necessary.

Decision Making

The rationale for implementing circumlaryngeal massage as described by Aronson[8] is as follows. Skillfully applied, systematic kneading of the extralaryngeal region is postulated to stretch muscle tissue and fascia, promote local circulation with removal of metabolic wastes, relax tense muscles, and relieve pain and discomfort associated with muscle spasms. The putative physical effect of such massage is reduced laryngeal height and stiffness and increased mobility. Once the larynx is "released" and range of motion is normalized, an improvement in vocal effort, quality, and dynamic range should follow. Circumlaryngeal massage helps patients become more aware of where they are holding tension. By being conscious of these laryngeal "trouble spots," the patient can begin to focus on relaxing them during self-massage, which can be undertaken daily. In a series of articles, Roy and others have evaluated the clinical utility of manual techniques as a primary approach for a variety of voice disorders including pMTD.[37–42] The results of these investigations suggest that most patients who were studied derived noticeable voice improvement, often within a single treatment session, using manual circumlaryngeal therapy.

Intervention

Session #1: Voice Therapy (Provided Within the Same Visit as the Evaluation)

The manual tension reduction technique (ie, circumlaryngeal massage) was undertaken according to Aronson's description.[8] The hyoid bone was encircled with the thumb and index finger, which were then worked posteriorly into the tips of the major horns of the hyoid bone. Pressure was applied in a circular motion over the tips of the hyoid bone. The procedure was repeated within the thyrohyoid space, beginning from the thyroid notch and working posteriorly. The posterior borders of the thyroid cartilage medial to the sternocleidomastoid muscles were located, and the procedure was repeated there. With the fingers over the superior border of the thyroid cartilage, the larynx was stretched downward and, at times, moved laterally. Sites of focal tenderness, nodularity, or tautness were deliberately given more attention. Gentle kneading or sustained pressure was focused over these sites and then released. The procedure began superficially, and the depth of massage was increased according to the degree of tension encountered and the tolerance of the patient. The clinician extended the technique into the medial and lateral suprahyoid musculature because excess tension and pain were encountered over those sites. The clinician encouraged the patient to "unhinge her jaw and assume a more relaxed jaw position." The immediate effects of massage were noticeable on the skin. A slight reddening and warming of the skin accompanied friction and circular stroking movements.

During the above procedures, Patient XX was asked to sustain vowels while both the clinician and the patient noted changes in vocal quality. The patient, as an active participant in the therapy process, was encouraged to continually self-monitor the type and manner of voice produced. Given her marked sensitivity to pressure in the laryngeal region, some discomfort during the procedure was unavoidable. Nonetheless, the clinician's goal was to sufficiently reduce tension without inducing reactive-reflexive muscle tensing because of pain. Improvement in voice was noted almost immediately and was combined with reductions in pain and laryngeal height. Such changes were suggestive of a relief of tension. The patient commented, "Even though it hurts, it still feels good." Over the course of approximately 20 minutes, the improved voice was extended from vowels to words (automatic serial speech, ie, counting, days of the week), to short phrases loaded with nasals (eg, "Many men in the moon," "one Monday morning"), to sentences and paragraph recitations, and then to conversation. Once sufficient tension was

released and the patient assumed a more normal laryngeal posture, progress was swift, with complete amelioration of the dysphonia. Following the procedure, Patient XX commented that the voice felt free of tension and effort.

On repeated laryngeal palpation, the sites of most severe tenderness were no longer apparent. Pain no longer radiated to the ears. The patient was warned that she could experience some mild laryngeal discomfort over the next 24 to 48 hours as a consequence of the intense massage but that this should resolve.

Patient XX was instructed in self-laryngeal massage techniques and encouraged to perform them twice daily and whenever she experienced any tightness or fatigue in the laryngeal region. She was scheduled for a follow-up visit in 1 month to assess progress and determine future management. Patient XX was instructed to contact the clinician should she experience any acute exacerbations. In the interim, the patient was encouraged to modify her work schedule to alleviate some of the situational stresses and to explore psychological counseling to acquire relaxation skills.

> In session #1, the author highlights that even when the clinician is applying manual therapeutic techniques, the patient is an active participant in the session rather than a passive recipient. This is critical for sustainable symptom improvement.

Session #2: Reassessment Due to Relapse/Acute Exacerbation

Patient XX contacted the clinician 2 weeks after her initial session with a *severe* strained dysphonia (with frequent aphonic breaks) that had begun suddenly a day earlier, which was Sunday. Until this exacerbation, the patient reported symptom-free voice for the 2-week posttreatment period. She indicated that her recent attempts at self-laryngeal massage were unsuccessful in modifying the voice. She denied any new situational conflicts,

Voice Therapy: Clinical Case Studies

stresses, or voice-use patterns that may have contributed to the onset but had not pursued counseling.

Using the GRBAS scale, her connected speech was now rated as Grade = 3, Roughness = 0, Breathiness = 2, Asthenia = 3, Strain = 3, reflecting a severe voice disturbance. The Cepstral Spectral Index of Dysphonia was calculated using the second and third sentences of the Rainbow Passage (CSIDR) using the ADSV (Pentax Medical, Montvale, NJ).[43]

Rigid and flexible videolaryngostroboscopy revealed an extraordinary sequence of laryngeal movements, most obvious during phonatory/laryngeal diadochokinesis (involving rapid abduction and adduction of vocal folds during repeated brief productions of the "ee" vowel). The laryngeal movement pattern was characterized by prephonatory supraglottic compression with complete obliteration of the view of true vocal folds by the overadducted ventricular folds. Phonatory initiation of the "ee" was preceded by _abduction_ of the left arytenoid complex while the right arytenoid remained adducted, producing an irregular-shaped posterior glottic and supraglottic gap. This paradoxical abduction of the left arytenoid during phonatory initiation appeared to represent a decoupling of symmetric ab- and adductory movements of the paired vocal folds typical of normal inspiration and voicing, respectively. While decoupling of the symmetrical (conjugate) movements of the paired vocal folds often characterizes unilateral vocal fold paralysis, the highly unusual sequence of asymmetric laryngeal movements observed above (within the context of normal vocal fold abduction during inspiration) was incompatible with unilateral vocal fold paralysis.

The clinician interpreted the dysphonia to be a more severe manifestation/exacerbation of the original muscle tension disorder. Manual circumlaryngeal therapy again was undertaken according to the previous description. Despite paralaryngeal tension and pain that were judged to be more severe than at the original visit, normal voice quality was again rapidly reestablished within a single treatment session. This time, however, the patient transitioned through several stages of decreasing vocal severity until normal voice was restored. One intermediate stage of dysphonia resembled the dysphonia she originally sought treatment for (ie, glottal fry). The pretreatment and posttreatment _sustained vowel_ acoustic analyses (same session) are displayed in Figures 4–1A and 4–1B, respectively. Her severely disturbed voice in the pretreatment analysis is replaced by a normal posttreatment voice. Likewise, auditory-perceptual and acoustic assessment of connected speech extracted from the second and third sentences of the Rainbow Passage also confirmed restoration of normal voice (ie, G0, R0, B0, A0, S0, and a CSIDR value of 20.4). Furthermore, posttreatment rigid videolaryngostroboscopy (same session) showed no evidence of the atypical and asymmetric arytenoid movement pattern and confirmed normal glottic and supraglottic symmetry and function. All vibratory parameters returned to within normal limits.

Once the voice was restored, a frank discussion ensued regarding the complex interplay of laryngeal muscle tension, life stresses, situational conflicts, and her apparently ineffectual coping strategies. She agreed that she needed to develop more pragmatic coping skills and that long-term maintenance of voice improvement probably would require supportive psychological counseling. Arrangements were made for her to return to her counselor.

Short-Term and Long-Term Follow-Up

The patient was reevaluated in the voice clinic at 3 and 6 months post treatment. On each occasion, she reported no further relapse. Initially post treatment, Patient XX completed self-laryngeal massage on a daily basis, then weekly, and eventually as needed. She returned to her psychologist for relaxation training and short-term cognitive behavioral therapy. By 6 months post treatment, she had discontin-

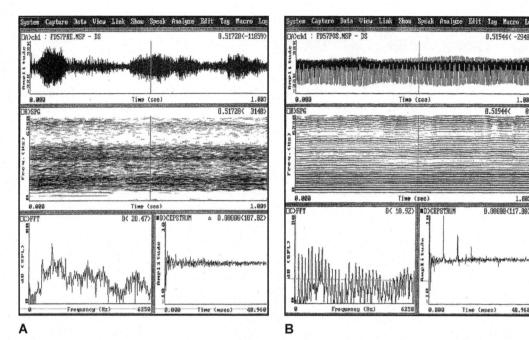

FIGURE 4–1. Acoustic analysis before (**A**) and after (**B**) manual circumlaryngeal therapy for the acute exacerbation (ie, recurrence). Each figure illustrates the middle 1-second segment extracted from the pre- and posttreatment sustained vowel /a/ productions, sampled at 25 kHz and acoustically analyzed using the Computerized Speech Lab (Pentax Medical CSL Model 4500, Montvale, NJ). (A) sound pressure waveform; (B) narrowband spectrogram of the preemphasized downsampled (12.5-kHz) waveform generated using a 36-Hz analyzing filter; (C) FFT (power spectrum) at the cursor location; (D) cepstrum power spectrum. The time axis is frequency and shows the dominant energy corresponding to the harmonic peaks in the spectrum. A prominent peak in the cepstrum is called the dominant harmonic, and its amplitude reflects the harmonic structure of the voice signal. Visual inspection of the pre- and posttreatment acoustic analyses confirms substantial improvement in spectral and cepstral characteristics. Improvement in harmonic intensity and structure following treatment is apparent in the posttreatment narrowband spectrogram (B) and power spectrum (C). The presence and amplitude of the dominant harmonic in the posttreatment cepstrum (D) substantiates these improvements.

ued counseling and self-laryngeal massage and had made many positive life and work adjustments. Contact by telephone approximately 2 years post treatment confirmed maintenance of therapy gains without any evidence of partial or complete relapse.

Summary

It is apparent from this case study that voice and musculoskeletal symptoms can be consequences of specific environmental triggers and stressors combined with individual differences in coping style. Therefore, understanding the contribution of laryngeal and extralaryngeal muscle dysregulation to these disorders is critical to proper diagnosis and selection of appropriate treatments. Manual techniques, including focal palpation, laryngeal reposturing maneuvers, and circumlaryngeal massage,[44,45] are valuable tools that augment the voice practitioner's diagnostic and treatment armamentarium.

> CASE STUDY 4.2
>
> **Boot Camp Voice Therapy for an Adult With Functional Dysphonia**
>
> Claudio F. Milstein and Michelle Adessa

Voice Evaluation

Case History

Patient TS, a 42-year-old cisgender female from rural Canada, presented to our clinic with a chief complaint of a 12-year history of on-and-off voice problems characterized by complete voice loss for extended periods of time. The triggers appeared to be URIs, after which she would have complete voice loss for weeks or months at a time. However, 4 years ago she had a severe bronchitis, after which she never recovered her voice. She has seen several physicians in the past, including lung, allergy, and otolaryngology specialists. She has undergone X-rays, CT scans of the neck and chest, swallow studies, pulmonary function tests, and laryngeal endoscopies, all of which were negative and did not reveal the etiology of her voice loss. Over the years, she was treated with courses of antibiotics and steroids, antireflux medications, asthma inhalers, and allergy control medications, but did not get benefit from any treatment modality. Access to a speech-language pathologist (SLP) with expertise in voice was limited in her hometown, but she had traveled to a larger city to pursue voice therapy. After many sessions of unsuccessful voice therapy, she was discharged.

TS revealed that several health care providers told her that "this was all in her head" and there was nothing that could be done for her. Per recommendation of one of the otolaryngologists, she consulted with a psychiatrist, but the evaluation was nonrevealing, finding her well adapted with no suspicion of psychogenic etiology for her voice problem. Friends suggested a trial of acupuncture and hypnosis, but neither of these helped. She went on elimination diets (gluten free and lactose free) for months at a time without benefit.

TS is married with 2 young children, ages 7 and 12. She describes her relationship as stable and loving, although her voice disability has put strains on the marriage, as her husband feels he has to do most of the parenting himself since she has difficulty communicating. TS and her husband have limited their social interactions, leading to depression in both her and her husband.

TS's medical history was unremarkable but significant for hypothyroidism, which is well controlled on levothyroxine, and seasonal allergies.

After a period of 6 months of unsuccessful workup visits, numerous specialists, medication, and therapy trials, TS gave up and felt relegated to a life with no voice. Four years later, she came across a YouTube video with a patient story that sounded similar to hers. In that video, the patient, who was also aphonic, had traveled to a specialized voice clinic, was diagnosed with a condition called functional dysphonia, and, after undergoing a brief laryngeal manipulation procedure, regained her voice. TS did not know if this is what she was experiencing but decided to travel across the country to the same clinic in hopes of getting some help. TS underwent a standard voice evaluation and a joint appointment with a well-established team of a laryngologist and a voice-specialized SLP. She brought all her previous medical records, which the team reviewed.

Auditory-Perceptual Evaluation

Perceptual evaluation revealed a complete aphonia, with a moderately strained whisper. The ratings on the GRBAS scale were as follows: Roughness = 0, Breathiness = 3, Strain = 2, Pitch = 3, Loudness = 3, Instability = 0 (rating scale: 0 = normal, 1 = slight, 2 = moderate, 3 = severe).

Laryngeal Imaging

Laryngoscopy with stroboscopic examination revealed a normal larynx with no evidence of inflammation or pathology. The range of motion of both vocal folds was within normal limits. During phonation, there was approxi-

4. Muscle Tension Dysphonia   117

mation of the anterior half of the vocal folds and no contact of the posterior half, with a large posterior glottic gap, moderate degree of compression of the false vocal folds (ventricular medialization), and no anteroposterior compression. No vibration of the vocal folds was observed.[46] Inhalation phonation yielded touch glottic closure with brief 2 to 3 seconds of true vocal fold vibration during videostroboscopy.

> The posturing of the vocal folds in this patient is often seen in primary MTD (pMTD)/functional aphonia patients. Normal-looking vocal folds are held in a stretched posture that prevents normal amplitude of lateral excursion and propagation of the mucosal wave due to the significant vocal fold tension and elongation. This is not indicative of loss of superficial lamina propria, presence of scar, or loss of pliability, but rather a functional manifestation of muscle tension sometimes referred to as hyperfunctional underclosure.

Manual Palpation

Upon palpation of the neck, the vertical height of the larynx was elevated with a tight coupling of the thyroid cartilage to the hyoid bone, and the mobility of the larynx and hyoid was impaired in the lateral to medial direction with palpation.

Stimulability

The patient was aphonic but stimulable for normal cough with cueing. Traditional stimulability tasks such as humming, sighing, and trilling were ineffective at facilitating improvement in perceptual voice quality in this patient.

> As seen in this case, traditional stimulability tasks are often ineffective in primary MTD (pMTD). In this case, the authors used vegetative tasks to demonstrate normal vocal fold function.

Impressions

TS had a prior history of long periods of voice loss (weeks or months) following URIs. The most recent period lasted for 4 years with complete inability to produce any voice. Her laryngeal examination showed no inflammation or pathology, and vocal fold motion was within normal limits. However, glottal closure was characterized by adduction of the anterior half of the vocal folds with severe splinting with phonation, leading to a large glottic gap in phonation attempts and absent vocal fold vibration. The diagnosis was consistent with functional dysphonia (also referred to elsewhere and in the introduction as pMTD) and TS was considered a good candidate for voice therapy with focus on laryngeal manual therapy techniques.

Plan of Care

Long-Term Goal. The patient will communicate consistently with normal voice quality.

Short-Term Goals:

1. The patient will increase consistency of full glottic closure pattern for all voicing activities.
2. The patient will decrease breathiness and achieve a resonant voice consistently in all phonatory activities.
3. The patient will implement manual strategies to rebalance laryngeal musculature to decrease upward pull of laryngeal elevators.
4. The patient will successfully implement self-treatment strategies to decrease vocal hyperfunction whenever needed to reset and restore normal voice quality.

Decision Making

Given the patient's distance from the center and the time and expense she had put forth to seek care, evaluation and therapy were conducted on the same day across multiple time points. Given the recalcitrant nature of the patient's voice complaint and extended period

118 Voice Therapy: Clinical Case Studies

of aphonia, as well as lack of improvement with traditional stimulability probes (humming, trilling), focusing therapeutically on unloading the musculature of the hyolaryngeal complex with laryngeal manual therapy was recommended. The goal to achieve normal voicing was threefold: (1) restore the neutral vertical height of the larynx, (2) increase flexibility and full range of motion of the hyolaryngeal complex musculature, and (3) achieve adequate vocal fold closure and vibration.

> This intense therapy paradigm has been referred to as boot camp voice therapy. Several therapy sessions are scheduled in a single day to create extensive opportunity for mastery experiences.

Intervention

The initial 1-hour session of therapy focused on laryngeal manipulation and reposturing to restore normal voicing.[23,37,47,48] During the first phase of treatment, the clinician was active, with the patient passive and silent as laryngeal manipulation was applied. With the patient seated in a chair, the clinician asked her to refrain from any conversational speech during the treatment. She remained silent as the clinician applied laryngeal reposturing maneuvers, including thyrohyoid pull-down, rocking the larynx medially and laterally, opening the tight coupling of the thyrohyoid space manually, and moving the head in rotation to unload neck muscles, specifically the sternocleidomastoid muscles. Once the musculature was rebalanced, the patient was instructed to produce an easy humming sound, trying to direct the focus away from the throat and into the front of the mouth, while manipulation continued. She was reminded not to speak during this, and just to follow the clinician's direct prompts. Using thyrohyoid pull-down, the patient achieved a brief vocalization, and this was reinforced over multiple

repetitions. Patient was asked to lean over with forearms on the upper legs and head dropping forward as the clinician applied gentle pressure and movement/shaking to the upper trapezius muscles. Patient was consistent with humming with clear sound 30% of the time using this distraction technique. Patient was reminded to not speak yet, just to follow the directions from the clinician. Next, the clinician guided the patient in vegetative tasks such as coughing and throat clearing to facilitate continued phonation. These did not result in better sound. Continuing with non-speech vocalizations, the patient was then asked to gargle. She was able to produce sound while gargling. Next, the patient was asked to sustain a vowel after a gargle; she was able to do this, but she demonstrated only minimal improvement and was not able to progress past this, as she could only sustain vowel production for a few seconds. Patient was then instructed in self-manipulation using the laryngeal manual therapy/manipulation techniques. The patient was left in a treatment room for 1 hour with instructions to work on the laryngeal manual therapy techniques herself without the clinician present.

> In addition to establishing normal voice quality, the goal is to develop the patient's self-efficacy to achieve and maintain normal voice. Building self-efficacy requires extensive mastery experience and development of an internal locus of control. In the pMTD population, this can be difficult to achieve in the traditional voice therapy paradigm (eg, being seen once a week or every other week with an hour of attention on the voice). In this case, the authors gave the patient an opportunity for self-practice by leaving her alone to practice laryngeal manual therapy. When scheduling boot camp therapy, it is important for clinicians to allow time for patient self-practice to build self-efficacy, in addition to treatment time with the clinician.

Later that same day, the patient came back after lunch for a second session of voice therapy. The patient was once again taken through laryngeal manipulation and non-speech vocalization with coughing/throat clearing facilitators and the gargling facilitator. Only through continuous gargling exercises was voice consistently elicited. With practice, the patient was able to sustain voicing during gargling, and with further practice, she was gradually able to continue voicing after swallowing the water and imitating "dry gargling." (See Video 6 Gargling as a Facilitating Technique by Milstein.) This took an entire session, and the patient was again left alone in an exam room with instructions to continue to practice voicing with and without gargling, but not attempting to talk.

A third session was conducted toward the end of the clinical day. This time, the patient was able to voice more consistently with sustained vowels. Tasks then moved through facilitated voicing with this hierarchical approach: sustained vowel, 1-syllable word, chanting, and pitch glides followed by automatic speech tasks including counting, days of week, and months of year, then chanting her name, her address, and her phone number. She was directed to follow instructions very specifically with no "off-the-cuff" chit-chat between tasks. If she had breathiness, roughness, or strain on these tasks, she was directed to move back one step in the hierarchical approach, retracing steps until she reached clarity of tone.

With this hierarchical approach, there was a rapid progression to better voicing. During this phase of treatment, the patient became more active and the clinician more passive. Tasks gradually shifted to sustained vowels, chanting, automatic speech, and finally conversational speech. Once the patient achieved normal voicing, she started crying. She was specifically instructed to continue talking throughout the emotional release to avoiding falling back into the strained whisper that she was accustomed to for 4 years. Once normal speaking was achieved consistently, to reinforce the normal voice, she was asked to intentionally return to aphonic/dysphonic voicing using the concept of negative practice. She was guided to focus her attention on "how it feels in your throat" when the voice is strained and compare it to the feeling when voice was normal. She was then guided into using the previously mentioned facilitating techniques without clinician intervention. This was done multiple times, switching between aphonia and normal voice, until the patient reported understanding how to reset her voice on her own.

Next, the patient was guided through tasks to reinforce carryover. The clinician accompanied the patient to the hospital cafeteria so that she could order food for herself, as this was something she was unable to do in the past and found very frustrating. She was able to interact with the cafeteria employee with a clear, strong voice and was able to be understood. Lastly, the patient called her children on the telephone as they were not able to accompany her on the long trip to the clinic. She was able to speak to them in a normal voice and was very happy and relieved. Her children were so happy to hear her voice.

The impact of this patient's voice problem on her quality of life was significant, as she could not communicate with her family, coworkers, and friends prior to attending this day of therapy. She found that simple tasks like going to the grocery store were daunting and embarrassing due to her severe dysphonia. She withdrew from communication and her husband described how he felt "almost not married," as he had to communicate with his children and was fully responsible for all parenting. He was so happy she could again express herself, but also thrilled that she was able to fully participate in parenting their children.

The patient was sent home with effective facilitating techniques for self-treatment. These techniques included manual adjustment of the larynx by rocking it medially and laterally, thyrohyoid pull-down, and gargling, the latter being the most effective reset for the patient. It was recommended that she practice these several times a day. The patient was instructed to reset the voice at the very first sign of voice quality change using the facilitating techniques. She was also instructed to direct family members to cue her to do so should she revert to dysphonic voice. Over time, it was recommended to decrease the frequency of using the facilitating techniques but to occasionally practice techniques to maintain self-treatment strategies should voice loss occur.

In our experience, these cases of functional dysphonia tend to respond rapidly to voice therapy intervention. This case took longer than most, with 3 voice therapy sessions conducted over a single day. Results were successful and the patient's condition did not recur.

At last update, the patient was happy with her regained normal vocal quality and able to maintain this over a 6-month period. When she got a URI in early autumn of the following year, she noticed some dysphonia but was able to reset this quickly using the techniques she learned in therapy.

Summary

This is a case of debilitating prolonged aphonia for over 4 years. Several health care providers told the patient that this was "all in her head," that she could talk if she really wanted to, or that a psychiatric intervention was needed. This made her feel very guilty. When told that there was nothing that could be done for her, she felt despair and hopelessness, believing that she would not ever be able to talk again.

This case highlights the fact that functional dysphonia remains a poorly understood and often misdiagnosed voice disorder. Once the disorder is correctly identified and the proper therapeutic approach is implemented, patients can rapidly regain voicing and quality of life can be significantly improved in a very short period of time. Manual techniques of laryngeal manipulation and repositioning, in conjunction with vegetative voicing tasks such as coughing, throat clearing and gargling, are recommended for treatment of this disorder and are valuable tools for all SLPs who treat voice disorders.

CASE STUDY 4.3

Flow Phonation to Treat a Teenager With Primary Muscle Tension Aphonia

Jackie L. Gartner-Schmidt

Voice Evaluation

Case History

Chief Complaint. Patient G's chief complaints are voice loss, vocal fatigue, and throat constriction when talking. She does not have any prior history of voice loss before this episode.

History. Patient G is a 15-year-old cisgender female high school student who reports a sudden onset of total voice loss approximately 3 months ago. This loss was precipitated by moving into her grandmother's house with her family while they saved money to buy a house of their own. Her grandmother would not let her bring her pet ferret, which angered Patient G. Her pet ferret meant the world to her. Furthermore, Patient G described the relationship between her and her grandmother as "two hoses pointed toward each other." She admits to being afraid of her grandmother and does not deny her grandmother's presence as the potential trigger to her voice problems.

Voice Evaluation. Clinical assessment was completed by the interdisciplinary team consisting of a fellowship-trained laryngologist and voice-specialized SLP.

Auditory-Perceptual Evaluation

The Consensus Auditory-Perceptual Evaluation of Voice (CAPE-V) was completed.[49] The overall severity of Patient G's voice using a visual analog scale was 95/100.

Patient Self-Assessment

Patient G's self-assessment of her overall voice problem was "severe" based on an ordinal scale (none, mild, mild-moderate, moderate, moderate-severe, severe), and her chief complaint included both the sound and feel of her voice. To quantify the effect of Patient G's perception of her voice handicap, the Voice Handicap Index–10 (VHI-10) was used.[50] Patient G's score was 36/40, which was above the normative value of a score of >11 being symptomatic of a voice problem.[51]

Vocal Effort. Patient G was also asked to rate her vocal effort from 0 (no vocal effort to produce voice) to 10 (extreme vocal effort to produce voice). She reported an 8/10.

Acoustic Analysis

The Analysis of Dysphonia in Speech and Voice (ADSV) system software (Pentax Medical, Montvale, NJ) from the Computerized Speech Lab (Pentax Medical, Montvale, NJ) with a Shure Beta-54 WBH54 head-mounted microphone was positioned at approximately a 45-degree angle from Patient G's mouth. Patient G was asked to read the all-voiced sentence "We were away a year ago" from the CAPE-V protocol. Although she was mostly aphonic, there were "moments" of voiced sound production to be assessed. Data reduction was used to provide measures of the Cepstral Spectral Index of Dysphonia (CSID).[52] The CSID is a multifactorial estimate of dysphonia severity and correlates with the labeled visual analog scales for severity used in the CAPE-V. The CSID was computed as 97, which corroborated the SLP's overall severity rating of 95/100 on the CAPE-V.

Aerodynamic Measures

The Phonatory Aerodynamic System (PAS) model 6600 (Pentax Medical, Montvale, NJ), with a customized protocol from previous work by Gartner-Schmidt, was used, which included reading the first 4 sentences of the Rainbow Passage to garner aerodynamic measures obtained in connected speech,[53] including number of breaths, duration of the passage, and mean airflow. Patient G took 12 breaths, used 60 mL/sec of airflow, and took 18 seconds to read the passage. All measures were abnormal using the adult normative values for phonatory aerodynamics in connected speech.[53] Patient G took more breaths, used less airflow, and had an increased rate of speech compared with patients without voice problems.

Stimulability Testing

Patient G was stimulable for voicing using lip bubbles, gargle phonation, and producing /u/ using biofeedback of egress of air created when producing the sound and felt on her finger held 1 inch from her mouth.

Laryngeal Imaging

The laryngologist visualized her larynx with videostroboscopy using a chip-tip flexible endoscope and reported no lesions and normal bilateral vocal fold motion. Flexible endoscopy was chosen because it allows visualization of speech during the exam. This examination also allows use of inhalation phonation (ie, breathing in while simultaneously phonating) as a stimulability test during videostroboscopy. The patient was able to demonstrate phonation using inhalation phonation, indicating both stimulability and pliability of the vocal folds. The patient was diagnosed with muscle tension aphonia (MTA), often referred to as functional aphonia or primary muscle tension dysphonia (pMTD).

Impressions

Patient G's severity of dysphonia was rated severe secondary to auditory-perceptual, acoustic and aerodynamic assessment, and her VHI-10 score of 36/40. Her prognosis for recovery with behavioral voice therapy was determined to be good secondary to a positive response to stimulability and her motivation for change. The expected frequency, duration, and goals were as follows: The SLP planned to initiate therapy using Flow Phonation, which the patient was expected to complete in 2 sessions based on her stimulability, voiced throat clear, and vocal communicator (a term used in Lessac Madsen Resonant Voice Therapy to reference carry over tasks for infusing resonant voice into conversation).[54] The duration of each session was set at approximately 45 minutes. The SLP and the laryngologist believed that this aphonic episode could have been precipitated by the patient's recent family living change and family dynamics, and the patient agreed. However, while acknowledging this, she did not believe she needed to be referred to a mental health professional. The patient's medical and speech history were otherwise unremarkable.

Decision Making

The SLP chose to pursue treatment with Flow Phonation in support of the concept of respiratory-laryngeal discoordination in patients with MTA or pMTD. Flow Phonation decreases "breath holding or holding back airflow" during voicing/speech by facilitating volitional control of unvoiced and phonatory airflow (breathy, flow, and pressed phonation).[55] The SLP also provided Patient G with a conceptual framework for reestablishing easy release of airflow while coordinating phonation and ultimately ending in conversational speech, so that if she relapsed, she could reinstate her own voice. Flow Phonation is a hierarchically based program of skill building from least (eg, phonemes, words) to most complex (eg, phrases, conversation). It establishes a bottom-up conceptual framework starting with reestablishing airflow release, a physiologic symptom from

---

Similar to the concepts highlighted in Case 4.2 of building self-efficacy and an internal locus of control, Gartner-Schmidt talks about providing Patient G with a conceptual framework for successfully managing her own voice.

---

lack of phonatory airflow in MTA. Patients with MTA often need a hierarchical-based program, as the maladaptive behaviors are embedded in conversational speech. Thus, connected speech must be deconstructed into its basic parts starting with airflow release.

Plan of Care

The long-term goal of therapy was for Patient G to maximize vocal effectiveness relative to her existing laryngeal disorder and to return to vocal activities of daily living (eg, functional voice communication). Initial short-term goals were as follows but expected to be altered based on session-to-session gains:

1. The patient will perform airflow release (unarticulated and articulated) on 10 trials at 80% accuracy as assessed by the clinician's auditory perception and patient corroborating vibrotactile sensations.
2. The patient will perform discriminatory practice between breathy, flow, and pressed phonation in both unarticulated and articulated tasks at 80% accuracy as assessed by the clinician's auditory perception and corroborated by the patient differentiating the sound and feel between the 3 respective voice productions.
3. The patient will perform clear speech in conversational speech at 80% accuracy as assessed by the clinician's auditory perception and patient corroborating vibrotactile sensations.

Intervention

After her initial evaluation, Patient G received 3 voice therapy sessions with a week in between the first 2 sessions followed by a month before the last session. The following is a summary of the basic skills of Flow Phonation. The 4 skill levels are represented in Table 4–1. Patients are asked to become aware of frontal energy/air-

Table 4–1. Skill Levels of Flow Phonation

Skill #1: Airflow Release	Skill #2: Breathy Phonation	Skill #3: Flow Phonation	Skill #4: Articulatory Precision
1. Unarticulated airflow	1. Unarticulated breathy phonation	1. Unarticulated flow phonation	Conversational speech
2. Articulated airflow	2. Articulated breathy phonation	2. Articulated flow phonation	

flow while feeling no throat tightness. Patients go through the hierarchy but, if problems recur, they go "down a step" until they reach functional performance. Also, patients can go back and forth between the steps as much as necessary, and because vocal balance is the goal, it does not matter if each step is used. Finally, this is not a programmatic approach to voice therapy; rather, it is conceptual. The reader is encouraged to invent new stimuli based on the concepts of Flow Phonation. The examples given are in no way exhaustive.

Flow Phonation Skills

Skill #1: Airflow Release—
Unarticulated Airflow

Gargling Technique. Patient G was first asked to do the gargle technique because that was the stimulability probe that enabled her to phonate in the initial assessment. Patient G was given a glass of water. The SLP modeled the gesture and Patient G was asked to produce plenty of bubbles with the water while bending her head back in the posture of a gargle. Patient G could gargle well, which represented the first step toward flow phonation, as gargling is merely airflow in a non-speech task. (See Video 6 Gargling as a Facilitating Technique by Milstein.) Having a patient gargle initiates airflow release without the maladaptive habits of extralaryngeal or intralaryngeal tensions. The head, chin, and elongated neck posture, characteristic of gargling, dissuaded Patient G from raising her larynx higher than it was at rest. In a gargling posture, a patient cannot make the hyolaryngeal sling tighter than it often already is. The posture also stretches the extrinsic laryngeal strap muscles.

/u/ Prolongation. Next, the clinician instructed Patient G to produce an /u/ without voicing. Patient G held a strip of facial tissue between her index and third fingers, approximately 2 inches from her nose. A voiceless /u/ is used because the lip contour for /u/ directs the airflow in a column from the lips and it is easy to move the tissue and hear a steady airflow stream. The cycle of inhalation followed by exhalation on a voiceless /u/ should be produced smoothly and without hesitation, resulting in consistently uplifted tissue. The goal is to achieve the task with minimal throat effort and a feeling of airflow "energy" at the lips. The SLP was careful not to use the word "blowing," which can connote effort, but rather instructed her "to release the air." Patient G was asked to take a breath and immediately exhale a sigh on a /u/. At first, the tissue only moved with the initial exhalation, but then the patient appeared to hold back her airflow; the tissue did not move. She did an audible semi-Valsalva maneuver as she stopped the airflow. The instruction was given again and this time the patient released the exhalation for a longer duration, but the exhalatory airflow sounds were jerky and inconsistent. Often, the SLP will tell her patients, "I want you to pretend that you have had a long day and that you are just letting out a nice, relaxed sigh but on the letter /u/." Patient G performed much better this time. Another technique to reduce tension is to ask patients to physically move (eg, sway their arms, flop forward) when sighing out a voiceless /u/-shaped sound. Linking physical release with airflow release can help many patients. (See Video 7 Flow Phonation by Gartner-Schmidt.)

Lip Bubbles. Wanting to capitalize on her success thus far, the SLP moved on to another airflow-inducing technique. She asked Patient G to do lip bubbles without voice. Patient G could lip bubble with the aid of placing her two index fingers on the corners of her lips. She lip bubbled for long and short durations. All the while, Patient G was asked if she could feel "airflow energy" at her lips and if her throat felt relaxed. Some patients find lip bubbles difficult to do; if so, they're asked to move on to another airflow-inducing task.

Voiceless Fricatives. Now that airflow was being released easily, Patient G was asked to sustain voiceless fricatives. She sustained /s/, /f/, and /sh/ easily with consistent airflow escape. The SLP asked her to do pitch (ie, formant frequencies) glides and sirens and to be loud and soft with the fricatives. All the while, Patient G was asked if she could feel airflow energy at her lips and if her throat felt relaxed.

Skill #1: Airflow Release— Articulated Airflow

Voiceless Phrases/Conversation. When it was apparent that Patient G could easily release unvoiced airflow, she was asked to articulate around the airflow. First, the SLP wanted to model articulated airflow (ie, efficient whisper), and second, she did not want Patient G to reinforce the old, strained whisper in between all her successful trials to establish airflow release. This is a very important instruction to a patient that should be said as follows: "I want you to move your tongue and lips around this steady stream of airflow like you have done so far." Having patients concentrate on airflow versus speech articulation may disentangle the possible maladaptive habits found in speech. The concept of airflow

should be front and center in Flow Phonation. So, keeping the facial tissue in the same position, as was done for the voiceless /u/, Patient G was asked to produce phrases with just airflow. The tissue should move with the airflow. It is important to note that certain phonemes will not allow the airflow to lift the tissue. However, phrases such as "Poo-loo-poo-loo-poo-loo" and "Who is Lou? Who is Sue? Who are you?" will allow this biofeedback. The SLP is encouraged to choose phonemes that allow the best airflow sensation. (For example, a word beginning with a /p/ phoneme allows the patient to feel more airflow at the front of the mouth than a word beginning with a /k/.) Within each phrase, Patient G was asked to connect each of the syllables or words together, so that no separation or pausing occurred.

At this juncture in the therapy, Patient G and the SLP communicated with each other in an easy, breathy, unvoiced whisper. Having the SLP whisper not only provides a proper model for whispering but can also be an indirect empathetic gesture. This stage of therapy is often a good time to interrupt the structured tasks of therapy and just talk. Furthermore, all patients are asked to adopt this easy, unstrained whispering in between sessions (eg, at home) if voice reinstatement is not achieved within the first few sessions.

> Here, Gartner-Schmidt encourages the patient to communicate in a whisper. In Case 4.2, Milstein and Adessa encourage the patient not to talk at all. Both methods aim to reduce the tendency to continue talking in a strained voice to help break the suboptimal motor pattern.

Skill #2: Breathy Phonation—Unarticulated

/u/ Prolongation. In this hierarchical step of therapy, phonation is gently coordinated with airflow. Patient G was asked to phonate while continuing to use the tissue as feedback. Patient G was told that the most important part of the exercise was to see and hear the airflow versus producing voice. Patient G was asked to take a breath and exhale on a breathy /u/ in a downward glide like a sigh. The tissue should move with the airflow. The tissue represents concrete evidence that the patient is using airflow. However, the sound she produced was breathy but unsteady and, at the end, she cut off her airflow, as evidenced by the tissue not moving. The SLP asked her to do the /u/ on just airflow alone to reestablish the easy feel and to see and feel the airflow on the tissue. Then, she tried again with sound and this time she was successful.

Voiced Lip Bubbles. Patient G was educated about the coordination of airflow with sound and was told that these exercises were merely coordinating her airflow with her sound generator. Next, she voiced lip bubbles and was very stimulable, producing a wonderful voice.

Voiced Gargle. The next instruction to Patient G was to add the gargle "sound" to the air bubbles, being careful not to use the word "voicing" so as not to introduce any anxiety-ridden verbiage. Patient G again was successful. The final step in the gargling technique was to have the patient slowly lower her chin while still gargling with sound. With some patients, once phonation is established with this technique, shaping the sustained gargle into speech is all that is needed. In general, whenever an SLP feels that a patient can jump right to conversational speech in the therapeutic process, the sooner the better. Unfortunately, Patient G was unable to transfer the voiced gargle to words. Thus, a hierarchical process of first establishing airflow, then airflow plus voicing, phonemes, words, phrases, and finally connected speech, was needed.

Skill #2: Breathy Phonation—Articulated

Cognate Pairs: Voiceless to Voiced Fricatives. Patient G was now asked to do a true vocal balancing technique; that is, to prolong an /s/ and seamlessly add voicing into the cognate /z/. Patient G was asked to pay attention to how little effort was needed to make a voice. She was asked to produce an /f/ into a /v/ and back and forth, as well as voiceless [th] to voiced [th] and [sh] to [dz]. Then she was asked to do pitch sirens while transitioning between the cognate pairs.

Phrases/Conversation. This is a very short section of Flow Phonation; namely, asking patients to converse in breathy phonation. This is very much like Confidential Voice Therapy (originally described by Colton et al, 1996)[56] but, because breathy phonation takes more effort than efficient voicing, this part of therapy is meant only to gradually introduce the patient to voicing with increased airflow. Patient G was told that she might need more breaths per phrase because of the breathiness. The same sentences as before were used, but voiced this time. Patient G was again reminded to feel airflow energy at her lips and see that her throat felt relaxed. She was asked to say, "Poo-loo-poo-loo-poo-loo" and "Who are you? Who is Lou? Who is Sue?" Often, patients skip Skill #2: Breathy Phonation and move right into Flow Phonation.

> More information on Confidential Voice Therapy can be found in Verdolini-Marston et al (1995).[57]

Skill #3: Flow Phonation—Unarticulated

/u/ Prolongation and the Kazoo Sound. Patient G was asked to prolong an /u/ like the breathy phonation stage but to make the sound louder and not breathy. Said differently, produce a nonbreathy sound, yet achieve the same movement of the tissue (airflow). Often, the only instruction a patient needs to go from breathy to flow phonation is to get louder if they are following the flow. Patient G successfully transitioned to flow phonation after spending much time simply doing pitch glides and sirens on /u/. She was then asked to contrast pressed and flow phonation styles on /u/.

First, she was asked to produce the /u/ again but not to allow any airflow to move the tissue. She was simply instructed to "hold her breath back." Then she was asked to produce /u/ using flow phonation, allowing the tissue to move but without the breathy voice quality. She also was asked to contrast the sensation and degree of effort for the different modes of phonation: breathy, flow, and pressed. It is very important to guide the patient toward feeling and hearing the difference between flow and pressed phonation.

Skill #3: Flow Phonation—Articulated

Cognate Pairs: Voiceless to Voiced Fricatives. Patient G was, again, asked to get louder when doing the seamless transition from the voiceless to voiced cognate pairs, and to do them on pitch glides. For example, on a siren, Patient G produced /s/→/z/→/s/→/z/, and so forth. This was also done on the other fricative cognates. This can be a difficult step for some patients when different pitches are being introduced, along with different articulatory postures and transitions from voiceless to voiced sounds. Patient G, with some practice, did well.

Phrases/Conversation. Patient G was then asked to say the same phrases in flow phonation and to contrast that with pressed phonation (explained as holding back her airflow, as evidenced by little tissue movement). Patient G did very well and discriminated not only between the difference in the 2 sounds (pitch lower and strained for pressed phonation) but also between the differences in feeling in the throat (constricted for pressed and open for flow phonation).

Skill #4: Articulatory Precision/ Clear Speech

An easy technique that seems to link cognition to flow phonation in speech is having patients concentrate on articulatory precision in their speech. The final key to using Flow Phonation in conversational speech is to allow articulation to facilitate the sensation of airflow energy at the front of the mouth as used in Conversation Training Therapy (see Case Study 3.1 by Gartner-Schmidt and Gillespie: Conversation Training Therapy [CTT] to Treat an Adult With Benign Midmembranous Lesions).[58,59] Patient G was encouraged to practice using Flow Phonation while maintaining awareness of articulatory activity first with sentences that include many phonemes known to have high anterior vibrotactile sensations. Patient G was asked to pretend that she was speaking clearly to a person who was hard of hearing while she said sentences loaded with phonemes with known anterior vibrotactile sensations (eg, "Freddy prefers French fries," "See Sammy slither in the grass," "Someone saw some fruit," "She saw sugar and spice," "Zane zoomed to Zurich").

Finally, Patient G and the SLP had a conversation about a topic chosen by Patient G. The only thing Patient G was asked to do was to use articulatory precision, monitoring airflow energy at the lips *without* any throat constriction. Without monitoring airflow, patients can be very precise in articulation but aphonic at the same time (with throat constriction). Patient G did well at using articulatory precision at the beginning of her phrases, but she often let her airflow drop at the end of linguistic strings, once again engaging in pressed phonation. This is a very common trait in North American English because of decreased pitch intonation contours at the ends of phrases. To counter this, she was asked to end every phrase with a voiceless /p/ to offset phonation with abducted vocal folds versus tightly adducted vocal folds. Patient G thought this was "very weird" but seemed to understand the rationale and was successful in monitoring the lack of flow at the ends of linguistic strings. She was encouraged to keep the energy up right until the end of phrases.

At the end of the session, Patient G's mother was invited into the session. She was ecstatic that her voice came back. However,

Table 4–2. Pre- and Posttherapy Outcome Measures

Outcome Measures	Initial Visit	Final Visit
VHI-10	36/40	3/40
Auditory-Perceptual Overall Severity	97/100	18/100
Cepstral Spectral Index of Dysphonia (CSID)	102	4
Number of Breaths in Rainbow Passage	12	5
Duration of Rainbow Passage (seconds)	18	23
Mean Airflow in Rainbow Passage	60 mL/second	170 mL/second

when she made that remark, the SLP quickly intervened with, "Your *voice production* came back." It was important for Patient G to think of herself as an active participant in voicing and not just a victim of her voice. This is a key meta-therapy goal in any type of therapy.[60]

Therapy Outcomes

Patient G was fully speaking normally after being aphonic for 3 months. Patient G was asked to return to therapy in 1 month to check for retention of her newly coordinated voice production. At that time, she was noted to still be speaking "fine."

Summary

Although this was the first time the patient had lost her voice production, her history and conversations led the SLP to believe that perhaps her aphonia may have been related to stress reactivity. Patient G wholeheartedly believed it and now knew the connection between voice and emotion. The SLP taught her that some people are "laryngoresponders" and may valve their stress through their larynx.[61] This can be normal. For now, flow phonation seemed to reestablish vocal balance and give her a conceptual framework for understanding how she could reinstate her voice if needed again. Her pre- and posttherapy outcome measures are represented in Table 4–2.

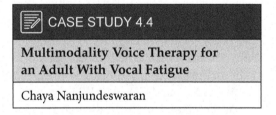

CASE STUDY 4.4

Multimodality Voice Therapy for an Adult With Vocal Fatigue

Chaya Nanjundeswaran

Voice Evaluation

The clinician obtained a case history, auditory-perceptual assessment, laryngeal imaging, and acoustic and aerodynamic measures during the clinical voice assessment.[62]

Case History

History of Voice Complaint. KS is a 25-year-old cisgender female, a trained singer, and the choral director at a high school for the past 4 years, with a gradual onset of voice problems starting about a year ago. She denies a specific precipitating factor but indicates that her vocal concerns have gradually progressed with her increased vocal demands. She indicated developing poor vocal habits and having difficulty maintaining her voice forward. Current complaints include drop in pitch in her speaking voice, glottal fry at the end of sentences, vocal effort, vocal fatigue, increased tension in her neck with voice use, and an occasional tickling sensation in her throat when speaking. Additional symptoms related to singing include increased effort and tension during singing. She reports that although she has had formal voice training, she was experiencing difficulty complying with the formal singing techniques. Additional complaints include experiencing a feeling of a lump or a sensation of something stuck in her throat. KS was enrolled in voice therapy about 3 years prior to this visit for similar complaints, received benefits with voice therapy, but reports having fallen through the cracks with her voice.

Medical History. KS has an existing problem of laryngopharyngeal reflux (LPR) and is on omeprazole (20 mg). In addition, KS experiences frequent nasal congestion and takes Zyrtec as needed. KS has diagnosed hypoglycemia but is not medically managed.

Vocal Hygiene. Hydration: 24 ounces of water per day, 4 caffeinated drinks per week. No history of smoking or alcohol use.

Vocal Demands. Patient KS is an active church choir member. She leads choir sessions every Wednesday night and Sunday morning. KS uses her voice constantly at work (about 90 minutes to 5 hours per day), as well as outside of work, and rates herself as being very talkative (9 on a scale of 1 to 10, with 1 being "least talkative" and 10 being "most talkative").

Quality-of-Life Impairment

The patient completed the VHI-10[50] and Vocal Fatigue Index (VFI),[63] with a score of 19/40 on the VHI-10 (threshold = 11).[51]

The VFI has 3 factors. Factor 1 indicates an avoidance of voice use, factor 2 indicates physical discomfort, and factor 3 indicates improvement or lack of improvement thereof with rest.[63]

VFI Factor 1: 42/44

VFI Factor 2: 12/20

VFI Factor 3: 12/12

KS scored high on factor 1 of the VFI, suggesting avoidance of voice use, and high on factor 2, indicating physical discomfort with voice use. Scores on factor 3 indicate that KS's vocal fatigue improves with voice rest.

Auditory-Perceptual Evaluation

The clinician administered the CAPE-V.[49] The evaluation revealed a mild dysphonia (an overall score of 20/100) characterized by roughness (40/100), strain (30/100), and low pitch (25/100). The ratings of strain and pitch were consistently present, while roughness was intermittently present at the end of a speaking task. Intermittent breath holding was also noted.

Manual Palpation Assessment

Palpation noted elevated laryngeal height and a tight thyrohyoid space with some tenderness to touch.

Laryngeal Imaging

A rigid videostrobolaryngoscope was used to evaluate the laryngeal anatomy and physiology. No obvious organic pathology was observed. Videostroboscopic evaluation revealed adequate bilateral arytenoid symmetry, increased vascularity of the true vocal folds, complete glottal closure, thick mucus on the free edges of the true vocal folds, increased medial compression, decreased amplitude of lateral excursion, diminished mucosal wave, and erythema and edema of the arytenoids and postcricoid area. Mild supraglottic compression was observed with the adduction of the false vocal folds.

Acoustic and Aerodynamic Assessment

All data were collected using the Medical Pentax CSL Model 4500 (Montvale, NJ) and the Pentax Medical PAS Model 6600 (Montvale, NJ). Results are documented in Table 4–3 A and B. Normative values are provided in Stemple et al (2020, pp. 220-221).[64]

Table 4–3. Initial Acoustic (**A**) and Aerodynamic (**B**) Assessment Measures

A.

	CAPE-V Sentences	Norms	Abnormal
Mean F0	181 Hz	193 Hz	X
Pitch Range	143-269 Hz		X
Intensity	61.5 dB SPL	68 dB SPL	
Dynamic Range	31.38 dB SPL	40 dB	X
Type of Voice	Type 1		

B.

	Results	Norms	Abnormal
Ps	7.53 cmH$_2$O	5.8 cmH$_2$O	X
Airflow	240 mL/sec	115 mL/sec	X

Stimulability

KS was stimulable for resonant voice exercises, including basic training gestures from Lessac-Madsen Resonant Voice Therapy (LMRVT)[54] such as humming on /m/, /n/, z/, words ("mom," "mime," "men"), and a phrase ("My mom made lemon muffins"). She also indicated increased ease of phonation following circumlaryngeal massage.

Impressions

KS presented with mild dysphonia and, based on stimulability and attitudes toward voice therapy, her prognosis was predicted to be good.

Plan of Care

KS was educated on the anatomy and physiology of the phonatory system. The therapist

> In this case, the author, Nanjundeswaran, practices in a graduate student clinic, and clinical frequency is often scheduled on a semester-to-semester basis for the student clinicians. Clinical practice patterns can vary by setting and patient availability, as seen in this case.

recommended that she increase hydration, continue to medically manage acid reflux, and initiate voice therapy. Therapy was recommended for 8 to 10 sessions twice a week for a period of 4 to 5 weeks.

Decision Making

The review of KS's history and results from the evaluation, including physiologic and videostroboscopic analysis, indicated that the primary source of the voice problem was the increased impact stress on the vocal folds during phonation as a result of an adducted hyperfunction pattern of voice use. With respect to voice production, the primary goals were to decrease impact stress between the vocal folds and to alleviate the adducted hyperfunction, thereby producing a well-balanced voice with decreased effort and decreased vocal fatigue with speaking voice.

Long-Term and Short-Term Goals (LTG and STG)

1. Improve overall vocal hygiene (LTG)
   - Increase knowledge and awareness of voice care, specifically knowledge of vocal hygiene (STG)

130 Voice Therapy: Clinical Case Studies

- Modify vocal behaviors in the patient's work environment to decrease vocal effort and vocal fatigue (STG)
2. Improve overall vocal efficiency (LTG)
   - Decrease the extralaryngeal muscle tension using stretches, circumlaryngeal massage, and flow phonation massage (STG)
   - Produce a resonant voice as an efficient and alternative mode of voice production to decrease impact stress of vocal fold vibration (STG)

Intervention: Voice Therapy

To decrease impact stress and alleviate hyperfunction, the clinician used an eclectic approach including voice care education, upper-body stretches, circumlaryngeal massage, and resonant voice with KS due to her presenting complaints. Voice care education related to anatomy and physiology of voice production, as well as impact of poor hydration and acid reflux on voice, improves buy-in to voice therapy. With the presenting complaint of vocal effort and fatigue and clinician evaluation of a tight thyrohyoid space, stretches and circumlaryngeal massage were recommended to relieve the sensation of effort and aid in ease of speaking. Resonant voice was recommended, as it is known to achieve a strong, clear voice with low effort and reduced impact of glottal closure during phonation by promoting a slightly abducted vocal fold posture during phonation.[65]

Patient Goals and Expected Outcomes. KS's functional goals were established during the first session of therapy:

- Produce her voice with less effort at the end of the day
- Experience less vocal fatigue with speaking voice
- Consistently use a forward voice to avoid a glottal fry at the end of the sentence
- Practice healthy voice use

Course of Treatment. Although KS was recommended to be seen for 8 to 10 sessions, she received a total of thirteen 50-minute sessions over a period of 2 semesters. Typically, patients are seen at the CSD student-led on-campus voice clinic over a period of 8 to 10 sessions, once a week. However, due to KS's work and choir schedule, treatment sessions were more spread out than usual. Treatment focus was divided into indirect voice care education and direct voice therapy.

Indirect Voice Care Education

Goals #1 and #2. Increase awareness and knowledge of voice care and modify vocal behaviors in the patient's work environment to decrease vocal effort and vocal fatigue.

In the first session of voice therapy, the SLP educated KS on the anatomy and physiology of voice production. The clinician discussed basic physiology of voice production, including the importance of adequate subglottic pressure and airflow. In vocal hygiene, the therapist addressed 3 important concepts, following the hygiene protocol as outlined in LMRVT[54] (see Case Study 3.7 by Orbelo, Li, and Verdolini Abbott: Lessac-Madsen Resonant Voice Therapy to Treat an Adult With Vocal Fold Nodules for more information on LMRVT). These concepts included (1) increasing hydration, (2) managing LPR, and (3) decreasing opportunities for phonotraumatic behaviors. Although the hygiene protocol for this client was based on LMRVT, the 3 main concepts addressed were individualized.

Increase Hydration. The clinician explained to KS the correlation between poor hydration, increased mucus on the vocal folds (as observed on videostroboscopy), and the increased effort to produce voice. Based on these discussions, KS was recommended to increase her water intake to about 64 ounces per day.

Manage LPR. KS was already on prescribed omeprazole. However, during the evaluation, KS indicated taking the medication after dinner. The clinician educated KS on the importance of taking the medication at the appropriate time (30 to 45 minutes before food). In addition, the therapist provided KS with tips to decrease acid reflux, including (1) not eating at least 3 hours prior to bedtime, (2) keeping her head elevated at night, and (3) monitoring a food diary to see if certain foods triggered more reflux symptoms than others.

Decrease Opportunity for Phonotrauma and Modify Work Environment. KS uses her voice frequently at an increased volume in her work environment. The clinician recommended the use of a vocal amplifier to control for vocal loudness, but KS did not feel comfortable using an amplifier at work. KS did not typically practice vocal warm-ups or cool-downs prior to or after her singing lessons at school. Vocal warm-ups and cool-downs help transition the mobility and flexibility of the vocal folds from speaking voice to singing voice and vice versa. KS was advised to incorporate some vocal warm-ups and cool-downs as part of her singing lessons with her students. In addition, the therapist educated KS on the importance of "vocal naps" (short periods of voice rest) and asked her to incorporate them periodically during her 7-hour workday.

Indirect voice therapy is an important part of an overall voice therapy plan. Since KS showed signs of dehydration and acid reflux, it was important to manage these factors, as they may be influencing increased impact stress on her vocal folds. In addition, there is a great demand on KS's voice in her work environment. It is important to modify certain vocal behaviors in her work environment to prevent phonotrauma prior to asking her to implement efficient voice strategies in voice therapy.

Direct Voice Therapy

Goal #3. Decrease extralaryngeal muscle tension using stretches, circumlaryngeal massage, and flow phonation.

KS demonstrated significant extralaryngeal tension in her neck that was directly related to the significant vocal effort to pro-

duce her voice. Upper-body stretches, specifically face and neck, used in LMRVT were part of every session routine. Stretches focused on relieving shoulder tightness by crossing the arms and tugging on the elbow, and on relieving jaw and tongue tightness by massaging the area around the zygomaticus major and minor with a yawn sigh. Additional strategies included massaging the back of the neck from the C2 to C5 area, neck rolls anchored with the thumb on the sternum and index finger on the chin, and stretching the sternocleidomastoid by using the opposite arm to stretch the neck to the side. Further, due to the presence of a knot and tightness in the thyrohyoid space, circumlaryngeal massage as outlined by Aronson (1990)[66] was used to release the thyrohyoid space. Circumlaryngeal massage generally begins by assessing the client's posture and stabilizing the client's head by placing the hand on the back of the head. The thyroid notch is located with a swallow and then the thumb and index finger are moved posteriorly toward the superior horns of the hyoid. A gentle circular and downward massage is applied from horns to the thyrohyoid space, and then the larynx is moved side to side and depressed. When in the depressed posture, the client is asked to hold the tongue out between the lips and hum.

To increase awareness of tension in the laryngeal area, the clinician asked KS to perform a series of tasks, alternating between voiceless and voiced sounds using flow phonation (see Case Study 4.3 by Gartner-Schmidt: Flow Phonation to Treat a Teenager With Primary Muscle Tension Aphonia for additional information on flow phonation).[67] A facial tissue was used as a visual feedback mechanism to indicate increased airflow and ease of phonation. Negative practice was used as part of this process as well. The therapist asked KS to voluntarily constrict her neck while producing the voiceless sound and preventing airflow; KS then let air flow consistently with the production of a voiceless sound and observed the difference in tension in the throat. Once KS achieved the target sensation in the voiceless sound, a voiced sound was introduced. Each time KS felt a constriction or tightness in her neck, she would pick up a facial tissue and practice achieving increased airflow and the target sensation. Since extralaryngeal tension seemed to be a primary cause of KS's vocal issues, it was important for KS to discriminate between constricted versus a relaxed throat and its effects on voice production.

Goal #4. Produce a resonant voice as an efficient and alternative mode of voice production to decrease impact stress of vocal fold vibration.

Impact stress seemed to be a primary reason for the patient's presenting voice complaints. To decrease impact stress, the goal was to train KS to produce an efficient and easy voice using a resonant voice production. Resonant voice (RV) has been well researched and documented to create a slightly abducted vocal fold configuration for most speech, thus alleviating vocal hyperfunction.[65] The LMRVT programmatic approach was used with KS to reduce impact stress.[54] The sequence included:

1. Exploring the basic training gesture (BTG) on voiced phonemes to produce a resonant voice in phoneme, word, phrase level, chanting, and conversational speech. During the exploration at the BTG and word level, negative practice was used to alternate between forward-focused voice production and voice from the throat. KS was asked to perceive the sensation between a forward-focused voice versus a voice from the throat. Initially during the sessions, KS had a difficult time perceiving her resonant sound. KS was directed to focus more on the feel and ease of production of voice (in BTG and at the word level) and less on the sound of the voice.

2. Following the ability to discriminate between the different voice production types, resonant voice was altered between voiced and voiceless production. KS could produce a resonant voice in the BTG and at word level (eg, easy production of hum on /m/, /n/, and /z/ and on words like "mom," "mine," "me," "nine," "name," and "Zane"). KS could produce resonant voice with ease in chanting at the phrase level. However, when speaking in a phrase or during conversation, it was difficult for KS to stay forward. The emphasis during such tasks and conversation was placed on the ability to identify when she dropped her voice to the throat and to bring it forward.

3. Due to the increased need to project her voice in school to her students, messa di voce (increasing and decreasing loudness using resonant voice) was also explored. Initially, all tasks were performed in a quiet clinic room. Toward the end of therapy, all exercises were performed in a classroom environment, with a specific emphasis on maintaining a loud conversation and staying forward. A sequence of messa di voce might look like this: starting with a hum on /m/ and going from soft to loud to soft, then on the word "mom" soft to loud to soft, then on phrases (eg, "hey you" or "good morning") or any functional phrases the client needed to use in the classroom.

KS's major complaint through her sessions was maintaining her voice forward and complying with therapeutic strategies in her work environment. Her major complaint was "I can feel it in my throat, but I continue to talk and sing."

Therapy Outcomes

Auditory-Perceptual Evaluation. KS's voice was rated as 10/100 for overall severity on the

CAPE-V with roughness at 20/100 and strain at 10/100. Pitch was judged to be within normal limits.

Acoustics Analysis. Posttherapy mean F0 was 200 Hz, and her average intensity was 69 dB SPL while reading CAPE-V sentences.

Patient Self-Assessment. KS's posttherapy score on the VHI-10 was 11/40. On the VFI, KS scored 22/44 for factor 1, 6/20 for factor 2, and 12/12 for factor 3. Her overall fatigue symptoms decreased.

Summary and Concluding Remarks

The clinician used an eclectic approach with KS to alleviate her voice symptoms. There was no underlying organic pathology resulting in her vocal symptoms. However, her increased vocal demands, increased impact stress, and hyperadduction resulted in an increased vocal effort to produce voice and significant vocal fatigue. Patient education on vocal hygiene and awareness, including increasing her hydration and controlling for acid reflux symptoms, decreased the tickle in her throat while speaking. In addition, resonant voice strategies helped decrease vocal effort and vocal fatigue with voice use.

KS 4 Years Later. KS returned to the clinic 4 years later after recognizing the recurrence of previous vocal symptoms, specifically vocal fatigue and a drop in pitch following a very busy school year and performance season. She indicated that she needed a refresher to set things right. This initiative from the patient highlights important factors that determine the success of voice therapy. Related to adherence to voice therapy, (1) voice therapy was made accessible to this patient and it was not hard, (2) the patient sought help again, and (3) the match matters—the clinician and the patient had a trusting relationship for the patient to follow through voice therapy.[68] Additional factors that emphasize the success of voice therapy include (1) appropriate and adequate patient education,[69] (2) increased awareness and responsibility to self-monitor,[68] and (3) good self-efficacy.[68]

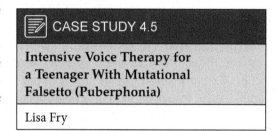

CASE STUDY 4.5

Intensive Voice Therapy for a Teenager With Mutational Falsetto (Puberphonia)

Lisa Fry

Voice Evaluation

Upon referral from a local otolaryngologist, I had the pleasure of seeing Patient AA, a 16-year-old-male, for a comprehensive voice evaluation for suspected mutational falsetto/puberphonia.

Case History

History of Voice Complaint. AA was accompanied to the session by his mother, who was present during the interview but left the room after historical information was obtained. Patient AA provided the majority of the background and historical information. He was reserved throughout the session, responding only briefly to direct questions and offering only limited detail in his comments.

AA's chief complaint was "high voice" and intermittent vocal fatigue at day's end. He could not recall the exact time of onset or any circumstances surrounding the onset but believed that the problem had been in existence for about 2 years. He reported that his voice did not really bother him and that he did not pay much attention to it. He stated that his mother was much more concerned about the problem than he was and that she was the primary instigator of the otolaryngology and voice therapy appointments. During history taking, AA was asked about his voice behaviors and if/when he had ever heard himself produce "another" voice. He indicated that he had heard this "other" voice from time to time. He recalled that this generally happened just upon waking in the morning. He stated that he generally makes only a few statements in this "other" voice before the high-pitched voice returns for the rest of the day.

Medical History. AA's medical history was significant for mild nasal allergies and acne. Current medications included an oral antibiotic for treatment of acne and an over-the-counter pain medication as needed for sports-related orthopedic pain/soreness.

Social History. AA is a sophomore at the local high school, where he participates in the school's junior varsity basketball team. He attends practice 4 or 5 times per week and does weightlifting 2 or 3 times per week. He reports great enthusiasm for the sport and indicates that most of his close friends at school are fellow members of the basketball team. When questioned about his school performance, AA described himself as "an OK student." He noted that he rarely speaks up in class and rarely talks with teachers apart from his coaches. He converses with close friends in the hallway before and after school and during breaks, but suggested that these hallway conversations are, at times, difficult, as he cannot project his voice over the hall noise. AA stated that his friends do not comment on his voice but indicated that when people meet him for the first time they often ask if he has a cold. AA lives at home with his parents and younger sister. He describes the home as quiet and uneventful. There are no smokers in the home. AA enjoys basketball, hanging out with friends, and attending church-related youth activities.

Laryngeal Imaging

The vocal folds were visualized using videostroboscopy with a 70-degree rigid videolaryngoscope. Vocal fold edges were smooth and straight bilaterally, and vocal fold coloration was normal. Abduction and adduction were normal and symmetrical bilaterally. Glottic closure was incomplete, characterized by a slight midline gap running the length of the folds. Amplitude and mucosal wave were mildly reduced bilaterally. The open phase of vibration predominated. The vocal folds were elongated and tense during all visualized phonatory attempts, preventing judgments at modal phonation.

Vocal Effort, Fatigue, and Pain

These parameters were assessed via patient interview. The patient reported a mild to moderate degree of vocal effort in conversation and a mild degree of vocal fatigue on days of heavy voice use (mostly weekends). He denied pain in the laryngeal region.

Quality-of-Life Assessment

The Voice Handicap Index (VHI)[70] was used to assess the impact of the voice concern on daily life. Scores were as follows: Functional Domain: 15/40; Physical Domain: 13/40; Emotional Domain: 17/40. Overall VHI score was 45/120, suggesting a moderate vocal handicap. Areas of specific concern for the patient included: "I am less outgoing because of my voice problem" and "The clarity of my voice is unpredictable."

Auditory-Perceptual Assessment

The CAPE-V[49] was used with an overall severity rating of 35/100, indicating a moderate dysphonia. AA consistently spoke in a falsetto voice. Intermittent pitch-breaks down into the modal register were observed. His voice quality was characterized by mild roughness, moderate breathiness, and mildly to moderately reduced loudness. A mild degree of strain was also present during voicing.

Manual Palpation Assessment

The clinician assessed laryngeal positioning and tension via manual palpation. The hyoid bone was positioned high in the neck. Thyrohyoid space was narrowed, and mild tenderness was reported with digital pressure in that region with minimal limitation of laryngeal lateralization upon manipulation.

Acoustic Assessment

The clinician used the Pentax Medical Computerized Speech Lab (Montvale, NJ) to acquire and analyze acoustic information regarding the voice. Normative data are derived from Baken and Orlikoff (1999)[71] and the Iowa Head and Neck Protocol.[72] Aerodynamic assessment was not available. See Table 4–4.

Stimulability

AA was able to produce a lower-pitched voice during vegetative tasks such as coughing, throat clearing, and laughing. Attempts to shape a throat clear into a prolonged [um] were minimally successful. The clinician was also able to garner consistent production of a lower-pitched, modal phonation with a glottal coup (hard throat-clearing behavior). However, the tone could not be sustained beyond the quick production during the attack phase. AA indicated he could hear the lower-pitched productions and was enthusiastic that he could achieve this sound volitionally.

Impressions

AA presents with a marked voice impairment as a result of mutational falsetto/puberphonia. He presents a good prognosis for recalibration to lower modal phonation following stimulability testing.

Plan of Care

It was expected that the patient would achieve the below goals in an extended treatment session (boot camp therapy) conducted immediately following the evaluation session:

1. AA will consistently achieve the lower-pitched voice after facilitating techniques. *Use of the hard glottal attack production. Production in back-and-forth exchange with the clinician.*
2. AA will extend use of the new pitch to increasingly complex linguistic contexts (syllables through conversation). *Use of chanting or monotone production (without inflection) will help to hold the proper laryngeal posture while extending the length of production slowly.*
3. AA will develop a plan for generalizing the new voice to new listeners and situations. *Open discussion between the clinician and patient. Create a hierarchy of settings where voice is required, from easiest to most concerning. Strategize ways of slowly extending use of the new voice from easy, familiar listeners on days 1 and 2 to more challenging listeners and settings on subsequent days. Work to have the new voice in use in all settings by day 3 or 4.*
4. AA will use the lower-pitched voice in all speaking contexts. *The patient will work through the designed hierarchy to begin using the voice in more and more settings.*

Table 4–4. Acoustic Assessment

	Rainbow Passage	Sustained Vowels	Norms
Mean F0	229.97 Hz	236.37 Hz	80-150 Hz
Mean Intensity	67.1 dB	68.0 dB	69-71 dB
Jitter	—	1.8%	<1%
Shimmer	—	7.2%	<5%
Noise-to-Harmonic Ratio	—	0.35%	<0.2%

5. AA will express satisfaction and comfort with his new speaking voice. *In a follow-up call, the SLP will discuss progress in using the voice and determine the patient's comfort with the new voice.*

> Boot camp voice therapy is a term used to describe intensive therapy delivered in a short period of time, often several hours in length over the course of 1 day. For another example of boot camp voice therapy, see Case Study 4.2 by Milstein and Adessa: Boot Camp Voice Therapy for an Adult With Functional Dysphonia. In this case by Fry, she uses and recommends an extended therapy session to begin immediately after the evaluation confirms mutational falsetto.

Decision Making

The size and positioning of the male larynx undergo marked changes in the short period of time we refer to as puberty, altering the physiology of phonation and requiring a new mechanism of laryngeal neuromuscular control. At the same time, anatomic changes bring about a significant reduction in fundamental frequency and, consequently, present a challenge to the individual's auditory feedback system. Most pubescent males proceed through these changes without difficulty, making the necessary motor and sensory adjustments without effort. However, in some males, the system does not adjust to the changing anatomy, and the individual persists in the higher pitch range. The use of a high-pitched voice beyond puberty in males has been commonly presented[4,15,66] and has taken on many names, including mutational voice, mutational falsetto, persistent falsetto, and puberphonia. The problem is most commonly observed in adolescent males in the months immediately following puberty when hormonal shifts bring about the changes described above. While rare, some cases extend beyond puberty into adulthood.

The voice of mutational falsetto is produced when the suprahyoid and cricothyroid muscles are contracted and the thyroarytenoid (TA) muscle is disengaged. The result is a tense laryngeal mechanism that is positioned high in the neck. The vocal folds are elongated and tense and exhibit decreased vibration and inadequate closure. This posture results in a high-pitched, weak, breathy voice, often accompanied by roughness and pitch breaks.

Mutational voice can be confirmed clinically in several ways. Throat clearing, coughing, laughing, and producing a hard glottal attack engages the TA muscles and dramatically lowers pitch into the modal register. Furthermore, digital manipulation of the larynx may reveal an elevated larynx that can be gently manipulated to a lower position with systematic digital manipulation of the thyroid cartilage.[66,73]

Several factors from this evaluation session suggested a positive prognosis and directed the speech pathologist in the most efficient course of treatment. First, while AA was less concerned about his voice deviation than his mother was, he indicated a willingness to participate in treatment. He stated that changing his voice may help him feel more comfortable around peers. In addition, AA's awareness of "another voice" on occasion suggested to the speech pathologist that he was aware of his ability to achieve a lower-pitched production and was likely willing to engage in methods to stabilize this tone.

The evaluation session was scheduled within a broad time frame, allowing the speech pathologist time to initiate treatment immediately following the evaluation. Due to the patient's interest and the clinician's availability, the decision was made to begin treatment immediately and to continue the treatment session until the desired voice was elicited and maintained in conversation with the clinician and the mother. While several options for treatment are available and effective, the speech pathologist considered two methods as best suited for this case. The first route of treatment would be to simply ask the patient if he could produce the "other voice" on command. If so, the speech pathologist would explain the physiology behind this second voice and use repeated trials to stabilize and then generalize the tone. If, however, the patient was unable to produce the "other voice" on command, a simple method would be used to engage the TA muscle (opposing the overactive cricothyroid) and position the larynx in the proper posture for voicing. Production of hard glottal attacks elicits TA engagement and facilitates the desired production.

Intervention

Intensive therapy included education, hard glottal attack productions to establish and stabilize the targeted pitch, and chanting to extend the tone to connected speech.

Background and Physiologic Rationale of Treatment

Patients with mutational voice possess abnormal laryngeal muscle *use* amid normal laryngeal *structure*. As the TA muscle (the muscular core of the vocal fold) is not actively engaged during voice production, the opposing cricothyroid elongates and tenses the folds, producing the characteristic falsetto quality.

The successful treatment of mutational falsetto begins with a thorough description of the anatomy and physiology of voicing and a discussion of how this changes at puberty. Images and a laryngeal model can support the explanation. The clinician reminds the patient that his laryngeal structures are normal and that his voice concerns are related to muscle *use* issues. The physiology of the mutational voice is shared. The patient is reassured that pubertal changes in laryngeal anatomy create challenges for the system and that he is not alone in his experience. Methods of facilitating proper muscle activity are reviewed; the rationale for each is explained.

After education is complete, production training begins. The goal is to establish consistent engagement of the TA during voicing. Production of a firm, hard glottal attack is one method of quickly triggering TA contraction and eliciting a lower-pitched production. Typically, the speech pathologist models the hard glottal attack. Hand motions and verbal cues can promote the production of the attack from the start. The patient is asked to imitate the clinician's production. If the patient is successful, continue rapid model-and-imitate productions of hard glottal attacks until the patient can consistently produce the low-pitched glottal attack without accidentally softening the onset and slipping into the falsetto tone. Once the patient successfully produces the hard glottal attack, the clinician and patient continue in a rapid back-and-forth exchange without much time lapse between attempts. If the patient is unable to produce the hard glottal attack at first, the clinician continues to model and use hand motions or descriptive terms (eg, "harder," "grunt") to elicit the firm glottal attack.

After the hard glottal attack is stabilized and the TA engaged, the clinician slowly progresses to more linguistically complex productions (from syllables to conversation). Use of a chanted style of production can be helpful as the patient learns to maintain TA engagement and keep the larynx in a lowered posture during longer and longer productions. Asking the patient to use intonation patterns too soon could cause the patient to lose the desired muscle pattern. Once the patient can produce connected speech in a monotone style, more normal intonation patterns can be slowly added. In addition, attention to the speech stimuli is important. Starting with all-voiced utterances helps the patient maintain the desired laryngeal posture; introducing a voiceless consonant too soon may result in an undesired shift in laryngeal position.

Most cases of functional falsetto (mutational falsetto) in the pubescent male can be managed in only 1 or 2 treatment sessions. In cases where the falsetto voice has been maintained over the course of many years, a few additional sessions may be necessary. A few guidelines regarding scheduling are generally followed. First, when clinic scheduling permits, it is helpful to arrange an extended block of time for the initial evaluation/treatment session, typically a 2- to 3-hour session for these cases. When more than 1 session is required, every attempt should be made to avoid a long period between sessions, as this may permit the patient to revert to previous vocal behaviors; arranging sessions on consecutive days is helpful.

Patient AA's Response to Intervention

After education, AA indicated an understanding of the voice goal and physiology underlying production. At this point, the speech pathologist spoke with AA about the "other voice" that he reported hearing at times. The clinician asked if AA could produce that voice on command. He made several attempts to produce the lower pitch without success. (Note: In some instances, this technique is sufficient to prompt the lower-pitched phonation, which can then be shaped into connected speech using the steps below.) As AA was unable to produce the lower pitch on command, a simple facilitating method—the hard glottal attack—was used. AA was asked to produce a hard, abrupt "ah." Initial attempts yielded breathy, high-pitched "ah's. The clinician requested a harder, louder tone, eventually asking the patient to press hard against her hands while attempting the abrupt "ah." With this, the glottal attack was produced, triggering a lower-pitched, fry-like phonation. The patient was instructed to repeatedly produce the glottal attack until the lower-pitched tone was stable. Once consistent hard glottal attacks were heard and the patient was able to identify the target pitch, the abrupt "ah" was sustained for longer periods of time. Eventually, the hard onset was faded; AA was able to sustain the "ah" for several seconds.

After the target tone had been stabilized, the tone was slowly extended into other speech contexts. First, the patient was asked to generalize the tone to other sustained vowels. Once that step was mastered, the clinician trained the patient in chanting all-voiced nonsense syllables (eg, /mamama/, /momomo/, /minimini/). Chanting syllables such as these permitted AA to extend the low-pitched voice to a variety of articulatory contexts without altering the newly acquired laryngeal posture for inflection or for production of a voiceless consonant. Consequently, the new voice became more stable.

AA continued chanting all-voiced productions through word, phrase, and sentence levels. Once mastered, AA progressed to producing voiced-voiceless syllables, words, phrases, and sentences in the context of a chanting style. Eventually, the chanting style was faded and the patient was able to gradually produce the new pitch with longer utterances with normal prosody. The patient was advanced through various readings and conversational topics.

Generalizing the Lower Pitch. Because of the dramatic nature of voice changes during treatment for mutational voice, transition of the voice outside of the therapy context can be challenging. Consequently, it is recommended that the clinician and patient discuss this challenge and develop a plan for generalizing the new voice. In the case of AA, the clinician asked, "What do you think others will say about your new voice?" to which AA replied, "They will be shocked. I don't know if they will like it." The clinician reassured the patient that, although the new voice was notably different, it was also quite pleasing and appropriate. To confirm this for the patient, digital recordings of the new voice were made and played back for the patient. After hearing only a few statements, AA expressed pleasure with the new voice, stating that it made him sound stronger and more confident. At this point, the clinician suggested that the patient create a hierarchy of persons and situations where the voice could be slowly introduced. The patient agreed to use the new voice with his immediate family and 2 close friends on the day of the session; he would be free to use his higher-pitched voice if he desired with other individuals on that day. The next day, AA would expand use of his new voice to include coaches and members of his team and members of his extended family. By the second day post therapy, AA would use the voice with teachers and with friends in the school hallway. Finally, by the third day following therapy, AA expected to use his lower-pitched voice in all situations.

> The author describes part of the therapeutic process that is vital to helping the patient generalize their voice. In this case, she encourages the patient to make a list of people he will feel comfortable using the new voice with and increasing the list of names over several days. The editors have used upcoming school holidays or vacations to help the patient gradually introduce the new voice that can be quite different from the voice that brought them into therapy.

With the above plan in place, the session drew to a close. The speech pathologist asked that the patient remain in the treatment area while she went to get his mother. Prior to taking the mother into the treatment area, the clinician took a few moments to prepare the mother for AA's new voice. Results of the session were discussed, and the speech pathologist asked that the mother not respond too dramatically to the new voice but that she simply make a few brief comments about the appeal of the new voice. Preparing the mother for the new voice and practicing her response reduced the likelihood that she would overreact and, thereby, cause the patient to be fearful of future interactions where he used the new voice with friends and family.

Refining the Lower-Pitched Voice. At the close of the session, AA's new voice possessed an element of glottal fry, suggesting that AA had lowered the pitch beyond the target and that some muscle imbalance was still present. To address this, an additional therapy session was recommended to refine the tone and to promote a proper, frontal tone focus. AA followed up 1 week following the initial visit; resonance training was used to correct tone focus.

> The author references the use of resonant voice therapy. Case 3.7 by Orbelo, Li, and Verdolini Abbott discusses a specific resonant voice therapy approach (LMRVT) and Case 3.3 by Murphy Estes discusses other resonant voice therapy tasks.

Therapy Outcomes

At the patient's follow-up visit, he had been using the lower-pitched voice in all contexts for several days. Consistent use of the voice and an increased comfort with the voice had resulted in a lessening of the fry and a more appealing voice quality. Pretreatment vocal features of pitch deviation, roughness, breathiness, and pitch breaks were not present. Nonetheless, an abbreviated program of resonant voice therapy was introduced. AA was given a program of daily resonance exercises to complete over the next 2 weeks.

Patient Self-Assessment. A follow-up call was placed to the patient 2 weeks later. AA reported doing well with the new voice and that the gravelly quality had dissipated. He expressed pleasure with the new voice and an increasing social confidence.

Summary and Concluding Remarks

Cases of mutational voice in young males are rewarding to patients and clinicians. Patients are encouraged as they experience normal voice production and improved social confidence after only a brief therapy period. Clinicians are rewarded by seeing the fruit of their labor in a short time. While the therapy experience is generally brief, the results of therapy give patients and clinicians a lasting interest in and respect for one another.

 CASE STUDY 4.6

Postsurgical Voice Therapy for a Child With Recurrent Respiratory Papillomatosis and Ventricular Phonation

Maia Nystrum Braden

Voice Evaluation

I had the pleasure of seeing a delightful, energetic 4-year-old boy, referred by the pediatric otolaryngologist, for a comprehensive voice evaluation. The patient presents with a history of recurrent respiratory papillomatosis.

Case History

Chief Complaint. Low, rough voice quality, present since child began speaking

Medical History. Patient LJ is a 4-year-old boy with a history of recurrent respiratory papillomatosis, first diagnosed at the age of 2 years. The child's mother reports that he had a "hoarse, rough," cry even as an infant. He had stridor, cough, and breathing difficulties, and was initially diagnosed with allergies, asthma, and acid reflux. He was treated for all 3 of these without improvement, and his parents became increasingly concerned. When he did not improve on medications, he was referred to a pediatric otolaryngologist, who completed laryngeal visualization and diagnosed recurrent respiratory papillomatosis. Over the past 2 years, he has had frequent surgeries, sometimes as often as once a month, to maintain his airway. While his breathing has been stable with surgeries, his voice quality never improved, and he was referred to the pediatric voice clinic for evaluation by the SLP and pediatric laryngologist.

Surgical History. Frequent (>25) surgeries, usually with cold instruments, sometimes with laser, to treat aggressive RRP. In the past 6 months, he has required 2 surgeries, representing a decrease in frequency.

Voice Use. LJ's mother describes him as a "typical" 4-year-old. He talks, engages in play noises, and sometimes yells. He is sometimes less talkative than she would expect, especially with unfamiliar listeners. She reports that he is sometimes hard to understand and has difficulty getting loud.

Speech Therapy History. He has never had speech therapy, and his mother denies any concerns with articulation or language.

Quality-of-Life Assessment

Due to age, quality-of-life assessment was completed by parent proxy using the Pediatric Voice-Related Quality of Life Assessment (P-VRQOL).[74] Score was 54/100. Higher scores are associated with higher (better) voice-related quality of life.

Auditory-Perceptual Assessment

The CAPE-V[49] was completed. The patient was noted to have an overall severity of 83 (severe), with severe roughness (88/100), mild breathiness (16/100), moderate-severe strain (67/100), abnormally low pitch for age and gender (92/100), and mildly reduced loudness (23/100). Other salient features included consistent apparent ventricular phonation, minimal pitch variability, and occasional diplophonia.

Acoustic and Aerodynamic Assessment

Acoustic data were gathered using the Pentax Medical Computerized Speech Lab (Montvale, NJ). The clinician held a microphone at 15 cm from the patient's mouth to acquire data. Due to the patient's young age, reading tasks were not completed. Instead, he was asked to repeat the CAPE-V sentences after the clinician and describe a picture. Acoustic norms were taken from Kent et al (2021),[75] Demirci et al (2021),[76] and Kent et al (2023).[77] Aerodynamic norms are not available for children under 6;0. Norms for children 6;0-11;0 are included for subglottal pressure (Psub),[78] and values for phonation threshold pressure (PTP) from a study on children age 4;0-17 are included.[79] See Table 4–5.

Laryngeal Imaging

Laryngeal imaging was completed using a pediatric flexible distal chip endoscope. The patient was positioned comfortably in his mother's lap. He was understandably upset but did participate in some vocalization. Full adduction and abduction of the arytenoid cartilages was observed. The airway was patent on resting breathing without residual papilloma in the glottis or subglottis. When viewed in the abducted position, vocal fold edges were smooth and straight, without visible evidence of scar or sulcus. There was a small amount of stippled-appearing lesions on the ventricular folds, but no evidence on the vocal folds. Vocal fold color was within normal limits without excessive vascularity, edema, or erythema.

On phonation, the true vocal folds could not be visualized due to the extreme level of secondary muscle tension to phonate as evidenced by complete adduction of the ventricular folds that obscured viewing of the true vocal folds. Stroboscopy was therefore not completed, as the aperiodic nature of phonation and the presence of ventricular fold vibration made laryngeal microphone tracking impossible.

Brief therapeutic probes were initiated during exam as tolerated, and on inspiratory phonation, the ventricular folds retracted, allowing for visualization of the true vocal folds. While closure could not be judged due to lack of stroboscopic imaging, there appeared to be adequate approximation.

Stimulability Testing

Dynamic assessment was conducted using therapy probes. Voicing with mild breathiness but without the severe roughness or apparent ventricular phonation was obtained using the following probes: inspiratory phonation, blowing bubbles with a straw in water, producing a very high pitch, and flow mode /u/ with a straw. During the evaluation, these did not generalize to words or sentences, but did become more consistent in sustained vowels with practice.

Table 4–5. Acoustic and Aerodynamic Assessment Measures

	Results	Norms
Mean F0 Sustained /a/ (Hz)	176.15 Hz	245.2 Hz (SD 25.48)
Mean F0 Connected Speech (Hz)	194.6 Hz Hz	218-274 Hz
CPP Sustained /a/ (dB)	0.644 dB	11.67 dB (SD 2.56)
L/H Ratio Sustained /a/	25.10	30.39 (4.52)
CPP All-Voiced Sentence (dB)	1.383 dB	5.39 dB (SD 0.418)
L/H Ratio All-Voiced Sentence	22.382	28.06 dB (SD 1.22)
PTP	5.63 cmH$_2$O	4.05 cmH$_2$O, SD 0.87
Psub	8.43 cmH$_2$O	No age-appropriate norms available; 8.69-10.05 cmH$_2$O ages 6.0 and older

Impressions

Patient LJ has severe dysphonia characterized by ventricular phonation. This likely represents maladaptive compensatory behaviors due to frequent and aggressive growth of recurrent respiratory papillomatosis. Vocal folds at this time appear free from disease, and stimulability testing indicated capacity for more typical voice.

Plan of Care

It is recommended that LJ be seen for 10 to 12 sessions of voice therapy, twice per week for 4 weeks, and then decreasing to once per week for 2 weeks, and once every 2 weeks for 1 month, with reassessment at the end of that time.

Long-Term Goal. LJ will produce true vocal fold phonation in 90% of connected speech with minimal clinician cues across 2 therapy sessions.

Short-Term Goal #1. LJ will discriminate ventricular phonation from true vocal fold voicing in 8/10 opportunities.

Short-Term Goal #2. LJ will produce true vocal fold phonation in sustained vowels following a clinician model and verbal cues in 8/10 opportunities.

Short-Term Goal #3. LJ will produce true vocal fold phonation in single words following a clinician model and verbal cues as needed in 8/10 opportunities.

Short-Term Goal #4. LJ will produce true vocal fold phonation in self-generated phrases and sentences with intermittent verbal reminders in 8/10 opportunities.

Decision Making

Understanding the Medical Condition. Recurrent respiratory papillomatosis (RRP) is a neoplasm caused by the human papilloma virus (HPV). It is most often caused by the subtypes of HPV6 and HPV11.[80] While HPV is relatively common, occurring in 75% to 80% of unvaccinated individuals, RRP is less common. There is a previously reported incidence of around 4.3 per 100,000 children and 1.8 per 100,000 adults.[81] With the availability of an HPV vaccine (Gardasil; Merck), incidence has decreased in recent years, but updated data are not available for the United States. RRP manifests as wartlike growths in the upper aerodigestive tract. These growths are particularly detrimental to breathing and voice. When growths occur on the vocal folds, they can cause voice disturbances ranging from mild to severe dysphonia.[82] Onset of disease can be classified as juvenile or adult. Juvenile onset RRP is thought to be contracted from the mother through transmission during delivery, and it is typically more aggressive than adult onset.[81]

Treatment of RRP in children relies on frequent surgical intervention. There are medications that show promise in slowing growth,[83,84] and vaccines have reduced the number of new cases in some places,[81] but there is no cure. Most children with RRP rely on frequent surgical treatments to remove the growths. Juvenile onset RRP is usually more rapidly growing than adult onset, and children with the papillomatosis have an average of 4.4 surgical procedures per year.[85] Surgical treatment varies depending on the location and extent of the disease and may be done with CO_2 laser, potassium titanyl phosphate (KTP) laser, cold instruments, and microdebrider. Rapid and variable growth and the need for frequent surgeries can result in constantly varying voice quality. There are no studies of voice therapy in children with RRP, likely because of the extremely variable presentation and course, and because of the necessary emphasis on airway. However, in addition to the effects of the lesions on vocal fold closure and pliability, individuals with RRP may experience maladaptive compensatory strategies. Voice therapy should be considered to manage both the primary dysphonia and secondary muscle tension and to teach strategies for producing optimal voice at all stages of disease.

Understanding the Role of Therapy in Pediatric RRP. Although LJ is young, it was determined that he was an excellent candidate for voice therapy. He had motivated and supportive parents, was stimulable for improvement with therapy probes, and followed instructions well. Structurally, although it would be easy to assume that his dysphonia was due to papilloma, this was not supported by the imaging. While pliability could not be assessed, there were no obvious lesions or tissue deficits. There is sometimes an assumption that young children cannot participate in voice therapy, but the literature does not support this. Studies of voice therapy effectiveness have included children as young as 3 years old and have demonstrated improvement with therapy.[86] When planning therapy for a child with RRP, timing of surgeries should be a consideration, as he may have fluctuating voice quality with RRP growth and with recovery from surgeries. However, at this time, he had no indication of present laryngeal disease, so no surgeries were planned. Therapy was recommended, and the family was in agreement.

Intervention

A holistic approach was used with a combination of indirect therapy and direct therapy.

Indirect therapy included child and parent education, rapport building, counseling regarding expectations and the impact of RRP and surgeries on the voice, and support in planning practice. Direct therapy included semi-occluded vocal tract (SOVT) exercises, flow phonation, and resonant voice therapy.

Session #1

The first session was focused on rapport building, stimulability probes, and auditory discrimination. Clinician/client/caregiver match is extremely important with all voice therapy patients, and especially so with young children. An interview with the parents and child helped to determine his interests so these could be built into the session. He enjoyed *Star Wars*, superheroes, and car racing, so these were incorporated. The clinician educated the parents on laryngeal function and on the patient's individual presentation. It was explained that while he *could* produce a near-normal voice, he did not know how to do so because the rapid growth/regrowth of the RRP often made phonation difficult. The clinician also provided education on voice at the child's level of understanding with a description of where his voice came from and how it worked. The clinician explained that he was using extra muscles that didn't need to work to make his voice, and his voice could be easier and clearer if he let those muscles "take a break." Next, voice exercises and probes were incorporated into a game of Candyland. With each turn, a different therapy probe was modeled, and he took a turn after attempting the sound. Probes included lip trills, inspiratory phonation, straw bubbles (phonation with a straw partially submerged in water), humming, and cues to use a high-pitched voice. (See Video 8 Lip Trills, Video 9 Inspiratory Phonation, and Video 10 Straw Bubbles by Braden.) All of these were successful in obtaining presumed true vocal fold voicing for approximately 1 second. Each time he achieved the target voice, the clinician and parent reacted with enthusiasm, encouraging him to continue.

> In this case, the vocal folds were essentially free of disease (RRP) at the time of the evaluation. However, LJ still used ventricular phonation to communicate, which is neither efficient nor considered normal phonation for a young child. Here, the author does an excellent job of guiding the clinician to think beyond the diagnosis to treat the child. The author is not treating RRP, but rather the secondary MTD that had developed due to the RRP. This muscle tension is not necessary when the vocal folds are free of disease, but it had become the habitual way of phonating. The editors of this text applaud the author for reminding the reader not to be deterred by the diagnosis before evaluating the patient to determine if there are other, more efficient and effective methods of phonation.

Once it was established that LJ was able to produce true vocal fold voicing, the clinician introduced an auditory discrimination task. The child helped named the target voice and the "old voice." He chose "Darth Vader Voice" to represent his "old voice" (characterized by ventricular phonation) and "Captain America Voice" to represent his new voice. Note that neither of these was intended to be "good" or "bad," but instead descriptive, and provided a more concrete representation for the child, as well as consistent language for the parent/caregiver to use. The clinician then modeled both voices and asked him to point to a picture of Captain America or Darth Vader based on the voice he heard. The parents were included in discrimination tasks as well, as they would be the primary source of feedback at home. Once he could reliably discriminate between ventricular and true vocal fold phonation in the clinician's voice, he was asked to identify whether his own voice was "Captain America" or "Darth Vader." This was done only in vowel sounds in the first session, as he had not yet consistently produced true vocal fold phonation in words or connected speech.

Home Practice. Home practice of lip trills, inspiratory phonation, and straw bubbles was assigned, with clear instructions to parents to provide feedback on accuracy.

Session #2

Session #2 focused on stabilization of vocalization, increasing respiratory/phonatory coordination, and moving into words. The facilitating techniques used in the previous session were reviewed to check for maintenance. He was consistently achieving brief periods of phonation (<1 second) using the facilitation techniques, but not sustaining for more than 1 second. With a cue to "use a higher, windy voice," he achieved a brief sustained /u/. A game with racing Hot Wheels cars was introduced to shape longer productions. He was cued to "make the sound go as long as the car goes," and the cars raced up and down a hallway. Using this strategy, he increased phonation time to 5 seconds. Cues based on flow phonation were employed during this activity.[87] He had not previously connected his breath with his voice, so cues to "feel the air come through your lips" and "make a smooth, windy voice" helped improve his voice production and respiratory/phonatory coordination. Straw phonation in water was also used, with the visual feedback of bubbles in water to demonstrate consistent use of airflow. He was given a straw and a cup of water, and the clinician modeled blowing bubbles while LJ imitated. When airflow was consistent, there was a steady stream of bubbles. The clinician then modeled adding voice and verbally reinforced his clear, true vocal fold phonation. As he became more consistent with these, pitch glides were added on both the straw bubbles and "windy /u/." Lip trills were introduced as another form of SOVT exercise.

True Vocal Fold Phonation in Single Words. As the sustained /u/ had been most effective in facilitating voice production, words containing the /u/ vowel were introduced. This was also done in a game activity (Memory). Modeling, verbal cues to use the "Captain America" Voice, and priming with a sustained /u/ all helped to establish voicing in words. (See accompanying Videos 8, 9, and 10 by Braden for demonstrations of lip trills, cup bubbles, and straw exercises with a child.)

Auditory Discrimination. LJ was asked to identify "Darth Vader" and "Captain America" productions in the clinician's voice during the game.

Parent Training. The parent was included in the game and asked to identify target and non-target productions in both child and clinician voice.

Home Practice. The SOVTs of straw bubbles, windy /u/, and lip trills were assigned. Practice with single words containing /u/ vowels was assigned as well.

Session #3

Indirect Therapy. The clinician provided education regarding next steps and moving toward generalization. Both parents and child were encouraged to practice every day to change old habits.

Direct Therapy. This began with SOVT exercises but progressed into words and connected speech as soon as LJ was able. Sessions began with a warm-up of SOVT exercises. These were practiced with a focus on straw bubbles (singing songs into a cup of water) and sustained /u/ with race cars, along with increasing control of fundamental frequency through pitch glides and "singing" using the straw bubbles.

Maintaining Voicing in Longer Utterances. /u/-loaded words were used as a basis for work in carrier phrases and sentences. These continued to be play based, including age-appropriate games such as Memory, Don't Break the Ice, and a *Star Wars*-themed board game. Therapy strategies used included direct modeling, verbal cues, and informative feedback on his accuracy. As accuracy increased, feedback was faded.

Negative Practice. To support the client's awareness and confidence, the clinician asked him to switch between his 2 voices in single words and sentences.

Sessions #4 to #6

LJ achieved true vocal fold voicing with improved respiratory/phonatory coordination, but voice quality was still mildly rough and breathy. Resonant voice therapy was introduced to improve the clarity of the sound, reduce effort, and optimize true vocal fold vibration.[65] Following a warm-up of SOVT exercises, he was introduced to resonant voice through humming. The clinician encouraged him to feel a "buzzy" vibration in his lips, nose, and mouth when he hummed. With a combination of focus on "buzzy" hum, higher pitch, and airflow, he obtained a voice with minimal roughness, breathiness, and strain. Resonant voice was trained following a flexible training pattern. Once the optimal voice was established in hums, single words containing /m/ and /u/ were introduced. The clinician

again encouraged him encouraged to feel the vibrations and the air. During these 3 sessions, practice was variable once the target was established to promote motor learning. Once he could consistently produce and identify his target voice in words, he was asked to make sentences, answer questions, and use the target voice in play. Cues consisted of models, verbal reminders, and attention cues to "feel the buzziness" and "use your 'Captain America' voice."

Home Practice. Parents were again involved in the session and trained to correctly identify and cue his target voice. Home practice consisted of SOVT exercises and practice of the target voice during play, shared book reading, and short conversations.

> It is well established that using principles of motor learning form the basis of much of voice therapy due to the need to adapt motor behaviors to establish efficient voicing. In this case, variable practice requires the patient to constantly confront novel situations to use the newly learned motor behavior.

Sessions #7 and #8

Moving Toward Independence and Generalization. Now that optimal voicing was established, the next step was to make this voice the "default" or "habit" voice. Each session began with a brief warm-up including straw bubbles, "windy" (flow mode) /u/, and single words to establish optimal voicing. Following this, he was asked to use his target ("Captain America") voice all the time. Sessions were spent in child-preferred activities, including board games, playing with cars, assembling a LEGO set, and playing with Star Wars action figures. Instead of moving strictly up the hierarchy, practice was variable. Some tasks involved a single word or a prolonged vowel, and some involved words, sentences, or connected speech. Following principles of motor learning, frequency of feedback was reduced, and feedback was primarily knowledge of

146   Voice Therapy: Clinical Case Studies

results (the clinician told him whether his production was accurate or not, but did not give extensive feedback on what details he needed to change). LJ was encouraged to self-evaluate and self-correct. When he did not do so spontaneously, the clinician reminded him to use his new voice, and he quickly adjusted.

> With increasingly better understanding of how people learn new motor patterns, SLPs are encouraged to reduce the constant use of feedback like "great job" or specifics of what to change, but rather to assess—does it feel the same or does it feel as easy? In this way, the patient determines if a response was a well-crafted production or if they could make it better. The clinician is not the decision maker.

Parents were included in therapy and trained in feedback to give at home.

Home practice included a daily warm-up to establish best voicing, with the remainder of home practice being in real-life situations (including play, shared book reading, and conversation).

Sessions #9 and #10

These sessions were less frequent than previous sessions, with 2 weeks in between them. Warm-ups were still used to achieve LJ's best voicing, but these sessions focused on using his target voice in situations as close to his daily life as possible. A friend was included to facilitate use of his voice with communication partners other than the clinician and parents. With parent permission, and accompanied by the parents, the clinician and patient went outside to a playground to use his target voice with more active play. While occasional reminders to use his "Captain America" voice were used, feedback was kept as sparse as possible to facilitate generalization.

Maintenance and Follow-Up. LJ's preschool teachers were provided with informa-tion regarding his voice therapy and strategies to help him with maintenance in the classroom. His parents reported confidence in helping him practice and with reminding him to use his target voice as much as possible.

Caveat Regarding the Nature of RRP and Voice Therapy

Due to frequent surgeries for removal of regrowth of RRP, he did return for "refreshers" of 1 to 3 sessions after a surgery, as he would occasionally revert to ventricular phonation. However, his return to target voice was rapid.

Summary

1. Do not assume the cause of a voice disorder based solely on history. This child had a known history of papilloma, so it could be assumed that his voice quality was due to the primary lesion. With careful probing, however, it was determined that he had capacity for better voicing and that the reason for his ventricular phonation was actually a secondary MTD. While MTD is not as common in children as in adults, it does occur, especially secondary to another cause for voice disorder.

2. Young children can participate in direct voice therapy and see benefits.

3. Involve relevant others. For children, the therapeutic relation is a triad of parent or caregiver, medical professional(s), and child. Caregivers are often responsible for carrying over therapy at home and should be trained and included in sessions.

4. Individualize therapy for the child. Including games and activities of high interest to the child, allowing them to provide vocabulary and input to name the voice, and engaging them directly in the process increases buy-in and engagement.

5. Voice therapy with a child often involves multiple approaches. In this case, indirect

therapy included education, counseling, parent training, and facilitation of carryover. Direct therapy included SOVT exercises, flow mode, and resonant voice.

> **CASE STUDY 4.7**
>
> **Interprofessional Assessment and Treatment for an Adult With Muscle Tension Dysphagia**
>
> Christina Kang Rosow

Evaluation

I had the pleasure of seeing this patient for a comprehensive evaluation of swallowing difficulties referred by the physician's assistant in the otolaryngology clinic. The patient was diagnosed with muscle tension dysphagia (MTDg).

Case History

Chief Complaint. Difficulty swallowing

History of Complaint. Patient W is a 46-year-old cisgender female who reported a gradual onset of dysphagia 2 years ago to all consistencies of food, worse with saliva and solid food consistencies. She reported fatigue of the neck muscles when eating or drinking.

She also reported having had a high fever 2 years ago accompanied by sore throat, odynophonia, occasional choking sensations, dysphonia, vocal strain, and a tickling sensation in the throat. Around the time she was ill, she also had high emotional stress, anxiety and a change in her job, and was completing a nursing degree. She reported worsening of her swallowing problem over the last 3 months. She went to the emergency department twice in the past 3 months due to difficulty swallowing as well as a persistent choking sensation. Patient W stated that the only thing that seemed to help was drinking alcohol or sucking on a cough drop.

Medical History. Patient W's medical history did not reveal any serious medical conditions. She denied a history of postnasal drip, allergies, and sinus infections. She did not smoke or drink alcohol. She consumed 64 ounces of water daily and 1 cup of coffee in the evening. She denied any history of eating disorders. She did not have any evidence of hearing loss. She reported having back and neck problems since being involved in a motor vehicle accident 8 years ago where she was "T-boned." On the day of the accident, she had an x-ray at the emergency department and was discharged with no further treatment recommendation.

Leading up to the onset of the swallowing problem, she reported having had severe stress for 8 years due to marital problems, which resulted in a divorce. Since her divorce, she has been taking medication for depression and anxiety. She briefly received psychotherapy after the divorce but discontinued. She did not find "talk therapy" helpful in dealing with the trauma of her divorce. She reported managing intermittent heartburn with over-the-counter antacids. She tried to eat "relatively healthy" but often ate just before bedtime whenever she worked late shifts.

Swallowing Assessments

Videofluoroscopic Swallow Study (VFSS)

No structural anomalies were noted in the upper aerodigestive tract. Oral, oropharyngeal, pharyngoesophageal, and esophageal phase of deglutition were normal as assessed by the Modified Barium Swallow Impairment Profile (MBSImP).[88] The patient initially exhibited a moderate fear of swallowing and frequently hesitated to initiate swallowing. This fear of swallowing initiation was successfully eliminated during videofluoroscopic swallow study (VFSS) by distracting her. She was instructed to watch the clinician's "conducting" hand gesture as a cue to swallow. She demonstrated no hesitation with distraction and verbalized that it was easier not to focus on the throat sensation when she swallowed. She maintained normal swallow initiation for the remainder of VFSS and was able to complete the test.

Gastroenterology Evaluation

Patient W was referred to the gastroenterology department and underwent a comprehensive gastroenterology evaluation including esophagogastroduodenoscopy (EGD) with normal findings and high-resolution esophageal manometry with stationary impedance with normal findings. She reported intermittent heartburn; therefore, she also underwent Bravo pH probe at the time of EGD. The test results did not indicate abnormal acid exposure, suggestive of absence of GERD. The gastroenterologist ruled out all causes for dysphagia to solid consistency by assessing for eosinophilic esophagitis, Schatzki's ring, peptic stricture causing esophageal mechanical obstruction, esophageal cancer, major esophageal motility disorders such as achalasia, esophagogastric junction outflow obstruction, distal esophageal spasm, Jackhammer esophagus, absent contractility, and hernia. Disorders affecting the esophagus such as pemphigoid and lichen planus were ruled out, as were potential neurological disorders that cause dysphagia.

Voice Evaluation

Patient W confirmed voice change secondary to her dysphagia complaint. She had a high-voice-demand job as a full-time nurse. She used her voice for about 8 to 10 hours per day, which involved teaching, educating patients, caring for people with hearing impairments, and parenting her own young children. She confirmed worsening voice quality with too much talking; however, she was more concerned about her swallow function than her vocal function.

Laryngeal Imaging

A videostrobolaryngoscopy was performed with the use of a high-definition fiber-optic distal-chip endoscope. The nasal cavity, nasopharynx, oropharynx, and hypopharynx were without masses or lesions. There was minimal evidence of nonspecific laryngeal inflammation, not suggestive of significant presence of reflux laryngitis. No vocal fold lesions were observed. Full mobility of the true vocal folds was appreciated with complete glottic closure. Vocal fold vibration was mildly reduced in amplitude and propagation of the mucosal wave. Vibration was aperiodic approximately 60% of the time. There were no masses or lesions within the visualized subglottis with a widely patent airway. With phonation, Patient W demonstrated a circumferential supraglottic compression, which reduced visibility of the glottis by at least 50%.

Acoustic and Aerodynamic Assessment

Acoustic data were gathered using the CSL (Pentax Medical, Montvale, NJ). A handheld Shure microphone was positioned at 15 cm from the mouth for data acquisition. Aerodynamic data were collected using the Pentax Medical PAS Model 6600 (Montvale, NJ) (Tables 4–6 to 4–9).

Stimulability Testing

The following probes yielded improvement in Patient W's symptoms:

1. A gentle circumlaryngeal massage was performed based on paralaryngeal assessment revealing (See Case Study 4.1: Manual Circumlaryngeal Techniques to Treat an Adult With Primary Muscle Tension Dysphonia) a severely reduced thyrohyoid membrane space and a moderately reduced lateral mobility of the thyroid cartilage. Upon completion of circumlaryngeal massage, the patient verbalized that it was "easier to swallow her saliva."
2. Resonant voice therapy[89] was also tried at the syllable and at /m/ initial word levels, and the patient achieved target resonant voice rather easily. (see Video 11 Resonant Voice Concepts by Kang Rosow)

The positive response from circumlaryngeal massage and easily achieved resonant voice were suggestive of rehabilitative potential.

Table 4–6. Pre- and Posttreatment Acoustic Measures

	Pretreatment	*Posttreatment*
F0: Sustained Phonation	218.53 Hz	249.44 Hz
F0: Conversation	177.78 Hz	178.93 Hz
F0: Variation	1.80%	0.99%
Noise-to-Harmonic Ratio	0.128	0.238
Jitter (in %)	2.01%	1.08%
Shimmer (in dB)	0.47 dB	0.23 dB
Pitch Range	75.51-679.21 Hz	52.72-896.77 Hz

Table 4–7. Pre- and Posttreatment Aerodynamic Measures

	Pretreatment	*Posttreatment*
Expiratory Volume	4.05 L	3.52 L
Maximum Phonation Time	11.92 sec	12.66 sec
Mean Peak Air Pressure	7.09 cmH_2O	5.99 cmH_2O
Mean Airflow During Voicing	0.41 L/sec	0.24 L/sec
Aerodynamic resistance	16.56 cmH_2O /L/sec	24.13 cmH_2O /L/sec
Mean SPL	84.18 dB	82.66 dB
Mean pitch	214.60 Hz	223.73 Hz

Table 4–8. Pre- and Posttreatment Patient-Reported Outcome Measures

	Pretreatment	*Posttreatment*
Eating Assessment Tool (EAT-10)	4	0
Voice Handicap Index (VHI-10)	27	20
Reflux Symptom Index (RSI)	17	11
Perceived Stress Scale (PSS 4)	7	9
Newcastle Laryngeal Hypersensitivity Questionnaire	14	17.4
Hospital Anxiety and Depression Scale	26	18
Dyspnea Index	22 with severe self-report	26 with moderate self-report

150 Voice Therapy: Clinical Case Studies

Table 4–9. Clinical Perceptual Measures: CAPE-V

	Pretreatment	Consistency	Posttreatment	Consistency
Overall Severity	24	Consistent	22	Intermittent
Roughness	15	Consistent	5	Intermittent
Breathiness	0	Consistent	0	Intermittent
Strain	34	Consistent	15	Intermittent
Pitch	28 reduced	Consistent	25	Intermittent
Loudness	35 reduced	Consistent	18	Intermittent
Resonance	Laryngeal tone	Consistent	Semi-oral tone	Consistent
Other Features	Glottal fry, breath holding, high clavicular breathing, fast rate of speech, speaking past her breath cycle	Consistent	Glottal fry	Intermittent

Impressions

The clinician observed muscle tension dysphagia (MTDg) and mild to moderately severe MTD. The patient demonstrated a good prognosis for rehabilitation. The patient expressed readiness and enthusiasm for therapy.

Plan of Care

Initiate voice therapy once a week for 8 weeks.

Long-Term Goal. Decrease excessive intrinsic and extrinsic laryngeal muscle activity during swallowing and communication events.

Short-Term Goals.

1. Independently utilize laryngeal massage as directed to facilitate free and flexible laryngeal and articulator function with 80% adherence.
2. Achieve 80% consistent implementation of low abdominal diaphragmatic breathing technique.

3. Achieve 80% consistent use of resonant voice therapy techniques across communication events.

Decision Making

Understanding Muscle Tension Dysphagia (MTDg). MTDg is an idiopathic swallowing problem described by Kang et al in 2016.[90] It is a patient-centered diagnosis that addresses a challenging group of patients who report a significant impact on quality of life due to swallowing difficulties, yet comprehensive assessment reveals **no** underlying etiology for the complaint. These patients often undergo multiple specialist evaluations with no diagnosis or treatment offered, thus resulting in increased anxiety and even fear of swallowing. As with its voice-related counterpart, muscle tension dysphonia, MTDg is thought to be a condition of muscle hyperactivity in the pharynx and the larynx. However, an improper or delayed diagnosis of dysphagia can have life-threatening consequences; therefore, a diagnosis of MTDg **must not** be made without a thorough laryngoscopic evaluation of the larynx and the pharynx, as well as assessment to rule out esophageal webbing, issues pertaining to the upper esophageal sphincter, and malignancies of gastroenterologic nature.[90,91]

As a diagnosis of exclusion, patients are defined as having MTDg if they have (1) swallowing difficulty as a primary complaint, (2) no physiologic and functional impairment evident on an instrumental swallow study, (3) no gastrointestinal and neurological causes of dysphagia, and (4) laryngeal function examination demonstrating significant laryngeal muscle tension. Patients are considered to have primary MTDg if they meet the above criteria and do not have any other contributing cause.

Patients are considered to have secondary MTDg if they meet the above criteria and have a contributing cause such as nonspecific laryngeal inflammation and/or a spectrum of muscle tension-based laryngeal disorders such as MTD, paradoxical vocal fold motion, chronic cough, chronic throat clearing, and globus pharyngeus.[90,91] The spectrum of muscle-tension-based laryngeal disorders may be evident during laryngoscopy in the form of the phonatory presence of plica ventricularis, medial-lateral supraglottic compression, and/or anterior-posterior supraglottic compression. Nonspecific laryngeal inflammation suggestive of presence of LPR may be evidenced by erythema or edema of the arytenoids, postcricoid region, and/or true vocal folds, as well as by interarytenoid pachydermia and hypopharyngeal wall cobblestoning.[90-93] Laryngoscopy may also reveal a hyperresponsiveness evidenced by increased adductory vocal fold movement during inspiration (>50% vocal fold adduction), quivering of the arytenoids, and/or excessive cough/gag.

Understanding the Combined Diagnosis of MTDg and MTD. Despite the patient presenting with a primary complaint of swallowing difficulty, she also presented with a mild to moderately severe dysphonia characterized by laryngeal tone focus and glottal fry. She demonstrated a significant phonorespiratory imbalance as evidenced by her tendency to hold her breath at length followed by shallow clavicular inhalation and speaking past her breath cycle. Her maladaptive phonatory function contributed to the maintenance of the excessive pharyngolaryngeal muscle tension with severely reduced thyrohyoid membrane space and a moderately reduced lateral mobility of the thyroid cartilage. Based on her aptitude for stimulability tasks, Patient W demonstrated good prognosis for rehabilitation aimed at unloading pharyngolaryngeal muscle tension that should eliminate her swallowing difficulty.

Plan of Care

During the initial evaluation, the clinician explained the potential causes of muscle tension dysphagia (MTDg) to solid consistencies. Although the patient did not feel that her voice was problematic, she verbalized understanding that her tendency to engage in laryngeal-focused voice may be one of the contributing factors that negatively affected her swallowing function. Patient W was scheduled for eight 50-minute therapy sessions 1 week apart, but she ultimately received only four 50-minute sessions over a 2-month period, noting she needed to cancel or reschedule many of the sessions due to scheduling constraints as a single mother with a full-time nursing job.

Intervention

Session #1

Short-Term Goal #1. Patient W exhibited visibly rigid strap muscles. Paralaryngeal assessment revealed a moderate rigidity of the upper trapezius, bilateral scalene, and bilateral sternocleidomastoid. The lateral mobility of the thyroid cartilage was moderately reduced.

Thyrohyoid space was severely reduced. The hyoid was placed posteriorly. The patient reported severe tenderness with palpation of the strap muscles. Circumlaryngeal massage was introduced with the goal of reducing extrinsic laryngeal muscle tension. The instructions were provided as follows:

- Submandibular massage: With index finger resting on chin, massage the space under the chin behind the jaw bone with the thumb. Keep the tongue relaxed inside the mouth. The goal is to have the area under the jaw "mushy."
- Massage the sternocleidomastoid muscles from the base of the earlobes down to the clavicle in circular motion. Also massage the scalene muscles by reaching across with the opposite hand.
- Place both hands on the thyroid cartilage and gently move it from side to side to gauge lateral mobility. Then gently push the thyroid cartilage to one side and hold for 30 seconds. Repeat on the other side.
- Find the thyroid notch (Adam's apple) with your index finger. With thumb and middle/index finger, slide horizontally back to thyrohyoid space. (Hint: Feel the slight indentation above the thyroid cartilage.) Massage the area clockwise in a small, circular motion.
- Using the same two fingers, with pressure, massage horizontally back and forth through the thyrohyoid space, making sure to come all the way forward where the space narrows by the thyroid notch.
- From the thyrohyoid space, glide down along the sides of the thyroid cartilage to the cricothyroid muscle. Reverse direction. Repeat multiple times.

Short-Term Goal #2. Patient W was instructed in a low abdominal diaphragmatic breathing technique to eliminate shallow clavicular breathing. She was instructed to exhale fully on /s/ phoneme by pulling her abdomen toward the spine. She was instructed to relax her abdomen when she could no longer produce the /s/ phoneme with exhalation, which resulted in circumferential rib cage and low abdominal expansion for diaphragmatic inhalation. She was told that the throat should feel wide and open, like the sensation of yawning, when engaging in diaphragmatic breathing.

Results of Session #1.

1. The patient reported 70% relief in swallowing difficulty after self-implementation of circumlaryngeal massage under clinical supervision. However, she complained of continued neck tightness and neck pain. Considering her past history of a motor vehicle accident, she was referred to physical therapy for assessment and treatment of possible delayed onset of pain after injury.

2. The patient demonstrated 50% competency in using low abdominal diaphragmatic breathing technique by the end of the session. She was cued to yawn frequently during the exercises to experience the sensation of open throat breathing.

Session #2

Short-Term Goal #3. Resonant voice therapy was initiated with the goal of reducing phonatory supraglottic muscle tension as observed during stroboscopic evaluation. Resonant voice therapy focuses on front-focused sound production with no perceivable laryngeal tension during phonation. The orofacial area feels "buzzy" while the throat feels "easy." The exercises were performed at the lip trilling, /m/ chanting, and /m/ initial word levels with emphasis on low abdominal diaphragmatic breathing.

Result of Session #2. The patient verbalized the ease of phonation during structured exercises and demonstrated an emerging resonant voice during spontaneous speech.

Session #3: Two Weeks Later

Patient W presented in good spirits and reported 90% improvement in her swallowing complaints at all times. She reported discomfort only with swallowing chicken. She started receiving physical therapy and chiropractic treatment by an outside provider to better accommodate her schedule. She reported a moderate improvement in her neck symptoms. In addition to physical therapy exercises, Patient W confirmed consistent implementation of the circumlaryngeal massage multiple times a day.

Paralaryngeal assessment revealed a moderate reduction in thyrohyoid membrane space. The clinician reviewed circumlaryngeal massage methods, which the patient performed with good technique via reverse demonstration.

With the goal of further reducing intrinsic laryngeal muscle tension with phonation while implementing low abdominal diaphragmatic breathing, Patient W was introduced to straw phonation exercises with water resistance, which were performed with a drinking straw in a cup half-filled with water. The patient initially made voiceless air bubbles in the cup with no difficulty; however, the air bubbles stopped when she attempted voicing on the /o/ vowel. She was asked to produce consistent air bubbles in the water while voicing. Although initially frustrated, she completed the task successfully with repeated trials with minimal clinical feedback. Water resistance was then taken away to segue into straw phonation without water, a semi-occluded vocal tract exercise task.[94] Patient W performed the exercises with emphasis on achievement of maximum orofacial vibratory tactile sensation. Once adequate technique was observed at modal pitch, pitch glides were introduced to stretch and contract the vocal ligaments.

There was a dramatic increase in oral tone focus observed following straw phonation exercises. Resonant voice therapy was performed at the lip trill, /m/ chanting, syllable, word, and sentence levels, which the patient performed with 90% accuracy independently by the end of the session. Patient W independently verbalized that she had been holding her breath during speaking as long as she could remember.

Session #4: One Month Later

Patient W returned for direct therapy after a monthlong absence and reported 100% efficiency in swallowing function. She demonstrated minimally rough voice quality with an oral tone focus. While she demonstrated glottal fry phonation intermittently and reported being aware of the habit, she also reported increased awareness of her tendency to hold her breath and noted that could contribute to the glottal fry. She had been working intensively in physical therapy for neck pain management and reported significant improvement in neck mobility and reduction in neck pain. She had also been receiving myotherapy per physical therapist recommendation and stated that it was helpful for pain management. She confirmed daily implementation of the circumlaryngeal massage and the resonant voice therapy exercises. Reassessment revealed an adequate thyrohyoid membrane presentation with good lateral mobility of the hyoid and the thyroid cartilage. Resonant voice therapy was performed at the conversational speech level with 90% accuracy and consistency. Patient W found the notion of "letting air come into the body by relaxing" helpful in reducing her breath-holding habit. She verbalized that she had the necessary tools to continue improving her voice and wished to be discharged from therapy, as her primary complaint of dysphagia had resolved to her satisfaction. She was assured that she may return for reassessment at any time.

Summary

Muscle tension dysphagia (MTDg) is a disorder of laryngeal muscle tension manifested as idiopathic functional dysphagia rather than as a voice or a breathing disorder.[90,91] A successful therapy outcome is dependent upon an individualized algorithm of care addressing all possible etiologies of the laryngeal muscle tension manifesting as a swallowing disorder: organic, physiologic, and emotional. Clinical experience has shown that an eclectic voice therapy approach targeting physiologic reduction of laryngeal muscle tension and reduction of laryngeal irritation via hygienic therapy provides best symptomatic relief.[95]

Patient W understood the multifactorial etiology of her disorder and took the initiative to address the physical and emotional aspects of her life that were previously neglected. After consulting her psychiatrist during a routine visit, she decided to undergo eye movement desensitization retraining (EMDR) therapy to manage her ongoing anxiety. Her remarkable aptitude for self-analysis and embracing challenges surely contributed to a successful recovery.

References

1. Hillman RE, Stepp CE, Van Stan JH, Zañartu M, Mehta DD. An updated theoretical framework for vocal hyperfunction. *Am J Speech Lang Pathol.* 2020;29(4):2254-2260. doi:10.1044/2020_AJSLP-20-00104
2. Morrison M, Rammage L. *The Management of Voice Disorders.* Singular Publishing; 1994.
3. Roy N, Ford CN, Bless DM. Muscle tension dysphonia and spasmodic dysphonia: The role of manual laryngeal tension reduction in diagnosis and management. *Ann Otol Rhinol Laryngol.* 1996;105(11):851-856. doi:10.1177/000348949610501102
4. Verdolini K, Rosen C, Branski R. *Classification Manual of Voice Disorders-I.* Lawrence Erlbaum; 2006.
5. Belafsky PC, Postma GN, Reulbach TR, Holland BW, Koufman JA. Muscle tension dysphonia as a sign of underlying glottal insufficiency. *Otolaryngol Head Neck Surg.* 2002;127(5):448-451. doi:10.1067/mhn.2002.128894
6. Halum SL, Koufman JA. The paresis podule. *Ear Nose Throat J.* 2005;84(10):624. doi:10.1177/014556130508401005
7. Roy N. Ventricular dysphonia following long-term endotracheal intubation: A case study. *J Otolaryngol.* 1994;23(3):189-193.
8. Aronson A. *Clinical Voice Disorders.* Thieme Medical Publishers; 1990.
9. Rammage LA, Nichol H, Morrison MD. The psychopathology of voice disorders. *Hum Commun Canada.* 1987;11(4):21-25.
10. Roy N, Bless D. Toward a theory of the dispositional bases of functional dysphonia and vocal nodules: Exploring the role of personality and emotional adjustment. In: Kent R, Ball M, eds. *The Handbook of Voice Quality Measurement.* Singular Publishing; 2000:461-480.
11. Roy N, Bless DM, Heisey D. Personality and voice disorders: A superfactor trait analysis. *J Speech Lang Hear Res.* 2000;43(3):749-768. doi:10.1044/jslhr.4303.749
12. Roy N, Bless DM, Heisey D. Personality and voice disorders: A multitrait-multidisorder analysis. *J Voice.* 2000;14(4):521-548. doi:10.1016/S0892-1997(00)80009-0
13. Koufman J, Blalock P. Vocal fatigue in the professional voice user: Bogart-Bacall syndrome. *Laryngoscope.* 1988;98(5). doi:10.1288/00005537-198805000-00003
14. Morrison MD, Nichol H, Rammage LA. Diagnostic criteria in functional dysphonia. *Laryngoscope.* 1986;96(1):1-8. doi:10.1288/00005537-198601000-00001
15. Morrison MD, Rammage LA. Muscle misuse voice disorders: Description and classification. *Acta Otolaryngol.* 1993;113(3):428-434. doi:10.3109/00016489309135839
16. Morrison M, Rammage L, Belisle G, Pullan C, Nichol H. Muscular tension dysphonia. *J Otolaryngol.* 1983;12(5):302-306.
17. Koufman JA, Blalock PD. Classification and approach to patients with functional voice disorders. *Ann Otol Rhinol Laryngol.* 1982;91(4):372-377. doi:10.1177/000348948209100409
18. Morrison M. Pattern recognition in muscle misuse voice disorders: How I do it. *J*

Voice. 1997;11(1):108-114. doi:10.1016/S08 92-1997(97)80031-8

19. Stepp CE, Lester-Smith RA, Abur D, Daliri A, Pieter Noordzij J, Lupiani AA. Evidence for auditory-motor impairment in individuals with hyperfunctional voice disorders. *J Speech Lang Hear Res.* 2017;60(6):1545-1550. doi:10.1044/2017_JSLHR-S-16-0282

20. Lieberman J, Rubin J, Harris S, Fourcin A. Laryngeal manipulation. In: Rubin J, Sataloff R, Korovin G, eds. *Diagnosis and Treatment of Voice Disorders.* 2nd ed. ThomsonDelmar; 2003:561-582.

21. Roy N, Bless D. Manual circumlaryngeal techniques in the assessment and treatment of voice disorders. *Curr Opin Otolaryngol Head Neck Surg.* 1998;6:151-155. doi:10.10 97/00020840-199806000-00002

22. Roy N. Functional voice disorders. In: Kent R, ed. *MIT Encyclopedia of Voice Disorders.* MIT Press; 2004:27-30.

23. Lieberman J. Principles and techniques of manual therapy: Application in the management of dysphonia. In: Harris T, Harris S, Rubin J, Howard D, eds. *The Voice Clinical Handbook.* Whurr; 1998:91-138.

24. Rubin JS, Blake E, Mathieson L. Musculoskeletal patterns in patients with voice disorders. *J Voice.* 2007;21(4):477-484. doi:10.10 16/j.jvoice.2005.02.001

25. Boone D, McFarlane S. *The Voice and Voice Therapy.* Allyn & Bacon; 2000.

26. Sapir S. The intrinsic pitch of vowels: Theoretical, physiological, and clinical considerations. *J Voice.* 1989;3(1):44-51. doi:10.1016/ S0892-1997(89)80121-3

27. Roy N, Nissen SL, Dromey C, Sapir S. Articulatory changes in muscle tension dysphonia: Evidence of vowel space expansion following manual circumlaryngeal therapy. *J Commun Disord.* 2009;42(2):124-135. doi:10.1016/j .jcomdis.2008.10.001

28. Articulatory L, Higgins MB, Schulte L. Vowel-related differences in laryngeal articulatory and phonatory function. 1998;41: 712-724.

29. McClean MD, Tasko SM. Association of orofacial with laryngeal and respiratory motor output during speech. *Exp Brain Res.* 2002;

146(4):481-489. doi:10.1007/s00221-002-1187-5

30. Dromey C, Nissen SL, Roy N, Merrill RM. Articulatory changes following treatment of muscle tension dysphonia: Preliminary acoustic evidence. *J Speech Lang Hear Res.* 2008;51(1):196-208. doi:10.1044/1092-4388 (2008/015)

31. Lawrence V. Suggested criteria for fibreoptic diagnosis of vocal hyperfunction. In: *Care of the Professional Voice Symposium;* London, UK; 1987.

32. Behrman A, Dahl LD, Abramson AL, Schutte HK. Anterior-posterior and medial compression of the supraglottis: Signs of nonorganic dysphonia or normal postures? *J Voice.* 2003;17(3):403-410. doi:10.1067/ S0892-1997(03)00018-3

33. Leonard R, Kendall K. Differentiation of spasmodic and psychogenic dysphonias with phonoscopic evaluation. *Laryngoscope.* 1999;109(2):295-300. doi:10.1097/00005537-199902000-00022

34. Sama A, Carding PN, Price S, Kelly P, Wilson JA. The clinical features of functional dysphonia. *Laryngoscope.* 2001;111(3):458-463. doi:10.1097/00005537-200103000-00015

35. Schneider B, Wendler J, Seidner W. The relevance of stroboscopy in functional dysphonias. *Folia Phoniatr Logop.* 2002;54(1):44-54. doi:10.1159/000048595

36. Desjardins M, Apfelbach C, Rubino M, Abbott KV. Integrative review and framework of suggested mechanisms in primary muscle tension dysphonia. *J Speech Lang Hear Res.* 2022;65(5):1867-1893. doi:10.10 44/2022_JSLHR-21-00575

37. Roy N, Bless DM, Heisey D, Ford CN. Manual circumlaryngeal therapy for functional dysphonia: An evaluation of short- and long-term treatment outcomes. *J Voice.* 1997;11(3):321-331. doi:10.1016/S0892-19 97(97)80011-2

38. Roy N, Leeper HA. Effects of the manual laryngeal musculoskeletal tension reduction technique as a treatment for functional voice disorders: Perceptual and acoustic measures. *J Voice.* 1993;7(3):242-249. doi:10.1016/S0 892-1997(05)80333-9

39. Van Lierde KM, De Ley S, Clement G, De Bodt M, Van Cauwenberge P. Outcome of laryngeal manual therapy in four Dutch adults with persistent moderate-to-severe vocal hyperfunction: A pilot study. *J Voice*. 2004;18(4):467-474. doi:10.1016/j.jvoice.2004.02.003

40. Awan SN, Roy N, Zhang D, Cohen SM. Validation of the Cepstral Spectral Index of Dysphonia (CSID) as a Screening Tool for Voice Disorders: Development of Clinical Cutoff Scores. *J Voice*. 2016;30(2):130-144. doi: 10.1016/j.jvoice.2015.04.009

41. Rezaee Rad A, Moradi N, Yazdi MJSZ, Soltani M, Mehravar M, Latifi SM. Efficacy of manual circumlaryngeal therapy in patients with muscle tension dysphonia. *Shiraz E Med J*. 2018;19(7):e64478. doi:10.5812/semj.64478

42. Aghadoost S, Jalaie S, Khatoonabadi AR, Dabirmoghaddam P, Khoddami SM. A study of vocal facilitating techniques compared to manual circumlaryngeal therapy in teachers with muscle tension dysphonia. *J Voice*. 2020;34(6):963.e11-963.e21. doi:10.1016/j.jvoice.2019.06.002

43. Dehqan A, Scherer RC. Positive effects of manual circumlaryngeal therapy in the treatment of muscle tension dysphonia (MTD): Long term treatment outcomes. *J Voice*. 2019;33(6):866-871. doi:10.1016/j.jvoice.2018.07.010

44. Kim J. Effects of laryngeal massage on muscle tension dysphonia: A systematic review and meta-analysis. 2021;32(2):64-74. *J Korean Soc Larygol Phoniatr Logop*. 2021;32(2):64-74.

45. Barsties V, Latoszek B, Watts CR, Hetjens S. The efficacy of the manual circumlaryngeal therapy for muscle tension dysphonia: A systematic review and meta-analysis. *Laryngoscope*. 2023;134(1):18-26. doi:10.1002/lary.30850

46. Tierney WS, Xiao R, Milstein CF. Characterization of functional dysphonia: Pre- and post-treatment findings. *Laryngoscope*. 2021;131(6):E1957-E1964. doi:10.1002/lary.29358

47. Roy N. Functional dysphonia. *Curr Opin Otolaryngol Head Neck Surg*. 2003;11(3):144-148.

48. Mathieson L, Hirani SP, Epstein R, Baken RJ, Wood G, Rubin JS. Laryngeal manual therapy: A preliminary study to examine its treatment effects in the management of muscle tension dysphonia. *J Voice*. 2009;23(3):353-366. doi:10.1016/j.jvoice.2007.10.002

49. Kempster GB, Gerratt BR, Abbott KV, Barkmeier-Kraemer J, Hillman RE. Consensus auditory-perceptual evaluation of voice: Development of a standardized clinical protocol. *Am J Speech Lang Pathol*. 2009;18(2):124-132. doi:10.1044/1058-0360(2008/08-0017)

50. Rosen CA, Lee AS, Osborne J, Zullo T, Murry T. Development and validation of the voice handicap index-10. *Laryngoscope*. 2004;114(9 I):1549-1556. doi:10.1097/00005537-200409000-00009

51. Arffa RE, Krishna P, Gartner-Schmidt J, Rosen CA. Normative values for the Voice Handicap Index-10. *J Voice*. 2012;26(4):462-465. doi:10.1016/j.jvoice.2011.04.006

52. Awan SN, Roy N, Jetté ME, Meltzner GS, Hillman RE. Quantifying dysphonia severity using a spectral/cepstral-based acoustic index: Comparisons with auditory-perceptual judgements from the CAPE-V. *Clin Linguist Phon*. 2010;24(9):742-758. doi:10.3109/02699206.2010.492446

53. Lewandowski A, Gillespie AI, Kridgen S, Jeong K, Yu L, Gartner-Schmidt J. Adult normative data for phonatory aerodynamics in connected speech. *Laryngoscope*. 2018;128(4):909-914. doi:10.1002/lary.26922

54. Verdolini Abbott K. *Lessac-Madsen Resonant Voice Therapy Clinician Manual*. Plural Publishing, Inc.; 2008

55. Sundberg J. Objective characterization of phonation type using amplitude of flow glottogram pulse and of voice source fundamental. *J Voice*. 2022;36(1):4-14. doi:10.1016/j.jvoice.2020.03.018

56. Colton R, Casper J, Hirano M. *Understanding Voice Problems*. Williams and Wilkins; 1996.

57. Verdolini-Marston K, Burke M, Lessac A, Glaze L, Caldwell E. Preliminary study of two methods of treatment for laryngeal nodules. *ISTM/2005 6th Int Symp Test Meas Vols 1-9, Conf Proc*. 1995;9(1):74-85.

58. Gartner-Schmidt J, Gherson S, Hapner ER, et al. The development of conversation

training therapy: A concept paper. *J Voice.* 2016;30(5):563-573. doi:10.1016/j.jvoice.2015.06.007

59. Gillespie AI, Yabes J, Rosen CA, Gartner-Schmidt JL. Efficacy of conversation training therapy for patients with benign vocal fold lesions and muscle tension dysphonia compared to historical matched control patients. *J Speech Lang Hear Res.* 2019;62(11):4062-4079. doi:10.1044/2019_JSLHR-S-19-0136

60. Helou LB, Gartner-Schmidt JL, Hapner ER, Schneider SL, Van Stan JH. Mapping meta-therapy in voice interventions onto the rehabilitation treatment specification system. *Semin Speech Lang.* 2021;42(1):5-18. doi:10.1055/s-0040-1722756

61. Helou LB, Welch B, Hoch S, Gartner-Schmidt J. Self-reported stress, trauma, and prevalence of laryngoresponders in the general population. *J Speech Lang Hear Res.* 2023;66(7):2230-2245. doi:10.1044/2023_JSLHR-22-00669

62. Roy N, Barkmeier-Kraemer J, Eadie T, et al. Evidence-based clinical voice assessment: A systematic review. *Am J Speech Lang Pathol.* 2013;22(2):212-226. doi:10.1044/1058-0360(2012/12-0014)

63. Nanjundeswaran C, Jacobson BH, Gartner-Schmidt J, Verdolini Abbott K. Vocal Fatigue Index (VFI): Development and validation. *J Voice.* 2015;29(4):433-440. doi:10.1016/j.jvoice.2014.09.012

64. Stemple JC, Roy N, Klaben KB, eds. *Clinical Voice Pathology: Theory and Management.* 6th ed, Plural Publishing; 2020:220-221.

65. Verdolini K, Druker DG, Palmer PM, Samawi H. Laryngeal adduction in resonant voice. *J Voice.* 1998;12(3):315-327. doi:10.1016/S0892-1997(98)80021-0

66. Aronson A. *Clinical Voice Disorders: An Interdisciplinary Approach.* Thieme; 1990.

67. McCullough G, Zraick R, Balou S, Pickett H, Rangarathnam B, Tulunay-Ugur O. Treatment of laryngeal hyperfunction with flow phonation: A pilot study. *J Laryngol Voice.* 2012;2(2):64. doi:10.4103/2230-9748.106980

68. van Leer E, Connor NP. Patient perceptions of voice therapy adherence. *J Voice.* 2010;24(4):458-469. doi:10.1016/j.jvoice.2008.12.009

69. Gartner-Schmidt JL, Roth DF, Zullo TG, Rosen CA. Quantifying component parts of indirect and direct voice therapy related to different voice disorders. *J Voice.* 2013;27(2):210-216. doi:10.1016/j.jvoice.2012.11.007

70. Jacobson BH, Johnson A, Grywalski C, et al. The Voice Handicap Index (VHI): Development and validation. *Am J Speech Lang Pathol.* 1997;6(3):66-69. doi:10.1044/1058-0360.0603.66

71. Baken R, Orlikoff R. *Clinical Measurement of Speech and Voice.* 2nd ed. Cengage Learning; 1999.

72. *Iowa head and neck protocols.* University of Iowa Healthcare. https://medicine.uiowa.edu/iowaprotocols/voice-clinic. Published 2018. Accessed June 20, 2023.

73. Roy N, Weinrich B, Gray SD, Tanner K, Stemple JC, Sapienza CM. Three treatments for teachers with voice disorders: A randomized clinical trial. *J Speech Lang Hear Res.* 2003;46(3):670-688. doi:10.1044/1092-4388(2003/053)

74. Boseley ME, Cunningham MJ, Volk MS, Hartnick CJ. Validation of the pediatric voice-related quality-of-life survey. *Arch Otolaryngol Head Neck Surg.* 2006;132(7):717-720. doi:10.1001/archotol.132.7.717

75. Kent RD, Eichhorn JT, Vorperian HK. Acoustic parameters of voice in typically developing children ages 4–19 years. *Int J Pediatr Otorhinolaryngol.* 2021;142:110614. doi:10.1016/j.ijporl.2021.110614

76. Demirci AN, Köse A, Aydinli FE, İncebay Ö, Yilmaz T. Investigating the cepstral acoustic characteristics of voice in healthy children. *Int J Pediatr Otorhinolaryngol.* 2021;148:110815. doi:10.1016/j.ijporl.2021.110815

77. Kent SAK, Fletcher TL, Morgan A, Morton M, Hall RJ, Sandage MJ. Updated acoustic normative data through the lifespan: A scoping review. *J Voice.* 2023. doi:10.1016/j.jvoice.2023.02.011

78. Weinrich B, Brehm SB, Knudsen C, McBride S, Hughes M. Pediatric normative data for the KayPentax phonatory aerodynamic system model 6600. *J Voice.* 2013;27(1):46-56. doi:10.1016/j.jvoice.2012.09.001

79. Hoffman MR, Scholp AJ, Hedberg CD, et al. Measurement reliability of phonation

threshold pressure in pediatric subjects. *Laryngoscope.* 2019;129(7):1520-1526. doi:10.1002/lary.27418

80. Derkay C, Bluher A. Update on recurrent respiratory papillomatosis. *Otolaryngol Clin North Am.* 2019;52(4):669-679.

81. Benedict JJ, Derkay CS. Recurrent respiratory papillomatosis: A 2020 perspective. *Laryngoscope Investig Otolaryngol.* 2021;6(2):340-345. doi:10.1002/lio2.545

82. Verma H, Solanki P, James M. Acoustical and perceptual voice profiling of children with recurrent respiratory papillomatosis. *J Voice.* 2016;30(5):600-605. doi:10.1016/j.jvoice.2015.06.008

83. Maturo S, Hartnick CJ. Use of 532-nm pulsed potassium titanyl phosphate laser and adjuvant intralesional bevacizumab for aggressive respiratory papillomatosis in children: Initial experience. *Arch Otolaryngol Head Neck Surg.* 2010;136(6):561-565. doi:10.1001/archoto.2010.81

84. Maturo S, Tse SM, Kinane TB, Hartnick CJ. Initial experience using propranolol as an adjunctive treatment in children with aggressive recurrent respiratory papillomatosis. *Ann Otol Rhinol Laryngol.* 2011;120(1):17-20. doi:10.1177/000348941112000103

85. Derkay C. Task force on recurrent respiratory papillomas: A preliminary report. *Arch Otolaryngol Head Neck Surg.* 1995;121(12):1386-1391.

86. Feinstein H, Verdolini Abbott K. Vocal fold lesions in children: A systematic review. *Am J Speech Lang Pathol.* 2021;30:772-788.

87. Stone R, Casteel R. *Intervention in Non-Organically Based Dysphonia.* CC Thomas; 1982.

88. Martin-Harris B, Brodsky MB, Michel Y, et al. MBS measurement tool for swallow impairment-MBSimp: Establishing a standard. *Dysphagia.* 2008;23(4):392-405. doi:10.1007/s00455-008-9185-9

89. Verdolini Abbott K. Lessac-Madsen Resonant Voice Therapy. In Stemple JC, ed: *Voice Therapy: Clinical Case Studies.* 2nd ed. Singular Publishing; 2000.

90. Kang CH, Hentz JG, Lott DG. Muscle tension dysphagia: Symptomology and theoretical framework. 2016;155(5):837-842. doi:10.1177/0194599816657013

91. Kang CH, Zhang N, Lott DG. Muscle tension dysphagia: Contributing factors and treatment efficacy. *Ann Otol Rhinol Laryngol.* 2021;130(7):674-681. doi:10.1177/0003489420966339

92. Koufman JA, Block C. Differential diagnosis of paradoxical vocal fold movement. *Am J Speech Lang Pathol.* 2008;17(4):327-334. doi:10.1044/1058-0360(2008/07-0014)

93. Patel NJ, Jorgensen C, Kuhn J, Merati AL. Concurrent laryngeal abnormalities in patients with paradoxical vocal fold dysfunction. *Otolaryngol Head Neck Surg.* 2004;130(6):686-689. doi:10.1016/j.otohns.2004.01.003

94. Titze IR. Voice training and therapy with a semi-occluded vocal tract: Rationale and scientific underpinnings. *Hear Res.* 2006;49(4):448-460.

95. Angadi V, Stemple J. New frontiers and emerging technologies in comprehensive voice care. *Perspect Voice Voice Disord.* 2012;22(2):72-79. doi:10.1044/vvd22.2.72

5

Glottal Gaps

Introduction

Aaron Ziegler

The valving action of the vocal folds (ie, phonatory closure pattern) causes disturbances in air pressure and transforms aerodynamic energy into acoustic energy, ultimately perceived as voice.[1] Two physiological mechanisms govern vocal fold closure during voicing. The first mechanism involves muscular contraction of intrinsic laryngeal muscles—namely, the lateral cricoarytenoid (LCA) and interarytenoid (IA) muscles—to draw the vocal folds together (ie, adduction) and narrow the space between them (ie, glottis). The second mechanism occurs as the membranous portion of the vocal folds (ie, mucosa) closes during self-sustained vibration. In a vocally healthy individual, the vocal folds fully approximate during voicing and spend roughly half of the vibratory cycle in a closing and closed phase. A problem with either or both valving mechanisms—that is, impaired vocal fold adduction or impaired vocal fold vibration—can lead to glottal dysfunction and dysphonia. This chapter illustrates the utility of voice therapy for glottal dysfunction in a collection of patient cases to help with decision making in patient care.[2]

Either in isolation or in combination, glottal dysfunction can arise from abnormal vocal fold structure, neurophysiological impairments, and abnormal volitional production of voice because of learned muscle tension patterns (Table 5–1). Together, they impair the vocal folds' aeromechanical valving action and result in inconsistent and incomplete closure of the vocal folds during voicing. The effects of glottal dysfunction are multidimensional, impacting fundamental frequency, vocal intensity, voice quality, and vocal endurance. Patients may demonstrate a breathy quality as minimum transglottal airflow increases or reduced vocal intensity as less aerodynamic energy converts to acoustic energy, both of which occur with poor valving action of the vocal folds. Roughness or diplophonia may be heard in the voice as the vocal folds demonstrate cycle-to-cycle variability or multiple modes of vibration, both of which can occur with a change in vocal fold tone or structure. As patients "work" to increase vocal fold closure during voicing, they may report that their voice fatigues quickly due to increased vocal effort. Discomfort with voicing may be a problem as patients increase activation of intrinsic and extrinsic laryngeal musculature to compensate for glottal dysfunction. This increased

Table 5–1. Classification Scheme for Glottal Dysfunction

Glottal Insufficiency: an anatomical or structural abnormality that results in a glottal gap between the vocal folds and insufficient vocal fold closure

> Examples: sulcus vocalis or scar, vocal fold atrophy, space-occupying vocal fold lesions (nodules, polyps, cysts, malignancies)

Glottal Incompetence: a neuromotor or physiological disorder that results in poor, "incompetent" movement and incomplete closure of the vocal folds

> Examples: cranial nerve X (vagus) deficits (ie, unilateral or bilateral, partial or complete; recurrent laryngeal nerve deficit, unilateral or bilateral, partial or complete; superior laryngeal nerve deficit of the external branch), myasthenia gravis, cerebral or brainstem tumors, cerebral vascular accidents

Glottal Mislearning: lack of capable vocal fold movement in the absence of anatomical vocal fold pathology, and without obvious neuromotor abnormality, that results in inadequate and inconsistent vocal fold closure

> Examples: primary muscle tension dysphonia, secondary muscle tension dysphonia

muscle tension to improve closure or tone typically increases fundamental frequency and perceptually raises the pitch of the voice.

The emerging corpus of evidence is mixed on the benefits of voice therapy. Successful management of glottal dysfunction with voice therapy depends on a number of factors, mainly related to the nature of the dysfunction. In cases of glottal insufficiency, loss of vocal fold tissue (ie, muscle atrophy and thinning of the lamina propria) precludes adequate vocal fold closure during voicing, and a space is present between the 2 concave-appearing vocal folds in the case of age-related vocal fold changes or, in the case of sulcus vocalis, a space in which the nature depends on the location and severity of lamina propria defect. Several approaches to voice therapy demonstrate benefit for glottal insufficiency.[3-5] Vocal Function Exercises (VFEs) and Phonation Resistance Training Exercises (PhoRTE®), for example, are effective voice therapy programs for patients whose glottal insufficiency is from mild-moderate age-related voice changes that occur in presbylarynges.[6-8] Case Study 5.2 by Ziegler and Hapner highlights the use of PhoRTE®

in age-related voice changes. Case Study 5.4 by Dietrich highlights the use of VFEs, while Case Study 5.1 by Bonilha and Desjardins highlights inspiratory muscle strength training (IMST) and voice therapy, and Case Study 5.3 by Lloyd and Murljacic discusses expiratory muscle strength training (EMST) in conjunction with voice therapy, all demonstrating promise for rehabilitation of presbyphonia.[9] In Case Study 5.6, Timmons Sund highlights the use of multimodality therapy via telehealth in the treatment of glottal incompetence due to unilateral vocal fold paresis in a singer.

Voice therapy whose goal is to improve quality, however, would likely be ineffective in restoring voice for a large glottal insufficiency associated with type 3 sulcus vocalis (ie, a loss of lamina propria all the way to the vocal ligament), for example. This glottal insufficiency results in a large space between the vocal folds and poor vibratory closure due to considerable stiffness of the vocal fold mucosa. In Case Study 5.7, Gillespie and Rosen discuss a patient with sulcus vocalis who attempts therapy but is unsuccessful in carryover into her vocally intensive life and requires vocal fold augmentation. As will be discussed, while not trying to improve voice quality, voice therapy can provide patients with improved voicing efficiency after surgery to correct a large glottal insufficiency thus reducing vocal effort and increasing vocal endurance.[10]

The success of voice therapy in cases of glottal incompetence also varies. Glottal incompetence refers to neuromotor or physiological disorders that result in "incompetent" vocal fold movement and incomplete closure of the vocal folds during adduction. Glottal incompetence is often due to complete or partial paralysis (ie, paresis) of one or both of the recurrent laryngeal nerves that leads to limitations in lateral-medial movement of the vocal folds (ie, incompetent vocal fold adduction). The vocal process of the paralyzed vocal fold would not approximate the vocal process of its nonparalytic, mobile counterpart. The size and nature of glottal incompetence depends on the degree to which the paralyzed vocal fold is positioned laterally. Voice therapy will benefit a patient with a complete vocal fold paralysis if the immobile vocal fold is in a median position.[11] The resulting glottal incompetence is minimal, and the glottal dysfunction is addressable with a favorable position of the immobile vocal fold. As will be discussed in the chapter cases, patients with glottal incompetence may be stimulable for improvement with voice therapy techniques. Although only one mobile vocal fold is necessary for voicing, the vocal folds must be approximated closely enough for vibration to occur. Patients who demonstrate small to moderate glottal incompetence are likely to respond better to voice therapy than those whose paralyzed vocal fold is positioned laterally and glottal incompetence is substantial. Accordingly, the role of voice therapy in glottal incompetence is typically part of a multidisciplinary approach to dysphonia management.[12,13] The multidisciplinary voice team must collaborate to maximally restore vocal function and achieve satisfactory treatment outcomes. In Case Study 5.5, Gutierrez and Hoffman discuss a case of a patient who needs both voice therapy and surgical intervention for effective voice use. Voice therapy in cases of vocal fold paralysis/paresis provides direct interventions that help patients adapt to voice changes as a result of glottal dysfunction, rather than developing hyperfunctional compensatory behaviors.[14] Early initiation of voice therapy may yield better treatment outcomes in cases of glottal incompetence due to unilateral vocal fold paralysis/paresis.[15,16]

> Ziegler uses the term glottal dysfunction to encompass glottal insufficiency, glottal incompetence, and glottal mislearning, with specific definitions and examples of each detailed in Table 5–1. In practice, many clinicians use the terms glottal insufficiency and glottal incompetence interchangeably, and this is observed throughout the cases of this chapter.

Case Studies

CASE STUDY 5.1

Inspiratory Muscle Strength Training to Augment Vocal Function Exercises in an Adult With Presbyphonia

Heather Bonilha and Maude Desjardins

Voice Evaluation

Case History

Mr. Fraco, a 68-year-old cisgender man, self-referred to the voice center with weak, breathy voice quality and difficulty speaking loudly or for extended periods. These issues affected his work, causing concerns about early retirement, and exacerbated communication problems with his partner, who had age-related hearing loss.

On reflection, the patient reported that signs of voice weakening began a year ago, initially impacting communication with his partner and now causing daily frustration. A recent comment from a fellow salesman about sounding like an old man prompted him to seek treatment. The medical history did not indicate surgical or viral causes. The patient had no smoking history, occasional alcohol consumption, and reported daily coffee and water intake. No comorbidities or medications were reported.

Voice Use. Like many older gentlemen, Mr. Fraco maintained a full-time job, as a salesman, with moderate to high voice use demands. He shared a fulfilling social life with his partner, enjoying gatherings with friends and family. However, due to the need to preserve his voice for work and struggles with background noise, he reluctantly started declining social invitations, leading to frustration. Maintaining an active lifestyle, Mr. Fraco and his partner embarked on weekend hikes with friends. He noticed a growing breathlessness while speaking during these outings but was unsure if it was related to his voice issue.

> Mr. Fraco is a pseudonym, as are all names in this text. "Fraco" means "weak" in Portuguese, a piece of information to make the reader smile.

Laryngeal Imaging

Rigid endoscopy with stroboscopy was performed to evaluate vocal fold structure and function across a range of pitch and loudness levels. As the patient presented with a slightly higher than expected pitch when speaking and reduced loudness, the clinician began the exam at these levels. Upon visualization, there was apparent bowing of the vocal folds (concave rather than straight vocal fold edges during inhalation) associated with a mild spindle-shaped glottal gap. Amplitude and mucosal wave appeared within normal limits (WNL) (60% and 60, respectively, as scored on

the Voice-Vibratory Assessment with Laryngeal Imaging [VALI]).[17] When the patient was instructed to phonate at a lower pitch (WNL for age and gender), the glottal gap was characterized as moderate. This indicates the increase in pitch was likely a compensatory strategy to achieve better vocal fold closure; however, the patient did not report volitionally using this strategy or awareness of increased pitch. During phonation at lower pitch (WNL for age and gender), amplitude and mucosal wave were larger than normal limits (80% and 80, respectively, as scored on the VALI), commensurate with the visualized vocal fold atrophy. Without the cricothyroid (CT) involvement during phonation at higher pitch levels, the reduced vocal fold integrity associated with atrophy was apparent. Further examination of the patient's laryngeal imaging sample revealed a predominantly open phase closure (on average, 86% of the cycle was open). The clinician next trialed this lower (WNL for age and gender) pitch with increased loudness after a larger breath, which resulted in a slightly decreased glottal gap. Mediolateral and anteroposterior supraglottic involvement were also noted during sustained phonation and were characterized as moderately severe (ratings of 3 on the VALI).

> As described in this case and in the introduction by Ziegler, increasing vocal fold tension via CT engagement is a subconscious but common compensatory strategy to reduce glottal gap. This compensation is often seen in patients with a glottal gap secondary to vocal fold atrophy or unilateral vocal fold immobility. When the patient disengages the CT muscles, the glottal gap may increase in size and yield a breathier voice.

Bowing Index. The Bowing Index (BI) was used to objectively measure vocal fold atrophy before and after treatment. BI is calculated using a formula described in previous literature,[18] which compares the maximum distance between the actual vocal fold edge and a hypothetical straight vocal fold edge to the length of the membranous vocal fold. For the right vocal fold, the BI was 8.64, and for the left vocal fold, it was 8.15. These values fall within 1 standard deviation of the mean BI for males with presbyphonia (mean = 10.07, SD = 5.10),[19] indicating moderate vocal fold atrophy.

Quality-of-Life Impairment

The clinician assessed the functional impact of the voice problem using 3 validated questionnaires. Mr. Fraco had a score of 15 on the Voice Handicap Index–10 (VHI-10) and a score of 10 on the Glottal Function Index (GFI), both above cutoff values for meaningful functional difficulties (11 and 4, respectively).[20,21] To get a more specific portrait of the voice problem's impact in various communication situations, Mr. Fraco filled out the Communicative Participation Item Bank General (CPIB) Short Form.[22] The score was 16 (best score = 30, worst score = 0), and answers revealed participation difficulties especially in situations involving long utterances and/or speaking durations.

Auditory-Perceptual Assessment

The patient received an overall score of 55/100 on the Consensus Auditory-Perceptual Evaluation of Voice (CAPE-V),[23] indicating a dysphonia of a moderate nature. Aberrant perceptual features identified in the voice included primary breathiness and secondary strain. Overall vocal loudness was noted to be below normal limits. Pitch of the voice was slightly above limits for age and gender. Resonance was focused in the laryngeal region. Respiration was primarily thoracic.

Acoustic and Aerodynamic Assessment

Table 5–2 displays Mr. Fraco's values for different acoustic measures, which were recorded using the Multi-Dimensional Voice Program Advanced (MDVP) and the Computerized Speech Laboratory (CSL) (Pentax Medical, Montvale, NJ). At pretreatment, voice quality during a sustained vowel (/a/) was characterized by a noise-to-harmonic (NHR) ratio WNL for elderly males and an amplitude perturbation quotient (APQ) slightly outside normal values.[24] Although reference values for smoothed cepstral peak prominence (CPPS) were not available for the patient's specific demographic group, vocal quality during reading was well below the normative range for vocally healthy adult speakers,[25] further corroborating the effects of age-related anatomical changes on laryngeal function. A sound pressure level of 62.9 dB was recorded during spontaneous speech, with a handheld microphone placed at 5.5 inches and 45 degrees from the patient's mouth.

Mr. Fraco's aerodynamic assessment was performed using the Voicing Efficiency program from the Phonatory Aerodynamic System (PAS) (Pentax Medical, Montvale, NJ). His

Table 5–2. Acoustic and Auditory-Perceptual Pretreatment and Posttreatment Measures

Timepoint	SPL in Spontaneous Speech (dB)	CPPS in Reading (dB)	NHR /a/	APQ /a/ (%)	Overall Severity (VAS 100 mm)
Preintervention	62.9	15.71	0.15	3.75	55
Postintervention	70.9	16.57	0.12	2.63	28
Reference Values	74.4 (SD = 3.5)	20.11 (SD = 1.27)	0.14 (SD = 0.02)	3.04 (0.37)	—

results were compared to normative data for elderly males[26,27] and revealed a mean airflow rate in the upper range, a subglottal pressure WNL, and a laryngeal resistance in the extreme lower range. Combined with the laryngeal imaging results, these values indicate a profile of glottal incompetence and suggest high respiratory effort to attain subglottal pressure WNL (Table 5–3).

Respiratory Assessment

Considering Mr. Fraco's older age, profile of glottal incompetence, and complaints of dyspnea during speech, the clinician performed a respiratory screening to assess whether decreased respiratory function could be a compounding factor in his voice symptoms, as has been shown in others seeking treatment for presbyphonia.[19] All respiratory assessments were performed by a speech-language pathologist (SLP) who had been trained accordingly by the department of pulmonology in the medi-cal center. Respiratory muscle strength was assessed with a handheld respiratory pressure meter (MicroRPM, MD Spiro, Lewiston, ME) by asking the patient to breathe in and breathe out as forcefully as possible into the device to obtain a correlate of maximal strength. The maximum inspiratory pressure (MIP) recorded suggested an inspiratory strength slightly below the reference value based on Mr. Fraco's age, sex, and weight, but not below the lower limit of normal (LLN).[28] A similar result was obtained for maximal expiratory pressure (MEP). Spirometry assessment was performed using a computer-based spirometer (KokoSx, NSPIRE Health, Longmont, CO) to screen for any substantial declines in pulmonary health. Results revealed a forced vital capacity (FVC) and forced expiratory volume in 1 second (FEV$_1$) slightly above 80% of predicted values based on the patient's profile, and a FEV$_1$/FVC ratio that was not suggestive of airflow limitation (Table 5–4).

Table 5–3. Aerodynamic Pretreatment and Posttreatment Measures

Timepoint	Mean Airflow (L/sec)	Mean Peak Air Pressure (cmH$_2$O)	Laryngeal Resistance (cmH$_2$O/L/sec)
Preintervention	0.31	7.00	22.58
Postintervention	0.14	6.26	44.71
Reference Values	0.15 (SD = 0.18)	6.31 (SD = 1.94)	38.11 (SD = 7.46)

Table 5–4. Respiratory Pretreatment and Posttreatment Measures

Timepoint	MIP (cmH$_2$O)	MEP (cmH$_2$O)	FVC (% predicted)	FEV$_1$ (% predicted)	FEV$_1$/FVC (% predicted)
Preintervention	77	189	87	86	97
Postintervention	114	196	88	89	99
Reference Values (LLN)	89.57 (48.57)	190.15 (119.15)	*Measures are already expressed as a percentage of expected values for age, sex, race, and height.*		

Stimulability

The patient was evaluated for stimulability for voice improvement during laryngeal videostroboscopy via the assessment of different pitch and loudness levels and different levels of respiratory muscle engagement during phonation. Trials demonstrated an ability to produce longer and louder phonation when taking a bigger breath; however, the patient reported fatigue after only a couple repetitions as well as increased perceived effort. Vocal quality remained breathy during most productions, with slight improvement. Stimulability trials for the treatment approach included briefly explaining the VFEs and having the patient attempt each of them. During trials, the clinician appreciated a reduced pitch range (especially on the lower end) and very short, sustained phonation (8 seconds); however, the patient was able to perform each task accurately after it was modeled.

Impressions

The patient presented with moderate presbyphonia and mildly reduced respiratory function. Prognosis for improvement was deemed good based on identified treatment targets (described in the next section). The patient was highly motivated and ready for intervention, perceiving potential for high benefit and minimal barriers.[29] The patient's self-efficacy for being able to accomplish the intervention tasks and believing that they would result in improvements indicated readiness for the Action stage of change.[30]

Plan of Care

At the conclusion of the evaluation, the patient was enrolled in weekly voice therapy to be reevaluated after 6 weeks. The long-term goal was to improve voice quality and loudness during speech, at an acceptable laryngeal and respiratory effort level, to allow for participation in work and social activities. The short-term goals were: (1) increase efficiency of inspiration during speech (greater depth and rapidity with less perceived effort) as well as expiratory control; (2) improve vocal fold closure; and (3) reduce the use of superfluous compensatory mechanisms (supraglottic activity) to decrease vocal effort and related fatigue. The clinician targeted these goals with a therapeutic approach including IMST, VFEs, conversational speech practice, and behavior modification techniques.

The treatment team did not target bringing pitch to WNL, as increased pitch was judged to be an adaptive compensatory strategy and the patient did not share complaints related to pitch. The clinician decided that, as treatment would progress, pitch as a possible treatment target if meaningfully associated with complaints of effort or fatigue would be revisited.

Decision Making

The major contributing factors to Mr. Fraco's voice problem included presbyphonia-related laryngeal changes, slightly reduced respiratory function, and high voice demands. The clinician elected to begin behavioral therapy after discussions with the laryngologist and the patient, who desired to try a noninvasive intervention before considering surgical procedures.

Two pathways as feasible targets for intervention were identified: improving vocal fold valving and improving respiratory muscle activity for voice. Therefore, the clinician had a reasonable expectation of improvement with behavioral treatment. Expectations for patient adherence to treatment were also strong due the patient's motivation and the planned treatment approaches that included explicit feedback on progress via objective measures to maintain patient engagement.

Treatment goals were chosen based on patient description of complaint and anatomical/physiological status as indicated by the evaluation. It was noted that both laryngeal-level presbyphonia and respiratory-level reduced function co-occurred. Thus, goals

> The reader is advised to be aware of all treatment options for presbyphonia and the role of voice therapy as a primary treatment option or as an adjunctive treatment to procedural/surgical intervention. Many variables influence treatment decisions, though no definitive paradigm has yet been developed at the time of writing this text. Further information about decision making for presbyphonia is available in this article by the co-editors and their collaborators, *Laryngologists' Reported Decision-Making in Presbyphonia Treatment.*[31]

Therapeutic Techniques. VFEs were chosen to improve vocal fold closure through enhanced thyroarytenoid (TA) function while promoting a vocal tract configuration that reduces compensatory hyperfunction.

> Stimulation of the TA muscles in rats has been shown to enhance TA function with increased density of neuromuscular junctions.[33] While not studied in humans, perhaps a similar effect may be achieved through strategic phonatory tasks.

related to directly targeting both vocal fold closure and improving respiratory function for speech were chosen.

The decision to focus on respiratory function in non-speech tasks during voice therapy sessions is controversial due to constraints that influence clinical voice practices (limited insurance coverage, the expectation of quick improvement, and increased clinical productivity requirements). Therefore, optimizing treatment time and providing strong justifications for interventions are crucial. Recent research has provided a better understanding of the respiratory demands for speech and has highlighted that targeting the respiratory system through voice-based exercises often achieves treatment goals satisfactorily and is generally more effective than nonspecific, low-effort breathing exercises (eg, diaphragmatic breathing) for most individuals with voice disorders.[32] However, certain patients with specific voice and respiratory conditions may benefit from dedicating time to high-effort respiratory training during treatment. For persons with presbyphonia, especially those with co-occurring age-related respiratory decline, there is some evidence to suggest that actively targeting improved respiratory muscle strength may be a valid use of time during a voice therapy session.[9]

IMST was selected to enhance the inspiratory phase of the respiratory cycle and increase subglottal pressure through greater natural recoil pressures, facilitating louder and longer phonation with reduced perceived effort. Targeting IMST aligns well with the naturally occurring strategy of older speakers, especially males, who compensate for age-related changes in the respiratory system by speaking at higher lung volumes.[34] Targeting the inspiratory muscles may also enhance control of the expiratory phase (where muscles of inspiration moderate elastic recoil for steady airflow for speech), which the clinician hypothesized would help Mr. Fraco produce longer utterances without feeling out of breath due to better airflow conservation. The rationale for choosing respiratory muscle strength training (RMST) rather than low-effort breathing exercises was based on evidence of increased capacity to generate respiratory muscle pressure in patients following a period of training, due to neuromuscular changes in the respiratory muscles.[35] Considering that the evaluation revealed a MIP below the reference value for Mr. Fraco's age, sex, and weight, the clinical reasoning was that increasing his ability to generate inspiratory pressures would allow him to make changes in his respiratory behavior for speech with less effort. Moreover, IMST would allow for task-specific generalization by combining resistive inspirations with voicing on the exhalation phase to facilitate transfer of the motor pattern to spontaneous speech.

Intervention

Course of Treatment

The patient participated in 6 weekly hour-long treatment sessions. Each session began with 15 minutes dedicated to discussing Mr. Fraco's progress, addressing challenges encountered during his weekly practice, taking measures, and adjusting training goals accordingly. The interventions consisted of 10 minutes of IMST, then 20 minutes of VFEs and 10 minutes of conversational speech practice, followed by 5 minutes of patient education.

Clinical Sessions

IMST preceded the VFEs in therapy sessions. This sequence is believed to not only exercise inspiratory muscles, but to also encourage the engagement of these muscles during the subsequent voice exercises, thus promoting transfer of the respiratory exercises to voice and enforcing a new motor pattern. The IMST exercises consisted of 5 sets of 5 breaths into an inspiratory pressure threshold trainer (POWERbreathe, Medic Plus) with a 1-minute break of rest breathing between each set for recovery. (See Video 12 Inspiratory Muscle Strength Training by Bonilha.) During each trial, the patient was instructed to breathe out and then forcefully inhale through the device using the mouthpiece and while wearing a nose clip. The trainer was set to offer a resistance to inspiration that corresponded to 75% of the patient's MIP, which was measured at each weekly session with the respiratory pressure meter. Some adjustments were made during the initial sessions to help Mr. Fraco achieve optimal training. First, the treating clinician noticed a lot of visible accessory muscle activity (especially in the sternocleidomastoid and trapezius muscles) as Mr. Fraco was working to overcome the resistance offered by the training device. To avoid the emergence of undesired compensatory respiratory behaviors, the patient was encouraged to relax his neck and shoulders as much as possible during the task. At first, Mr. Fraco was not able to overcome the resistance while using this more relaxed posture and, therefore, the threshold was reduced to 60% of his MIP. This allowed him to get a sense of the target motor pattern prior to gradually increasing the resistance back to 75%. Once the resistance was overcome and air flowed through the device, the patient was instructed to continue inhaling for a couple of seconds prior to breathing out. There was no resistance at expiration.

VFEs broadly followed the 4-step protocol by Stemple[36] (for additional information, see Case Study 3.6 by Stemple: Vocal Function Exercises to Treat an Adult With Undifferentiated Phonotrauma and Video 5 Vocal Function Exercises by Stemple). The clinician slightly adapted the protocol to promote forward resonance and used the following stimuli for each step: (1) sustain "mi," (2) glide from low to high on "whoop," (3) glide from high to low on "boom," and (4) sustain "moo" on sequentiall pitches (C-D-E-F-G). During training of the VFEs and in subsequent practice, attention was given to achieving a forward-focused voice quality.

During the conversational speech portion of the treatment session, the clinician engaged the patient in dialogue and prompted him to pay attention to his forward-focused voice quality and loudness. The patient reported that this part of the session was particularly valuable as he was able to practice breathing and speaking in a facilitative setting and could better understand how to incorporate changes into his daily life.

Additional therapeutic techniques of evoking mastery experiences and providing feedback on progress toward goals were used to maintain and improve self-efficacy. The measures taken at each treatment session, particularly MIP measurements, were critical to both tracking treatment outcomes and incentivizing patient adherence. This objective measure of progress, combined with a sense that performing the VFEs felt easier after a session of IMST, helped the patient connect the physiological goals of the exercises to functional results. This relationship became even more obvious when Mr. Fraco started noticing changes in his daily vocal activities, including an ability to more easily increase loudness and less vocal fatigue at the end of a workday or family dinner.

Home Practice

The patient practiced twice daily at home, completing IMST exercises followed by 2 sets of VFEs. IMST exercises involved 5 sets of 5 breaths with 1-minute breaks between sets. To ensure accuracy in home practice, the patient received a recording of the VFEs. A practice log was provided for Mr. Fraco to track his sessions and share practice details with the clinician.

Posttreatment

Mr. Fraco showed continuous improvement throughout the treatment. By the end of the sixth week, his voice quality had significantly improved and vocal effort had reduced to a satisfactory level. Voice quality, as judged on a scale of 0 to 100, improved from 55/100 before treatment to 28/100 after treatment. This improvement was supported by enhanced CPPS during connected speech, as well as decreased NHR and APQ values during sustained vowel production. Additionally, Mr. Fraco's habitual loudness during spontaneous speech increased from 62.9 dB to 70.9 dB.

The positive effects on vocal quality and loudness can be attributed to physiological changes in both the laryngeal and respiratory systems.[37] While laryngeal imaging showed only minor changes in bowing, analysis of phase closure during sustained phonation revealed a reduction in the open phase of the vocal fold vibration (from 86% to 80%), accompanied by reduced supraglottic activity. It is reasonable to speculate that the improvement in vocal fold closure—confirmed by a reduced mean airflow rate and increased laryngeal resistance—was partly driven by the availability of a more constant subglottal pressure to sustain vibration during the whole phonation duration, with less need for compensatory supraglottic involvement. This mechanism of action is consistent with the noted increase in MIP at posttreatment. There was no improvement in pulmonary function measures, which was expected as the patient did not have insufficient vital capacity for voicing but rather did not efficiently use his respiratory muscles during speech.

Improved scores on self-assessment questionnaires further confirmed the functional impact of the treatment. Mr. Fraco's VHI-10 score was 10, GFI score was 4, and CPIB score was 23 at posttreatment. He demonstrated high adherence to home exercises, missing only 2 home sessions over the 6-week period. This strong adherence can be attributed to the significant impact of his voice problem on his life, his belief in the intervention approach, and continual feedback on his progress.

Need for Additional Treatment. The patient was eager to continue his home exercise routine in hopes of continuing to improve (or at least maintain) function. The patient did not want to contemplate medialization interventions at this time. Recognizing that a long-term structured exercise program might be discouraging, the clinician suggested Mr. Fraco engage in activities like joining a choir to sustain laryngeal and respiratory function. He expressed enthusiasm for this idea, reminiscing about his positive experiences in a choir during childhood.

Clinician Reflections

Although it is controversial and not our typical practice, there are cases where dedicating time in voice therapy sessions to non-voicing techniques is justified. Specifically, for patients with weakened respiratory muscles or the need to compensate for incomplete vocal fold closure, incorporating respiratory exercises that evoke measurable respiratory improvements can be an important part of our clinical toolbox. The patient showed strong motivation and adherence to the treatment, both in the clinic and at home. This may be attributed to the patient's perceived severity of the voice problem, the perceived benefits of the intervention approach, and the use of clinical methods that provided mastery experiences and feedback to boost self-efficacy.

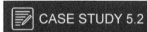

CASE STUDY 5.2

Phonation Resistance Training Exercises (PhoRTE®) to Treat an Adult With Presbyphonia

Aaron Ziegler and Edie R. Hapner

Voice Evaluation

A comprehensive voice evaluation with acoustic and aerodynamic assessment was completed on referral of the physician for a diagnosis of presbylaryngis with glottal insufficiency and resulting presbyphonia.

Case History

The patient is a 75-year-old cisgender Caucasian female who lives with her husband in an English-speaking home and presents to the interprofessional voice clinic with complaints of difficulty being loud and increased vocal effort, as well as a persistent rough voice quality and occasional aphonic voice breaks. She describes voice production as effortful and strained, which leads to increased vocal fatigue with prolonged voice use. She describes a dry cough that seems to worsen when speaking. The onset of her voice problem was 6 months prior to being seen in the clinic, and her symptoms are reported to be gradually worsening. She denies any signs or symptoms of an upper respiratory infection or other illness at the onset of voice difficulties. On a self-rating scale of 1 to 7 for innate talkativeness and loudness (where 1 is "quiet and introspective" and 7 is "loud and talkative"), the patient rates her degree of talkativeness as 6 and her degree of loudness as 4.5.[38]

Medical History. The patient previously sought the evaluation of several community otolaryngologists and reported being treated with nasal steroids and nasal irrigation for her cough and an H2 blocker for reflux, though she denied symptoms of reflux and reported no relief from any of these treatments.

The patient's past medical history was significant for hyperlipidemia, for which she was being treated with Lipitor. This medication has no known effects on voice. She has not had any relevant surgeries to the head or neck or those that would be related to these voice complaints. Review of systems was otherwise unremarkable and cranial nerves II to XII were grossly intact. She denies shortness of breath with exertion but occasionally feels winded with prolonged speaking. She denies dysphagia.

The patient has always been a nonsmoker and only very occasional drinker. Water intake is reportedly minimal (about 8 ounces per day) in addition to 2 cups of coffee per day. She denies any exposures to dust or chemicals known to cause cough or impact the voice.

Social History. The patient works as a part-time instructor at a culinary arts school, which requires her to project her voice to large groups over several 60- to 90-minute courses, 3 to 4 days a week. She reports intermittent use of amplification at work when this equipment is working properly. The patient notes that her voice problems have negatively affected her work, forcing her to reduce the number and duration of classes she teaches. She describes that people have trouble hearing her when teaching and that she is frequently asked to repeat herself.

Laryngeal Imaging and Physician Referral

The referring physician's report was accompanied by a video copy of the laryngeal videostroboscopic examination for the clinician to review. The physician noted bilateral vocal fold atrophy with prominent vocal processes and patulous ventricles. Glottal closure was marked by teardrop anterior closure during complete adduction and mild bowing during complete abduction, both common findings in patients with vocal fold atrophy. The mucosa was healthy but there was evidence of reduced amplitude of lateral excision with stiffer mucosa at the midmembranous phonatory edges bilaterally. The physician noted that in the examination, the patient was stimulable for change with increased loudness and increased pitch and therefore referred her for voice therapy as the first line of treatment.[31] The physician noted that bilateral vocal fold injections could be considered if the patient did not achieve the desired voice outcome after therapy.[39] The physician was not concerned about the patient's hearing impacting her voice complaints, as she passed a hearing screening at 0.5, 1, and 2 kHz at 40 dB conducted by the audiologist in their office.[40]

> Chapter 2 discusses the importance of communication with the referring physician. While the physician's Plan A for this patient was to refer to voice therapy, the physician also noted and likely told the patient that, "If therapy does not achieve the desired response, an augmentation can be considered." Physicians are obliged to discuss all treatment options with the patient, and it is important for the SLP to understand these options, the frequency and duration of therapy that is likely needed to achieve desired results, and the timing of the physician follow-up. This is especially important if the SLP and physician do not work in close proximity. Being aware of Plan B allows the SLP to knowledgeably discuss collaborative care and improve treatment outcomes.

Patient-Reported Outcome Measures (PROMs)

The Aging Voice Index (AVI)[41] was self-administered to assess the patient's perception of the impact of the voice disorder on her quality of daily life. AVI scores range from 0 to 92 with higher values indicating an increased impact to the quality of daily life. Her AVI score was 40, indicating she perceives that her voice disorder has a negative impact on the quality of daily life. Other pertinent PROMs were:

- **Cough Severity Index[42]:** 15/40 (threshold = 3)
- **Dyspnea Index[43]:** 5/20 (threshold = 3)
- **Voice Problem Impact Scales (VPIS)[44]:**
  - 6/7 work life/daily activities
  - 6/7 social life
  - 3/7 home life
  - 4/7 overall
- **Reported Edmonton Frail Scale (REFS)[45]:** Total score: 7/18, which results in a profile of "apparently vulnerable to frailty"
- **OMNI Vocal Effort Scale (OMNI-VES)[46]:** 5/10 during the evaluation and 10/10 at worst, which she describes as occurring on days with significant talking, eg, teaching classes or going out to a noisy restaurant

Auditory-Perceptual Assessment

The CAPE-V[23] was administered. Overall CAPE-V score was 28/100, indicating dysphonia of a mild-moderate nature. Aberrant perceptual features identified in the voice include asthenia, mild breathiness, strain, and roughness. Overall vocal loudness was reduced in quiet conversation. Pitch of the voice was WNL for age and gender but with occasional use of a pitch in the lower end of her modal register. Resonance was focused in the epilaryngeal region, giving the perception of a strained voice. Respiration was primarily abdominal-thoracic. However, the patient held her breath during reading and conversational speech and often dropped into her expiratory reserve volume at the end of breath groups.

Loss of air and inefficient respiratory phonatory coordination are all consistent with complaints of shortness of breath (SOB) during talking and with studies on speech breathing in the elderly, characterized by an increased number of inhalations and placement of pauses/breaths at linguistically inappropriate boundaries.[19,47]

Manual Palpation Assessment

Muscle tension was rated on a 0 to 5 scale where 0 = no tension and 5 = most tension. Results indicated increased perilaryngeal muscle tension with accompanying discomfort with palpation at the thyrohyoid space, most notably:

- 3/5 tension at the thyrohyoid space with report of discomfort
- 2/5 tension at the base of tongue/suprahyoid region without report of pain
- 4/5 laryngeal height as assessed by palpation of the hyoid
- 3/5 restriction of lateralization of thyroid cartilage bilaterally

Acoustic and Aerodynamic Assessment

All data were gathered utilizing the Pentax Medical Computerized Speech Laboratory (CSL) with Multi-Dimensional Voice Program (MDVP) 6600, Analysis of Dysphonia in Speech and Voice (ADSV), Real-Time Pitch Analysis, and the PAS (Pentax Medical, Montvale, NJ). Norms utilized represent information from the Instrumental Voice Assessment Profile.[48] An omnidirectional headset microphone (Shure SM 48) and Extech sound level meter (SLM) were placed at a 45-degree angle at 2 cm from the mouth for data acquisition.[49] Results of the assessment are detailed in Tables 5–5 and 5–6. Normative data for acoustic measures are derived from Patel et al (2018), Awan (2011), Huber and Darling White (2017), Sperry and Klich (1992), and Eckel and Boone (1981).[48,50–53] Normative data for aerodynamic measures are derived from Huber and Darling-White (2017), Sperry and Klich (1992), Eckel

and Boone (1981), Garcia-Rio et al (2009), Simões et al (2010), Kim and Sapienza (2006), Pessoa et al (2014), and Lewandowski et al (2018).[51,53–58]

Stimulability

The patient was stimulable for improvement in voice quality and increased vocal loudness when utilizing low abdominal breathing during forced expiratory flow maneuvers (ie, the clinician modeled and prompted the patient to say, "Hey, you" or "Hey, taxi" in a louder voice).

Confidence and Commitment to Therapy

When asked how important it was to her to complete voice therapy on a scale of 1 to 10, with 10 being most important, the patient rated both the importance of and her commitment to participating in therapy at this time as a 9/10.

> The Transtheoretical Model (TTM) of behavior change, described by van Leer et al (2008) as it applies to voice therapy, conceptualizes the stages patients may traverse when making significant changes to their life for vocal health and healing.[59] Here, the authors of this case use a tool often discussed in TTM, the readiness ruler, to address confidence and the importance of making those needed changes. Hapner presents the use of the ruler exercise in chapter 3 of Behrman and Haskell's third edition of *Exercises for Voice Therapy* by Plural Publishing.[60]

Impressions

The patient presents with mild-moderate dysphonia with vocal characteristics consistent with presbyphonia. Voice quality is stimulable for change using louder conversational speech.

Prognosis for the Use of Voice Therapy

The patient appeared to be an excellent candidate for voice therapy. Positive prognostic

172 Voice Therapy: Clinical Case Studies

Table 5–5. Pre- and Posttreatment Acoustic Assessment

	Norms 60+ Years	Pretreatment Results	Posttreatment Results	+ Indicates Improvement
Voice Task: Sustained "ah"				
Cepstral Peak Prominence (CPP)	F 10.7 ±1.6 M 13.0 ±1.7	9.9 dB	10.3 dB	+
CPP Standard Deviation (SD)	F 0.4 ±0.2 M 0.6 ±0.2	0.7 dB	0.6 dB	+
L/H Spectral Ratio	F 33.0 ±4.3 M 38.1 ±6.0	28.09 dB	29.1 dB	+
L/H Spectral Ratio SD	F 1.0 ±0.3 M 1.3 ±0.6	1.2 dB	1.1 dB	+
CPP Fundamental Frequency (F0)	F 210.4 ±22.7 M 110.9 ±16.0	200 Hz	205 Hz	+
CPP F0 SD	F 2.4 ±5.2 M 0.7 ±0.3	2.2 Hz	1.9 Hz	+
Maximum Phonation Time (MPT)	61-70: F 18.0 ±2.5 M 26.0 ±1.2 71-80: F 22.0 ±1.4 M 23.0 ±1.7 81-90: F 20.0 ±1.2 M 21.0 ±1.5	12 seconds	18 seconds	+
Voice Task: Pitch glides on "ah"				
Physiological Frequency Range (max-min)	F 130-750 M 90-550	150-400 Hz	150-500 Hz	+

indicators included high level of commitment, recent onset, positive response to stimulability tasks, and a vocal condition that is known to respond to voice therapy. Negative prognostic indicators included low awareness of voice use patterns. The patient indicated that her long-term goal was to improve loudness and decrease vocal fatigue so she could remain effective in the classroom and enjoy socializing with family and friends.

Plan of Care

Voice therapy was recommended as the first line of treatment for this patient. The patient was enrolled in a series of 4 therapy sessions over 2 months with each session 45 to 60 minutes in length. Goals of therapy include:

Long-Term Goal. Improve the patient's ability to communicate effectively in all life situations including occupationally, socially, and at home.

Table 5–6. Pre- and Posttreatment Aerodynamic Assessment

	Norms 60+ Years	Pretreatment Results	Posttreatment Results	+ Indicates Improvement
Voice Task: Rainbow Passage (first 4 sentences)				
Duration of Reading	F/M 24.97 ±3.43****	45 sec	25 sec	+
# of Breaths per Passage	F/M 5.64 ±1.83****	7	4	+
Mean Flow Rate (MFR) at Typical Loudness	F/M 100-220 mL/sec	250 mL/sec	220 mL/sec	+
Voice Task: /pa/ 5× at typical pitch and loudness				
Subglottal Pressure (P_{sub})	F 8.0 ±4.3 M 6.7 ±1.9	7 cmH_2O	8 cmH_2O	+
Phonation Threshold Pressure (PTP)	4.22 ±1.02 cmH_2O	6.65 cmH_2O	5.0 cmH_2O	+
Voice Task: s/z ratio* **				
s Duration 20 sec z Duration 13 sec Ratio	<1.40	20 S/13 Z 1.538	20 S/18 Z 1.11	+
Dynamic Range (max-min)	Impaired <40 dB SPL	58-78 20 dB SPL	60-90 30 dB SPL	+
Spirometry				
Peak Expiratory Flow	F 150 M 174	180 L/sec	220 L/sec	+
Forced Vital Capacity (FVC)	F 2.3 ±0.5 L M 3.5 ±0.6 L	2.5 L	2.5 L	
Forced Expiratory Volume 1st Sec (FEV_1)	F 1.8 ±0.4 L M 2.6 ±0.5 L	1.7 L	1.8 L	
FEV_1/FVC	F 78.9 ±5.6 M 76.8 ±5.5	90%	90	
Maximal Inspiratory Pressure (MIP)	60-69: F 75.1 ±8.0 M 92.7 ±8.0 70-83: F 65.3 ±8.0 M 76.2 ±6.0	58 cmH_2O	60 cmH_2O and increased to 65 cmH_2O with adjuvant IMST	+

continues

Table 5–6. *continued*

	Norms 60+ Years	Pretreatment Results	Posttreatment Results	+ Indicates Improvement
Maximum Expiratory Pressure (MEP)	60-69: F 82.5 ±3.5 M 94.5 ±3.6 70-79: F 57.8 ±4.7 M 71.0 ±4.5 80-89: F 45.3 ±6.0 M 62.3 ±5.0	57 cmH$_2$O	57 cmH$_2$O	

Norms: Garcia-Rio et al (2009); Simões et al (2010); Kim & Sapienza (2006); Pessoa et al (2014); Sperry & Klich (1992); **Huber & Darling-White (2017); ***Eckel & Boone (1981); ****Lewandowski et al (2018)

Short-Term Goals. Complete a systematic series of evidence-based exercises known as Phonation Resistance Training Exercises (PhoRTE®) over a 3-month period to achieve the following goals:

1. Reduce vocal effort for conversational speech in all communication situations
2. Increase vocal loudness for conversational speech in all communication situations
3. Increase vocal endurance to allow her to teach 90-minute cooking courses once per week

Decision Making

PhoRTE® was selected because of its high-intensity nature, which has demonstrated the potential to effectively treat the voice decline in presbyphonia.[7,8] The program uses respiratory phonatory voice exercises akin to progressive resistance training, which, in the exercise science literature, demonstrates positive changes in muscular force production and endurance so people can better act out activities of daily living.[61,62] Four mechanisms incorporated into PhoRTE® support achievement of the suggested outcomes:

1. Increased subglottal pressure through increased expiratory muscle activity and generation of higher alveolar pressures will lead to increased vocal loudness.
2. Increased subglottal pressure from increased laryngeal resistance as a result of increased TA and LCA muscle activity will lead to increased vocal loudness. The theory is that increased subglottal pressure to overcome the added laryngeal resistance from increased vocal fold adduction and intrinsic vocal fold tension will further increase vocal loudness.
3. Increased amplitude of vocal fold excursion with greater subglottal pressures will provide another mechanism for promoting improved glottal closure as the vocal folds close with greater recoil forces.
4. The use of a megaphone mouth shape during production of the vowel /a/ will maximize phonatory efficiency and help to recalibrate phonatory effort.

All of these physiological changes will allow a speaker to vocalize safely and without vocal effort. Phonotrauma is not a concern in people with presbylaryngis with incomplete glottal closure.[63]

5. Glottal Gaps

> PhoRTE® is not intended as a treatment for patients with phonotrauma and should not be used when patients present with phonotrauma or a predominant closed phase of vibration. PhoRTE® was specifically designed and studied to address glottal insufficiency as a result of presbyphonia. In the case of presbylaryngis, there is either incomplete glottal closure or reduced vocal fold collision forces due to a shorter closed phase. Therefore, producing a louder, more exuberant voice with efficient laryngeal postures and without extralaryngeal muscle tension does not result in hard glottal contacts that would be concerning for phonotrauma in this population.

Intervention

The patient completed 4 individual voice therapy sessions approximately once every 3 weeks for 45 minutes per session.

Session #1

The initial session consisted of determining the individualized SPL target for the 5 PhoRTE® voice exercises.

Establishing the Target Loudness

The clinician set up a C-weighted SLM at 12 inches from the patient's mouth using a ruler to consistently standardize the distance for measurement (Figure 5–1). The clinician measured the sound floor of the room, asking the patient to sit quietly and allow the SLM to record the room loudness. The loudness of the room should be at least 10 dB below the patient's comfortable vocal loudness to prevent the Lombard Effect.[64] The clinician completed the PhoRTE® protocol for developing the starting target loudness at 50 to 60% of the patient's overall dynamic dB SPL range.

This patient was able to use the National Institute for Occupational Safety and Health (NIOSH) sound level meter app on her phone when practicing PhoRTE® at home. If the patient cannot use a smartphone app to measure loudness, the use of the OMNI-VES with 6 circled ("somewhat hard") has been found to be an acceptable alternative to measuring loudness (Figure 5–2). When a patient is prompted to complete the tasks using a somewhat hard effort, it is akin to working at a moderate level of exercise using the Borg scale.[65]

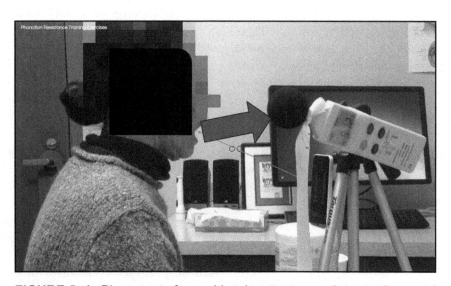

FIGURE 5–1. Placement of sound level meter to mouth to monitor vocal loudness.

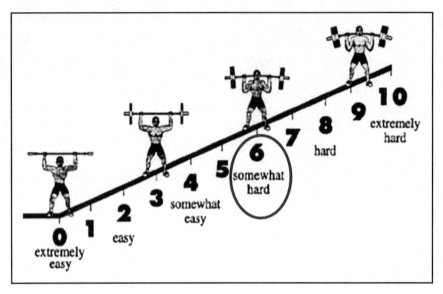

FIGURE 5–2. OMNI-Vocal Effort Scale level 6, "somewhat hard."

Developing Proper Vocal Form

Next, the clinician taught the patient to use low abdominal breathing gestures by relaxing the abdominal musculature to allow natural expansion on inhalation and engaging the abdomen in exhalation, especially at end expiratory level. In this exercise, the clinician asked the patient to sit quietly in a chair while monitoring the movement of her abdomen below the belly button with her hand as she completed a minute of quiet breathing. Then, the clinician asked the patient to breathe in through the mouth (people breathe in and out of the mouth when speaking) and exhale on prolonged /ʃ/. The goal of the task was to develop the ability to use and monitor low abdominal breathing by observing that the belly expands with inhalation and returns inward during slow exhalation. The sensation of work of the abdominal muscles should occur at the end of the breath group, indicating the use of breath at the end expiratory level of the cycle.

Introducing PhoRTE®

The final part of session #1 consisted of teaching the patient the 5 PhoRTE® voice therapy exercises using either the SLM set to the target loudness or the OMNI-VES at an effort level of 6 to complete:

1. 10 repetitions of energized and sustained phonation on /a/
2. 10 repetitions of energized ascending and descending pitch glides over the entire pitch range on /a/
3. 10 patient-specific functional phrases using an energized "calling" voice completed once each
4. 10 phrases from exercise #3 in a commanding voice of "authority" completed once each
5. Conversational exchange in an energized voice production for 2 to 3 minutes.
(See Table 5–7 and Video 13 Developing Proper Form for PhoRTE® by Ziegler and Hapner.)

At the end of the first session, the clinician explained that, similar to physical exercise, it is expected to take 3 to 4 weeks for the patient to feel change as the vocal mechanism adapts to the overload of vocal exercise demanded of it and becomes a more efficient voice production mechanism. The patient was asked to contact the clinician should she expe-

5. Glottal Gaps   177

Table 5–7. PhoRTE® Voice Therapy Exercises

Exercise #1: Phonatory Respiratory Isotonic	Prolonged /a/ at target loudness/effort
Exercise #2: Eccentric-Concentric Cricothyroid Contraction	Glide from loudest to highest note in range and back to lowest note at target loudness/effort 5×, then reverse 5x gliding highest to lowest to highest note in range
Exercise #3: Phonatory Respiratory Power Endurance	Produce functional phrases at target loudness/effort in a calling voice
Exercise #4: Phonatory Respiratory Power Endurance	Produce functional phrases at target loudness/effort in voice of authority
Exercise #5: Phonatory Respiratory Muscular Endurance	Using target loudness/effort, engage in conversational speech for 30 seconds to 2 minutes

rience any prolonged discomfort (daily with practice for over 5 days). The patient received the PhoRTE® charting logs to track progress, written instructions on how to complete the daily home practice program, and a recording with audio demonstrations of the exercises. The clinician asked the patient to perform the 5 exercises of the PhoRTE® voice therapy program once daily, 6 days a week, with 1 day of no practice. Then, at the start of week 2 when she restarted exercising again after her day off, she was to increase her vocal loudness target per her established PhoRTE® protocol for increasing vocal load/demands. She was counseled that it would feel harder to complete the exercises the first 3 to 4 days each week, but by days 5 and 6, she should once again feel it was becoming easier to produce all 5 exercises. She was told that it was like increasing the size of weights when working out at the gym—as the vocal mechanism gets stronger, the exercises will feel easier until she increases the vocal demand/loudness target once again.

Session #2

The second voice therapy session, 2 weeks later, started with a review of how the patient was doing. She reported that her friends had recently told her they thought she sounded

better. The patient and clinician reviewed the PhoRTE® charting logs. The clinican reassessed the patient's vocal range and target loudness, and the patient demonstrated the PhoRTE® voice exercises with her newly established loudness targets, ensuring she was using good vocal form with the increased vocal demands. She was reminded that PhoRTE® should never make her cough or cause a sore throat. If so, she was likely using improper vocal form, such as hard glottal attacks or too great of a loudness increase. The patient adjusted her form with increased loudness, and the clinician provided feedback on the execution of the exercises to optimize patient production and maximize patient benefit. These included opening her mouth with a dropped jaw, ie, megaphone mouth shape.

Session #3

The third voice therapy session, 2 weeks later, started with a review of how the patient was doing. She reported that all her friends now comment that they can hear her even in noisy restaurants and, importantly, she has returned to teaching 3 to 4 classes a week. She reported that she does use amplification consistently with teaching and that she had the cooking school purchase a hands-free headset microphone for her to use during teaching. The patient and clinician reviewed the PhoRTE® charting logs from the prior 2 weeks of home practice. The clinician reassessed the patient's vocal range and target loudness, and the patient demonstrated the PhoRTE® voice exercises with her newly established loudness targets, ensuring she was using good vocal form with the increased vocal demands. She was counseled to continue the protocol for 2 more weeks, after which she will undergo instrumental testing and stroboscopy.

Session #4

At the fourth therapy session appointment (2 weeks later, occurring on week 6), the patient reported satisfaction with her treatment. She stated her voice had improved since completing 6 weeks of the PhoRTE® voice therapy program, and she believed the program caused positive changes in her voice. In addition, she experienced a substantial reduction in perceived phonatory effort to the extent that voice production was now comfortable (rating of 4/10 on the OMNI-VES). Her voice quality also improved, as evidenced by an overall severity on the CAPE-V of 11/100; the clinician perceived little to no roughness or strain in the patient's voice and increased loudness during conversational speech. Acoustic and aerodynamic assessment revealed clinically meaningful changes. Average vocal intensity increased to 72.8 dB SPL. The patient's dynamic range expanded due to an increase in maximum vocal intensity. The NHR ratio value decreased, suggesting an improved vocal quality. Functionally, the patient reported few requests to repeat herself and resumed teaching at her regularly scheduled times (see Figure 5–3, Table 5–5, and Table 5–6).

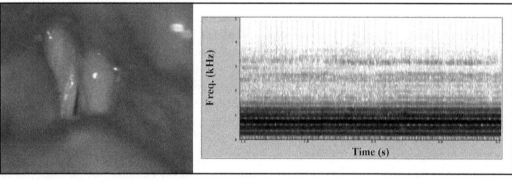

A

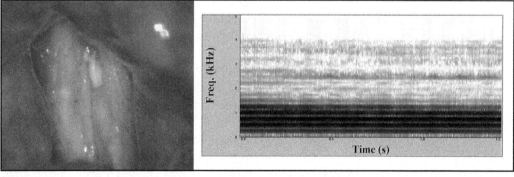

B

FIGURE 5–3. Pre- (**A**) and posttreatment (**B**) vocal fold adduction and spectrographic signal.

During laryngeal videostroboscopy, there were no detectable changes to the original physician's laryngeal examination, with the exception of much-reduced supraglottal hyperfunction. The patient was counseled that often we do not see changes to the size of the glottal gap but there is increased endurance, less effort to produce voice, increased loudness and improved quality of life, and therefore the assumption is that our current level of instrumentation for vocal fold imaging is just not able to detect the physiologic changes. The patient was counseled to schedule a follow-up with her physician and that this clinician would send the physician a full report and copy of the videostroboscopy.

The patient and clinician then worked to implement the PhoRTE® maintenance protocol. A telephone follow-up was scheduled at 3 months, 6 months, and 9 months to determine maintenance of a stronger, less effortful voice.

CASE STUDY 5.3

Expiratory Muscle Strength Training and PhoRTE® to Treat an Adult With Presbyphonia

Adam Lloyd and Maria Murljacic

Voice Evaluation

Chief Complaint. Soft, quiet voice that "sounds dry"

Case History

History of Voice Complaint. The patient is a 71-year-old cisgender woman who was previously known to our practice from 4 years prior when she was treated for chronic refractory cough and compensatory muscle tension dysphonia (MTD) after upper respiratory infection. At that time, she was successfully treated with in-person behavioral cough suppression therapy, voice therapy, an antireflux diet, and lifestyle modifications over the course of 3 months.

The patient now presents with complaints of a soft, quiet voice that "sounds dry" and has slightly worsened over the course of 6 months. Her husband is concerned about her voice and encouraged her to return for a reassessment. Her voice symptoms include difficulty projecting, decline in voice quality over the course of the day, and neck soreness and tension. The patient reported that her voice sounds intermittently hoarse, increasing in severity at the end of the day. She stated: "My voice isn't a strong voice, it's a small voice." She denied difficulty swallowing or breathing as well as denied symptoms of reflux. She reported that she was otherwise in good health. The patient reported no medical comorbidities and does not take any prescription medications. She noted that the cough that she was previously treated for has been under control.

Voice Use. The patient indicated that she was retired and not using her voice as much as she had previously and said that her husband is her main communication partner.

Social History. The patient was a former smoker, 1 pack per day for 8 years, but quit approximately 40 years ago. She drinks alcohol at most once per week, 2 cups of caffeinated beverages per day, and approximately 32 ounces of water per day. She describes her stress levels as 5/10, where 1 is "no stress" and 10 is "severe stress."

Laryngeal Imaging

Laryngeal videostroboscopy was performed transnasally with a flexible distal chip laryngoscope.

Salient Examination Findings. True vocal folds were fully mobile bilaterally. The right vocal fold was mildly bowed and without specific lesions. The left vocal fold was mildly bowed and without specific lesions. Glottic closure during phonatory tasks was intermittently incomplete with a very slender midline glottal gap. The amplitude and mucosal wave were intact bilaterally. Phase symmetry was normal. There were no exophytic or ulcerative lesions within the remainder of the lar-

180 Voice Therapy: Clinical Case Studies

ynx. There was moderate anterior, posterior, and lateral supraglottic compression with increased phonatory effort.

Quality-of-Life Impairment

The VHI-10[66] was completed with a total score of 18/40 (threshold for abnormal score = 11)[20] (Table 5–8).

Auditory-Perceptual Assessment

The CAPE-V[23] was administered (Table 5–9). An overall CAPE-V score of 45/100 indicated dysphonia of a moderate nature. Aberrant perceptual features identified in the voice included intermittent breathiness, intermittent roughness, and consistent strain. Overall vocal loudness was noted to be reduced and described as soft. Pitch of the voice was WNL for age and gender. Resonance was WNL. Respiration was primarily abdominal-thoracic. There was intermittent consistent asthenia and intermittent pitch instability.

Acoustic Assessment

All acoustic data were gathered utilizing the KayPentax CSL 4500 (Pentax Medical, Montvale, NJ) (Table 5–10). ADSV software was utilized for the assessment. Norms utilized represent information from the corresponding references.[67–71] A handheld Shure micro-

Table 5–9. Consensus Auditory-Perceptual Evaluation of Voice (CAPE-V) Results

CAPE-V Parameter	Clinician Rating
Overall Severity	45; intermittent
Roughness	35; intermittent
Breathiness	45; intermittent
Strain	30; consistent
Pitch	0; appropriate consistent
Loudness	30; soft consistent
Resonance	Normal
Additional Characteristics	20; asthenia (weakness) consistent
	45; pitch instability intermittent

Table 5–8. Patient Responses on the Voice Handicap Index–10

VHI-10 Question	Rating
My voice makes it difficult for people to hear me.	2
People have difficulty understanding me in a noisy room.	3
My voice difficulties restrict my personal and social life.	2
I feel left out of conversations because of my voice.	2
My voice problem causes me to lose income.	0
I feel as though I have to strain to produce voice.	2
The clarity of my voice is unpredictable.	2
My voice problem upsets me.	2
My voice makes me feel handicapped.	1
People ask, "What's wrong with your voice?"	2
Total	18

Table 5–10. Acoustic Assessment Results

Acoustic Parameter	Patient Data	Female Normative Data; Mean (SD)	X Indicates Abnormal
Maximum Phonation Time	17.01 sec	60-89 years; 20.02 (6.58)[67]	
Mean CPP F0 Sustained Vowel	212.377 Hz	60-89 years; 191.90 (23.79)[67]	
CSID Sustained Vowel	22.210	>17.68: dysphonic[68]	X
Mean CPP F0 All-Voiced Sentence	206.235 Hz	60+ years; 178.92 (19.71)[69]	X
CSID All-Voiced Sentence	11.346	>24.3: dysphonic[70]	
SPL dB	65.8 dB	Older age; 74.0 (4.2)[71]	X

phone was placed 12 inches from the mouth for data acquisition. A handheld digital SLM (CEM sound level meter, DT-85A) was used to collect SPL. It was held at a 45-degree angle with a 12-inch mouth-to-microphone distance. Results of the assessment were as follows.

Impressions

The patient presented with mild dysphonia characterized by breathy, strained quality with normal resonance in structured tasks and conversation. Based on the CAPE-V perceptual analysis, she was found to have an overall severity of 45/100, with the dysphonic quality occurring intermittently. Her self-perceived voice quality of life as measured by the VHI-10 was slightly outside the normal range. Her laryngeal function studies (acoustic and aerodynamic assessment) were generally WNL or less than 1 standard deviation from the mean. Videostroboscopic examination revealed bowing of the edges of the vocal folds and an intermittent small glottic gap. Findings were consistent with presbyphonia resulting in glottic insufficiency and contributing to patient perceived hypophonic vocal quality. The laryngologist observed presbylaryngis and the SLP observed presbyphonia with compensatory extralaryngeal maladaptive muscular compression disorder (secondary MTD). Follow-up for

voice therapy was recommended to work to balance respiration, phonation, and resonance.

Proposed Plan of Care

The clinician recommended voice therapy once per week for 4 to 8 weeks, with 30-minute sessions. The frequency of services was to increase or decrease depending on the patient's progress.

Long-Term Goal. Achieve vocal quality and function that meets the patient's communicative needs

Short-Term Goals. Included but not limited to:

1. Decrease secondary MTD through targeted relaxation breathing, mindfulness, and body stretches
2. Increase expiratory muscle strength and respiratory force generation through strength training with EMST
3. Decrease vocal effort, increase vocal endurance, and improve vocal loudness and clarity with the use of systematic voice therapy targeting the respiratory and phonatory decline experienced with presbyphonia

Decision Making

This patient presented with a hypophonic voice disorder consistent with noted glottic insufficiency, self-perceived weak vocal quality, and clinician-perceived breathy voice with pitch instability. She also presented with supraglottic hyperfunction that was likely compensatory. The clinician determined that voice therapy would be the most appropriate modality of treatment, targeting improving respiratory muscle strength and breath coordination, to support clarity of voice as well as work to reduce compensatory muscle tension. The decision to offer and pursue therapy was a consensus between the voice-specialized SLP and laryngologist, who jointly evaluated the patient on the same day. The decision was to use RMST—in this case, EMST—as the primary modality to improve respiratory muscle strength and breath coordination.

Intervention

The patient underwent a total of 8 voice therapy sessions over the course of 3 months via telehealth. Below are the therapy protocols that were used, including goals and progress made.

Goal #1

Goal #1. Reduce or eliminate extrinsic laryngeal and submandibular tension across speaking tasks

Therapeutic Technique. Laryngeal manual therapy.[72] Specific exercises included: circular massage of the sternocleidomastoid muscles, kneading of the supralaryngeal area, massage of the hyoid bone, and depression of the larynx with fingers on the superior border of the thyroid cartilage.

Goal #1 was introduced during the first therapy session. Prior to completing laryngeal massage, the clinician noted mild-moderate rigidity of the suprahyoids and base of tongue muscles, moderate rigidity of the CT musculature, and moderate to severe rigidity of the thyrohyoid space on palpation. Crepitus was also appreciated. After completing laryngeal massage for 4 minutes, mild reduction in rigidity was noted, and the thyrohyoid space

rigidity decreased to moderate. The patient reported a relaxation response and was educated regarding self-massage and reposturing. Throughout the massage, and in teaching the patient the technique, the clinician emphasized maintaining a relaxed and lowered laryngeal posture during phonation as well as a sensation of relaxation in the throat region. The clinician instructed the patient to complete home exercises of circular massage of the thyrohyoid space and downward manipulation/massage of lateral thyroid cartilage. She met goal #1 at session 4 and continued to practice independently.

Goal #2

Goal #2. Increase force generation of the expiratory muscles (MEP) for voice production

Therapeutic Techniques. RMST using the EMST 150, a pressure-threshold EMST device, was utilized.[9] As a note to the reader, there are 2 methods of RMST. One method involves using a resistance trainer such as the Breather, whereby one breathes through holes that decrease in diameter, with the philosophy that smaller holes require increased resistance to the airflow. Unfortunately, these types of trainers are not accurate in ensuring specific expiratory pressures, as changes to airflow velocity can compensate for smaller diameters such that higher pressures are not necessarily achieved. We recommend avoiding resistive trainers in voice therapy when the goal is strength training. The other method, pressure threshold training, utilizes a spring-loaded membrane that requires greater and greater generation of subglottal pressures to open the membrane; these are true strength training devices. The EMST 150 is well calibrated to allow for more accurate measurement of increasing expiratory muscle strength.

Goal #2 was introduced during the third session. The standard training level is 80% of MEP. Prior to using the EMST device, the clinician first determined the patient's MEP by using a digital respiratory manometer. This required the patient to exhale into the manometer as forcefully as possible without straining. The patient's MEP was 69 cmH$_2$O. Based on this, their starting pressure threshold was set at 55 cmH$_2$O (80% of MEP). From there, the patient was encouraged to continue to practice at a moderate effort level increasing the pressure threshold when effort began to feel easy. At first, the patient required cueing to slow the rate of her repetitions, establishing a full lip seal when blowing through the device. She was cued to inhale with the device outside of her mouth, immediately seal her lips around the device, and blow hard and fast into the device for 1 second. She was encouraged to bring her attention to contracting her abdominal region and rib cage during exhalation. She was instructed to hold her cheeks in with her nondominant index finger and thumb while holding on to the device with her dominant hand, being mindful not to obstruct the flow of air through the device. Additionally, she was encouraged to take 5-second breaks between repetitions and 1-minute breaks between sets for a total of 5 sets of 5 breaths. The clinician explained to the patient that she could split the sets up if needed (eg, 2 sets of 5 breaths in the morning, 3 in the evening). The full EMST protocol was completed over the course of 4 weeks, after which the patient continued to practice maintenance. The patient completed 5 sets of 5 breaths, 5 days per week for 4 weeks. At subsequent therapy sessions, the clinician began each session by checking in on how the EMST protocol was going for the patient. She completed 2 sets of 5 breaths with the clinician, who adjusted the pressure threshold and the technique as needed. In 4 weeks, she was able to increase her pressure threshold training level to approximately 90 cmH$_2$O. During the last therapy session, MEP increased to 113 cmH$_2$O. The clinician then instructed her to continue to practice at this level for 2 days per week, using 5 sets of 5 breaths for maintenance indefinitely. (See Video 14 Using the EMST 150 Device by Lloyd.)

Goal #3

Goal #3. Maintain a well-balanced body alignment and posture and reduce the impact of tension in the shoulders, neck, back, and face, 90% of the time over 2 consecutive sessions

Therapeutic Techniques. Mindfulness and body alignment[73,74]

Seated Abdominal Breathing. The clinician instructed the patient to sit comfortably and erect in a chair with both feet on the ground. The SLP emphasized relaxing the abdomen and rib cage and allowing the breathing to be natural and easy. The clinician also encouraged the patient to notice the natural expansion and contraction of the abdomen and rib cage during inhalation and exhalation. This was performed for approximately 2 minutes.

Body Scan. After performing the seated abdominal breathing, the patient performed a body scan exercise for about 2 minutes. While in a seated position, the clinician instructed the patient to close her eyes and breathe comfortably. Next, they instructed her to bring her attention to the sensations in her body (scanning) from the tip of her toes to the tip of her fingertips and top of the head. During the scan, the clinician encouraged her to continue to breathe slowly and try to relax any tight areas with each exhalation.

Stretches. While breathing slowly, the patient was directed to gently stretch her neck in all comfortable directions, right and left, front and back, and in a half and/or full circle. The clinician directed her to spend at least 3 breaths in each position and longer if she was feeling soreness.

Goal #3 was introduced during the first therapy session. Each voice therapy session began with approximately 5 minutes of relaxed breathing, body scanning, and light and easy stretches. Basic mindfulness, relaxation, and stretching exercises were used to facilitate a reduced sensation of tension, strain, and effort associated with compensatory MTD. At the end of the course of therapy, the patient was independent with these practices and encouraged to practice them daily. The patient consistently noted a relaxation response after practicing the exercises.

Goal #4

Goal #4. Improve perceived vocal clarity, stability, and loudness through the use of PhoRTE® [8] (see Case Study 5.1 by Ziegler and Hapner for a complete description of PhoRTE® voice therapy which includes 5 distinct exercises and methods to accurately determine target loudness and Video 13 Developing Proper Form for PhoRTE®)

Goal #4 was introduced at session #3 and practice continued through session #8. The patient was careful to avoid hyperfunction during these athletic vocal exercises. The clinician emphasized improving the balance of expiratory airflow and laryngeal resistance by increasing the perceptual loudness and effort. The patient used the Decibel X application for iPhone during therapy sessions and in her home practice to track intensity during treatment. Prior to collecting intensity measures, the clinician worked with the patient to ensure a quiet environment, which was the same across data collection, and mouth-to-microphone distance was established with a ruler at 12 inches. The patient increased her average intensity during functional phrases from 65 dB to 73 dB from the first to last therapy sessions. The patient was encouraged to take a mindful inhalation and sustain phonation by increasing energy and effort of the exhalation without straining. The clinician gave the patient home exercises to practice once per day, 10 repetitions of each exercise.

Posttreatment Outcomes

At the last treatment session, the patient's maximum phonation time had increased to 17 seconds (12 seconds at baseline). Perceptual voice clarity and loudness improved throughout the course of therapy. The VHI-10 and CAPE-V assessment were found to have returned to normal levels (Tables 5–11 and 5–12). There was an 8-dB increase in SPL, indicating a normal vocal intensity. Lastly, there was a 44-cmH$_2$O increase in MEP after undergoing EMST, indicating an increased expiratory muscle strength.

Table 5–11. Posttreatment Voice Handicap Index–10 Results

VHI-10 Question	Before	After
My voice makes it difficult for people to hear me.	2	1
People have difficulty understanding me in a noisy room.	3	1
My voice difficulties restrict my personal and social life.	2	1
I feel left out of conversations because of my voice.	2	1
My voice problem causes me to lose income.	0	0
I feel as though I have to strain to produce voice.	2	2
The clarity of my voice is unpredictable.	2	2
My voice problem upsets me.	2	0
My voice makes me feel handicapped.	1	1
People ask, "What's wrong with your voice?"	2	1
Total	18	10

Table 5–12. Posttreatment CAPE-V Results

CAPE-V Parameters	Before	After
Overall Severity	45; intermittent	20; intermittent
Roughness	35; intermittent	0; intermittent
Breathiness	40; intermittent	20; intermittent
Strain	30; consistent	14; consistent
Pitch	0; appropriate consistent	0; appropriate consistent
Loudness	30; soft consistent	0; appropriate consistent
Resonance	Normal	Normal
Additional Characteristics	20; asthenia (weakness) consistent 40; pitch instability intermittent	None

The patient reported that her voice sounded clearer in general, but it did decline somewhat with usage. She stated that when she incorporated the voice therapy techniques, the clarity of her voice and loudness increased, but it felt like an effort to maintain this. The patient stated that although her voice was not perfect, people could hear and understand her better and she no longer needed to repeat herself all the time. When asked what therapy technique she believed helped her to achieve the best voice, she stated, "It's all about the airflow." The clinician instructed the patient to continue to practice PhoRTE® in the maintenance mode, EMST maintenance, and mindful relaxation and stretching daily. The clinician also encouraged her to follow up as needed if symptoms changed, regressed, or worsened.

Clinician Reflection

As with all cases of presbylaryngis, the voice team determines the most appropriate recommendations based on multiple objective and subjective data. Of most importance is the patient's perceptions of their voice difficulty and how their life is affected. In this case, because the bowing and glottic insufficiency were not severe, the clinician recommended starting with voice therapy as described above. The decision to use laryngeal massage and mindful relaxation was to help reduce compensatory muscle tension, which the patient responded well to. EMST was used to increase expiratory muscle strength, potentially supporting the generation of a louder voice. PhoRTE® was also chosen to improve respiratory phonatory coordination, aiding in reducing vocal effort, increasing endurance, and potentially supporting the generation of a louder voice.

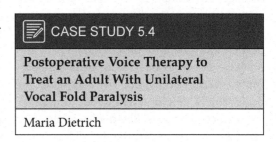

CASE STUDY 5.4

Postoperative Voice Therapy to Treat an Adult With Unilateral Vocal Fold Paralysis

Maria Dietrich

Voice Evaluation

Chief Complaint. Hoarseness and vocal fatigue

The patient was referred by her surgeon for a voice evaluation for a left unilateral vocal fold paralysis following thyroid surgery. The surgeon discussed the possibility of a vocal fold augmentation on the left side to medialize the vocal fold. The patient wanted to wait for the voice evaluation before making a decision regarding treatment.

Case History

History of the Voice Problem. Patient SJ is a 39-year-old cisgender woman with a complaint of gradually worsening dysphonia since her thyroid surgery for a large benign mass 4 months ago. At her 3-month follow-up appointment with the surgeon, the vocal fold paralysis persisted. Abnormalities of the crico-arytenoid joint were ruled out. The voice disorder was deemed iatrogenic in nature and was linked to injury of the patient's left recurrent laryngeal nerve during thyroid surgery. At the time of the voice evaluation, SJ described her voice as extremely hoarse and weak, and she complained that she had to push her voice. Her voice reportedly becomes occasionally aphonic after a speaking-intensive day. Current voice complaints include dysphonia worsening with use, increased vocal effort, vocal fatigue at the end of the day, diminished projection, and shortness of breath during speaking and during exertion. In addition, SJ reported having occasional swallowing difficulties with liquids, but she has become more careful and able to manage these difficulties. SJ reported no major voice problems prior to her surgery.

Medical History. The patient's medical history was otherwise unremarkable. She did not have any previous relevant surgeries apart from a tonsillectomy, nor any trauma to the head or neck. She rarely suffered from upper respiratory infections. She denies issues with allergies, reflux, or pulmonary disease. The patient takes thyroid medication.

Social History. Patient SJ is married with no children and works in human resources. She does not smoke and used to exercise 2 times per week. She reportedly drinks about 32 ounces of water and 2 cups of coffee or caffeinated tea per day. Her job is speaking-intensive and includes speaking one on one, on the telephone, to small groups, or while holding seminars with up to 25 employees. Prior to her thyroid surgery, she recalls occasional vocal fatigue, but she denied having had any longer-lasting voice problems. SJ relies on her voice for work, and she has become increasingly worried that she might lose her job due to her ongoing voice problems. Over the past month, there were a few days that she had to call in sick because of her dysphonia. She had to stop running and playing tennis because of shortness of breath. Overall, she has become increasingly frustrated that her dysphonic and weak voice limit her participation in professional, social, and recreational activities.

Auditory-Perceptual Assessment

The CAPE-V[23] was used to rate the patient's voice quality. SJ presented with a severe dysphonia with an overall score of 66/100 consistently characterized by severe breathiness (80/100), moderate roughness (36/100), severe vocal asthenia (88/100), and severe strain (66/100). Loudness was severely reduced (71/100) and pitch was mildly increased (15/100). Respiration was clavicular.

Laryngeal Imaging

A videostroboscopic examination was performed with a 70-degree rigid endoscope and without the use of a topical anesthetic. The VALI[17] was used to rate vocal fold structure and function. The left vocal fold was immobile and fixed in the paramedian to intermediate position, causing an incomplete vocal fold closure pattern with a dominating open phase. A plane difference (vertical level) of the vocal folds was not seen. The affected vocal fold had a severely reduced mucosal wave (rating 20/100) and vibrated only irregularly (0%), resulting in aperiodicity as seen on stroboscopy. Furthermore, supraglottic antero-posterior (rating 2/5) and medial (rating 3/5) compression of the ventricular folds was observed during phonation consistent with secondary MTD in response to the underlying glottal insufficiency. The vocal folds and posterior larynx were free of lesions and irritation, and structure and function of the unaffected vocal fold was unremarkable.

Patient-Reported Outcome Measures
- Voice Handicap Index (VHI)[75]: 88/120 (severe)
- Vocal Fatigue Index (VFI)[76]: 33/44 (vocal fatigue, high), 12/20 (physical discomfort, high), and 4/12 (recovery from fatigue, lower worse). Scores were abnormal.[77]
- Adapted Borg CR10 for Vocal Effort Ratings: 4/10, somewhat severe vocal effort[78]

Manual Palpation Assessment
Perilaryngeal muscle tension was assessed and rated normal, mild, moderate, or severe.

- Tension at the thyrohyoid space with/without report of pain: mild, with pain
- Tension at the base of tongue/suprahyoid region with/without report of pain: moderate, with pain
- Restriction of lateralization of thyroid cartilage bilaterally: normal

Acoustic and Aerodynamic Assessment
The patient's voice was analyzed using ADSV (Pentax Medical, Montvale, NJ) software.

Normative data are from ADSV[50] and Murton et al (2020).[79] An AKG C520 headset microphone was placed at a 45-degree angle at 4 cm from the corner of the mouth for data acquisition. Results of the assessment were as follows (Table 5–13).

Further, the patient's voice fundamental frequency and vocal intensity ranges were reduced at the top of the range. A pitch glide on /i/ was recorded (semitone range 26, female norm untrained 32) and the patient was asked to produce /a/ as quietly and as loudly as possible (intensity range 23 dB, female norm untrained 43).

Phonatory airflow and subglottic pressure as derived from intraoral pressure were assessed using the PAS (Pentax Medical, Montvale, NJ) and their respective norms.[67] The patient was asked to repeat 3 sets of 5 /pi/ syllables (Table 5–14).

Stimulability
The patient was not sufficiently stimulable for voice improvement utilizing twang voice (eg, facilitated by words "maybe" and "back") or resonant voice.

Impressions
The patient presented with a severe dysphonia characterized by a predominantly breathy voice quality with moderate roughness. The prognosis is limited by the large glottal gap

Table 5–13. Pretreatment Cepstral Measures

	Sustained Vowel /a/	All-Voiced Sentence
Mean CPP (dB)	5.06	2.62
SD CPP (dB)	0.44	0.81
Mean L/H Ratio (dB)	33.04	25.69
SD L/H Ratio (dB)	0.84	2.75
Mean CPP F0 (Hz)	248.49	229.97
SD CPP F0 (Hz)	1.67	16.95
CSID	27.57	81.92

188 Voice Therapy: Clinical Case Studies

Table 5–14. Pretreatment Aerodynamic Assessment

	Results	Norms	X Indicates Abnormal
Mean Airflow During Voicing (mL/s)	380.0	100.0 (50.0)	X increased
Subglottic Pressure (cmH_2O)	11.4	5.40 (1.37)	X increased
Laryngeal Resistance (cmH_2O/mL/sec)	29.1	68.20 (53.08)	X decreased

(paramedian to intermediate vocal fold position) during phonation.

Plan of Care

The voice evaluation supports a temporary vocal fold injection laryngoplasty preceded by 1 session of voice therapy and followed by voice therapy for 10 sessions, once a week. The impression and plan of care were discussed with the patient and questions answered.

Long-Term Goal. The patient will participate in social and professional activities without feeling vocally restricted.

Short-Term Goals:

1. Provide education and psychoeducation about the laryngeal mechanism
2. Produce efficient voicing by appropriately balancing airflow and subglottal pressure
3. Train resonant voice to project without vocal strain

Decision Making

From the results of the laryngeal exam and voice assessment, it became clear that the patient's ability to produce a voice that is functional in daily life was limited. There is a risk that compensatory laryngeal hyperfunction will be carried over following the injection procedure. The temporary injection will improve voice immediately and will create a window of time to reset vocal habits. As her voice quality will fluctuate when the injection is wearing off or immediately after injection,

a structured voice exercise program such as VFEs will be essential to maximize vocal efficiency and to stabilize voice production with improved vocal technique. The synergy of early injection medialization laryngoplasty and early voice therapy aims to optimize vocal function in the long term.

Intervention

The patient decided to have the vocal fold injection procedure. The transnasal endoscopic vocal fold augmentation was scheduled as an outpatient office procedure. Voice therapy was scheduled once before the injection, with the remainder of the sessions after the injection. A vocal fold injection with Juvéderm into the left membranous vocal fold was performed successfully. Juvéderm is a hyaluronic acid-based injectable and is a temporary filler that lasts 4 to 6 months.

There are multiple hyaluronic acid-based injectables, as well as other materials, available for injection augmentation with varying duration of effectiveness. Duration of effect for hyaluronic acid products is impacted by the interaction of a variety of factors, including crosslinking and viscosity. It is incumbent on the SLP to communicate with the laryngologist regarding expected duration of benefit for the purposes of therapy planning and accurate patient counseling.

Preoperative Voice Therapy

Short-Term Goal #1. Education and psychoeducation about the laryngeal mechanism

Session #1. In the first voice therapy session prior to the injection procedure, the patient learned about vocal fold structure and function in accessible ways using images, videos, and her own assessment records. She also took a video of her laryngeal exam with her phone. The clinician reviewed the condition of vocal paralysis and the many options to treat glottal incompetence medically (injection laryngoplasty) and surgically (medialization thyroplasty). In addition, the clinician explained and visualized the condition of MTD. Due to SJ's speaking-intensive job, current pattern of MTD, and added stress with insecurity about voice quality, psychoeducation was an important additional treatment component. Together, the clinician and patient explored how she reacted to stress. She said that she would generally tense up in her head and neck during stress with occasional headaches. Vocally, she would get slightly louder and angry. Since the thyroid surgery, she felt that voicing was a battle and a gamble and that she pushed her voice to exert control. When she could not be heard and understood well, she became frustrated and increased her vocal effort even more to produce as much voice as possible. She used to have a strong voice and was rather talkative (7/10, where 1 means "quiet listener" and 10 means "extremely talkative"). Now, SJ noticed that triggers for laryngeal tension included when she sensed others were frustrated with her voice. She also noticed that she would automatically increase muscular tension when in "presentation mode" or when she was excited or annoyed about something. The clinician and patient explored, using (attempt of) breath holding as an example, how rising tension during stress strains the laryngeal muscles in the neck and changes respiration to shallow breathing.

Postoperative Voice Therapy

Short-Term Goal #2. Produce efficient voicing by appropriately balancing airflow and subglottal pressure

Session #2. As expected, SJ's voice quality improved after 1 week following vocal fold injection. Most importantly, she had a louder voice again. However, vocal endurance reportedly remained mildly limited, and she had a tendency for hard glottal attacks, which put her at continued risk for vocal fatigue. Her voice quality was mildly rough and strained. Given her vocal demands, SJ was asked to create a weekly chart of all vocal activities performed when she was awake. The clinician introduced vocal explorations to increase awareness of laryngeal function. The clinician guided the patient to practice contrasts of breathy, easy, and hard glottal onsets. (See Video 17 Contrasting Glottic Onset Types by Bond.) Then, practice advanced to contrasts of flow phonation and pressed voice using a tissue held between the index and middle finger as a biofeedback tool for airflow during vowel production modulated into words. The visual biofeedback helped her to form an appreciation for balancing airflow and pressure for voice for speech. The resonant humming gesture was introduced and explored. Finally, practice was advanced to clear speech using crisp articulation of consonants, while reducing vocal effort, to facilitate her intelligibility in noisy environments. An affirmative resonant hum was weaved into conversational speech.

To address vocal health and hygiene, an ultrasonic handheld inhaler was recommended to use with saline to address her sensations of frequent vocal tract dryness.

Session #3. The clinician and patient identified peak times of heavy voicing regarding both amount and type. She was advised to avoid scheduling vocally intensive meetings back to back, to schedule quiet work times several times a day, to avoid large group sessions at the end of the day, and to allow for rest and recovery before, during if possible (5-10 minutes), and after presentations of a duration of 1 hour or longer. The clinician guided the patient to look for phases where voicing went well and analyze those that were challenging.

To release tension in the perilaryngeal muscles and base of tongue, the clinician introduced progressive muscle relaxation to improve muscle tone in the patient's face, neck, and upper body by increasing and releasing tension. Then, the patient moved on to loosen vocalization by pounding gently on the chest or shaking the belly up and down while sustaining the vowel /a/ in unison, paying attention to a relaxed articulation posture. SJ started noticing the difference between a nearly complete bodily relaxation during voicing facilitated by playfulness versus compensatory respectively habitual vocal effort during voice production. She further realized how much control she had over her voice production patterns. Her task was to capture this whole-body experience of letting voice pass through her body and to memorize it. Her new visualization was supposed to be an open, easy, and effortless voice, as in a resonant voice. At the end of the session, SJ was introduced to the VFE training program to facilitate adoption of a voice production pattern with an efficient interplay of airflow and subglottal pressure for voicing. (See Case Study 3.6 by Stemple: Vocal Function Exercises to Treat an Adult With Undifferentiated Phonotrauma and Video 5 Vocal Function Exercises by Stemple.)

Session #4. The following sessions started with gentle stretches for the neck and face (eg, tilting head and stretching neck, yawning, massaging tongue muscles under the chin with knuckles) and progressive muscle relaxation exercises, which the patient could perform periodically throughout the day. Through increased awareness of vocal demands, SJ adjusted her work routine so that it was functional. When meeting with friends, she was advised to consider the location and the demands on her vocal system. If she found herself in a noisy environment, she was advised to sit close to her communication partners and to limit the time she would speak over background noise.

The patient really struggled to practice VFEs on the prescribed pitches despite help with audio recordings on her phone. Therefore, the clinician quickly took the exercises out of the prescribed context and emphasized quality instead of meeting the requirement of all 5 pitches. SJ improved the "ol" buzz but needed frequent feedback to further improve the vocal tract gesture. At the beginning, imitating the clinician worked best. The clinician also acted as a model for resonant voice during a conversational stretch at the end of the session.

> Dietrich describes the patient's difficulty with pitch matching. Initially, audio supports were used, but when this problem solving did not sufficiently correct the issue, Dietrich encouraged the patient to take the exercises "out of the prescribed context" to reduce cognitive load. The clinician used increased feedback and modeling to shape the resonant sound. Practicing exercises in poor form is unlikely to yield improvement. Taking time to assist the patient with achieving optimal form (open resonatory tube), as described here, will better ensure benefit from the exercises.

Session #5. The patient continued work with VFEs and, after achieving optimal form, she was able to hold out a note in exercise #4 for 35 seconds. In exercises #2 and #3, pitch glides on "ol" became smoother with improved supportive airflow. Despite problems with pitch accuracy, the patient was asked to practice the exercises twice a day as much as possible.

Short-Term Goal #3. Train resonant voice to project without vocal strain

Session #6. The patient improved the quality of VFEs once again and was able to practice in a self-guided manner. Resonant voice in conversational speech was made a specific target in voice therapy as soon as session #2. First, awareness for resonance was built to facilitate generalization of resonant voice to conversational speech. Resonant voice therapy is a well-known and well-researched voice therapy approach to produce a voicing pattern that is easy and efficient through minimum phonatory effort. The bonus is a louder voice. (For more information, see Case Study 3.7 by Orbelo, Li, and Verdolini Abbott: Lessac-Madsen Resonant Voice Therapy to Treat an Adult With Vocal Fold Nodules.) Practice started with the self-exploration of vibrations in the face and establishment of a basic humming gesture. The patient intuitively hummed, but time was taken each session to raise the bar and fine-tune her humming. Thinking of something tasty, for example, helped to make the production more natural. Automatizing this gesture in conversational speech was next. Using cueing, the patient became increasingly proficient in employing an optimal hum and using a hum to ease into phrases, so that cues could be faded. SJ quickly became adept at switching back and forth between her regular conversational voice, vocal fry, and resonant voice. The skills were honed with funny and animated poems where the patient was asked to connect words as much as possible and to linger on voiced consonants to stay in resonant mode. Brief audio recordings of the patient during therapy with time for feedback helped to hone the patient's vocal and auditory skills. The clinician created phone audio files with resonant voice exercises, as well as video clips that demonstrated the exercises. In particular, the patient appreciated the video examples to model her own vocal performance at home. SJ noticed that resonant voice remarkably improved her vocal endurance and voice quality, and she was very pleased that she was able to turn on resonant mode when needed.

In total, SJ participated in six 45-minute therapy sessions over an 8-week period. After the injection procedure, the sessions were held weekly.

Therapy Outcomes

The follow-up visit was scheduled 1 week after the last therapy session, which was 7 months after the thyroid surgery and 10 weeks after the vocal fold augmentation procedure. The previously severe dysphonia significantly improved to a mild dysphonia with mild vocal fatigue and vocal effort, as outlined in more detail as follows.

Auditory-Perceptual Assessment. The patient presented overall with a mild dysphonia (6/100) and consistent mild breathiness (4/100), roughness (15/100), asthenia (2/100), and strain (3/100) on the CAPE-V. Loudness and pitch were appropriate for age and gender.

Laryngeal Imaging. The videostroboscopic examination confirmed the continued presence of a left vocal fold paralysis. However, glottal closure with a predominant closed phase was present during modal phonation, which is likely due to the injectable still being present. The mucosal wave of the affected vocal fold remained reduced (rating 20/100), and vocal fold periodicity was still

> Materials used for vocal fold injection augmentation have variable life spans. Dietrich mentions that the follow up videostroboscopy was completed 10 weeks after the injection. Most injectable materials have at least a 3-month life span, so observing that the material was still present and notable in the examination is not surprising. The next steps for the patient will likely be dependent on how long the injectable endures in the vocal folds. Once the material is fully absorbed, the glottal gap typically returns, with a decline in voice quality. In this case, the benefit of the injectable wore off as expected, and the physician suggested a repeat injection. Another option for durable improvement in voice quality is a medialization laryngoplasty (thyroplasty).

irregular (0%). Significant secondary MTD characterized by supraglottic compression was not observed (anteroposterior rating 0/5 and medial rating 1/5).

Self-Reported Voice-Related Quality of Life, Vocal Effort, and Vocal Fatigue:

- VHI: 30/120, mild
- VFI: 13, 5, and 7 per subscale, indicating mild problems
- Adapted Borg CR10 for Vocal Effort Ratings: 2/10, slight vocal effort

Manual Palpation Assessment. Perilaryngeal muscle tension was assessed and was rated normal without pain for the thyrohyoid space, base of tongue/suprahyoid region, and lateralization of the thyroid cartilage.

Acoustic and Aerodynamic Assessment. Post therapy, the acoustic data were within the normal range. Mean Cepstral Peak Prominence (CPP) F0 (Hz) improved (sustained /a/ 231.1 Hz, SD 0.8; all-voiced sentence 186.7 Hz, SD 4.9) in that the baseline tendency for a slightly elevated pitch declined. The Cepstral Spectral Index of Dysphonia (CSID), which correlates with the auditory-perceptual evaluation of voice, improved significantly. The improvement was especially noticeable at the sentence level, which is more ecologically valid than the sustained vowel production (sustained /a/ 4.88, all-voiced sentence 5.58). The measures of CPP (dB) and low/high spectral (L/H) ratio (dB) contributed to overall improvement. Mean phonatory airflow (160 mL/sec), subglottic pressure (7.64 cmH$_2$O), and laryngeal resistance (43.24) were in the normal range matched for age and sex posttreatment.

Summary and Concluding Remarks

The outcome of voice therapy was excellent, and the patient was quite pleased with the sound and feel of her voice. The vocal fold augmentation procedure improved vocal fold closure immediately, but ultimately the patient's commitment to the treatment program helped her to better understand her vocal condition, to balance vocal function, and to monitor an easy and efficient voice in daily life, being prepared for the ups and downs as the injection material wears off. Approximately 6 months after the vocal fold injection, which was about 1 year after onset of vocal fold paralysis, a follow-up visit was scheduled that included laryngeal needle electromyography (EMG). The rationale was to evaluate the status of innervation in the left vocal fold and to discuss long-term treatment options as the effect of the vocal fold injection would have largely subsided. The instrumental evaluations showed that the left vocal fold paralysis persisted and that vocal fold closure was mildly incomplete. The laryngologist suggested a repeat vocal fold injection to maintain good results and encouraged the patient to seek voice therapy as needed.

CASE STUDY 5.5

Interprofessional Treatment for an Adult With Unilateral Vocal Fold Paresis

Desi Gutierrez and Matthew Hoffman

Voice Evaluation

Chief Complaint. Dysphonia, vocal fatigue, decreased pitch range, decreased volume

This patient was seen in an interprofessional model with the SLP and laryngologist. She presented with a diagnosis of left vocal fold paresis and suspected superior laryngeal nerve (SLN) injury.

Case History

History of Voice Complaint. Patient XZ is a 45-year-old cisgender woman who reports sudden onset of voice changes after her left thyroid lobectomy 3 months ago. Immediately after surgery, she reported her voice sounded raspy, breathy, and low in pitch and volume, especially with yelling. Her symptoms have slightly improved since onset. Voice quality worsens at the end of day with associated increased effort and soreness. Voice rest and hot tea marginally improve her voice. Her symptoms significantly impact her professional and personal life. Today is her first evaluation by a laryngologist or SLP. She has a history of asthma and multinodular goiter, which was the impetus for her thyroid surgery. Per surgical documentation, the recurrent laryngeal nerve (RLN) was intact at the conclusion of the operation. The SLN was not specifically identified during the procedure. She denies preoperative dysphagia or dysphonia.

Voice Use. The patient reports extremely high occupational voice demands as a department trainer for an insurance company. She talks on the phone and conducts Zoom meetings 3 to 4 times per week. She also has very high personal and social voice demands. She describes herself as "a very talkative person" and leads women's self-defense classes weekly, which requires her to yell. She does not use amplification for leading class or an external microphone for Zoom calls.

Laryngeal Imaging

Laryngeal videostroboscopy was performed transnasally with a flexible distal chip videolaryngoscope. The exam revealed no lesions or masses. Right vocal fold motion was normal. The left vocal fold had decreased motion, resting at paramedian position, and mild concavity of the medial edge. There was no vocal fold lengthening with an upward glissando. There was significant mediolateral supraglottic hyperfunction, with right greater than left false vocal fold hyperfunction. Glottic closure was incomplete with about a 1-mm gap. Phase asymmetry was present, with aperiodic vibration at higher frequencies.

Patient-Reported Quality-of-Life Impairment

- VHI-10[66]: 33/40 (threshold = 11)[20]
- Dyspnea Index (DI)[43]: 20 (threshold = 3)
- Eating Assessment Tool (EAT-10)[80]: 0 (threshold = 3)

Auditory-Perceptual Assessment

The CAPE-V was administered.[23] The patient was determined to have an overall CAPE-V score of 78/100, indicating severe dysphonia. Aberrant perceptual features included breathiness, strain, and roughness. Overall vocal loudness was noted to be mildly reduced. Pitch of the voice was slightly decreased for age and gender, with minimal pitch variability in conversation or pitch glides. Reduced phonatory airflow was noted, and resonance had posterior tone focus.

Manual Palpation Assessment

Muscle tension was assessed and rated on a visual analog scale where 0 = no tension and 100 = most tension. Results indicated:

- 69/100 tension at the thyrohyoid space
- 58/100 tension at the base of tongue (BOT)/suprahyoid region
- 52/100 tension at the submandibular region
- Patient had no report of pain or tenderness with palpation

Stimulability

The patient was marginally stimulable for a change in voice quality and not stimulable for change in pitch utilizing semi-occluded vocal tract exercises (SOVTEs; eg, lip trills, /v/) and exuberant voicing.

Impressions

This is a 45-year-old female with severe dysphonia and complaints of vocal fatigue and decreased vocal volume after thyroid surgery 3 months ago. The patient demonstrates inefficient voice use patterns, posterior tone focus, increased strain, low volume, and limited physiological pitch range. Based on the recency of her nerve injuries, it is unclear to what degree she may experience spontaneous return of vocal fold motion. She is highly motivated to participate in behavioral therapy; however, she is not stimulable for changes in quality or pitch range, which is a poor prognostic factor for voice therapy alone.

Plan of Care

The SLP and the laryngologist discussed the above findings with the patient. Therapy was deferred at this time in favor of initial vocal fold injection augmentation, per the laryngologist. The clinicians decided to reevaluate the patient for voice therapy postoperatively.

Intervention 1: Procedure

A transoral injection augmentation was performed in the clinic. The patient was seated in the sniffing position. Topical lidocaine with oxymetazoline was applied intranasally. Benzocaine was applied intraorally. The flexible endoscope was passed transnasally to visualize the larynx. Topical lidocaine was applied to the glottis during sustained phonation via an Abraham cannula. Restylane was then loaded onto the curved orotracheal injector and passed transorally, targeted to the posterolateral true vocal fold. A gentle medial convex contour was achieved. The patient was placed on 1 day of voice rest postinjection.

Reevaluation Highlights

Patient XZ returned for a 1-month postprocedural laryngoscopy and voice evaluation. She reported an 80% improvement in her voice. She has been able to return to regular voice use at work, but she continues to have vocal fatigue after a few hours of talking and is unable to yell. Laryngeal videostroboscopy revealed no changes to vocal fold mobility. Glottic closure was now characterized as complete. An overall CAPE-V score of 24/100 indicated mild dysphonia. Aberrant perceptual features identified in the voice included strain and roughness. Overall vocal loudness was noted to be WNL. She demonstrated minimal pitch variability in speech or pitch glides. The patient was stimulable for improved voice quality with SOVTEs but not stimulable for pitch change.

Acoustic Assessment

All data were gathered remotely using Phonalyze (https://phonalyze.com), a web portal that patients can access with their smartphones and that utilizes Praat software. Norms are derived from a literature review examining optimal norms for remote acoustic voice analysis.[81] Patients recorded themselves using their own smartphones, placed 12 inches from their mouth. Results are documented in Tables 5–15 through 5–18.

Impressions and Plan

Despite improvement from her injection augmentation, Patient XZ continues to demonstrate inefficient voice use patterns and limited physiological pitch range. Acoustic assessment reveals high pitch variability in sentences and passage reading; however, this is likely due to roughness rather than an actual ability to modify her pitch up by 80 Hz. She is motivated to participate in behavioral therapy and now stimulable for change in quality. The patient

Table 5–15. Physiological Pitch Range

Hertz	Notes	Semitone Range	Semitone Range Norms (SD)	Abnormal
182–215	F#3–A3	4	32 (10)	X

5. Glottal Gaps   195

Table 5–16. CPP Sustained Vowel

Sustained Vowel /a/	Value	Norms (SD)	Abnormal
Mean F0 (Hz)	177	210.4 (22.7)	X
Mean F0 SD (Hz)	7	2.37 (5.24)	
CPP	27.49	N/A	N/A
CPPS	18.53	15.08 (2.04)	X

Table 5–17. CPP All-Voiced Sentence

Voiced Sentence: "We were away a year ago."	Value	Norms (SD)	Abnormal
Mean F0 (Hz)	183	197.90 (16.70)	
Mean F0 SD (Hz)	80	33.17 (5.82)	X
AVQI	6.19	2.60 (0.67)	X
CPP	19.18	N/A	N/A

Table 5–18. CPP Rainbow Passage

Rainbow Passage: Sentences 1-5	Value	Norms (SD)	Abnormal
Mean F0 (Hz)	175	197.90 (16.70)	X
Mean F0 SD (Hz)	56	33.17 (5.82)	X
CPP	16.24	N/A	N/A
CPPS	10.34	7.59 (0.73)	X

will schedule 4 sessions of voice therapy, with further sessions as needed.

Long-Term Goal. The patient will demonstrate improved ease and quality of voice production with 80% accuracy into conversational speech independently with self-corrections.

Short-Term Goals:

1. The patient will implement amplification devices to reduce vocal fatigue during Zoom meetings and self-defense classes as measured by patient report.
2. The patient will demonstrate improved coordination of breathing and phonation with improved oral resonance in brief conversation with 80% accuracy.
3. The patient will demonstrate projection and natural prosody without strain in role-play scenarios with 80% accuracy.

Decision Making

Based on her evaluation, Patient XZ had 2 problems that contributed to her dysphonia. First, she had a glottal gap as a result of her paresis, which impaired her ability to approximate her vocal folds and generate adequate subglottic pressure to achieve sustained vocal fold oscillation. Vocal fold paresis can be treated initially with procedural/surgical intervention or voice therapy. Key factors driving treatment decisions include degree of glottic insufficiency, stimulability for improvement with therapy, and presence of thin-liquid dysphagia. This patient had incomplete closure even with compensatory supraglottic hyperfunction and was not stimulable for improvement with behavioral intervention. In this setting, initial procedural optimization to facilitate glottic closure, followed by postprocedural voice therapy to optimize coordination of respiration and phonation, was warranted. Injection augmentation is the primary procedural intervention for new-onset vocal fold paresis, and a variety of injectables can be used. This patient presented with improved glottic closure as a result of the injection augmentation but continued to push and strain during voicing. This persistent compensatory hyperfunction is common in the setting of a paresis after injection augmentation, and voice therapy has been used to improve subjective and objective measures of voice quality after injection augmentation in patients with vocal fold mobility impairment.[82]

Another factor that contributed to her continued dysphonia is her suspected SLN injury, as evidenced by limited ability to increase pitch. Laryngeal electromyography (LEMG) of the CT muscles is the gold standard to assess SLN function.[83] However, diagnostic indicators include an inability to alter pitch and, in the case of this patient, strain with even slight intonation and while yelling. On laryngeal imaging, some suggest that SLN injuries can manifest as deviation of the epiglottic petiole to the side of weakness dur-

ing high-pitched phonation[84] or axial rotation of the anterior commissure toward the side of weakness during rapid alternating adduction/abduction tasks.[85] Both voice therapy and injection augmentation are commonly prescribed for SLN injury; however, outcomes are more variable and harder to predict than for RLN injury.[83,86]

Considering the above, therapy aimed to (1) improve her coordination of respiration and phonation to decrease strain and (2) work within her limited pitch range to achieve loud voicing and natural prosody to convey emotions. This was achieved with a combination of approaches that target more forward resonance in normal and loud speech (ie, SOVTEs, Conversation Training Therapy, megaphone mouth posture) and by using volume and duration as a surrogate for pitch emphasis in various scenarios.

Intervention 2: Voice Therapy

Therapy began with a review of evaluation results, anatomy and physiology of voice production as related to Patient XZ's diagnosis and complaints, her goals, and time commitment required to achieve her goals. She was bothered by the tight sound and feel of her voice, vocal fatigue at the end of the day, and her inability to yell or emote. The patient was encouraged to reflect on the improvements since the injection augmentation while acknowledging that she needs behavioral intervention to decrease compensatory strain, which was previously required to produce any voice. Importantly, she was counseled on duration of the injectate, as significant decline in vocal quality during therapy may indicate return of glottic insufficiency. When this occurs, communicating with the laryngologist can allow for repeat examination and consideration of repeat injection augmentation if needed while awaiting potential return of nerve function. Education regarding the role of therapy for SLN injuries was also provided. Evidence is limited that therapy can lead to expanded pitch range and

SLN regeneration,[82] so although expanding her range will be targeted, the primary goal of therapy is to optimize her voice within her limited pitch range.

> As the case study authors point out, there are several options for injectables to use in augmentation. Most differ by pliability and duration of effect, ranging from about 3 to 12 months depending on the injectable. In this case, the authors indicate that the patient may need a repeat injection while waiting to see if the nerve recovers. Recovery, when it happens, can take between 6 and 12 months. Most surgeons counsel their patients to wait the 6 to 12 months to determine if the nerve will heal on its own or if the motion difficulties are permanent before recommending more durable treatments such as thyroplasty.

Short-Term Goal #1. The patient will implement amplification devices to reduce vocal fatigue during Zoom meetings and self-defense classes as measured by patient report. In session #1, Patient XZ was introduced to assistive technology to decrease vocal fatigue and the need for loud voicing. The clinician recommended an external microphone for her daily Zoom calls and a personal external amplification system for her self-defense classes, as the classroom does not have an amplification system. She purchased both devices before her second session. She had difficulty avoiding straining even with amplification, but she had slightly less vocal fatigue at the end of each meeting and class.

> Using amplification efficiently is not always intuitive for a patient. Sometimes, people continue to experience vocal effort even with amplification. The clinician can teach the patient to use amplification to increase vocal loudness while also minimizing vocal strain and effort.

Short-Term Goal #2. The patient will demonstrate improved coordination of breathing and phonation with improved oral resonance in brief conversation with 80% accuracy. In her first session, Patient XZ was introduced to SOVTEs to improve phonatory airflow and oral resonance while reducing strain. She began on an /f/ to establish easy airflow. Initially she demonstrated a forceful burst of air with head movement. With prompts to "let the air flow," she was able to decrease the intensity of her breath. She added her voice to produce a /v/ and was prompted to attend to the vibrations on her lips. She was able to feel the vibrations and noted how easily her voice came out. She was then prompted to maintain this easy feeling and clear voice in glides throughout her pitch range. As she approached the limits of her range, she reintroduced some strain and forward head movement. After a few minutes of independent practice, she was able to reduce strain and maintain easy phonation through her pitch range.

Tasks were then advanced to words beginning with /v/ (eg, "van," "viable," "view," "vest") and using /v/ to assist in the onset of phrases (eg, "v-Good morning," "v-I'm fine," "v-I'm on my way"). Adding this linguistic complexity resulted in her resonance becoming more posterior. As she practiced these words, she tended to say each word or phrase quickly, without feedback or taking a breath, repeating it until it sounded or felt right. To help her decrease her speaking rate and promote forward resonance, she was introduced to principles of Conversation Training Therapy (CTT). (For more information on CTT, see Case Study 3.1 by Gillespie and Gartner-Schmidt: Conversation Training Therapy [CTT] to Treat an Adult With Benign Midmembranous Lesions.) She was prompted to decrease her rate and speak crisply and clearly. She was able to feel the most forward resonance on the phrase "tip of the tongue and the teeth," which became somewhat of a mantra for her moving through therapy. With these techniques, she immediately progressed to the conversation level, maintaining forward resonance with minimal cueing. She benefited from negative practice to feel the harsh difference between her new "teeth voice" and her "throat voice." (See Video 2 Clear Speech and Negative Practice by Gillespie.)

This concluded her first session. Her homework included going through the /v/ hierarchy as needed or simply repeating "tip of the tongue and the teeth" to create a more forward sound, then using that voice for at least 30 to 60 seconds several times per day during reading or conversation. She was also tasked with gliding through her pitch range on /v/ several times throughout the day, especially before a meeting, martial arts class, or speaking engagement.

At her second session, her ability to find and maintain her forward resonance was fairly strong during structured activities; therefore, the majority of her second session was spent solidifying her "teeth voice" in conversation. She was able to return to her clear voice with the repetition of "tip of the tongue and the teeth," but this was not feasible to reset her voice in daily life. She was encouraged to brainstorm phrases she already says frequently that could function as a new mantra. She had difficulty identifying any phrases, but the clinician identified that she often asked, "You know what I mean?" at the end of sentences. She practiced this phrase with her "teeth voice" and was able to use it to maintain forward resonance and avoid pitch drop and fry at the end of her sentences. She also benefited from vocal resets midsentence on SOVTEs, which she was able to achieve by decreasing her rate and prolonging consonants in accordance with CTT, and from resonant communicators (eg, "mhm," "umm") in accordance with resonant voice therapy techniques.

At her third session, she reported that she felt confident maintaining her forward voice in conversation, but felt it was inflexible, as she had to sit upright and lean forward to achieve her voice. She was prompted to talk with her

"teeth voice" and gently sway her torso. She initially had difficulty but was able to stabilize her voice after a few minutes of practice. She slowly advanced to more complex movements, including shrugging her shoulders, shaking her head, moving her arms, walking around her room, and doing light aerobic exercise. By her fourth session, she felt confident that she was able to maintain her "teeth voice" in the majority of daily life, with only an occasional need to return to /v/ to reset her voice.

Short-Term Goal #3. The patient will demonstrate projection and natural emotional prosody without strain in role-play scenarios with 80% accuracy. During her second session, she was introduced to projection with a megaphone posture. She was prompted to take a full breath, maintain a relaxed open mouth, and say a strong "ah" without pushing out her voice. After initially pushing and straining her voice, she was able to achieve a clear, strong "ah" with prompts to "ease off it." She was advised to practice sparingly (~5 "ah"s per day) as she acclimated to this posture. At her third session, she progressed to words beginning with /ɑ/ (eg, "on," "option," "olive," "aunt"), words containing /ɑ/ (eg, "job," "drop," "water," "conduct"), and then short phrases beginning with /ɑ/ or /aɪ/ (eg, "Olive oil," "Options everywhere," "I'm over here," "I have one").

After she established her ability to project without strain, she was introduced to 3 methods to add emphasis to a sound or word: increasing pitch, increasing volume, or increasing vowel duration. Typically, when she added emphasis, she relied on increasing pitch, which increased strain. Therefore, she had to rely on increasing volume and duration to give similar prosody to her speech. These concepts were combined to practice the following natural phrases in her fourth session:

What are you doing?!	*This is too hot!*	*Wait for me!*
You'll never believe this!	*I'm over here!*	*Center! (for her classes)*

She had most difficulty with phrases with /i/ and /ɪ/ sounds, but she benefited from cues to relax her jaw and tongue. After she practiced each phrase a few times, she role played with the clinician to capture her emotions in various scenarios. For example:

Patient: "Wait for me! [breath] Wait for me! [breath] Wait for me!"

Clinician: "You're hiking with your husband and son, but you have to stop to tie your shoe. After you finish, you see that they are several yards ahead of you."

Patient: "Wait for me!"

Often, the phrase after the scenario was more strained and she reverted to increasing pitch for emphasis. By the end of the session, she demonstrated a strong understanding of concepts and by her fourth session, she was able to maintain a loud voice with emotional prosody without increasing pitch or strain in structured activities.

Posttreatment Outcomes

At her 1-month posttherapy laryngoscopy and voice evaluation, Patient XZ exhibited several improvements. She reported gaining confidence and comfort using her "teeth voice" and now only occasionally strains to get loud. Laryngeal videostroboscopy revealed no changes to vocal fold mobility. Glottic closure was characterized as complete with touch closure. Overall CAPE-V score was 6/100, indicating WNL voice quality. Aberrant perceptual features identified in the voice included slight, inconsistent strain and roughness. She continued to demonstrate limited pitch variability in conversation and pitch glides.

Patient XZ's acoustic assessment revealed an increase in her physiological pitch range from 33 to 109 Hz, or 4 to 9 semitones. This did not result in a perceptual change in her pitch range during speech, but it allowed her increased flexibility in pitch. Without LEMG, we are unable to confirm if therapy encouraged SLN regeneration or if this is the result of improved coordination of respiration and phonation. Her acoustic measures revealed that her previously high pitch variability during sentence and passage reading, which was likely due to roughness, returned to WNL. She had negligible change in her Acoustic Voice Quality Index (AVQI), CPP, and CPPS measures. Patient XZ planned to return to the clinic in 6 months, or sooner if her voice begins to deteriorate. If she does not have improved motion or tone in her left vocal fold, she may benefit from a repeat injection augmentation or, if she has persistent issues with glottic incompetence up to a year after injury, permanent procedural options such as medialization thyroplasty can be considered. She should continue to use her therapy techniques and may benefit from a review of therapy concepts at that time.

 CASE STUDY 5.6

Multimodality Teletherapy for an Adult Avocational Singer With Unilateral Vocal Fold Paresis

Lauren Timmons Sund

Voice Evaluation

I had the pleasure of seeing this patient for a comprehensive voice evaluation referred by a community laryngologist. The patient was diagnosed with dysphonia secondary to a left vocal fold paresis and compensatory muscle tension.

Case History

Chief Complaint. Voice changes status post thyroidectomy

History of Voice Complaint. Patient DJ is a 46-year-old cisgender woman with sudden onset of voice problems 4 years ago status post total thyroidectomy for thyroid cancer. The patient is a licensed marriage and family therapist as well as an avid avocational singer. She reports voice cracks, instability, and raspy quality in both speaking and singing. Voice is raspier when she is tired or has been using her voice a lot. She reports reduced range with loss of highest pitches, loss of control in falsetto, and reduced ability to belt. The patient has not received the services of an SLP for this problem in the past.

The patient reports high voice demands as a therapist and singer. She sings commercial/contemporary Christian music primarily and was a music worship leader at her church for many years before the onset of voice problems. She still occasionally leads worship at church, but she has mostly let others take over due to her voice problems and this upsets her, as music is reportedly an important emotional and spiritual outlet for her.

Laryngeal Imaging

Laryngeal videostroboscopy was performed transnasally with a flexible distal chip video-laryngoscope.

Salient Examination Findings. No supraglottal or hypopharyngeal masses. Full abduction and adduction of right vocal fold. Mildly reduced abduction and adduction of the left vocal fold. Small, anterior glottic gap with touch closure (reduced duration of closed phase). Moderate anterior-posterior and mediolateral supraglottic compression with reduced false fold squeeze on the left. Intermittent phase asymmetry. Mucosal wave was intact bilaterally with WNL amplitude and periodicity.

Quality-of-Life Impairment

1. VHI-10[66]: 20/40 (threshold = 11)[20]
2. Voice Catastrophization Index[87]: 28/52
3. Voice Problem Impact Scales (VPIS)[44] where 1 = no impact and 7 = profound impact, the patient reported the following:
   a. Impact on work life or daily activities: 4/7

b. Impact on social life: 3/7
c. Impact on home life: 3/7
d. Impact of voice overall: 5/7

Vocal Effort, Fatigue, and Pain

The OMNI-VES was completed. The patient reported that vocal effort was 3/10 (easy-somewhat easy) during the evaluation and 8/10 (hard) at worst, occurring in singing or at the end of a workday.

Auditory-Perceptual Assessment

The CAPE-V[23] was administered. The patient had an overall score of 23/100, indicating a dysphonia of a mild nature. Aberrant perceptual features identified in the voice included intermittent roughness. Overall vocal intensity was noted to be WNL. Pitch of the voice was WNL for age and gender in connected speech. There were pitch breaks and strained quality in ascending pitch glides. Maximum pitch range was reduced compared to expected range given singing experience, and the patient confirmed reduced pitch range compared to healthy baseline. Resonance was focused in the laryngeal region. Respiration appeared to be primarily abdominal-thoracic.

Manual Palpation Assessment

Muscle tension was assessed and rated on a 0 to 5 scale where 0 = no tension and 5 = most tension. Results indicated:

- 3/5 tension at the thyrohyoid space without report of pain on palpation
- 2/5 tension at the base of tongue (BOT)/suprahyoid region without report of pain
- laryngeal height was WNL as assessed by palpation of the hyoid bone
- 2/5 restriction of lateralization of thyroid cartilage bilaterally

Acoustic and Aerodynamic Assessment

Acoustic and aerodynamic assessment were completed using the Pentax Computerized Speech Lab (CSL) and PAS (Pentax Medical, Montvale, NJ) using recommendations from

Patel et al (2018).[88] Results were largely WNL, consistent with the auditory-perceptual assessment of a mild dysphonia. Maximum fundamental frequency was reduced compared to the patient's reported baseline. Results are detailed in Table 5–19 and Table 5–20 with normative data compiled from Zraick et al (2012), Goy et al (2013), Kent et al (2023), Siupsinskiene and Lycke (2011), Sanchez et al (2014), Buckley et al (2023), and Lewandowski et al (2018).[26,71,89–93]

Stimulability Testing

The patient was stimulable for reduced roughness in semi-occluded /u/ prolongations with patient-reported low vocal effort.

Impressions

The patient presents with mild dysphonia in the context of unilateral vocal fold paresis, which limits communication, daily activities, and participation. The dysphonia is characterized by intermittent roughness with posterior

Table 5–19. Acoustic Assessment Results

	Results	Normative Data Cisgender Females				Outside Norms
		Younger		Older (60+)		
Connected Speech: Frequency						
Mean F0: Rainbow Passage (Hz)*	195.78	181	226	151	248	
F0 SD: Rainbow Passage (Hz)*	43.3	34	57	27	52	
Mean F0: Conversation (Hz)	215.38, SD: 35.15					
Sustained Phonation /a/: Frequency						
Mean F0 (Hz)*	218.87	191	211	189	211	X
Range: Max F0 (Hz)*	775	363	683	231	502	
Range: Min F0 (Hz)	140	117.69		130		-
Range (in octaves)	2.5	1.85	3.05	1.85	3.05	-
Connected Speech: Intensity						
Mean SPL: Rainbow Passage (dB)*	70.56	62	73	60.8	71.7	
Sustained Phonation /a/: Intensity						
Mean SPL (dB)*	73.34	68.9	80.2	68.7	79.5	
ADSV Sustained Vowel CPP (dB), SD	12.518, 0.581	8.09				
ADSV Rainbow Passage CPP (dB), SD	6.024, 4.173	5.04				

Voice Therapy: Clinical Case Studies

Table 5–20. Aerodynamic Assessment Results

	Results		Normative Data			1SD Form Mean	Outside Norms
			F 18-39	F 40-59	F 60+		
Vital Capacity (L)	3.68		**2.87**	**2.85**	**2.09**	X	
		SD	0.69	0.78	0.63		
MFR (L/sec): Vowel (mean airflow during voicing)	0.123		**0.13**	**0.15**	**0.11**		
		SD	0.06	0.07	0.06		
MFR (L/sec): Rainbow Passage First 4 Sentences	0.175		**0.15**	**0.16**	**0.14**		
		SD	0.05	0.05	0.05		
Duration (sec)	21.22		**20.95**	**23.15**	**24.97**		
		SD	2.06	2.67	3.43		
Breaths (#)	3		**4.38**	**4.72**	**5.64**		
		SD	1.44	1.73	1.83		
Psub (cmH$_2$O) (mean peak air pressure)	7.8		**5.4**	**5.88**	**7.78**		
		SD	1.37	2.06	4.23		
PTP (cmH$_2$O): Quietest Modal (mean peak air pressure)	4.59						

locus of resonance in connected speech with strain and pitch breaks in falsetto register and reduced pitch range.

Plan of Care

Treatment with voice therapy was recommended and deemed medically necessary. The patient appeared to be a good candidate for therapy. Positive prognostic indicators included patient-reported motivation to engage in voice therapy and favorable response to stimulability testing. Negative prognostic indicators included dysphonia secondary to persistent vocal fold paresis now 4 years status post thyroidectomy. Given the time elapsed since the initial injury, further recovery of vocal fold motion is not expected; however, optimizing coordination of voice subsystems and reducing compensatory muscle tension can be addressed behaviorally to improve voice quality, voice function, and voice-related quality of life. The patient elected to begin voice therapy with the following plan:

Long-Term Goal. Optimize coordination of voice subsystems and increase vocal endurance to improve voice quality, voice function, and voice-related quality of life

Frequency. 4 to 6 sessions of 45 to 60 minutes each, twice monthly

Short-Term Goals:

1. VFEs to improve vocal endurance, vocal stability, and reliability through optimizing coordination of voice subsystems
2. Vocal tract shaping using nasal twang to optimize resonance with low vocal effort throughout the frequency range, especially in high modal register and when transitioning between TA-dominant phonation and CT-dominant phonation
3. Utilize additional SOVTEs to optimize glottal postures, stabilize respiratory phonatory coordination, and improve vocal precision throughout the frequency range

Decision Making

The laryngologist did not recommend vocal fold injection augmentation as the first line of treatment because the patient had relatively good glottal closure and some stimulability for better voice during the laryngology exam. Therefore, the laryngologist suspected the patient may be a candidate for voice therapy and referred the patient to the SLP to evaluate therapy candidacy. In this clinician's experience, singers who suffer from vocal fold paresis or hypomobility often completely stop singing after the nerve injury due to an experience of devastation when hearing the change in voice quality or due to fear of inducing further injury. Even in cases in which vocal fold motion eventually recovers completely, singers can continue to experience voice problems due to persistent compensatory muscle tension, deconditioning, aging, or a combination of these. In this patient's case, she had sung daily prior to her injury and had nearly eliminated all singing after the injury. Her voice problem was due, in part, to the vocal fold paresis but presumably also to disuse from reduced singing and muscle tension secondary to the voice change following the injury. The intermittent roughness was perceived to be secondary to poor respiratory phonatory coordination in the context of vocal fold asymmetry, and strain in high TA dominant phonation was perceived to be due to suboptimal resonance leading to supraglottic hyperfunction. Often, improving respiratory phonatory coordination, resonance, and vocal endurance can improve the voice even when hypomobility is present. Therefore, an approach was taken to directly target vocal endurance using VFEs and to directly target coordination of respiration, phonation, and resonance within the context of daily voice use, both singing and speaking. In this clinician's experience, it is helpful to start with VFEs, explaining to the patient that the goal is to first rebuild vocal endurance after a period of injury and deconditioning, then refine voice coordination for specific tasks (eg, singing, conversation) after improving endurance. Typically, the patient will notice marked improvement after the use of VFEs for this purpose but will still have specific deficits that can more easily be identified. For example, patients can more easily specify distinct problems such as breaks in register transition or roughness in a certain range versus a general complaint of "I've lost my singing voice" or "I can't sing anymore."

Intervention

Voice therapy was conducted via synchronous telepractice using a video-enabled, HIPAA-compliant platform. The patient participated in 6 sessions of voice therapy over the course of 3 months.

Session #1

Goal #1. Use VFEs to improve vocal endurance, vocal stability, and reliability by optimizing coordination of voice subsystems.

204 Voice Therapy: Clinical Case Studies

Patient DJ was trained in completing VFEs to capitalize on the use of the semi-occlusion for impedance matching, optimizing glottal configuration, improving balance among the subsystems of voice, and increasing vocal endurance. (For further information, see Case Study 3.6 by Stemple: Vocal Function Exercises to Treat an Adult With Undifferentiated Phonotrauma and Video 5 Vocal Function Exercises by Stemple.) The clinician first guided the patient to feel a sensation of anterior vibrations on a /mimimi/ chant at comfortable pitch and loudness to establish forward resonance and low vocal effort. The task was then transitioned to quiet sustained /mi/ with forward focus on F4 for maximum duration (VFE #1—warm-up). DJ benefitted from cues for an abdominal-thoracic preparatory breath to achieve a maximum duration of 14 to 15 seconds. The clinician then trained DJ in the kazoo buzz /u/ sound with narrow, round /u/ lips and more open /o/ posture inside the mouth. This kazoo buzz /u/ posture was implemented for exercises #2, ascending glides (stretch), and #3, descending glides (contraction). In exercise #4 (strength/power exercises), the patient sustained phonation on C4 to G4 on the kazoo buzz /u/ for a range of 11 to 24 seconds. Initially, DJ demonstrated vocal instability due to inconsistent airflow in exercises #2 through #4 on the kazoo buzz. The clinician provided cues for round lip posture and instructed the patient to hold a finger up in front of her mouth to feel the airflow. Self-monitoring of airflow on the patient's finger resulted in a significant improvement in vocal stability and eliminated pitch breaks that were initially present in pitch glides (exercises #2 and #3). (For more information on flow phonation, see Case Study 4.3 by Gartner-Schmidt: Flow Phonation to Treat a Teenager With Primary Muscle Tension Aphonia.)

Importantly, the clinician counseled the patient on frequency of practice. The clinician described that research on VFEs is typically conducted with participants completing the program twice per day. However, in this clini-cian's experience, it is rare for patients in the clinical setting to achieve this frequency and, when they don't, they often feel defeated. The patient was advised that, anecdotally, nearly all patients complete the program only once per day, 5 to 7 days per week, and these patients still get better. With this information and considering her own schedule, the patient made an informed decision to set her goal as practicing once daily, 6 days per week. She reported she would attempt twice per day when possible to give herself "an extra pat on the back." However, if she only achieved once per day, she would "feel accomplished."

Session #2 (Two Weeks Later)

Goal #1. *VFEs.* Patient DJ reported she had practiced her exercises for the first few days but then had been unable to practice due to a family emergency that had since been resolved. She requested review of her technique for VFEs to ensure optimal practice, which was provided. The clinician also educated the patient further on improving precise laryngeal coordination for exceptional voice demands after 4 years of minimal singing. This clinician likes to describe this process as adjusting to a "new instrument":

Recalibrating your voice after injury and disuse is like learning to play an instrument that has changed. You haven't forgotten how to sing, but the instrument you're playing has changed. Think about a talented concert pianist who can play every note from memory with their eyes closed. If you moved some of the piano keys by even a millimeter, that incredible pianist would suddenly play all the wrong notes. But they still know how to play piano! The instrument has just changed. If the pianist practices on that new piano with the shifted keys, they'll adjust and start playing beautifully again. Your voice— your instrument—has changed. It will take some time and effort to acclimate to your new instrument. Importantly, your voice will likely not be exactly the same as it was 4 years ago, but that is to be expected. Even in the absence of injury, your voice would have changed slightly over the course of 4 years, though at a slow rate that you may not have noticed. Despite this, acclimating to your new instrument can greatly improve your voice production because you still know how to sing.

Following this discussion, the clinician and patient collaboratively developed a plan to implement VFEs for 1 month to improve vocal endurance and stability. At the next appointment, the patient will identify remaining voice concerns, and additional exercises will be introduced to address any remaining voice deficits.

Session #3 (Four Weeks Later)

Goal #1. *VFEs.* Patient DJ demonstrated VFEs for the clinician to assess accuracy and progress. MPT ranged from 20 to 25 in exercises #1 and #4 and there were no voice breaks in pitch glides for exercises #2 and #3. There was mild breathiness in kazoo buzz /u/ tasks, and this was subtly improved with cues to increase forward resonance.

Goal #2. *Vocal tract shaping using nasal twang to optimize resonance with low vocal effort throughout the frequency range, especially in high modal register and when transitioning between TA-dominant phonation and CT-dominant phonation.* Patient DJ reported particular concern that her voice still cracked when "belting," which is high-intensity modal/TA dominant phonation. The clinician utilized nasal twang for vocal tract shaping to increase aryepiglottic narrowing for a "clearer" sound with low vocal effort. Nasal twang and aryepiglottic narrowing are both concepts discussed in Estill Voice Training.[94,95] Stimuli for this began with "nyeah" on a 3-note scale, 1-2-3-2-1. This resulted in improved clarity and stability of voice production and reduced vocal effort reported by the patient. The task was then advanced to gradually reduce nasality and expanded to additional syllables, "nyah" and "nee." (See Video 15 Anchoring and Twang to Reduce Vocal Effort by Timmons Sund.)

The patient's home program was to continue with VFEs once daily (to be completed first and used as a warm-up), followed by 5 to 10 minutes of nasal twang tasks with gradual fading of nasality.

Session #4 (Two Weeks Later)

Patient DJ reported continued use of VFEs plus nasal twang exercises for 10 minutes daily and noted her voice is improving. She even started recording music this past week. She reported she still notices voice breaks and strain in her register transition around B4 to C5.

Goal #1. *VFEs.* Maximum phonation time increased to 23 to 29 seconds across VFE #1 and #4. Resonance, loudness, and voice quality were appropriate across tasks and further cueing was not needed. Since the patient had experienced improved vocal stability with VFEs and enjoyed these exercises, the clinician advised the patient she could expand exercise #4 to include additional pitches, both below C4 and above G4. The patient decided to expand exercise #4 to include A4 to C5 (C4-C5 total). This clinician frequently expands the pitch range for exercise #4 with singers once they are comfortable with VFEs, if they report benefit.

Goal #2. *Vocal tract shaping.*

Goal #3. *Utilize additional SOVTEs to optimize glottal postures, stabilize respiratory phonatory coordination, and improve vocal precision throughout the frequency range.* The clinician introduced tasks to reduce strain and voice breaks in the patient's register transition from TA-dominant to CT-dominant phonation. First, semi-occluded lip trills were used on pitch pattern 3-5-1 across the range of F3 to F5. The clinician provided cues to maintain steady airflow and to "shift tension from the throat" to other parts of the body. The Estill concept of "anchoring" was used for this purpose.[94] The clinician described the following:

Anchoring is the idea that we need stability in the large muscles of our body to best support the fine motor movement in the larynx without excess strain. As an example, think about handwriting. We use our hands and fingers for fine motor movement, but we rest a larger part of our body, our arm, on the table to stabilize the hand and fingers. If we don't rest our arm on the table, then we end up with more tension in our hand (and our handwriting isn't as good).

To achieve anchoring, the patient was guided to feel her feet connected to the floor and add a slight push in her feet/toes when approaching a pitch that she anticipated straining on. Typically, this will be the highest pitch. In the 3-5-1 pattern, DJ attended to anchoring particularly on pitch 5. Use of anchoring resulted in reduced strain as reported by the patient, as well as improved voice quality per the clinician's auditory perception. Lip trills were then advanced to resonant voice prolongations /m/-, /v/-, and /n/-initial syllables on a variety of pitch patterns. Use of nasal twang was incorporated when strain was heard or vocal effort was reported. Over the course of the session, voice breaks were eliminated and the patient reported reduced vocal effort.

Since the patient was improving as desired, the clinician began to discuss an eventual transition to a singing teacher when discharged from voice therapy. It is often helpful to start this conversation early so it can continue across several sessions, if needed, and so the patient understands the difference between voice rehabilitation and habilitation.

Estill Voice Training is an approach to vocal skill development that aims to isolate control of different components of the vocal mechanism. These elements are known as voice figures and can be combined in various ways to achieve different voice and resonant qualities. The method was first developed by Jo Estill, a singer and vocal pedagogue. While not originally created for use in voice therapy, elements of the program can be thoughtfully incorporated into a comprehensive, physiologically robust voice therapy plan.

Session #5 (Two Weeks Later)

Patient DJ reported that her voice had been "so good" that she is auditioning for a televised singing competition tonight. She reported continued intermittent strain, but this usually resolves with use of her voice exercises.

Goal #2. *Vocal tract shaping.*

Goal #3. *SOVTEs.* Resonant voice (/v/, /m/, /n/), SOVTEs (lip trills), and twang ("nyeah") tasks were continued to establish respiratory phonatory coordination and forward resonance with reinforcement of low vocal effort. In the range of F3 to F5, DJ reported vocal comfort and demonstrated favorable oral/forward resonance when provided with minimal clinician cueing. Helpful cues included aiming the voice toward the top lip or nose, increasing mouth aperture for "megaphone" mouth shape in the "nyeah" belting context, and anchoring with "feet to floor."

The clinician and patient discussed vocal pacing for the rest of the day given the patient's audition later that night. The patient was advised to minimize intensive practice during the day. Although her voice had significantly improved, she still had vocal fold paresis and there was concern for vocal fatigue that could negatively impact her performance.

The clinician and patient additionally continued the conversation on preparing for discharge and transitioning to a singing teacher.

Session #6 (Two Weeks Later) and Discharge

Patient DJ reported her voice function had been "very good" since she was last seen, and she was pleased with the progress. She had several upcoming performances. Patient DJ reported her voice seemed back to her healthy baseline.

The clinician reassessed voice quality, stability, and flexibility throughout the physiological frequency range to determine if there were any remaining impairments to be addressed in voice therapy. In vowels and lip trills, voice quality was clear through E5.

Minor strain was perceived on the /a/ vowel in the falsetto register. Cues were provided for vowel modification, which resulted in reduction of auditory-perceptual strain. The clinician recommended further work on vocal tract shaping and vowel modification in voice lessons since this was a concern related to habilitation versus rehabilitation for this patient.

Follow-up measures:

- CAPE-V: 11/100 with intermittent roughness at the ends of utterances (improved from 23/100)
- OMNI-VES: 1/10 (improved from 3/10 during the evaluation and 8/10 at the end of a workday)

Patient DJ completed 6 sessions of voice therapy in 3 months, with improved voice quality and function per clinician and patient measures. The clinician and patient discussed this progress and agreed on readiness for discharge with a transition to a singing teacher. Follow-up with the referring laryngologist was recommended. The patient was advised that her motion asymmetry due to vocal fold paresis would likely be stable compared to pretherapy since this was an old nerve injury. However, this should not be a concern given the functional voice improvements.

Concluding Remarks

This case demonstrates the benefit of a consistent vocal fitness routine, even in the presence of a mild, long-standing vocal fold paresis. In this clinician's experience, singers who have been away from singing, regardless of reason, can benefit from a dedicated vocal endurance routine to rebuild stamina and rapport with their voice. VFEs work well for this purpose given the focus on vocal precision and stability, forward resonance, and full pitch range. The addition of skill-specific exercises (eg, targeting register transitions, pitch agility) is often more successful after improving baseline stamina and vocal control. This case also demonstrates the benefit of involving the patient in goal setting and the development of a home practice program.

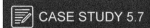

CASE STUDY 5.7

Interprofessional Treatment for an Adult With Sulcus Vocalis

Amanda I. Gillespie and Clark A. Rosen

Voice Evaluation

Sarah underwent a comprehensive, interdisciplinary voice evaluation that consisted of an auditory-perceptual, acoustic, and aerodynamic voice evaluation; patient-perceptual evaluation of voice handicap; and laryngeal imaging with rigid stroboscopy.

Case History

History of the Voice Problem. Sarah, a 36-year-old cisgender female, presented with complaints of severe dysphonia that worsened with prolonged or loud voice use. She reported her voice problems began 12 years ago and had been gradually worsening since onset. While her voice quality was never "normal," she described more severe dysphonia with voice use and with seasonal changes. For the last 5 years, she had used her voice professionally as an elementary school teacher. Prior to that, she worked in the restaurant industry with substantial voice demands. Her past medical history included laryngopharyngeal reflux disease and migraines. Her past surgical history was significant for microsuspension laryngoscopy at an outside hospital to remove bilateral vocal fold lesions 11 years ago. She reported that although her voice improved temporarily after that surgery, it never completely returned to normal and began deteriorating within a few months. She never participated in voice therapy, nor had she ever received consultation by an SLP. She continued to work after

Voice Therapy: Clinical Case Studies

her voice surgery but was currently on medical leave due to severe dysphonia impacting her ability to teach a full day of classes.

Voice Hygiene. Sarah reported drinking approximately 4 bottles of water and 2 cups of coffee per day. She had a remote history of social tobacco use. Her job as an elementary school teacher caused frequent changes to the quality of her voice, and it is notable that she reported that she does not use amplification.

Auditory-Perceptual Evaluation

An SLP perceptually evaluated Sarah's voice with the CAPE-V.[23] Her overall voice severity was rated at 72/100 on a visual analog scale of 100 equal intervals, and was described as rough, breathy, strained, and with a lower than normal pitch for her age and sex.

Patient Self-Assessment

Sarah reported that her voice problem had a moderate to severe effect on her daily life and that she experienced severe vocal fatigue. She scored 36/40 on the VHI-10,[66] indicating a high degree of self-perceived vocal handicap.[20]

Acoustic Analysis and Aerodynamic Measures

Sarah underwent an acoustic and aerodynamic voice assessment as a part of her initial clinic evaluation. Acoustic evaluation was completed using the Pentax computerized speech lab (Pentax Medical, Montvale, NJ), ADSV program. Cepstral analyses of connected speech (all-voiced sentence, "We were away a year ago") revealed a cepstral peak prominence (CPP) of 3.74 dB and a cepstral-spectral index of dysphonia (CSID) score of 42. These values all indicated an acoustic voice signal outside the normal range.[8] Importantly, cepstral measurements are sensitive to microphone type, mouth-to-mic distance, and vocal intensity, among other factors. Therefore, gold-standard normative data that can be applied across patients and clinics do not exist. Some general guidelines for interpretation of patient outcomes are included in Table 5–21.[70,96]

Table 5–21. Acoustic Normative Values

Measure	Normative Referent Value
CPP in sustained vowel	11.08 dB
CPP in connected speech	5.42 dB
CSID in connected speech	24

The authors remind the reader that it is important to know details about microphone type and mouth-to-mic distance, as these factors influence acoustic results. Many clinicians who treat dysphonic patients use CPP to demonstrate change within the same patient, but it is important to use the same microphone, same distance to the microphone, and same stimuli when comparing results.

Aerodynamic evaluation of consonant-vowel repetitions (/pipipipipi/) revealed greater than normal mean translaryngeal airflow (237 mL/sec) and estimated subglottal pressure (Psub) values (9.01 cmH$_2$O). In connected speech reading of the first 4 sentences of the Rainbow Passage, Sarah took 6 breaths in 25 seconds of reading and had a mean translaryngeal airflow of 241 mL/sec. Normal values for healthy speakers are 5 breaths in 23 seconds and mean phonatory airflow of 160 mL/sec.[58] These voice laboratory values, including the patient-perceptual measurements, are consistent with those found in individuals with sulcus vocalis.[97,98]

Stimulability Testing

After objective measures were obtained and results explained to the patient, the SLP proceeded to test Sarah's ability to modify her voice production in response to therapeutic cues.[99] SOVTEs were trialed. Sarah was able to achieve perceptually easier voicing when phonating through a straw in water and modulating her pitch in slow ascending and descending glides. Resonant voice basic training gestures were trialed next. The basic training gesture is a strategy introduced by Verdolini Abbott in Lessac-Madsen Resonant Voice Therapy (LMVRT) wherein a patient sustains a phoneme (often a nasal consonant) in a word or short phrase to focus on the articulatory sensations. In this case, isolated nasal sounds (hum) resulted in an increase in perceptual voice clarity, and Sarah reported feeling anterior oral and facial sensations during the production but was not able to maintain the clarity into single words or short phrases. (For further information on LMRVT, see Case Study 3.7 by Orbelo, Li, and Verdolini Abbott: Lessac-Madsen Resonant Voice Therapy to Treat an Adult With Vocal Fold Nodules.)

Laryngeal Imaging

Sarah's laryngeal function was evaluated with rigid laryngeal stroboscopy. Mucosal waves of both true vocal folds were decreased. Vocal fold closure was short, and an elliptical closure pattern and aperiodic vibratory activity were seen. Right true vocal fold sulcus deformity of the vocal fold was diagnosed, causing glottal incompetence. Flexible laryngoscopy was performed to assess vocal fold motion and observe laryngeal behaviors associated with connected speech. This revealed normal vocal fold motion and secondary compensatory MTD.

Impressions

Sarah presents with a voice disorder characterized by high self-perceived voice handicap and abnormal acoustic measures that correspond to aperiodic vibration visualized on stroboscopic laryngeal imaging. She phonates with high translaryngeal airflow that corresponds to her stroboscopic findings of incomplete glottal closure. Her medical diagnosis is a sulcus deformity of the true vocal fold. She demonstrates moderate stimulability for

voice improvement with behavioral strategies. Her prognosis for improvement with voice therapy alone, however, is guarded given her laryngeal anatomy, high occupational voice demands, and only moderate stimulability for change. On the other hand, she is motivated and states willingness to adhere to therapeutic recommendations.

Plan

It is recommended that Sarah proceed with a behavioral trial of voice therapy. Her long-term goal is to rehabilitate her vocal functioning for full participation in vocal activities of daily living. Short-term goals include reducing secondary muscle tension through vocal exercises using an SOVTE approach. Should this initial goal be successful, additional short-term goals to reduce tension and improve vibratory function in extemporaneous connected speech will be pursued. A reassessment should occur following 4 sessions of voice therapy, or sooner based on progress and the treating SLP's discretion. If voice goals are not met with voice therapy alone, surgical intervention will be considered.

Decision Making

Sulcus denotes a groove or furrow, and when a groove/furrow occurs along the vibrating edge of the vocal fold (free edge) *and* disrupts mucosal vibration, it is called a sulcus deformity of the vocal fold. If a linear depression occurs along the vocal fold free edge *without* disruption of the mucosal wave (called a physiologic sulcus vocalis or Ford type 1), no treatment is required.[100] Sulcus deformity of the vocal fold results in a loss of lamina propria with an invagination of the epithelium down to the vocal ligament (sulcus vergeture, Ford type 2). This pathologic change can also be found with significant deposition of scar tissue within the subepithelium space, resulting in sulcus vocalis (Ford type 3)[101] (Figure 5–4). Stroboscopically, pathologic sulcus deformity of the vocal fold causes vocal fold stiffness,

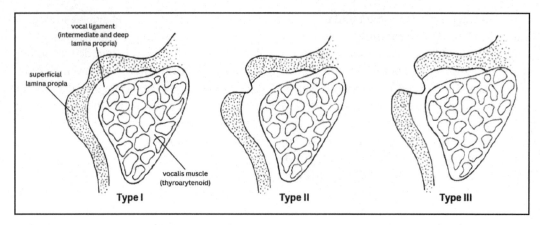

FIGURE 5–4. Ford classification for sulcus.

reduced mucosal wave, a "bowed" appearance of the vocal fold of the affected side(s), and glottal incompetence.[97,98]

Sulcus deformity of the vocal fold(s) is often a severe vocally limiting pathology, and despite aggressive treatment, full recovery of normal vocal function is rare.[98] Sulcus deformity of the vocal fold is most commonly treated with surgery.[100] Voice therapy is rarely successful as a sole treatment for sulcus. However, in many situations, patients have developed maladaptive voicing behaviors to compensate for the phonatory defects caused by the sulcus. In those cases, voice therapy can play a complementary role in improving overall voice technique and assisting in rehabilitation of vocal function in individuals with sulcus.[97] It is imperative that a team approach, combining the expertise of a laryngologist and a voice-specialized SLP, be utilized in the management of patients with sulcus deformity of the vocal fold. It is also critical that the treating SLP knows the limits of voice therapy for a patient with sulcus and knows when discharge from therapy is appropriate.

Based on Sarah's objective and subjective evaluation, a team approach including initial trial voice therapy, followed by reevaluation to determine the need for surgical intervention, was recommended. Voice therapy was considered a trial given Sarah's laryngeal examination revealing a sulcus deformity of the vocal fold (sulcus vergeture, Ford type 2) and her minimal to moderate response to stimulability probes. The plan for the voice therapy trial was continued stimulability testing with a goal of realizing a voice therapy strategy with the greatest likelihood of improving her speaking voice technique to optimize Sarah's voice production given her laryngeal disorder. The physician-SLP team thought Sarah may eventually require surgical treatment given the severity of her pathology and her voice demands and expectations. Voice therapy prior to surgery would also improve laryngeal biomechanics to prevent postoperative phonotrauma and assist with postoperative healing.

Intervention

Respiratory-Phonatory Coordination Training
Sarah began voice therapy 2 weeks after her initial clinic evaluation. The first session was dedicated to continued stimulability testing; that is, discovering techniques that improved both the sound and feel (eg, effort, pain, fatigue) of Sarah's voice. During that first session, the SLP noted that Sarah demonstrated excessive clavicular movement with respirations. She was frequently out of breath by the middle of phrases, but attempted to continue phonating, breathing when linguistically, but

not physiologically, appropriate. Sarah was instructed to slow her respiratory rate, reduce clavicular movements and the use of accessory muscles when breathing, and allow relaxation of abdominal musculature for free, uncontrolled abdominal movement during speaking. The SLP had Sarah place her hand on her abdomen to remain mindful of abdominal and not accessory muscle movements during phonation. She instructed Sarah to take small sips of air during speech whenever a pause or punctuation point occurred. Sarah was able to achieve this with minimal SLP cueing by the end of the session.

Resonance Training

During the evaluation, resonant voice techniques such as production of prolonged nasal consonants after inhalation successfully decreased her vocal fatigue and discomfort as well as modestly improved her voice quality. Sarah was also trained in SOVTEs, including phonating through straws of varying sizes.[102] These exercises further helped eliminate the tension and reduce the effort she experienced during phonation. In the first therapy session, these exercises were reviewed and coupled with a slowed respiratory rate and a focus on abdominal muscle relaxation and natural movements with breathing. These techniques were trained in a series of vocal warm-ups and cool-downs. Sarah was instructed to warm up her voice before any period of prolonged vocal activity and to cool down her voice after any voice use lasting longer than 10 minutes. Specifically, she was to focus on small nasal inhalations and prolonged exhalations with vocal output alternating between lip trills and nasal (/m/, /n/, /ng/) and /z/ phonemes (see Video 8 Lip Trills by Braden). These vocalizations were encouraged on single pitches and with small ascending and descending pitch glides. The purpose of the exercises was to bring awareness to anterior vibrations felt during resonant voice production and to relieve vocal effort and strain.[103] All of the exercises were recorded on Sarah's smartphone and provided in a paper handout for her to practice at home. It was recommended that she practice in short sessions (3-5 minutes) 3 or 4 times daily.

Course of Treatment

Sarah returned weekly for additional 45-minute voice therapy sessions. In the second session, the warm-up and cool-down exercises were reviewed. The SLP then guided Sarah to carry the anterior vibrations and ease of voicing experienced with resonant voice phonemes in the warm-up to short phrases containing frequent nasal sounds (eg, "My mom made money," "Many men were mining," "Gene is a lean mean machine"). Sarah had difficulty maintaining forward resonance as her rate of speech increased, so a slower rate was recommended, allowing her more time for conscious awareness of proprioceptive feedback from the resonant voice exercises. Next, treatment focused on blending phonemes between words to encourage flow of phonation. Sarah and the SLP practiced these techniques, coupled with resonant voice therapy, in conversation. The SLP produced the target techniques in conversation to provide a model to help guide Sarah's productions. In addition, Sarah used "negative practice," a technique that encouraged her to alternate between the target technique and the "unbalanced" former voice technique. This exercise helped Sarah gain more control over her productions and increased her self-efficacy in her ability to self-correct in conversation. (See Video 2 Clear Speech and Negative Practice by Gillespie.)

At the start of the third voice therapy session, Sarah reported less vocal effort when focused on therapy techniques. She was able to practice in conversation with her family and was even able to read 3 books to her children before bed without vocal fatigue or worsening dysphonia. She reported she felt encouraged about her vocal progress, was looking forward to returning to work, and had ordered amplification to assist her classroom voice use.

The third session was spent working with the trained techniques in conversational speech, as well as with simulated occupational voice use (ie, classroom teaching). Sarah was able to independently produce the target voice techniques in conversation as well as with simulated teaching. It was determined then that Sarah would try these techniques in the real-life classroom.

Sarah returned to the clinic 1 month later. She reported that even with conscious implementation of the techniques in the classroom, she was experiencing severe dysphonia and debilitating vocal fatigue. At that time, it was recommended she discontinue her behavioral treatment sessions and return to the clinic for a repeat interdisciplinary evaluation.

Follow-Up

On the recommendation of the SLP, Sarah returned to the voice clinic for follow-up assessment, which yielded the following results:

Patient Self-Assessment. Her VHI-10 score was reduced from 36 to 25/40, a clinically meaningful decrease, indicating that Sarah perceived improvement in voice production.

> A 2017 study by Misono et al found that the minimal important difference on the VHI-10 is 6 points, indicating that a reduction by 6 points represents a meaningful improvement in quality of life.[104]

Acoustic Analysis and Aerodynamic Measures. As is often the case, the patient's perceived voice improvement was not evident by the acoustic and aerodynamic analyses that were still outside the normal range. This is not an unusual finding in individuals with sulcus vocalis and glottal incompetence.

While it is not unusual for some voice evaluation components to improve and others to even worsen following treatment, based on Sarah's subjective complaints and inability

to continue in her profession because of her voice problem, the voice care team determined now was the appropriate time to offer surgical treatment, with realistic expectations discussed in detail. Sarah's voice complaints can be grouped as (1) increased voice effort and decreased volume and (2) decreased voice quality. Conceptually, the former is thought to be due to the glottal incompetence and the latter due to disruption of the mucosal wave. This approach is helpful from a surgical option perspective. Vocal fold augmentation (via injection or medialization laryngoplasty) can assist with the effort/volume issues, and surgery to enhance mucosal wave may assist with voice quality. One surgery to alter mucosal wave is called a Gray's mini-thyrotomy. This involves a surgical implantation of a vibratory enhancement (often autologous fat) material into the subepithelial space.[98,105] See Table 5–22 for further information on surgical options for glottal incompetence and mucosal vibration pathology.

> A variety of vocal fold injectables exist at the time of this text's publication, with even more in development. Several different hyaluronic acid-based fillers are available with variable duration effect, some up to a year in the vocal folds. Duration of effect for hyaluronic acid products is impacted by the interaction of a variety of factors, including crosslinking and viscosity. Renuva is a cosmetic filler that uses a fat extracellular matrix and may have augmentation effects lasting longer than a year, which is being investigated at the time of this writing.[106]

The SLP reviewed with Sarah the various categories of surgical treatment including risks, benefits, and expected symptom improvement. Sarah elected to start with vocal fold augmentation/medialization because it is reliable and would address the effort and

Table 5–22. Surgical Options for Glottal Incompetence and Mucosal Vibration Pathology

I. Surgeries for Glottal Incompetence

A. Vocal Fold Injection/Augmentation

Materials (approximate duration of augmentation)

- Carboxymethylcellulose ("gel") (1-2 months)
- Hyaluronic acid (2-3 months depending on formulation)
- Calcium hydroxylapatite (CaHA) (12 months)
- Autologous fat (permanent if survives first 30 days)
- Silk/HA (unknown)

Injection Techniques/Approaches (anesthesia)

- Microlaryngoscopy (general)
- Per-oral ("awake"—local/sedation)
- Thyrohyoid ("awake"—local/sedation)
- Cricothyroid ("awake"—local/sedation)
- Transthyroid ("awake"—local/sedation)
- Flexible laryngoscope endoscopic ("awake"—local/sedation)

B. Laryngeal Framework Surgery

- Medialization laryngoplasty (AKA type I thyroplasty); common materials: Gore-Tex, Silastic, CaHA
- Arytenoid adduction
- Adduction arytenopexy
- Cricothyroid approximation (type IV thyroplasty)
- Cricothyroid subluxation

II. Surgeries for Enhancement of Mucosal Vibration Pathology (Vocal Fold Scar and Sulcus Deformity)

A. Gray's mini-thyrotomy; common materials: autologous fat, fascia

B. Microlaryngoscopy with fat graft implantation

C. Vocal fold steroid injection (best for acute and subacute setting)

---

fatigue complaints. Sarah underwent bilateral medialization laryngoplasty (thyroplasty) with Gore-Tex® implants. This surgery resulted in less vocal effort and less voice loss with significant voice demands (VHI-10 score of 14). Given that she had experienced many years of dysphonia and that the surgery and voice therapy had allowed her to resume her teaching duties without restriction, she elected to have no further treatment that would address her mucosal wave abnormality due to her sulcus deformity.

> For detailed information on Gore-Tex® bilateral thyroplasty with images of the surgery, see Rosen et al (2024).[107]

Summary and Concluding Remarks

Sulcus deformity of the vocal fold(s) is a sulcus or groove in one or both true vocal folds. It may be contained in the mucosa or extend into the vocal ligament. Sulcus deformity of the vocal fold(s) can be congenital or occur as a result of surgical resection of vocal fold lesions or repeated injury to the lamina propria of the vocal fold(s). Vocal fold lesions can develop as a result of glottal incompetence caused by sulcus. In addition, vocal fold lesions can also mask a sulcus.

Sulcus deformity of the vocal fold is a challenging disorder for both the patient and voice care team. This case represents a classic presentation of the disorder and highlights the importance of a team approach in successful treatment of a patient with sulcus vocalis. The voice therapy techniques presented in this case were chosen not for the specific diagnosis but because of their appropriateness in ameliorating the specific patient's unique voice physiology and voice complaints, including vocal effort and fatigue.

In concordance with current voice therapy literature, more therapeutic time was spent in direct (voice production) than indirect (voice hygiene) instruction. Due to the patient's severe dysphonia and laryngeal disorder, more therapy time was dedicated to voice exercise than to spontaneous conversation. Transfer to conversational speech is often the most difficult component of voice therapy for patients. Therefore, it is imperative that the SLP devote significant therapy time to this ecologically valid task. However, some voice problems are severe enough that considerable time must be spent finding and practicing a voice technique that improves the sound quality and feel of the patient's voice. These patients and their disorders, in the end, are likely not amenable to voice therapy alone. This point was well illustrated by the case presented here and has been stated elsewhere in the literature.[5]

The current case represents one in which voice therapy served as a first-line, conservative approach to vocal rehabilitation, as well as an adjuvant to surgical treatment in a patient with glottal incompetence caused by sulcus deformity of the vocal fold. Voice therapy as initial treatment allowed the voice care team to evaluate Sarah's adherence to voice therapy recommendations, as well as her ability to modify her vocal techniques and behaviors. This information helped the team make decisions about her ability to manage her voice with future surgeries. Sarah's vocal effort was relieved and her sound quality moderately improved with the use of relaxed abdominal breathing and resonant voice techniques. As was demonstrated by this case, not all diagnoses and physiologic presentations are appropriate for voice therapy alone. It is imperative that the laryngologist and SLP establish a respectful working relationship to provide optimal, complementary care of these difficult patients.

References

1. Titze IR. Regulating glottal airflow in phonation: Application of the maximum power transfer theorem to a low dimensional phonation model. *J Acoust Soc Am.* 2002;111(1):367-376. doi:10.1121/1.1417526
2. Rosen CA, Mau T, Remacle M, et al. Nomenclature proposal to describe vocal fold motion impairment. *Eur Arch Otorhinolaryngol.* 2016;273(8):1995-1999. doi:10.1007/s00405-015-3663-0
3. Oates JM. Treatment of dysphonia in older people: The role of the speech therapist. *Curr Opin Otolaryngol Head Neck Surg.* 2014;22(6):477-486. doi:10.1097/MOO.0000000000000109
4. Avellaneda JC, Allen JE. Vocal fold sulci—What are the current options for and outcomes of treatment? *Curr Opin Otolaryn-*

gol Head Neck Surg. 2021;29(6):458-464. doi:10.1097/MOO.0000000000000770

5. Bick E, Dumberger LD, Farquhar DR, et al. Does voice therapy improve vocal outcomes in vocal fold atrophy? *Ann Otol Rhinol Laryngol.* 2021;130(6):602-608. doi:10.1177/0003489420952464

6. Gorman S, Weinrich B, Lee L, Stemple JC. Aerodynamic changes as a result of Vocal Function Exercises in elderly men. *Laryngoscope.* 2008;118(10):1900-1903. doi:10.1097/MLG.0b013e31817f9822

7. Ziegler A, Verdolini Abbott K, Johns M, Klein A, Hapner ER. Preliminary data on two voice therapy interventions in the treatment of presbyphonia. *Laryngoscope.* 2014;124(8):1869-1876. doi:10.1002/lary.24548

8. Belsky MA, Shelly S, Rothenberger SD, et al. Phonation Resistance Training Exercises (PhoRTE) with and without expiratory muscle strength training (EMST) for patients with presbyphonia: A noninferiority randomized clinical trial. *J Voice.* 2023;37(3):398-409. doi:10.1016/j.jvoice.2021.02.015

9. Desjardins M, Halstead L, Simpson A, Flume P, Bonilha HS. Respiratory muscle strength training to improve vocal function in patients with presbyphonia. *J Voice.* 2020;36(3):344-360. doi:10.1016/j.jvoice.2020.06.006

10. Rosen C. Vocal fold scar: Evaluation and treatment. *Otolaryngol Clin North Am.* 2000;33(5):1081-1086.

11. Kaneko M, Sugiyama Y, Mukudai S, Hirano S. Effects of voice therapy for dysphonia due to tension imbalance in unilateral vocal fold paralysis and paresis. *J Voice.* 2022;36(4):584.e1-584.e6. doi:10.1016/j.jvoice.2020.07.026

12. Simpson CB. Glottic insufficiency: Vocal fold paralysis, paresis, and atrophy. In Rosen CA, Simpson CB, eds: *Operative Techniques in Laryngology.* Springer; 2008:29-35.

13. Walton C, Carding P, Flanagan K. Perspectives on voice treatment for unilateral vocal fold paralysis. *Curr Opin Otolaryngol Head Neck Surg.* 2018;26(3):157-161. doi:10.1097/MOO.0000000000000450

14. Walton C, Conway E, Blackshaw H, Carding P. Unilateral vocal fold paralysis: A systematic review of speech-language pathology management. *J Voice.* 2017;31(4):509.e7-509.e22. doi:10.1016/j.jvoice.2016.11.002

15. Miyata E, Miyamoto M, Shiromoto O, et al. Early voice therapy for unilateral vocal fold paralysis improves subglottal pressure and glottal closure. *Am J Otolaryngol Head Neck Med Surg.* 2020;41(6):102727. doi:10.1016/j.amjoto.2020.102727

16. El-Banna M, Youssef G. Early voice therapy in patients with unilateral vocal fold paralysis. *Folia Phoniatr Logop.* 2014;66(6):237-243. doi:10.1159/000369167

17. Poburka BJ, Patel RR, Bless DM. Voice-Vibratory Assessment With Laryngeal Imaging (VALI) form: Reliability of rating stroboscopy and high-speed videoendoscopy. *J Voice.* 2017;31(4):513.e1-513.e14. doi:10.1016/j.jvoice.2016.12.003

18. Omori K, Kojima H, Slavit DH, Kacker A, Matos C, Blaugrund SM. Vocal fold atrophy: Quantitative glottic measurement and vocal function. *Ann Otol Rhinol Laryngol.* 1997;106(7 Pt 1):544-551. doi:10.1177/000348949710600702

19. Desjardins M, Halstead L, Simpson A, Flume P, Bonilha HS. Voice and respiratory characteristics of men and women seeking treatment for presbyphonia. *J Voice.* 2022;36(5):673-684. doi:10.1016/j.jvoice.2020.08.040

20. Arffa RE, Krishna P, Gartner-Schmidt J, Rosen CA. Normative values for the voice handicap index-10. *J Voice.* 2012;26(4):462-465. doi:10.1016/j.jvoice.2011.04.006

21. Bach K, Belafsky P, Wasylik K, Postma G, Koufman J. Validity and reliability of the glottal function index. *Arch Otolaryngol Head Neck Surg.* 2005;131:961-964. doi:10.1016/j.jvoice.2024.04.004

22. Baylor C, Yorkston K, Eadie T, Kim J, Chung H, Amtmann D. The communicative participation item bank (CPIB): Item bank calibration and development of a disorder-generic short form. *J Speech Lang Hear Res.* 2013;56(4):1190-1208. doi:10.1044/1092-4388(2012/12-0140)

23. Kempster GB, Gerratt BR, Abbott KV, Barkmeier-Kraemer J, Hillman RE. Consensus auditory-perceptual evaluation of voice: Development of a standardized clinical protocol. *Am J Speech Lang Pathol.* 2009;18(2):124-132. doi:10.1044/1058-0360(2008/08-0017)

24. Castellana A, Carullo A, Astolfi A, Puglisi GE, Fugiglando U. Intra-speaker and inter-speaker variability in speech sound pressure level across repeated readings. *J Acoust Soc Am.* 2017;141(4):2353-2363. doi:10.1121/1.4979115

25. Sauder C, Bretl M, Eadie T. Predicting voice disorder status from smoothed measures of cepstral peak prominence using Praat and analysis of dysphonia in speech and voice (ADSV). *J Voice.* 2017;31(5):557-566. doi:10.1016/j.jvoice.2017.01.006

26. Zraick RI, Smith-Olinde L, Shotts LL. Adult normative data for the KayPentax phonatory aerodynamic system model 6600. *J Voice.* 2012;26(2):164-176. doi:10.1016/j.jvoice.2011.01.006

27. Melcon M, Hoit JD, Hixon TJ. Age and laryngeal airway resistance during vowel production in women. *J Speech Hear Res.* 1992;35(2):309-313. doi:10.1044/jshr.3502.309

28. Enright P, Kronmal R, Manolio T, Schenker M, Hyatt R. Respiratory muscle strength in the elderly. Correlates and reference values. Cardiovascular Health Study Research Group. *Am J Respir Crit Care Med.* 1994;149(2):430-438.

29. Rosenstock IM, Strecher VJ, Becker MH. Social learning theory and the health belief model. *Health Educ Q.* 1988;15(2):175-183. doi:10.1177/109019818801500203

30. Prochaska JO, Velicer WF. The transtheoretical model of health behavior change. *Am J Health Promot.* 1997;12(1):38-48. doi:10.4278/0890-1171-12.1.38

31. Timmons Sund L, Cameron B, Johns MM, Gao WZ, O'Dell K, Hapner ER. Laryngologists' reported decision-making in presbyphonia treatment. *J Voice.* 2024;38(3):723-730. doi:10.1016/j.jvoice.2021.10.008

32. Desjardins M, Bonilha HS. The impact of respiratory exercises on voice outcomes: A systematic review of the literature. *J Voice.* 2019;34(4):648.e1-648.e39. doi:10.1016/j.jvoice.2019.01.011

33. McMullen CA, Butterfield TA, Dietrich M, et al. Chronic stimulation-induced changes in the rodent thyroarytenoid muscle. *J Speech Lang Hear Res.* 2011;54(3):845-853. doi:10.1044/1092-4388(2010/10-0127)

34. Huber JE, Spruill J. Age-related changes to speech breathing with increased vocal loudness. *J Speech Lang Hear Res.* 2008;51(3):651-668. doi:10.1044/1092-4388(2008/047)

35. Ramírez-Sarmiento A, Orozco-Levi M, Güell R, et al. Inspiratory muscle training in patients with chronic obstructive pulmonary disease: Structural adaptation and physiologic outcomes. *Am J Respir Crit Care Med.* 2002;166(11):1491-1497. doi:10.1164/rccm.200202-075OC

36. Stemple JC, Lee L, D'Amico B, Pickup B. Efficacy of Vocal Function Exercises as a method of improving voice production. *J Voice.* 1994;8(3):271-278. doi:10.1016/S0892-1997(05)80299-1

37. Desjardins M, Halstead L, Simpson A, Flume P, Bonilha HS. The impact of respiratory function on voice in patients with presbyphonia. *J Voice.* 2022;36(2):256-271. doi:10.1016/j.jvoice.2020.05.027

38. Bastian RW, Thomas JP. Do talkativeness and vocal loudness correlate with laryngeal pathology? A study of the vocal overdoer/underdoer continuum. *J Voice.* 2016;30(5):557-562. doi:10.1016/j.jvoice.2015.06.012

39. Brown HJ, Zhou D, Husain IA. Management of presbyphonia: A systematic review of the efficacy of surgical intervention. *Am J Otolaryngol Head Neck Med Surg.* 2020;41(4):102532. doi:10.1016/j.amjoto.2020.102532

40. Park JH, Chae M, An YH, Shim HJ, Kwon M. Coprevalence of presbycusis and its effect on outcome of voice therapy in patients with presbyphonia. *J Voice.* 2022;36(6):877.e9-877.e14. doi:10.1016/j.jvoice.2020.09.030

41. Etter NM, Hapner ER, Barkmeier-Kraemer JM, Gartner-Schmidt JL, Dressler EV, Stemple JC. Aging Voice Index (AVI): Reliability and validity of a voice quality of life

scale for older adults. *J Voice*. 2019;33(5):807. e7-807.e12. doi:10.1016/j.jvoice.2018.04.006

42. Shembel AC, Rosen CA, Zullo TG, Gartner-Schmidt JL. Development and validation of the cough severity index: A severity index for chronic cough related to the upper airway. *Laryngoscope*. 2013;123(8):1931-1936. doi:10.1002/lary.23916

43. Gartner-Schmidt JL, Shembel AC, Zullo TG, Rosen CA. Development and validation of the Dyspnea Index (DI): A severity index for upper airway-related dyspnea. *J Voice*. 2014;28(6):775-782. doi:10.1016/j.jvoice.2013.12.017

44. Castro ME, Sund LT, Hoffman MR, Hapner ER. The Voice Problem Impact Scales (VPIS). *J Voice*. 2024;38(3):666-673. doi:10.1016/j.jvoice.2021.11.011

45. Rolfson DB, Mujumdar SR, Tsuyuki RT, Tahir A, Rockwood K. Validity and reliability of the Edmonton Frail Scale. *Age Ageing*. 2006;35(5):526-529. doi:10.1093/ageing/afl023

46. Shoffel-Havakuk H, Marks KL, Morton M, Johns III MM, Hapner ER. Validation of the OMNI vocal effort scale in the treatment of adductor spasmodic dysphonia. *Laryngoscope*. Published online October 12, 2018. doi:10.1002/lary.27430

47. Hoit JD, Hixon Th. J. Age and speech breathing. *J Speech Hear Res*. 1987;30(3):351-366. doi:10.1044/jshr.3003.351

48. Patel RR, Awan SN, Barkmeier-Kraemer J, et al. Recommended protocols for instrumental assessment of voice: ASHA expert panel to develop a protocol for instrumental assessment of vocal function. *Am J Speech Lang Pathol*. 2018:1-19.

49. Titze IR. Workshop on acoustic voice analysis: Summary statement. *National Center for Voice and Speech*. 1995:1-36.

50. Awan SN. *Analysis of Dysphonia in Speech and Voice (ADSV): An Application Guide*. KayPentax; 2011.

51. Huber JE, Darling-White M. Longitudinal changes in speech breathing in older adults with and without Parkinson's disease. *Semin Speech Lang*. 2017;38(3):200-209. doi:10.1055/s-0037-1602839

52. Sperry EE, Klich RJ. Speech breathing in senescent and younger women during oral reading. *J Speech Hear Res*. 1992;35(6):1246-1255. doi:10.1044/jshr.3506.1246

53. Eckel FC, Boone DR. The S/Z ratio as an indicator of laryngeal pathology. *J Speech Hear Disord*. 1981;46(2):147-149.

54. Garcia-Rio F, Dorgham A, Pino JM, Villasante C, Garcia-Quero C, Alvarez-Sala R. Lung volume reference values for women and men 65 to 85 years of age. *Am J Respir Crit Care Med*. 2009;180(11):1083-1091. doi:10.1164/rccm.200901-0127OC

55. Simões RP, Deus APL, Auad MA, Dionísio J, Mazzonetto M, Borghi-Silva A. Maximal respiratory pressure in healthy 20 to 89 year-old sedentary individuals of central São Paulo State. *Rev Bras Fisioter*. 2010; 14(1):60-67. doi:10.1590/s1413-35552010000100010

56. Kim J, Sapienza C. Effects of expiratory muscle strength training with the healthy elderly on speech. *Commun Sci Disord*. 2006;11(2):1-16

57. Pessoa IMBS, Neto MH, Montemezzo D, Silva LAM, Andrade AD de, Parreira VF. Predictive equations for respiratory muscle strength according to international and Brazilian guidelines. *Braz J Phys Ther*. 2014; 18(5):410-418. doi:10.1590/bjpt-rbf.2014.0044

58. Lewandowski A, Gillespie AI, Kridgen S, Jeong K, Yu L, Gartner-Schmidt J. Adult normative data for phonatory aerodynamics in connected speech. *Laryngoscope*. 2018;128(4):909-914. doi:10.1002/lary.26922

59. van Leer E, Hapner ER, Connor NP. Transtheoretical model of health behavior change applied to voice therapy. *J Voice*. 2008; 22(6):688-698. doi:10.1016/j.jvoice.2007.01.011

60. Behrman A, Haskell J. *Exercises for Voice Therapy*. 3rd ed. Plural Publishing; 2020.

61. Narici MV, Maffulli N. Sarcopenia: Characteristics, mechanisms and functional significance. *Br Med Bull*. 2010;95(1):139-159. doi:10.1093/bmb/ldq008

62. Chodzko-Zajko WJ, Proctor DN, Fiatarone Singh MA, et al. Exercise and physical

activity for older adults. *Med Sci Sports Exerc.* 2009;41(7):1510-1530. doi:10.1249/MSS.0b013e3181a0c95c

63. Titze IR. Human speech: A restricted use of the mammalian larynx. 2017;4(11):135-141. doi: 10.1016/j.jvoice.2016.06.003

64. Castro C, Prado P, Espinoza VM, et al. Lombard effect in individuals with non-phonotraumatic vocal hyperfunction: Impact on acoustic, aerodynamic, and vocal fold vibratory parameters. *J Speech Lang Hear Res.* 2022;65(8):2881-2895. doi:10.1044/2022_JSLHR-21-00508

65. Scherr J, Wolfarth B, Christle JW, Pressler A, Wagenpfeil S, Halle M. Associations between Borg's rating of perceived exertion and physiological measures of exercise intensity. *Eur J Appl Physiol.* 2013;113(1):147-155. doi:10.1007/s00421-012-2421-x

66. Rosen CA, Lee AS, Osborne J, Zullo T, Murry T. Development and validation of the Voice Handicap Index-10. *Laryngoscope.* 2004;114(9 I):1549-1556. doi:10.1097/00005537-200409000-00009

67. Zraick RI, Smith-Olinde L, Shotts LL. Adult normative data for the KayPentax phonatory aerodynamic system model 6600. *J Voice.* 2012;26(2):164-176. doi:10.1016/j.jvoice.2011.01.006

68. Awan SN, Roy N, Jetté ME, Meltzner GS, Hillman RE. Quantifying dysphonia severity using a spectral/cepstral-based acoustic index: Comparisons with auditory-perceptual judgements from the CAPE-V. *Clin Linguist Phon.* 2010;24(9):742-758. doi:10.3109/02699206.2010.492446

69. Nishio M, Niimi S. Changes in speaking fundamental frequency characteristics with aging. *Folia Phoniatr Logop.* 2008;60(3):120-127. doi:10.1159/000118510

70. Awan SN, Roy N, Zhang D, Cohen SM. Validation of the Cepstral Spectral Index of Dysphonia (CSID) as a screening tool for voice disorders: Development of clinical cutoff scores. *J Voice.* 2016;30(2):130-144. doi:10.1016/j.jvoice.2015.04.009

71. Goy H, Fernandes DN, Pichora-Fuller MK, Van Lieshout P. Normative voice data for younger and older adults. *J Voice.* 2013;27(5):545-555. doi:10.1016/j.jvoice.2013.03.002

72. Mathieson L, Hirani SP, Epstein R, Baken RJ, Wood G, Rubin JS. Laryngeal manual therapy: A preliminary study to examine its treatment effects in the management of muscle tension dysphonia. *J Voice.* 2009;23(3):353-366. doi:10.1016/j.jvoice.2007.10.002

73. Brown CK, Vazquez J, Metz SM, McCown D. Effects of an 8-week mindfulness course in people with voice disorders. *J Voice.* Published online November 15, 2023. doi:10.1016/j.jvoice.2023.10.031

74. Lloyd A, Hoffman-Ruddy B, Silverman E, Jeffrey LL. Vocal yoga: Applying yoga principles in voice therapy. *J Sing.* 2017;73(5):511-518.

75. Jacobson BH, Johnson A, Grywalski C, et al. The Voice Handicap Index (VHI): Development and validation. *Am J Speech Lang Pathol.* 1997;6(3):66-69. doi:10.1044/1058-0360.0603.66

76. Nanjundeswaran C, Jacobson BH, Gartner-Schmidt J, Verdolini Abbott K. Vocal Fatigue Index (VFI): Development and validation. *J Voice.* 2015;29(4):433-440. doi:10.1016/j.jvoice.2014.09.012

77. Nanjundeswaran C, van Mersbergen M, Banks R, Hunter E. Vocal Fatigue Index in teachers using Mokken analysis. *J Voice.* 2023;37(2):298.e1-298.e9. doi:10.1016/j.jvoice.2020.12.053

78. van Leer E, van Mersbergen M. Using the Borg CR10 physical exertion scale to measure patient-perceived vocal effort pre and post treatment. *J Voice.* 2017;31(3):389.e19-389.e25. doi:10.1016/j.jvoice.2016.09.023

79. Murton O, Hillman R, Mehta D. Cepstral peak prominence values for clinical voice evaluation. *Am J Speech Lang Pathol.* 2020;29(3):1596-1607. doi:10.1044/2020_AJSLP-20-00001

80. Belafsky P, Mouadeb D, Rees C, et al. Validity and reliability of the Eating Assessment Tool (EAT-10). *Ann Otol Rhinol Laryngol.* 2008;117(12):919-924. doi:10.1177/000348940811701210

81. Schneider SL, Habich L, Weston ZM, Rosen CA. Observations and considerations for

implementing remote acoustic voice recording and analysis in clinical practice. *J Voice*. 2024;38(1):69-76. doi:10.1016/j.jvoice.2021.06.011

82. Jeong GE, Lee DH, Lee YS, et al. Treatment efficacy of voice therapy following injection laryngoplasty for unilateral vocal fold paralysis. *J Voice*. 2022;36(2):242-248. doi:10.1016/j.jvoice.2020.05.014

83. Orestes MI, Chhetri DK. Superior laryngeal nerve injury: Effects, clinical findings, prognosis, and management options. *Curr Opin Otolaryngol Head Neck Surg*. 2014; 22(6):439-443. doi:10.1097/MOO.000000 0000000097

84. Roy N, Smith ME, Houtz DR. Laryngeal features of external superior laryngeal nerve denervation: Revisiting a century-old controversy. *Ann Otol Rhinol Laryngol*. 2011;120(1):1-8. doi:10.1177/0003489411 12000101

85. Roy N, Barton ME, Smith ME, Dromey C, Merrill RM, Sauder C. An in vivo model of external superior laryngeal nerve paralysis: Laryngoscopic findings. *Laryngoscope*. 2009;119(5):1017-1032. doi:10.1002/lary .20193

86. Kaneko M, Hitomi T, Takekawa T, Tsuji T, Kishimoto Y, Hirano S. Effects of voice therapy on laryngeal motor units during phonation in chronic superior laryngeal nerve paresis dysphonia. *J Voice*. 2018;32(6):729-733. doi:10.1016/j.jvoice.2017.08.026

87. Shoffel-Havakuk H, Chau S, Hapner ER, Pethan M, Johns MM. Development and validation of the Voice Catastrophization Index. *J Voice*. 2019;33(2):232-238. doi:10 .1016/j.jvoice.2017.09.026

88. Patel R, Awan S, Barkmeier-Kraemer J, et al. Recommended protocols for instrumental assessment of voice: American Speech-Language-Hearing Association expert panel to develop a protocol for instrumental assessment of vocal function. *Am J Speech Lang Pathol*. 2018;27(3):887-905.

89. Kent SAK, Fletcher TL, Morgan A, Morton M, Hall RJ, Sandage MJ. Updated acoustic normative data through the lifespan: A scoping review. *J Voice*. Published online March 18, 2023. doi:10.1016/j.jvoice .2023.02.011

90. Siupsinskiene N, Lycke H. Effects of vocal training on singing and speaking voice characteristics in vocally healthy adults and children based on choral and nonchoral data. *J Voice*. 2011;25(4):e177-e189. doi:10 .1016/j.jvoice.2010.03.010

91. Sanchez K, Oates J, Dacakis G, Holmberg EB. Speech and voice range profiles of adults with untrained normal voices: Methodological implications. *Logop Phoniatr Vocol*. 2014;39(2):62-71. doi:10.3109/1401 5439.2013.777109

92. Buckley DP, Abur D, Stepp CE. Normative values of cepstral peak prominence measures in typical speakers by sex, speech stimuli, and software type across the life span. *Am J Speech Lang Pathol*. 2023;32(4):1565-1577. doi:10.1044/2023_AJSLP-22-00264

93. Lewandowski A, Gillespie AI, Kridgen S, Jeong K, Yu L, Gartner-Schmidt J. Adult normative data for phonatory aerodynamics in connected speech. *Laryngoscope*. 2018; 128(4):909-914. doi:10.1002/lary.26922

94. Estill J, McDonald Klimek M, Obert K, Steinhauer K. *Estill Voice Training Level 1: Figures for Voice Control Workbook*. Estill Voice Training Systems International, LLC; 2005.

95. Estill J, McDonald Klimek M, Obert K, Steinhauer K. *Estill Voice Training Level 2: Figure Combinations for Six Voice Qualities Workbook*. Estill Voice Training Systems International, LLC; 2005.

96. Watts CR, Awan SN. Use of spectral/cepstral analyses for differentiating normal from hypofunctional voices in sustained vowel and continuous speech contexts. *J Speech Lang Hear Res*. 2011;54(6):1525-1537. doi:10.1044/1092-4388(2011/10-0209)

97. Giovanni A, Chanteret C, Lagier A. Sulcus vocalis: A review. *Eur Arch Otorhinolaryngol*. 2007;264(4):337-344. doi:10.1007/ s00405-006-0230-8

98. Welham NV, Choi SH, Dailey SH, Ford CN, Jiang JJ, Bless DM. Prospective multi-arm evaluation of surgical treatments for vocal fold scar and pathologic sulcus vocalis.

Laryngoscope. 2011;121(6):1252-1260. doi: 10.1002/lary.21780

99. Gillespie AI, Gartner-Schmidt J. Immediate effect of stimulability assessment on acoustic, aerodynamic, and patient-perceptual measures of voice. *J Voice.* 2016; 30(4):507.e9-507.e14. doi:10.1016/j.jvoice.2015.06.004

100. Ford CN, Inagi K, Khidr A, Bless DM, Gilchrist KW. Sulcus vocalis: A rational analytical approach to diagnosis and management. *Ann Otol Rhinol Laryngol.* 1996;105(3):189-200. doi:10.1177/000348949610500304

101. Hantzakos A, Dikkers FG, Giovanni A, et al. Vocal fold scars: A common classification proposal by the American Laryngological Association and European Laryngological Society. *Eur Arch Otorhinolaryngol.* 2019;276(8):2289-2292. doi:10.1007/s00405-019-05489-3

102. Titze IR. Voice training and therapy with a semi-occluded vocal tract: Rationale and scientific underpinnings. *Hear Res.* 2006; 49(2):448-460.

103. Verdolini K, Druker DG, Palmer PM, Samawi H. Laryngeal adduction in resonant voice. *J Voice.* 1998;12(3):315-327. doi:10.1016/S0892-1997(98)80021-0

104. Misono S, Yueh B, Stockness AN, House ME, Marmor S. Minimal important difference in Voice Handicap Index-10. *JAMA Otolaryngol Head Neck Surg.* 2017;143(11): 1098-1103. doi:10.1001/jamaoto.2017.1621

105. González-Herranz R, Hernandez García E, Granda-Rosales M, Eisenberg-Plaza G, Montojo Woodeson J, Plaza G. Improved mucosal wave in unilateral autologous temporal fascia graft in sulcus vocalis type 2 and vocal scars. *J Voice.* 2019;33(6):915-922. doi:10.1016/j.jvoice.2018.06.013

106. O'Dell K, Bhatt N, Gao W, Markarian A, Johns MM. Novel use of allograft adipose matrix (Renuva) for vocal fold augmentation: Safety and efficacy. Virtual Poster presented at: *Annual Meeting of the American Laryngological Association; May 15, 2020.*

107. Rosen CA, Simpson CB, Postma GN, Amin MR. Gore-Tex® medialization laryngoplasty. In: Rosen CA, Simpson CB, eds. *Operative Techniques in Laryngology.* Springer Cham; 2024:415-422.

6

Movement Disorders Affecting the Voice

Laryngeal Dystonia, Vocal Tremor, and Parkinson's Disease

Introduction

Katherine L. Marks

Laryngeal dystonia, vocal tremor, and Parkinson's disease are all movement disorders that can negatively impact the voice, as well as a person's voice-related participation, functioning, and quality of life. Many individuals with these disorders present to the clinic seeking voice care. This chapter includes clinical cases related to treatment of laryngeal dystonia, vocal tremor, and Parkinson's disease.

Laryngeal Dystonia

Laryngeal dystonia (LD), a rare focal dystonia of the laryngeal musculature, affects approximately 1 in every 100,000 people.[1] In recent years, the term "laryngeal dystonia" replaced what had historically been called "spasmodic dysphonia."[2] The latter term, still used in

some clinical contexts, reflects the voice quality associated with laryngeal spasms, whereas "laryngeal dystonia" more accurately classifies the disorder within the dystonia framework.

LD is a neurological disorder in which the laryngeal muscles spasm during connected speech. LD is task-specific: Spasms occur during phonation, but not during innate vocal tasks (eg, crying, laughing, whispering, or singing/humming).[1] Common subtypes include adductor (AdLD), abductor (AbLD), and mixed LD.[2] AdLD accounts for roughly 82% of LD cases.[3] In AdLD, adductory laryngeal muscles spasm during phonation, with signs most apparent on voiced phonemes. Spasms result in the perception of a strained, strangled voice quality, with elevated patient-reported vocal effort.[4] AbLD is a rarer subtype characterized by spasms of the posterior cricoarytenoid muscles, causing intermittent breathy voice breaks primarily on voiceless phonemes. In mixed LD, abductor and adductor muscles spasm during phonation, causing both hyperadductory and breathy spasms. Approximately 33% of individuals with LD also present with dystonic tremor[3] (see Case Study 6.3 by Timmons Sund: Tele-therapy Without Medical Management for an Adult With Abductor Laryngeal Dystonia and Vocal Tremor). In some instances, spasms occur with rhythmic regularity, creating a pattern of phonatory breaks nearly indistinguishable from severe vocal tremor.[5]

LD, particularly AdLD, is often misdiagnosed as muscle tension dysphonia (MTD). Their similar presentations, combined with the rarity of LD, leads to diagnostic delays.[2] Poor interrater agreement and classification among voice experts led to the development of consensus-based attributes for LD identification.[6] Due to acoustic and phoneme-specific attributes of LD, speech-language pathologists (SLPs) make important contributions toward a differential diagnosis. Videostroboscopy is used to rule out other pathology, but it is rare that spasms are captured. Instead, clinicians often rely on auditory perception to discern features differentiating AdLD, AbLD, vocal tremor, and MTD.

Patient-reported outcomes validated specifically for LD include the Communication Participation Item Bank[7] and the OMNI Vocal Effort Scale (OMNI-VES).[4] Few clinically feasible quantitative (acoustic and aerodynamic) measures are specific to LD. Acoustically, higher levels of cepstral peak prominence (CPP) reflect a lower amount of noise in the signal. Aerodynamically, LD is characterized by increased subglottal pressure, laryngeal resistance, and phonation threshold pressure.[8] Acoustic discontinuities in speech signals (phonatory breaks, frequency shifts, aperiodicity, and creak) are specific to AdLD, differentiating it from MTD.[9] However, manual labels of acoustic discontinuities are time consuming and not clinically feasible. Acoustic measures that have differentiated AdLD from MTD in the research literature include the Cepstral Spectral Index of Dysphonia (CSID), the long-term average spectrum, and automated estimates of creak.[10]

As LD is a neurological condition, voice therapy alone is typically not recommended, except for instances in which a person declines other treatment (see Case Study 6.2 by Stemple: Voice Therapy Without Medical Management for an Adult With Adductor Spasmodic Dysphonia). However, voice therapy to unload compensatory tension is often recommended as an adjunct to other treatments (see Case Study 6.1 by Hapner and Johns: Medical and Behavioral Management for an Adult With Laryngeal Dystonia–Adductor Type). The most widely used treatment for LD is botulinum toxin (eg Botox®) injections into the affected laryngeal muscles. This produces denervation, temporarily causing muscle fibers to atrophy.[5] Within 2 to 3 days, an initially breathy voice emerges with reduced spasms and lasts approximately 2 weeks, after which the voice becomes stronger and spasms continue to be reduced.[11] As treatment effects dissipate, spasms gradually return, indicating need for a repeat injection. Physicians often dose using trial and error and typically have patients document their duration of breathiness and improved voice to inform dosing adjustments. Alternative treatments include surgical approaches for laryngeal remodeling (eg, selective laryngeal denervation-reinnervation or type 2 thyroplasty with implant) and off-label medications (eg, beta-blockers, benzodiazepines, or anticonvulsants), with mixed results.[2]

Vocal Tremor

Tremor is characterized by regular, involuntary movements of muscles, resulting in near-rhythmic oscillation of one or more body parts. Vocal tremor is perceived as unstable or shaky due to structural oscillations.[11] Researchers have characterized the clinical phenotypes of vocal tremor using consensus-based tremor classification criteria. Phenotypes include dystonic tremor, tremor in Parkinson's disease, essential tremor, and isolated vocal tremor.[12]

Dystonic tremor is difficult to diagnose and can co-occur with LD. Unlike essential or isolated vocal tremor, dystonic tremor is task specific (ie, only occurs during speech production and is specific to phonemic context) and may decrease with a sensory trick, such as placement of a nasoendoscope. Treatment with botulinum toxin may improve dystonic tremor but may only decrease the amplitude of essential/isolated vocal tremor.[5]

Essential vocal tremor, characterized by co-occurring action tremors in the upper limbs, typically begins subtly and progresses over time. Isolated vocal tremor occurs in the absence of other body tremors.[12] Both types often variably involve muscles of the phonatory system beyond intrinsic laryngeal muscles (eg, extrinsic laryngeal, pharyngeal, and palatal muscles), in addition to articulatory and respiratory muscles. Patients with either type may present with regular oscillations of frequency and/or amplitude and often report increased vocal effort. Compensatory vocal hyperfunction is common as the body attempts to stabilize the vocal tract. Symptoms typically present across phonatory activities and often during quiet respiration.[5]

A neurologic examination of the upper extremities, gait, head, and neck may identify additional body tremors or reveal signs of Parkinson's disease, such as bradykinesia or cogwheeling.[5] A cranial nerve test can be used to assess sensory and motor function and document the presence or absence of tremor in articulatory and respiratory structures. Nasoendoscopy can be used to assess tremor of the soft palate, pharynx, and/or larynx during quiet breathing, sustained phonation tasks, syllable repetitions, and connected speech tasks. Tremor affecting the larynx can present as vertical, abductory, adductory, or lengthwise oscillations.[12]

Medication is usually the first recommended treatment of essential or isolated vocal tremor and can include beta-blockers, anticonvulsants and, less frequently, benzodiazepines or antidepressants.[5] Botulinum toxin injections to the affected laryngeal muscles may reduce the amplitude of a horizontal laryngeal tremor. Voice therapy may benefit patients reporting increased vocal effort or fatigue, demonstrating vocal hyperfunction, and/or displaying stimulability for decreasing tremor perception in connected speech (see Case Study 6.4 by Barkmeier-Kraemer: Reducing Voicing Duration to Treat an Adult With Vocal Tremor). Voice therapy may also be recommended for singers or other professional voice users with vocal tremor (see Case Study 6.5 by Bond: Multimodality Voice Therapy for an Adult Classical Singer With Vocal Tremor). Deep brain stimulation (DBS) may be recommended if tremor is unresponsive to other treatments (see Case Study 6.6 by DiRenzo: The SLP's Role in Deep Brain Stimulation for Vocal Tremor).

Parkinson's Disease

Parkinson's disease (PD), the second most common neurological disease, affects over 5 million people worldwide.[13] PD is characterized by muscular rigidity, tremor, bradykinesia, and postural instability, resulting from depleted dopamine in the substantia nigra.[14] Disease progression is insidious, with subtle speech and voice impairments presenting up to a decade before hallmark motor deficits.[15] These changes often go undiagnosed in early disease stages, likely attributed to natural aging.[14] Once considered solely a basal ganglia disease, PD involves multiple neurotransmitter pathways throughout the central and peripheral nervous systems. Lewy pathology is a neuropathological hallmark of PD and has been discovered in the main pharyngeal sensory nerves and alpha-synuclein pathology in the tongue, pharynx, larynx, and upper esophagus.[16] These finding may provide an avenue for the development of novel therapies in PD.

A neurologist often diagnoses PD through comprehensively examining medical history, clinical presentation, neurological imaging, and medication trials.[14] Voice clinicians assess using videoendoscopy, which often reveals vocal fold bowing and glottic insufficiency, resulting in breathy voice quality. Tremor is present in 55% of patients with idiopathic PD, typically involving the strap muscles that produce vertical laryngeal movements.[5] Other findings can include hypopharyngeal secretions, decreased sensation, diminished cough reflex, and dysphagia.[14] Ninety percent of individuals with PD develop hypokinetic dysarthria, which affects multiple subsystems of speech and swallowing, resulting in decreased vital capacity as well as impaired tidal breathing and speech breathing.[14] Laryngeal effects include impaired prosody with monopitch and monoloudness, as well as rigidity. These deficits result in hypophonia and lower subglottal pressures.[17] Acoustically, patients may present with high average fundamental frequency (F0) in connected speech, reduced variability in fundamental frequency, decreased intensity, and decreased harmonics-to-noise ratio. Articulatory impairments may include imprecise articulation and reduced range of movement with smaller vowel space areas. Resonatory deficits may include velopharyngeal incompetence, causing perceived hypernasality or cul-de-sac resonance. Combined, these deficits tend to impact intelligibility.[14]

Dopaminergic medications are commonly used to treat motor symptoms of PD. These medications do not affect the underlying disease process and may include side effects of dystonia, dyskinesias, confusion, and on-off effects.[18] Speech improvements are not typically appreciated with dopaminergic medications.[14] Global motor improvements have been demonstrated following DBS surgery, though the impact on speech remains unclear.[14]

Speech therapy is the most effective treatment for communication deficits in PD. Historically, rate-control approaches (eg, pacing boards and applications) benefited individuals with accelerated speech. Biofeedback devices (eg, sound level meters or other devices) may target reduced loudness[18] (see Case Study 6.7 by Huber: Maintaining Gains From Voice Therapy Using the SpeechVive for an Adult With Parkinson's Disease). Exuberant voice therapy programs using external cues exist specifically for treating speech in PD.[14] Lee Silverman Voice Therapy (LSVT)-LOUD aims to improve vocal fold adduction and intelligibility through cues for loud voicing and maximum effort across sustained phonation and connected speech tasks.[19] LSVT-LOUD involves an intense regimen of four 1-hour sessions per week for 4 weeks. Significant increases in sound pressure level and fundamental frequency variability have been found immediately after treatment and at 6- and 12-month follow-ups, as well as improved Voice Handicap Index and United Parkinson's Disease Rating Scale (UPDRS) scores.[20] SPEAK OUT!, another program developed specifically for PD, cues patients to speak with intent.[18] Like LSVT-LOUD, SPEAK OUT! requires intense 45-minute sessions, though the number of sessions depends on patient progress. Significant increases in vocal intensity have been found immediately after treatment and at 6- and 12-month follow ups.[21] Behavioral speech treatments in PD provide short-term benefits, though effects lessen over time.[14] As such, maintenance programs help patients retain their gains through LOUD for Life (LSVT), SPEAK OUT! refreshers, and LOUD crowd group sessions.

Case Studies

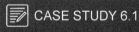

CASE STUDY 6.1

Medical and Behavioral Management for an Adult With Laryngeal Dystonia–Adductor Type

Edie R. Hapner and Michael M. Johns III

Background

Interprofessional practice (IPP) denotes the collaborative efforts of multiple healthcare professionals in treatment. IPP has been shown to improve patient-centered care and treatment outcomes.[22] Voice centers around the United States have adopted IPP, though the model for this care is not homogenous across centers.[23] In this case, the patient was seen by a laryngologist and SLP at the same appointment. Following joint history taking, the physician completed the general medical examination and head and neck examination. The SLP completed a motor speech evaluation, a comprehensive voice evaluation, and an acoustic and aerodynamic assessment. The laryngeal imaging examination was completed by the SLP but was jointly reviewed by the laryngologist and SLP. The team then met to discuss findings and develop a suggested plan of care to present to the patient. The physician discussed all the treatment options with the patient and a shared decision was made for the plan moving forward. The following represents the medical documentation from the physician and SLP jointly in one note. Generally, the physician's and SLP's notes are written separately, however, for the benefit of this case presentation to highlight the collaborative care by both the physician and SLP, the evaluation note is written together.

Voice Evaluation (Written by the SLP and MD as a Team Note)

We had the privilege of completing a comprehensive voice evaluation including physician medical assessment, behavioral and qualitative assessment of voice and resonance, laryngeal videostroboscopy, and laryngeal function studies.

Case History

Ms. Smith, a 56-year-old cisgender female, presented for evaluation with suspected AdLD (ICD-10 R49.0, J38.5, R49.8, R25.1). She was evaluated in the interprofessional voice center by both the laryngologist and SLP together and separately during this appointment.

Chief Complaint. Difficulty with specific words that seem to get "stuck," especially those

that begin with vowels or /h/. Occasional normal sound during laughter or short, automatic speech, including but not limited to responses such as "yes," "no," or "maybe." Voice and fluency improve with drinking alcohol and decline in noisy situations, over the telephone, while in the drive-thru, and when under stress.

History of the Problem. The patient presents a 5-year history of dysphonia that gradually increased in severity over the first 6 to 8 months but has been stable the past 4 years. The voice problem significantly impacts her ability to work as an 11th-grade history teacher. Her students often ask her if she is nervous or upset. She has previously seen 3 other otolaryngologists and received diagnoses including chronic laryngitis, gastroesophageal reflux disease (GERD), laryngopharyngeal reflux (LPR), and stress-induced voice disorder. She has been treated with several courses of antibiotics, steroids, and proton pump inhibitors without improvement. The previous otolaryngologist who diagnosed her with stress-induced MTD referred her for voice therapy. She was seen at another facility for 28 voice therapy visits over 3.5 months. She was able to achieve a clearer tone during therapy, but she frustrated both herself and the SLP when she was unable to carry over the clearer voice outside of therapy. That otolaryngologist had suggested that perhaps there was some unconscious stressor in the patient's life that she was not dealing with and recommended that she see a psychiatrist. During her own Google search, she came across information about the interprofessional voice center and made an appointment to be seen.

General Medical Examination
(Completed by the Laryngologist)

On physical examination, the patient appeared healthy and was breathing comfortably in no acute distress. Vital signs showed that the patient was afebrile, pulse was 82, respirations were 14, and blood pressure was 146/91. The patient had a normal gait. Upper and lower extremity examination demonstrated full muscular strength and normal sensation. No hand tremor or joint cogwheel rigidity was noted. Reflexes were 2+. Respiratory examination showed clear breath sounds with full inspiration and normal forceful expiration.

> Deep tendon reflexes are involuntary muscle contractions in response to a specific stimulus. A rating of 2+ indicates a brisk response, which is considered normal.

Head and Neck Examination
(Completed by the Laryngologist)

The patient's voice had a severe strained and strangled quality, making her difficult to understand. The neck was supple without skin lesions, thyromegaly, lymphadenopathy, or masses. There was moderate symmetrical tenderness upon palpation in the thyrohyoid region. Cranial nerves II through XII were grossly intact, eye movements were full, and head and neck muscle strength were normal. Otoscopy demonstrated clear external auditory canals and intact tympanic membranes with aerated middle ear spaces. Hearing was grossly normal. Anterior rhinoscopy showed healthy mucous membranes without masses or obstruction of the nasal cavities. Oral cavity and oropharyngeal examination demonstrated moist mucous membranes without lesions. Palatal rise and gag reflex were normal. Indirect laryngoscopy was somewhat limited by the gag reflex, but there were no gross masses and vocal fold mobility appeared normal.

Motor Speech Evaluation (Completed
by the Speech-Language Pathologist)

Motor speech evaluation indicated a normal oral mechanism with intact articulatory precision. On vowel prolongation, there was a frequent delayed onset time with strained-strangled phonation noted. Laryngeal diadochokinesis was marked with difficulty with initiation on rapid repetitions of the vowel

/a/. Repetition of multisyllabic words such as "Methodist," "Episcopal," and "no ifs, ands, or buts" (https://www.asha.org/practice-portal/clinical-topics/) demonstrated intact syllabic order but with fluency issues related to glottal stops on voiceless-voiced phoneme chains.

Auditory-Perceptual Assessment

The Consensus Auditory-Perceptual Evaluation of Voice (CAPE-V) [24] was administered per protocol, and the patient was asked to count from 60 to 65 and from 80 to 85 and to read sentences that were either voiced consonant and vowel laden or were voiceless consonant laden.[6] The consensus CAPE-V score by the laryngologist and SLP was 84/100, indicating a dysphonia of a severe nature. Aberrant perceptual features identified in the voice included roughness, pitch breaks, phonation breaks, and strain. Glottal stops on vowel-initial words were consistently present. The patient noted more difficulty with counting 80 to 85 than 60 to 65 and on the voiced consonant- and vowel-laden sentences, eg, "We were away a year ago." There was laryngeal/pharyngeal focused resonance with base of tongue tension that dampened the intensity of sound output.

Laryngeal Imaging

Laryngeal Imaging was performed using a transnasal distal chip flexible laryngoscope with videostroboscopy for detailed motion and mucosal assessment in addition to dynamic assessment of the palate, nasopharynx, base of tongue, posterior pharyngeal walls, and larynx. The endoscopic examination was performed by the SLP and reviewed by both the laryngologist and SLP. Results indicated that palatal closure was complete on repetitions of /ʃ/, /z/, and [kitkat]. Pharyngeal squeeze was symmetric bilaterally. There were no pharyngeal or laryngeal masses noted. The laryngeal mucosa appeared healthy. Arytenoid motion showed full adduction and abduction that was symmetrical and brisk bilaterally.

As has been noted in the literature regarding dystonic voices, following topical anesthesia and during the examination, the patient's voice improved significantly and allowed for enough sustained phonation to complete the stroboscopic examination.[25]

Utilizing the Voice-Vibratory Assessment With Laryngeal Imaging (VALI)[26] to assess stroboscopic findings at modal pitch (185-192 Hz), results indicated:

1. Glottal closure: Complete
2. Amplitude of lateral excursion: Normal at 30% bilaterally
3. Mucosal wave: Normal at 40% of the superior surface of the folds bilaterally
4. Vertical level: On plane
5. Nonvibrating portion: None present
6. Supraglottic activity: Clearly present anterior-posterior compression that occasionally obscured viewing of the vocal folds during phonation
7. Free edge contour: Normal/straight bilaterally
8. Phase closure: Nearly equivalent with occasions of increased open phase
9. Phase symmetry: 20% of the time asymmetry noted
10. Regularity: 50% of examination regular due to the presence of complete glottal stops impacting the vibratory cycle

Vocal Effort, Fatigue, and Pain

The patient rated her vocal effort using the OMNI-VES,[4] a visual analog 0 to 10 scale where 0 = "extremely easy" to produce voice and 10 = "extremely hard" to produce voice. The patient reported that vocal effort was 7/10 during speaking and 10/10 at worst, occurring in noisy situations, on the telephone, while in the drive though, and when under stress.

Patient-Reported Quality-of-Life Measures

1. Voice Handicap Index-10 (VHI-10)[27]: 38/40 (threshold = 11)[28]

2. Cough Severity Index[29]: 0/40 (threshold = 3)
3. Dyspnea Index[30]: 3/20 (threshold = 3).
4. Voice Problem Impact Scales (VPIS)[31]: 6/7 work/daily activities, 6/7 social, 3/7 home, 6/7 overall

Aerodynamic Measures

Aerodynamic measures of syllable repetition have been suggested for use in differential diagnosis.[32] To complete this task, the patient was fitted with a standard face mask connected to a commercially available pneumotachograph and pressure transducer. Results of the assessment can be found in Table 6–1 with normative data from Barkmeier and Case (2000)[32] and Patel et al (2018).[33]

Acoustic Analysis

A headset microphone was placed at a 45-degree angle at 2 cm from the mouth to acquire acoustic information per standards recommended in the American Speech-Language-Hearing Association (ASHA) Instrumental Voice Assessment Protocol (IVAP).[33] The noise floor for the testing room was measured at 40 dB. The results of the assessment were abnormal, including decreased maximum phonation time of 5 seconds (norms 12-15+ seconds for females). Results of the testing indicated a voice type 3, with chaotic or random signal acquisition and high relative average perturbation. This indicated that time-based acoustic data such as jitter and shimmer were not a reliable source of information and that CPP and perceptual assessments should be used for assessment. Results are documented in Table 6–2.

Stimulability Testing

During trial therapy, the patient was stimulable for improvement in voice quality using chant talk, high-pitched productions, vegetative vocal tasks, and whispering. Geste antagoniste (GA)[34] is a term used to describe the improvement in speech/voice in people with dystonia

228 Voice Therapy: Clinical Case Studies

Table 6–1. Aerodynamic Assessment

Aerodynamic Measures	Results	Norms	X Indicates Abnormal
Vital Capacity (L) (expiratory volume)	5 L	4-6 L	
MFR (mL/sec): Vowel (mean airflow during voicing)	130 mL/sec	Norms = 177-187 mL/sec	X
PTP (cmH_2O): Quietest Modal	8.56 cmH_2O	4.22 +/− 1.02	X
Laryngeal Resistance (cmH_2O/L/sec)	55.20 cmH_2O/L/sec	32-45 cmH_2O/L/sec	X

Table 6–2. Acoustic Assessment

	Rainbow Passage: Results	Sustained Vowel: Results	Norms	X Indicates Abnormal
Mean F0 (Hz)	185 Hz	199 Hz	M 121-163 Hz F 200-266 Hz	X
SD (Hz)	45 Hz	18 Hz	<29.1 Hz	X
Physiological Pitch Range (Hz)	158-459 Hz		M 90-550 Hz F 130-750 Hz	X
CPP in Sustained Vowel /a/	**Results**		**Norms**	**X Indicates Abnormal**
CPP (dB)	5.23 dB		F 10.74, M 13.03	X
CPP SD (dB)	4.0 dB		F 2.37, M 0.75	
Mean CPP F0 (Hz)	199 Hz		F 210.37, M 110.89	
CPP F0 SD (Hz)	18 Hz		F 10.74, M 0.75	
CSID	58		F 4.43, M 3.58	

using accents, singing, or a high pitch.[35] GA is considered a confirmatory sensory trick in dystonia. In other words, if the patient can use sensory tricks to improve the voice, then it is likely confirmatory of AdLD rather than MTD alone.

Assessment

The patient's presentation is consistent with AdLD with moderate to severe compensatory MTD.

Plan of Care

The patient will receive Botox® type A injections into the laryngeal adductor muscles (thyroarytenoid-lateral cricoarytenoid [TA-LCA] complex) with voice therapy 4 to 6 weeks postinjection following the first injection only, for a maximum of 4 sessions, either once every week or every 2 weeks over 2 months.

Long-Term Goal. The patient will regain the ability to communicate at work and in social settings by reducing the impact of the glottal stops using Botox® injections and postinjection voice therapy to reduce any residual compensatory MTD.

Following discussion of the diagnosis and recommended treatment plan, the physician and SLP answered the patient's questions about the disease. They explained that the problem was a focal dystonia, a benign neurologic condition that results in uncontrolled spasms of the laryngeal muscles responsible for vocal fold adduction (primarily the thyroarytenoid and lateral cricoarytenoid muscles). The patient asked what caused the condition and was told that the exact cause is unclear but that it is felt to result from an abnormality in the neural networks of the brain and the basal ganglia.[36] The patient was then told that alternative diagnoses of MTD or vocal tremor can present similarly to or simultaneously with AdLD. She was advised that the assessment tasks confirmed that she did not present with vocal tremor nor MTD as a primary diagnosis, but rather as a compensatory MTD (secondary

MTD; see Chapter 4 Introduction by Nelson Roy).

The physician counseled the patient that Botox® injections for LD have been shown to be the most effective in reducing voice breaks and improving quality of life for patients.[37] He told her that Botox® is a neurotoxin that blocks the nerves' ability to make muscles contract. When Botox® is injected into a target muscle, it impairs the release of neurotransmitters from the nerve endings at the neuromuscular junction, which effectively paralyzes or significantly weakens the muscle and prevents muscle contraction. Botox® acts temporarily, with effects lasting from 3 to 6 months. Consequently, repeated injections are necessary for long-term treatment. The injections usually are given to an awake patient in the outpatient setting, utilizing laryngeal electromyography (LEMG) for accurate guidance into the laryngeal adductor muscles. Usually, a starting dose of 1.25 U to 2.5 U is used, either unilaterally or bilaterally, in the thyroarytenoid muscles.

The SLP went on to tell the patient that the effects of injection appear after 24 to 48 hours. There is a fairly typical clinical course following injection that is important for patients to understand. Approximately 48 to 72 hours following injection, patients begin to notice a gradual weakening of their voice. This can range from mild breathiness to whispered voice and can be accompanied by mild dysphagia for liquids. The breathy period usually lasts for 1 to 2 weeks and is based on the patients response to the toxin injected. Patients usually can manage the dysphagia with conservative techniques such as using a slower rate of drinking especially for thin liquids, using a nectar-thick consistency for liquids, and performing a slight chin tuck or effortful swallow on drinking liquids. After 1 to 2 weeks, the patient's voice begins to return and gradually gains strength with dramatic reduction in the voice breaks, improved fluency, and less vocal effort. This therapeutic period typically lasts 2 to 3 months. Following this, the patient will begin to notice voice breaks returning as the effects of the injection wear off, and a repeat injection is scheduled.

The SLP and laryngologist explained that Botox® dosing for AdLD is an art and is based on the individual patient's needs and results from prior treatments. The breathy period following injection can be very bothersome to patients. This can be minimized by using lower-dosed (0.625-1.25 U) bilateral injections, performing unilateral injections, or using false vocal fold injections as described below. Because Ms. Smith would need to travel a long distance to receive her injections, the laryngologist told her that some patients want to maximize the duration of the effect, so they tolerate a longer breathy period in favor of longer-lasting effects. In these situations, a higher dose that provides the least amount of side effects can be used. The physician explained that there is another less commonly used injection method treatment of AdLD.[38] This method requires viewing the larynx during injection and using a higher degree of topical anesthesia prior to the injection of higher doses of Botox®. He said that doses of 5.0 to 7.5 U, via a transthyrohyoid approach, are injected into the submucosal plane of the ventricular folds. The benefit of this injection is generally little to no side effects like breathy voice or dysphagia; however, the injection is believed to have a shorter life span of generally 10 weeks.

The patient asked about medications that could be used for treatment. She was told that there are no medications that have demonstrated any long-term benefit. Benzodiazepines, such as diazepam, help some patients for short periods, but the risk of dependency from chronic use was discussed as well as the goal of avoiding the routine use of such medications. Some medications have limited utility specifically for vocal tremor, such as beta-blockers (eg, propranolol) and antiepileptics (eg, primidone), but these have not been shown to be effective for isolated LD.[39]

The patient asked about surgical treatments and the physician discussed recurrent laryngeal nerve section, recurrent laryngeal nerve avulsion, and the newer selective laryngeal adductor denervation and reinnervation (SLADR).[40] He explained that the former two were limited by frequent recurrences of voice breaks, typically do not have long-term benefits, and may be complicated by permanent breathiness to the voice. The latter is a newer procedure that may be effective in patients who respond well to botulinum toxin injections, but it has not become widely utilized for AdLD largely due to lack of long-term data regarding its effectiveness.

> There have been some promising studies in the use of sodium oxybate for short-duration (4+ hours) reduction in glottal stops and vocal strain in people who report their voice improves when they drink alcohol (alcohol responsive). However, the use of sodium oxybate has important factors to consider, including not being able to drive while on the drug, dosing difficulty, and the cost of the drug. The reader is encouraged to review more information regarding sodium oxybate in Simonyan et al (2021).[2]

Last, Ms. Smith asked how long she could receive Botox® treatment, and the team explained that repeated dosing can be performed for long periods of time. They told her that many patients have had successful treatment with Botox® for nearly 2 decades.

Decision Making

At the time of writing, Botox® injections for LD remain the gold standard and primary/first-line treatment of AdLD. There is a small body of literature that discusses the use of voice therapy post injection to help recalibrate voice use to be less effortful and to work with the glottal stops rather than anticipate and respond to the stops.[41] Voice therapy should not need to be done after every injection, but rather only once to help the patient best utilize the postinjection paretic period for optimal efficient voice.

Intervention

Botox® Injections

This patient received a starting dose of 1.25 U into each thyroarytenoid muscle. As expected, no voice changes occurred for the first 48 hours. She then experienced a weak and breathy voice with very mild dysphagia for liquids that was most noticeable in the first week following treatment and waned by the second week. She returned to the clinic 1 month following injection with a significantly improved voice. She did notice some vocal strain and occasional voice breaks that were still causing some voice fatigue and a brief course of voice therapy was recommended.

Voice Therapy

Voice therapy took place over 4 sessions spaced 1 week apart, beginning week 4 post-injection.

Short-Term Goal #1. The patient will increase kinesthetic awareness of compensatory muscle tension in the chest, shoulders, jaw/face, and laryngeal/pharyngeal areas of the vocal mechanism. The rationale for this goal lies in the frequency of extralaryngeal muscle tension utilized by those with AdLD to overcome the excessive strain of sound production prior to treatment. Despite the use of Botox®, the patient continued to utilize preinjection compensatory muscle tension. Scanning techniques in Lessac-Madsen Resonant Voice Therapy (LMRVT) (see Case Study 3.7 by Orbelo, Li, and Verdolini Abbott: Lessac-Madsen Resonant Voice Therapy to Treat an Adult With Vocal Fold Nodules), laryngeal massage (see Case Study 8.8 by Schneider and Courey: Perioperative Management for an Adult Jazz Singer With a Vocal Fold Cyst), myofascial release (see Case Study 8.3 by Le-

Borgne: Myofascial Release for an Adult Touring Musical Theater Performer With Vocal Fatigue), and progressive relaxation (see Case Study 6.2 by Stemple: Voice Therapy Without Medical Management for an Adult With Adductor Spasmodic Dysphonia) are useful to meet this goal.

Short-Term Goal #2. The patient will reduce effortful production of speech. Despite the use of Botox® injections and the reduced glottal closure, the patient continued to use preinjection effortful voicing behaviors. The rationale for this goal was to teach the patient to use less subglottal pressure and more of a continuous flow phonation during sound production. Treatment began with use of semi-occluded vocal tract exercises to balance the resonators and amplify the sound intensity of phonation. Using the OMNI-VES to self-assess level of vocal effort and then to progressively reduce effort to level 2 to 3/easy allowed the patient to gain an internal locus of control of the vocal effort expended for voicing. Once the patient realized that she could produce phonation of a normal loudness by using an open vocal tract through resonant voice therapy, semi-occluded vocal tract exercises, and Conversation Training Therapy, she was able to implement a speaking style with less phonatory effort, thus decreasing vocal fatigue and encouraging a smoother phonatory style. See the following for additional information on each technique: Case Study 3.3 by Murphy Estes: Multimodality Voice Therapy to Treat an Adult Female Opera Singer With a Vocal Fold Pseudocyst; Case Study 8.4 by Muckala: Voice Recalibration With the Cup Bubble Technique for an Adult Country Singer With Chronic Phonotrauma; and Case Study 3.1 by Gartner-Schmidt and Gillespie: Conversation Training Therapy (CTT) to Treat an Adult With Benign Midmembranous Lesions.

Short-Term Goal #3. The patient will improve coordination of respiration and phonation. Pre-injection, the patient tended to hold her breath to overcome the vocal spasm.

After injection, the patient continued to hold her breath, often producing words on expiratory reserve volume. Additionally, with the increase in glottal gap because of Botox®, the patient had less glottal valving and had difficulty efficiently coordinating respiration and phonation for longer phrases. Therefore, the patient was encouraged to use shorter breath groups. Treatment began with low abdominal breathing, stressing awareness of the onset of abdominal muscle contraction during exhalation. The next step was to add phonation to the low abdominal breathing, encouraging the patient to use voiceless fricative prolongation of /ʃ/, /f/, and /s/ to avoid the laryngeal valve effort. Next, she was instructed to do pulsed productions of voiceless fricatives /ʃ/, /f/, and /s/. She was then instructed to repeat the tasks with voiced fricatives /ʒ/, /v/, and /z/. The task progression continued by using sentences of increasing length and instructing the patient to use shorter breath groups with brief replenishing breaths in conversation. The patient was reminded that breathing for speech used mouth breathing and that replenishing breaths were those low abdominal mouth breaths just large enough to replenish the air expended for the prior sentence.

Summary and Concluding Remarks

The impact of Botox® injections on quality of life is very personal and is usually dependent on the effectiveness of the injections, the vocal demands of the patient, and the environmental support of the patient. As a teacher, the patient was often plagued with balancing the breathy, whispered immediate postinjection voice and the vocal demands of teaching. She tried to coordinate injections a few days before the winter semester break, right before spring break, during the quieter months of summer when she did not teach, and a few weeks before the school year began. But, even with all the planning, she often felt her life was ruled by her injections. The SLP encouraged her to attend a local Dysphonia International (formerly National Spasmodic Dysphonia Association; www.dysphonia.org) support group. In the group, the patient found camaraderie, support, and a wealth of resources from people who had lived with AdLD, undergone Botox® injections, and tried a plethora of adjunctive treatments.

 CASE STUDY 6.2

Voice Therapy Without Medical Management for an Adult With Adductor Spasmodic Dysphonia

Joseph C. Stemple

Voice Evaluation

Case History

Patient VV, a 57-year-old cisgender female high school English and drama teacher complaining of dysphonia, was referred to the voice center for an interdisciplinary evaluation by her colleague, the SLP serving in the school where they both worked. She had been symptomatic for 3 years and had consulted 3 physicians and 1 SLP, and each provider diagnosed her problem as MTD.

> Diagnostic delays are not uncommon in laryngeal dystonia/spasmodic dysphonia. One study found that it can take up to 4.43 years and 3.95 physicians to be accurately diagnosed with AdLD[42]

Medical History. The patient's medical history was unremarkable as related to this problem.

Social History. Patient VV lived alone and described herself as extremely independent and outgoing. She had taught for 34 years and stated that she "lived to teach." By the time of the initial evaluation, she was emotionally upset, confused, and full of self-doubt. She had independently sought the counsel of a psychologist who, unfortunately, was not familiar with laryngeal dystonia and who supported the notion that the problem was "all in my head." She had developed lesson plans and teaching techniques that minimized her own classroom speaking, but she suffered with these teaching modifications. Previously, she had been honored as an outstanding educator and she was convinced that she had become less than effective in the classroom.

Away from school, this normally outgoing individual had withdrawn and, for at least 18 months, lived a reclusive existence. She refused to see friends and totally avoided the telephone. The two things most dear to her, teaching and friendships, had been taken from her because of her voice disorder.

History of Voice Complaint. The voice problem began in the fall 3 years prior to the examination. It manifested as dysphonia that persisted following an upper respiratory infection. When the dysphonia persisted for several weeks, she sought the opinion of an otolaryngologist, who prescribed antibiotics 3 times over a 4-month period. As the symptoms worsened, hesitations began "shutting off" her voice, requiring her to speak with increased effort. She reported that teaching was causing her to be physically fatigued because of the effort it took to speak. She was exhausted at the end of a school day. Some days, her abdominal muscles would become sore from straining to produce a voice. During the 2 subsequent years, she sought the opinion of 2 more physicians, one of whom prescribed more medication, while the other recommended psychological counseling. An SLP new to Patient VV's school heard her speak and thought the patient presented with the symptoms of AdLD. She then suggested that the patient be seen by the voice center for evaluation.

SLP Evaluation

The speech pathologist performed 3 roles during the initial session: *evaluator* to confirm the presence of AdLD, *educator* to teach the patient what was known about the disorder, and *treatment planner* to attempt to remediate the disorder. The team laryngologist confirmed that Patient VV presented with adductor type laryngeal dystonia of moderate severity. Initial observations were that phonation was characterized by intermittent glottal stops and glottal fry phonation as well as a flat, monotonous inflection pattern. It was evident from the physical appearance of neck and shoulder tension and facial expression that she was very tense, nervous, upset and, by self-report, depressed.

Auditory-Perceptual Assessment

The patient demonstrated normal phonation when humming or singing or when speaking in lilting accents. She loved to read aloud from the writings of the American dramatist Tennessee Williams because the higher-pitched rhythm of the US southern dialect reduced her effort to talk and improved the voice quality. She could laugh normally and felt that her voice was "near normal" when she talked to her cat. The patient also thought that her voice quality was improved following ingestion of wine. This led her to sample tranquilizers, which did not improve her voice quality.

On phonemically loaded sentences frequently used to evaluate the presence of laryngeal dystonia, the patient demonstrated glottal stops on voiced phonemes and reported voice was less effortful on phrases loaded with voiceless phonemes. Table 6–3 illustrates common phrases used to identify laryngeal dystonia and to differentiate adductor- and abductor-type.

During the clinical assessment, the clinician noted that Patient VV produced voice with increased vocal and respiratory effort manifesting as pressed voice quality, disordered breathing with breath holding, a back

Table 6–3. Phrases Loaded With Voiced or Voiceless Phonemes

Voiced Phonemes	Voiceless Phonemes
The dog dug a new bone.	Keep Tom at the party.
We mow our lawn all year.	Sam usually takes coffee with sugar.
The waves were rolling along.	Put the cookies in the tin.
We rode along Rhode Island Avenue.	He saw half a shape mystically cross a simple path at least fifty or sixty steps across from his sister Kathy's house.

resonatory focus, and often a low pitch in what appeared to be an attempt to overcome the intermittent spasms.

Laryngeal Imaging

All stroboscopic observations were within normal limits. Despite demonstrating a very mild head tremor, which is not an unusual co-occurrence with laryngeal dystonia,[43] there was no visual evidence of tremor in the palate, pharynx, base of tongue, glottis, or supraglottis using the Vocal Tremor Scoring System[44] (see Case Study 6.6 by DiRenzo: The SLP's Role in Deep Brain Stimulation for Vocal Tremor).

It is well recognized that the symptoms of laryngeal dystonia are not typically seen on laryngeal imaging examinations. Due to the significant aperiodiciy that occurs due to intermittent vocal spasms, videostroboscopy is not an optimal diagnostic tool to *confirm* the disorder. However, it is appropriate to rule out other factors that could impact vocal fold vibration. Plain light laryngeal examinations are useful to rule out motion asymmetries or other incidental findings prior to initiating treatment for this disorder.[6,25]

Assessment

Given the normal appearance of the laryngeal examination as well as the absence of other neurological deficits including extremity tremor, dysarthria and/or dysphagia, and presence of increased difficulty with phrases laden with voiced phonemes, the presence of glottal stops on voiced phonemes, and comments about improved voice with alcohol consumption, the interprofessional team determined the patient was likely presenting with AdLD.

Decision Making

The clinician discussed treatment options including the gold-standard treatment for AdLD using injections of botulinum toxin (Botox®), other modalities for treatment (see Case Study 6.1 by Hapner and Johns: Medical and Behavioral Management for an Adult With Laryngeal Dystonia–Adductor Type), voice therapy, and no treatment. Patient VV was distressed to learn that treatments would produce only symptom relief, not cure the disorder, and require repeat injections every 2 to 4 months. She was not interested in newer modalities, so the clinician focused the discussion on Botox® injections to reduce the severity of adductor spasms versus functional voice therapy designed to eliminate secondary muscle tension (though with less evidence for treatment of of this disease). The patient

Intervention

Patient VV was given information regarding laryngeal dystonia provided by the Dysphonia International website, previously known as the National Spasmodic Dysphonia Association (NSDA) (http://www.dysphonia.org), which included resources to read further about the disease and its treatment options, research-based information and, importantly, support groups in her area to connect with other people with her disease.

Voice Therapy

During the first session, stimulability tasks identified the vocalization styles that Patient VV could perform well with fair consistency. These included:

- humming and singing
- speaking at a higher pitch
- speaking with a slight Southern accent
- speaking to her cat (higher-pitched baby voice sound)

> These tasks are examples of *geste antagoniste*, sensory tricks that temporarily reduce the severity of dystonic postures or movements. Additionally, some improvement may be attributed to cricothyroid-dominant phonation at higher pitches rather than thyroarytenoid dominance (as typically used in speech).

The first step in therapy was to demonstrate the degree of tension, even at rest, in the voice-producing structures. To raise this awareness, the clinician taught VV techniques of progressive relaxation and performed laryngeal massage and surface electromyographic (sEMG) biofeedback.[45-47] Progressive relaxation involves teaching the patient to alternately tense and relax individual body parts from the forehead to the toes to raise awareness of overall body tension. Following this exercise, laryngeal massage focused on reducing tension specific to the laryngeal area of the neck (see Case Study 4.1 by Roy: Manual Circumlaryngeal Techniques to Treat an Adult With Primary MTD). Finally, the patient underwent 2 sessions of EMG biofeedback. Using surface electrodes placed on each side of the thyroid lamina, the patient monitored muscle tension levels while alternately tensing and relaxing the neck muscles. These methods permitted her to gain awareness and control of her laryngeal area tension.

> Opinions vary in the literature regarding the use of sEMG to identify or monitor laryngeal muscle tension. The most recent study at the time of this edition's publication is by Wang and Yiu (2024). The reader is encouraged to review this article and its findings to learn more.[48]

Phonatory tasks then were added to this newly relaxed state by utilizing a slightly higher pitch and a less pressed phonation. Vowels, consonant-vowel-consonant combinations, and phrases of different lengths were progressed along a continuum of difficulty.[49] Although the spasms persisted, the clinician and the patient noted that frequency and severity decreased. Phrases were incrementally lengthened, and the patient was trained to speech breathe with decreased tension (see Case Study 4.3 by Gartner-Schmidt: Flow Phonation to Treat a Teenager With Primary Muscle Tension Aphonia). Often, patients with AdLD create increased laryngeal tension with inappropriate breathing patterns. Training them to take a breath before running out of air can reduce this tension. In addition, the patient deemed it acceptable to use a more forwardly placed, slightly nasal tone focus and allow a slightly breathy phonation. In addition, she felt comfortable in slightly overinflecting her phonation patterns of pitch and loudness, which also decreased the severity of the spasms. Longer phrases utilizing these techniques were then expanded into paragraph readings with and without phrase or breath markers and finally into practiced conversational speech. Because of VV's background in drama, she felt comfortable in experimenting with these techniques, and the entire therapy program was completed within 6 weeks.

Posttreatment Outcomes

The spasms persisted as expected but were perceived only as occasional hesitations during speech production. This result may be considered the patient's baseline level of spasticity. The patient learned to let her voice flow through and past the hesitations without redeveloping the previous maladaptive laryngeal and respiratory postures. Eliminating these compensatory behaviors proved adequate for this patient. She chose not to pursue Botox® injections. Prior to discharge, the patient was advised that her voice may continue to fluctuate or even decline in the months and years to come and that she should seek follow-up care to reconsider the possibility of Botox® injections should concerns arise in the future.

Summary and Concluding Remarks

This patient presented with a classic case of AdLD. The severity of her voice production was exacerbated by her attempt to compensate for the presence of the spasms with laryngeal and respiratory muscle tension, low resonance posture, and lowered pitch. While behavioral voice therapy will not eliminate vocal spasms, the techniques applied successfully reduced the maladaptive behaviors, thus decreasing effort to speak and improving overall voice production.

CASE STUDY 6.3

Teletherapy Without Medical Management for an Adult With Abductor Laryngeal Dystonia and Vocal Tremor

Lauren Timmons Sund

Voice Evaluation

Case History

Chief Complaint. Quiet voice with increased vocal effort

History of Present Illness. I had the pleasure of seeing this patient for a comprehensive voice evaluation referred by the laryngologist as part of an interprofessional voice evaluation. The patient was diagnosed with dysphonia due to AbLD, vocal tremor, and vocal fold atrophy. The patient was previously seen by a neurologist, who observed vocal tremor without other concerning neurological signs or symptoms and referred the patient to our voice center.

History of Voice Complaint. Patient FR is a 68-year-old cisgender woman with gradual onset of voice problems starting several years ago without a known inciting event. Symptoms include a quiet voice with increased vocal effort and occasional vocal instability with difficulty "making sounds come out." She reports her voice has always been relatively quiet, but it is quieter now than it used to be. The patient has not received the services of an SLP for this problem in the past.

Patient FR previously worked as a clinical psychologist and has been retired for 3 years. She reports moderate voice use with family and friends. Others ask her to repeat herself more frequently compared to several years ago. She lives with her husband, who has hearing loss, and she reports she often needs to repeat herself when talking to him.

Laryngeal Imaging

Laryngeal videostroboscopy was performed transnasally with a flexible distal chip videolaryngoscope. There were no supraglottal or hypopharyngeal masses. There was full abduction and adduction of both vocal folds. The VALI[26] was used to assess vibratory parameters as documented in Table 6–4.

Quality-of-Life Impairment
1. VHI-10: 28/40[27]
2. Voice Catastrophization Index: 42/52[50]
3. VPIS[31] where 1 = no impact and 7 = profound impact; the patient reported the following:
   a. Impact on work life or daily activities: 4/7
   b. Impact on social life: 6/7 (related to being asked to repeat herself)
   c. Impact on home life: 6/7 (related to being asked to repeat herself)
   d. Impact on voice overall: 5.5/7

Vocal Effort, Fatigue, and Pain
The OMNI-VES[4] was completed. The patient reported that vocal effort was 6/10 (somewhat hard) during the evaluation and 8/10 (hard) at worst, occurring when repeating herself or in background noise.

Auditory-Perceptual Assessment
The CAPE-V[24] was administered. The patient was determined to have an overall CAPE-V score of 44/100, indicating a dysphonia of a moderate nature. Aberrant perceptual features identified in the voice included breathiness with breathy breaks, strain, and instability/tremulous quality. Overall vocal loudness was reduced. Pitch of the voice was within normal limits. Resonance was focused in the epilaryngeal region. Locus of respiration was primarily thoracic, and breath holding was noted.

Phonetically loaded sentences for assessing LD were administered. Breathy breaks were perceived most prominently in the voiceless consonant sentences. The patient reported her vocal effort was higher in the voiceless consonant sentences as well. (See Case Study 6.2 by Stemple for examples of phonetically loaded sentences.)

Table 6–4. VALI Findings

Stroboscopy Parameter	Findings
Free Edge Contour	Concave bilaterally
Glottal Closure	Complete
Phase Closure	Open phase predominates
Mucosal Wave	Approximately 60% excursion bilaterally
Amplitude	Approximately 60% excursion bilaterally
Nonvibrating Portion	None
Supraglottic Activity	2 (mild) anterior-posterior and mediolateral compression
Vertical Level	On plane
Phase Symmetry	90% symmetrical
Regularity (Periodicity)	80% periodic
Other Features	Tremor at the level of the true vocal folds. No palatal or pharyngeal tremor.

238   Voice Therapy: Clinical Case Studies

Manual Palpation Assessment

Muscle tension was assessed and rated on a 0 to 5 scale where 0 = no tension and 5 = most tension. Results indicated:

1. 2/5 tension at the thyrohyoid space with report of tenderness on palpation
2. 2/5 tension at the base of tongue (BOT)/ suprahyoid region without report of pain
3. Laryngeal height within normal limits as assessed by palpation of the hyoid
4. 2/5 restriction of lateralization of thyroid cartilage bilaterally

Stimulability

With cues to increase loudness following a clinician model, the patient was able to demonstrate a mild increase in loudness. Vocal tremor was still present.

Patient Education

The SLP and laryngologist discussed the difficult nature of treating AbLD with vocal tremor. Commonly, treatment for abductor spasms includes botulinum toxin injections into the posterior cricoarytenoid muscles,[51] whereas botulinum toxin injections into the thyroarytenoid muscles are used to treat vocal tremor.[5] The physician additionally discussed medications, such as propranolol for vocal tremor.[39]

Impressions

The patient presents with moderate dysphonia that limits communication, daily activities, and participation. Dysphonia is characterized by breathiness with breathy breaks in phonemically loaded contexts, vocal tremor, reduced loudness, and strain. The patient demonstrated minimal-moderate ability to increase vocal loudness. Following counseling regarding medical treatments, the patient reported she is not ready to pursue medication or botulinum toxin injections. Given stimulability and the SLP's perception of strain with suboptimal respiratory phonatory coordination, voice therapy was recommended to improve volitional control of voice subsystems to optimize vocal efficiency, reduce vocal effort, and improve the ability to increase vocal loudness for certain contexts.

Plan of Care

Voice therapy was recommended. The patient appeared to be a fair to good candidate for voice therapy. Positive prognostic indicators included patient-reported motivation to engage in voice therapy and mild favorable response to stimulability testing. Negative prognostic indicators included the diagnoses of AbLD and vocal tremor as the etiology for her dysphonia, which are conditions that will not resolve with voice therapy. However, optimizing coordination of voice subsystems and reducing compensatory muscle tension can be addressed behaviorally. This can reduce vocal effort and the perceptibility of tremor in conversational speech (see Case Study 6.4 by Barkmeier-Kramer: Reducing Voicing Duration to Treat an Adult With Vocal Tremor). The patient elected to begin voice therapy with the following plan:

Long-Term Goal. Improve coordination of voice subsystems to reduce vocal effort and optimize communication

Frequency. 4 to 6 sessions of 45 to 60 minutes each, twice monthly

Short-Term Goals:

1. Establish abdominal-thoracic locus of respiration to optimize participation in tasks for respiratory phonatory coordination
2. Trial Phonation Resistance Training Exercises (PhoRTE)®[51] to increase vocal loudness with emphasis on respiratory phonatory coordination (see Case Study 5.2 by Ziegler and Hapner: Phonation Resistance Training Exercises [PhoRTE®] to Treat an Adult With Presbyphonia)
3. Flow phonation as an alternative for addressing respiratory phonatory

coordination and/or resonant voice for addressing forward resonance if PhoRTE® response is suboptimal (see Case Study 4.3 by Gartner-Schmidt: Flow Phonation to Treat a Teenager With Primary Muscle Tension Aphonia)

Decision Making

Patient FR's voice problem was due to AbLD with vocal tremor, both of which are neurological conditions, and underlying vocal fold atrophy. The combination of abductor breathy breaks with vocal tremor is relatively rare and is difficult to treat. While breathy breaks can be treated with botulinum toxin injections (Botox®) to the posterior cricoarytenoid muscles, vocal tremor is often treated with Botox® to the thyroarytenoid muscles. Patient FR was counseled on options for procedural intervention (Botox®), as well as medications to treat tremor (propranolol), but she reported she was hesitant to try these medical interventions. Though voice therapy cannot cure either LD or vocal tremor, voice therapy can improve coordination of the voice subsystems and reduce maladaptive compensatory behaviors.[53] In this case, the patient was observed to hold her breath with a high locus of respiration, and the SLP perceived that some improvement in voice could be achieved through voice therapy to increase effectiveness of daily communication. Due to the breath holding, the first short-term goal pertained to abdominal-thoracic locus of respiration. The patient was stimulable for increased vocal loudness without strain in exuberant voice trials on short phrases, following a clinician model to determine stimulability for change due to her underlying vocal fold atrophy. For this reason, PhoRTE® was selected to improve coordination of respiration, phonation, and resonance in the context of a louder voice.[54] Flow phonation and resonant voice were considered as alternative methods for improving respiratory phonatory coordination (see Case Study 4.3 by Gartner-Schmidt: Flow Phonation to Treat a Teenager With Primary

Muscle Tension Aphonia), though less favored by the clinician since they do not "power up" the presbyphonic voice in the same way as PhoRTE®.

Intervention

Voice therapy was conducted via synchronous telepractice using a video-enabled, HIPAA-compliant platform. The patient participated in 4 sessions of voice therapy over the course of 3 months, with the first 3 sessions about 2 weeks apart and the final session 1 month later.

Session #1

Goal #1. *Establish abdominal-thoracic locus of respiration to optimize participation in tasks for respiratory phonatory coordination.* Patient FR was guided to place her hands on her abdomen. She was then cued to maximally exhale on /s/ to feel abdominal excursion during a reflexive replenishing breath following maximum exhalation. The patient consistently felt this abdominal excursion after several trials. She was then cued to attend to the sensation of abdominal squeeze at the end of maximum exhalation to access expiratory reserve volume. Verbal cues were provided to keep the shoulders relaxed during this technique. The technique was expanded to include exhalation on /z/ to add a phonatory component.

Goal #2: *Use PhoRTE® to increase vocal loudness with emphasis on respiratory phonatory coordination.* Once the abdominal-thoracic locus of respiration was established and clavicular engagement was extinguished, PhoRTE® tasks were trialed. Patient FR initially demonstrated a posterior locus of resonance with strain on tasks #1 and #2, strong sustained /a/ and strong pitch glides on /a/, respectively. The clinician used a redirection to help the patient develop optimal form, a hallmark of PhoRTE® voice therapy, rather than eliminating the use of exuberant voice therapy. The clinician used resonant exercises to shape correct form with reduced strain, then returned to exuberant therapy with PhoRTE®. (See Video 13 Developing Proper Form for PhoRTE® by Hapner and Ziegler.)

Elements of resonant voice were utilized to correct the locus of resonance. The clinician guided the patient through /hm/ prolongations and /m/-initial consonant-vowel chants (eg, /mimimi/ and /mumumu/) with cues to attend to sensations of anterior vibrations on the lips while gradually increasing loudness. Contrastive practice was used to shift between feeling vibrations on the lips versus tension in the throat. The clinician prompted the patient to describe and label the contrasted voices. The patient labeled the target voice the "face voice" and the contrasted voice the "throat voice." She noted that it was easier to be louder using the "face voice," whereas her voice felt "constricted" when she tried to use the "throat voice" loudly. Once the patient consistently demonstrated "face voice" versus "throat voice," the clinician cued her to try exercises #1 and #2 of PhoRTE® again with /m/-initial /ma/ rather than /a/ to initiate the production with forward resonance. Performance on sustained /ma/ at modal pitch improved considerably, while moderate strain remained present in pitch glides. Maximum phonation time for /ma/ in a strong voice was 4 seconds. The clinician then advanced the patient to PhoRTE® exercise #3, functional phrases in a strong, "calling voice." Patient FR achieved the target voice with increased loudness, reduced breathiness, and forward resonance in 3- to 4-word functional phrases with maximal cues for taking a preparatory breath, using crisp/clear speech, and envisioning her mouth as a megaphone to keep forward resonance.

Session #2 (Two Weeks Later)

Patient FR reported practicing her "projected face voice" by consciously taking a breath before speaking. She also noted that when she gets anxious, her voice "tightens up" and becomes much worse in quality.

Goal #3. *Use flow phonation as an alternative for addressing respiratory phonatory coordination and/or resonant voice for addressing forward resonance if PhoRTE® response is suboptimal.* To address the patient's concerns of throat tightening when anxious, a resonant voice "reset" was recommended, using the /hm/ prolongations and /m/-initial chants as taught in the first session. With /mʌm/ chant, vocal tremor was more apparent and voice was more strained. In shorter productions of /hm/ and /hma/ in descending glides, the patient felt a release of tension in the throat, and vocal tremor was less obvious. The patient was counseled to use this strategy as a vocal reset as needed and to focus more on the feel of the voice than the sound.

Goal #2. The patient continued with elements of PhoRTE® as well as flow phonation and resonant voice tenets to shape the target voice. In functional phrases in the "calling voice" (PhoRTE® #3), the patient benefited from cues for a preparatory abdominal breath and crisp/clear speech to increase loudness and intelligibility. As would be expected, sustained phonation tasks highlighted the presence of vocal tremor. The patient reported it bothered her to hear the tremor, but she also wanted to participate in a voice program that would improve her endurance. The clinician and patient decided together to create a program that combined maximum duration tasks for endurance, pitch glides for pitch flexibility, and connected speech tasks for generalization of her louder target voice. This program was based on the tenets of PhoRTE® with patient-specific modifications. The patient selected the following maximum duration tasks after trialing several options:

- Sustained, strong /ma/ (as in PhoRTE® #1): 5 repetitions
- Strong, resonant voice counting chant of increasing length (ie, the patient counted aloud for as long as possible): 5 repetitions

These 2 tasks were selected because they allowed for addressing respiratory phonatory coordination in sustained duration without highlighting the tremor as much as in other sustained vowels.

For pitch flexibility, the clinician used /ma/ ascending and descending glides, with the patient plugging her ears to alter auditory feedback and mask tremor. The patient demonstrated favorable pitch range regardless of occluding her ears, but she noted that she did not perceive her tremor as much when plugging her ears, which she preferred.

Exercise #3 of PhoRTE®, functional phrases in a strong, "calling voice," were used as the connected speech task.

Session #3 (Two Weeks Later)

Patient FR reported doing her voice exercises regularly. When talking in conversation, she is trying to be more conscious of her breath and articulating crisply. She perceives this is of benefit to her.

Goals #2 and #3. Patient FR demonstrated favorable forward resonance in /hm/-sigh context (resonant voice vocal resets for use when voice feels "tight," especially when anxious). The clinician assessed the patient's performance of the voice exercise program as follows:

- **Exercise #1.** Strong /ma/ maximum duration. Maximum duration was 3 seconds, with voice fading into breathiness between 2 and 3 seconds. Patient reported she did not necessarily feel like she was running out of breath, but that she could not keep the sound going. The clinician perceived this to be a potential abductor break in phonation, which is involuntary. Since performance on this task was not improving after consistent practice, nor did it seem to be benefiting the patient, the clinician elected to eliminate this exercise moving forward.
- **Exercise #2.** Counting on a single pitch. At the previous session, the patient was

able to count from 1 to 7 on a single breath. Today, she was able to count to 9 in 3 out of 5 attempts. Resonance and quality were favorable. The patient was encouraged to continue with this exercise.
- **Exercise #3.** /ma/ on a pitch hill up and down. Favorable pitch range was observed with mild tremor. The patient continued to use bilateral ear occlusion to reduce her perception of vocal tremor.
- **Exercise #4.** Functional phrases in a strong/projected voice. With consistent use of abdominal-thoracic inhalation, the patient achieved oral resonance without breathy breaks. There was mild tremor that did not detract from intelligibility in the functional phrase context.

Session #4 (Four Weeks Later)

Patient FR reported consistent use of her voice exercise routine, about 5 days per week, as well as intentional use of strong, crisp speech in conversation.

Patient FR demonstrated favorable improvement on exercise #2 (counting on a single pitch). She was able to count to 10 in 100% of attempts with favorable voice quality and resonance. She continued to demonstrate favorable pitch range with exercise #3 (/ma/ on a pitch hill up and down in a strong voice with bilateral ear occlusion). In exercise #4, the patient demonstrated a strong, resonant voice with crisp/clear speech. There was mild tremor and intermittent breathy breaks. Practice of target voice in conversation revealed additional breathy breaks. However, the patient reported she was able to talk with a reduction in the sensation of "tightness" that she felt in her throat before starting voice therapy. The patient reported that the most important achievement for her was that she could call out functional phrases clearly now. This allowed her to get her husband's attention at home, making it is easier to have a conversation with him after getting his attention.

The CAPE-V was readministered. The patient was determined to have an overall CAPE-V score of 29/100, indicating a dysphonia of a moderate nature. Aberrant perceptual features identified in the voice included intermittent breathy breaks and instability/tremulous quality. Overall vocal loudness was mildly reduced. Pitch of the voice was within normal limits. Resonance was focused in the oral region. Locus of respiration was primarily abdominal-thoracic.

The OMNI-VES was completed. The patient reported that vocal effort was 3/10 (easy to somewhat easy) in most contexts.

Therapy Outcomes and Conclusions

There was mild improvement in auditory-perceptual voice quality following voice therapy. Specifically, the patient presented with a reduction in strain and improved ability to increase vocal loudness when desired. As would be expected, breathy breaks and vocal tremor were not eliminated. The patient reported a reduction of vocal effort in general and an improved ability to manage "throat tightness" when anxious.

The SLP discussed the variety of medical options available for tremor and atrophy, including botulinum toxin injections and injection augmentation. Patient FR reported she was not interested in any procedures and that she was presently satisfied with the improvements achieved in voice therapy. She reported that she might consider vocal fold injection augmentation in the future if her voice became quieter/weaker due to vocal fold atrophy (see Case Study 5.5 by Gutierrez and Hoffman: Interprofessional Treatment for an Adult With Unilateral Vocal Fold Paresis).

In this case, the SLP provided patient education and supportive counseling about the patient's diagnosis, available treatment options, and expected prognosis with each modality. Though botulinum toxin injections are presently considered the "gold standard" for treating AbLD, the patient reported this was not suitable for her. While the clinician may have favored procedural management, patient autonomy, informed decision making, and *shared* decision making are critical. Importantly, declining procedural intervention did not mean that treatment was withheld. Rather, the SLP provided physiologically based strategies to optimize communication while managing patient expectations and, ultimately, the patient was extraordinarily satisfied with her results.

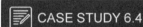

CASE STUDY 6.4

Reducing Voicing Duration to Treat an Adult With Vocal Tremor

Julie Barkmeier-Kraemer

Voice Evaluation

Case History

History of the Problem. Ms. Jones is a 73-year-old cisgender female with a gradual onset of her voice problem beginning 10 years ago. She noticed that her voice became increasingly shaky and that others had increased difficulty understanding her. At the time of experiencing onset of a shaky speaking voice, Ms. Jones was also a member of her church choir. She reported increasing difficulty controlling her upper pitch ranges and excessive vibrato that made her voice stick out in the choir. This worsened the more she tried to modify her vibrato during singing. She eventually stopped participating in choir because of her embarrassment about her excessively shaky voice.

Medical History. Ms. Jones has a medical history of essential tremor diagnosed at the age of 52 years after 3 years of worsening bilateral tremor in her hands affecting her ability to hold objects such as a pen, cup, or eating utensils. Ms. Jones was prescribed propranolol to control her hand tremor; this medication helped reduce her hand tremor for improved function during daily living activities. However, her shaky voice continued to progressively worsen. Additional medical diagnoses include hypertension and seasonal allergies that are controlled by taking Allegra as needed.

Ms. Jones reported that she consumes 48 to 64 ounces of water daily in addition to 3 cups of decaffeinated coffee or a can of decaffeinated soda. She also reported consuming a nightly cocktail that reportedly improves her voice symptoms. Ms. Jones reported smoking 1 pack per day of cigarettes for 15 years, but she quit when she turned 30 years old. She sleeps an average of 5 hours nightly and uses Ambien twice weekly to help her sleep. She denied snoring and has not been told that she snores.

Social History. Ms. Jones was widowed 3 years ago and retired from teaching 8 years ago. She has 4 adult children all living nearby with whom she frequently interacts. Ms. Jones remains active in her church and volunteers to serve meals to the elderly in their homes through the local Meals on Wheels program.

Auditory-Perceptual Examination

The CAPE-V[24] was completed. Specific ratings of Ms. Jones's voice quality are shown in Table 6–5.

She was judged to exhibit a moderately severe amount of strain and vocal tremor during sustained phonation of /a/ and /i/. The vocal tremor was perceived as mild to moderate during sentence reading and conversation in addition to a mild degree of breathiness. Vocal tremor was noted as most evident during production of sentences or phrases loaded with voiced phonemes such as "We mow our lawn all year" or "Momma makes lemon jam." The overall severity of Ms. Jones's voice across all tasks was judged as moderately abnormal.

Laryngeal Imaging

A distal chip nasoendoscopic examination was completed to evaluate the sensorimotor function of the velopharynx, pharynx, base of tongue, and larynx.[1,2,33] Due to the possibility of dystonia, no topical anesthesia was used to minimize the impact of sensory tricks on signs of dystonia other than the presence of the scope.[1,2] Assessment of velopharyngeal function demonstrated normal valve function during speech and swallowing tasks. A low amplitude and fast frequency soft palate oscillation occurred during sustained phonation of /s/ and /f/. However, during sustained phonation of /a/, the soft palate exhibited a slower and moderately severe amplitude of vertical oscillation.

Views of the pharynx and larynx showed bilateral mobility of the vocal folds during sniffing and phonation tasks. In addition, tremor was observed in the base of tongue, bilateral pharynx, and larynx during both speech and quiet breathing tasks as follows.

During sustained phonation of /a/ and /i/ at comfortable pitch and loudness, a small amplitude oscillation of the base of the tongue occurred in the anterior-posterior direction. During these same tasks, the larynx exhibited mild to moderate adductory-abductory (ie, horizontal) oscillation of the arytenoid cartilages and vocal folds; this was also observed during quiet breathing associated with inspiratory respiratory cycles.

During sustained phonation of /a/ and /i/ across all pitch and loudness levels, mild rhythmic oscillatory constriction and relaxation of the bilateral pharyngeal walls occurred. During sustained phonation of /a/ and /i/ at comfortable pitch and loudness as well as comfortable pitch produced softly and at a low pitch, mild to moderate degrees of rhythmic horizontal oscillation of the vocal and ventricular folds occurred. During sustained phonation at high pitch, the vocal folds exhibited incomplete approximation along their length (considered normal) with increased approximation of the arytenoid cartilages that occluded views of the cartilaginous folds. Oscillation of the laryngeal structures was reduced during voicing at high pitches for both vowels. During sustained

244 Voice Therapy: Clinical Case Studies

Table 6–5. Pre- and Posttreatment Measures

Measure	Pretreatment	Posttreatment	Normal Values
Consensus Auditory-Perceptual Evaluation of Voice (CAPE-V)			
Overall Severity	55 mm (moderate)	23 mm (mild)	0
Roughness	25 mm (mild) vowels only	9 mm (mild) vowels only	0
Breathiness	24 mm (mild) sentences and conversation	24 mm (mild) sentences and conversation	0
Strain	55 mm (moderate) vowels only	14 mm (mild) vowels only	0
Pitch	0	0	0
Loudness	0	0	0
Vocal Tremor	52 mm (moderate) for vowels and 35 mm (mild to moderate) for sentences and conversation	35 mm (mild to moderate) for vowels and 15 mm (mild) for sentences and conversation	0
Resonance	Normal	Normal	Normal
Acoustic Measures			
Laryngeal Diadochokinetic Rate (syllables/sec)	4	4	4-7 syllables/sec
Average F0 During /a/	247 Hz	200 Hz	189 Hz (169-209 Hz)
	70 dB SPL	68 dB SPL	50-70 dB SPL
CPPs During Sustained /a/	10 dB	12 dB	11.7 + 1.8 dB
F0 During Rainbow Passage	194 Hz	204 Hz	155-334 Hz
F0 SD During Rainbow Passage	49 Hz	40 Hz	44 Hz
dB SPL During Rainbow Passage	66 dB	69 dB	50-70 dB SPL
CPPs During Rainbow Passage	6.5 dB	6.7 dB	6.6 + 1.2 dB

Table 6–5. *continued*

Measure	Pretreatment	Posttreatment	Normal Values
Maximum F0 Range	555 Hz (104-659 Hz)	690 Hz (105-795 Hz)	978 (131 (+16)-1109 (+189))
Maximum dB SPL Range	38 dB SPL (61-99 dB SPL)	40 dB SPL (59-99 dB SPL)	37 dB SPL (+3.67)
F0 Modulation Rate	8 Hz	8 Hz	0
F0 Modulation Extent	3%	2%	0
dB SPL Modulation Rate	6 Hz	6 Hz	0
dB SPL Modulation Extent	24%	20%	0
Articulation Rate (syllables/sec)	2.9	4.5	5
Aerodynamic Measures			
Average airflow	0.34 LPS	0.18 LPS	0.1-0.2 LPS
Average intraoral pressure	13 cmH_2O	11 cmH_2O	6.4 (+1.9) cmH_2O
Laryngeal resistance	38 cmH_2O /LPS	61 cmH_2O /LPS	29-47 cmH_2O /LPS
Voice Handicap Index (VHI)			
Total Score (out of 120)	107	42	<18
Functional Subscore (out of 40)	36	18	
Physical Subscore (out of 40)	31	11	
Emotional Subscore (out of 40)	40	13	

phonation of /a/ and /i/ at comfortable and low pitches, the vocal folds exhibited a mild degree of rhythmic lengthwise oscillation. During loud phonation of both vowels, severe oscillatory overclosure of the vocal folds occurred, associated with increased squeezing of the supraglottal structures resulting in voice stoppages.

A summary of tremor-based visual-perceptual ratings is displayed in Table 6–6. The summation of these observations demonstrated tremor involving all of the visible upper airway structures in addition to varied degrees of tremor affecting intrinsic and extrinsic laryngeal musculature. Horizontal vocal fold tremor appeared most prominent and severe,

Table 6–6. Visual-Perceptual Ratings of Tremor

Nasoendoscopy Task	Degree of Tremor by Structure and Task								
	Soft Palate			Pharynx			Vertical Larynx		
	Mild	Moderate	Severe	Mild	Moderate	Severe	Mild	Moderate	Severe
Sustained /a/ Comfortable Pitch/Loudness		X		X			X		
Sustained /a/ Comfortable Pitch, Loud				X					X
Sustained /a/ Comfortable Pitch, Soft				X					
Sustained /a/ High Pitch				X					
Sustained /a/ Low Pitch				X				X	
Sustained /i/ Comfortable Pitch/Loudness		X		X			X		
Sustained /i/ Comfortable Pitch, Loud				X					X
Sustained /i/ Comfortable Pitch, Soft				X					
Sustained /i/ High Pitch				X					
Sustained /i/ Low Pitch				X				X	
Connected Speech									
Sustained /s/ and /f/	X								
Quiet Breathing									

Nasoendoscopy Task	Vocal Folds: Horizontal			Vocal Folds: Lengthwise			Base of Tongue		
	Mild	Moderate	Severe	Mild	Moderate	Severe	Mild	Moderate	Severe
Sustained /a/ Comfortable Pitch/Loudness		X		X			X		
Sustained /a/ Comfortable Pitch, Loud			X						
Sustained /a/ Comfortable Pitch, Soft		X							
Sustained /a/ High Pitch	X								
Sustained /a/ Low Pitch		X		X					
Sustained /i/ Comfortable Pitch/Loudness		X		X			X		
Sustained /i/ Comfortable Pitch, Loud			X						
Sustained /i/ Comfortable Pitch, Soft		X							
Sustained /i/ High Pitch	X								
Sustained /i/ Low Pitch		X		X					
Connected Speech		X							
Sustained /s/ and /f/									
Quiet Breathing	X								

248 Voice Therapy: Clinical Case Studies

suggestive of adductory vocal fold musculature being most severely affected within the larynx.

Tracking of the fundamental frequency was slightly off during use of stroboscopic lighting, making it difficult to judge mucosal wave motion, particularly with oscillations of the laryngeal structures occurring during sustained phonation. Full approximation of the membranous vocal folds was observed to occur at comfortable pitch and loudness with a posterior gap between the cartilaginous folds at comfortable and low pitches. During quiet breathing, the medial edge of the vocal folds exhibited a slightly concave shape with prominent vocal processes suggestive of typical age-related vocal fold tissue changes.

A moderate to severe amount of anterior-posterior squeezing was observed throughout the examination. Articulatory rate during connected speech tasks was reduced during sentences loaded with voiced speech sounds associated with increased occurrence of vocal tremor and laryngeal oscillations.[55] In contrast, vocal tremor was not as perceptible during production of sentences loaded with voiceless speech sounds associated with absent laryngeal oscillation.[55]

Acoustic Measures

As shown in Table 6–5, Ms. Jones exhibited normal diadochokinetic testing[56,57] (repetition of a glottal stop paired with /a/ as quickly and completely as possible for 7 seconds), indicating adequate valve function of the larynx. During sustained phonation of /a/ (see Table 6–5), Ms. Jones exhibited a slightly elevated F0 for her age with slightly increased noise levels (ie, CPP measures).[58–60] Ms. Jones exhibited a reduced maximum F0 range, although maximum intensity range (dB SPL) was within normal limits.[61]

Measures of the nearly rhythmic modulation of F0 and SPL were completed on a representative 2-second duration midsegment of sustained phonation of /a/. As shown in

Table 6–5, the larger extent of voice modulation appeared related to SPL modulation compared to F0 modulation. In addition, articulation rate was measured[62,63] from the CAPE-V sentences and shown to be significantly slower (ie, 2.9 syllables/second) than normal (ie, 5 syllables/second). Prolongation of voiced speech sounds was perceived to occur associated with slower articulation rate.

Aerodynamic Measures

Airflow and intraoral pressures were obtained during the vowel portion and consonant portion, respectively, during repetition of /pi/ at comfortable pitch and loudness at approximately 1.5 syllables per second.[64] As shown in Table 6–5, Ms. Jones showed elevated average airflow and intraoral pressure values, resulting in normal laryngeal resistance.[65] Thus, the elevated intraoral pressure likely offset the elevated average airflow to provide a normal measure of laryngeal resistance.

Patient Self-Assessment

The Voice Handicap Index (VHI)[66] was administered to determine the degree of impact Ms. Jones's voice problem had on her daily life. Ms. Jones's scores on the VHI indicated severe impact of her voice problem across functional, physical, and emotional areas of her life (see Table 6–5).[67]

Impressions

Ms. Jones exhibited signs and symptoms consistent with a moderate vocal tremor due to essential tremor syndrome. Nasoendoscopy showed tremor affecting the soft palate, bilateral pharyngeal walls, base of tongue, and bilateral larynx. Ms. Jones was determined to be a good candidate for modification of voicing duration as a speaking strategy during voice therapy. This was determined based on the observation that tremor was observed to predominantly affect the larynx and that vocal tremor was less severely prominent during connected speech, particularly during production of sentences loaded with voiceless speech sounds. Further, Ms. Jones was shown to speak at a slower articulatory rate characterized by prolongation of voiced speech sounds.

Plan of Care

Speech Therapy Recommendation. Speech therapy was recommended with focus on reduction of voicing duration to "hide" vocal tremor[63,68,69] and easy voice onset to offload excessive laryngeal tension during speaking with secondary benefit of reducing tremor amplitude (ie, severity) in affected upper airway musculature to achieve the following short-term goals.

Goal #1. Ms. Jones will utilize increased expiratory effort and easy voice onset during speaking to reduce excessive levels of upper airway/laryngeal muscle activation and improve coordination of respiration with phonation.

Goal #2. Ms. Jones will speak with shorter voicing duration using a "staccato-like" voicing pattern in addition to inserting pauses intermittently rather than prolonging voicing to reduce the opportunity for listeners to perceive vocal tremor during conversation.

Frequency and Duration of Treatment. Ms. Jones was recommended to complete eight 1-hour weekly therapy sessions over the course of 2 months.

Long-Term Goal. Incorporate generalized speaking strategies using Ms. Jones's personalized prosodic style of speaking while maintaining utilization of the respiratory apparatus as the energy source for speech in addition to reduced voicing duration and pauses that reduce perception of vocal tremor. To evaluate successful generalization of therapy-based speaking strategies, Ms. Jones was scheduled to return for a follow-up session at 3 months following completion of therapy to determine the need for a refresher course of therapy.

Decision Making

Ms. Jones exhibits signs and symptoms consistent with vocal tremor that is most likely a clinical feature of her diagnosis of essential tremor syndrome.[12,70,71] Ms. Jones demonstrated lessening of the perception of vocal tremor during connected speech, in general, and during production of sentences loaded with voiceless speech sounds compared to voice-loaded speech sounds, resulting in the impression of a moderate vocal tremor severity.[55] Further, Ms. Jones exhibited a slowed articulation rate associated with prolongation of voiced speech sounds, giving opportunity to hear her vocal tremor.[72] Thus, training Ms. Jones to speak with shortened voicing duration and strategic use of pauses could reduce the opportunity for listeners to perceive her vocal tremor. In addition, Ms. Jones exhibited supraglottal squeezing indicative of increased laryngeal muscle activation during speaking, perhaps as a strategy for controlling the tremor perturbation during speaking. Thus, easy voice onset and increased utilization of the respiratory apparatus may reduce muscle activation levels contributing to supraglottic constriction; increased respiratory drive may also reduce or offload tension of the throat and articulatory muscles affected by tremor in the upper airway causing Ms. Jones's vocal tremor.[73]

While many people choose to use medical treatments for essential voice tremor, other patients choose not to use medical procedures or do not experience sufficient symptom improvement with treatments such as botulinum toxin injections, injection augmentation, or medications like propranolol. The literature documents that there is often a lack of improvement with these medical procedures and medications.[73] In this case, the author documents a comprehensive behavioral voice therapy treatment to reduce the symptoms of essential voice tremor.

Intervention

During sessions #1 and #2, the clinician first instructed Ms. Jones on tasks that facilitated improved use of the respiratory apparatus to drive voice production (Goal #1). This was achieved by instructing Ms. Jones to take a deep breath and then shush the clinician loudly (see Table 6–7, sessions #1 and #2). After repeating this activity accurately 3 times, Ms. Jones was instructed to try to sustain the /ʃ/ sound while alternatively making it loud twice during continued exhalation. Next, a voiced fricative was selected (either /v/ or /z/) to repeat the same pattern. Then, a series of easy voice onset tasks was used to facilitate airflow at speech initiation while practicing shortened production of voiced sounds (Goal #2) (see Table 6–7). At the end of the first session, Ms. Jones was instructed to use this technique to say, "Hi!" using a shortened voicing duration on a daily basis (Goal #2). (See Video 16 Shortened Voicing Duration for Vocal Tremor by Barkmeier-Kraemer.) Sessions #2 and #3 addressed Goal #1 by practicing increased use of airflow and expiratory musculature. This was achieved by using one of the tasks from the Casper-Stone Flow Phonation approach to encourage Ms. Jones to lose all of her air with low-effort speaking each time she says a number as she counts from 1 to 10. This can then be performed with 2 numbers spoken at a time (see Table 6–7, sessions #2 and #3). In addition, easy voice onset and shortened vowel duration were practiced during single- and 2-syllable words and then /h/-loaded phrases. For these sessions, Goal #2 was achieved by asking Ms. Jones to provide 3 daily phrases on which she could practice shortened voicing duration and pause insertion every day. During session #4, Ms. Jones expanded her application of Goals #1 and #2 using novel and increasingly more challenging speech stimuli with /h/-loaded words, phrases, and sentences. As Ms. Jones mastered /h/-loaded sentences, she began practicing transfer of shortened voicing duration and easy voice onset while speaking all-voiced single- and 2-syllable words. She also began to monitor her use of the strategies she learned during one 2-minute conversation daily to encourage transfer to conversation. Sessions #5 and #6 focused on practicing the same skills on progressively more difficult all-voiced words, phrases, and sentences and then on sentences with mixed types of speech sounds. She then began self-monitoring accuracy in using the shortened voicing duration and pause insertion during two 2- to 5-minute conversations. Sessions #7 and #8 added practice of strategies during paragraph reading and increasingly longer durations of self-monitoring during daily conversations to encourage transfer to daily communication situations. Finally, Ms. Jones was recorded during her accurate production of all-voiced tasks at the end of each session so that she could use her audio recording of the therapy exercises during daily practice. The clinician also gave her an exercise log with a summary of the exercises and a weekly chart to log her daily practice.

Therapy Outcomes

Posttherapy measures reported here were completed during the eighth therapy session.

Auditory-Perceptual Examination. The CAPE-V was readministered. As shown in Table 6–5, Ms. Jones showed a reduction in overall severity associated with reduced perception of vocal tremor during sentences and conversation contexts.

In addition, Ms. Jones exhibited reduction of strain and roughness during sustained phonation of vowels. Finally, Ms. Jones did not prolong voiced speech sounds associated with slowed articulation rate and enhanced perception of vocal tremor pretreatment.

Nasoendoscopic Imaging. The findings of the nasoendoscopic evaluation were similar to those observed pretreatment in the form of identifying the location and patterns of the structures exhibiting oscillation associated with production of vocal tremor. However,

Table 6–7. Voice Therapy Tasks by Session

Treatment Task	Method
Session #1	
Facilitation of Respiratory Drive During Speech: Voiceless	Take a deep breath and say /ʃ/ loudly as though shushing someone. Repeat this 3 times. Next, take a breath and sustain /ʃ/. As you sustain this sound, alternate making it loud and then soft by pushing harder with your breath 2 times during the exhale. (Caution: Correct production is characterized by continuous exhalation that is pulsed rather than stopping the airstream in between pulses.)
Facilitation of Respiratory Drive During Speech: Voiced	Take a deep breath and say /v/ or /z/ (pick the one that is easiest to say) loudly. Repeat this 3 times. Next, take a breath and sustain /v/ or /z/. As you sustain this sound, alternate making it loud and then soft by pushing harder with your breath 2 times during the exhale so that it sounds like a motor revving.
Easy Voice Onset During Single Syllables	Take a breath before you say each of the following sounds. As you say each sound, begin with an audible "h" sound followed by the vowel sound produced with the shortest possible duration. ("Huh," "Ha," "Hoe," "Who," "He," "Hey")
Easy Voice Onset During Single-Syllable Words	Take a breath and then say each of the following words using the same audible "h" sound as before, but use a staccato style of speaking to produce a shortened vowel and then the final speech sound. ("Heck," "Hook," "Hoop," "Hiss," "Hack," "Hope," "Hut," "Heat," "Hate")
Daily Phrase Activity	Each day, practice greeting others by saying, "Hi!" using an audible "h" sound and a shortened voiced portion as practiced on the exercises.
An exercise log sheet and audio recording were provided to Ms X to use during her home practice	Instructed to practice these exercises 2-3 times daily
Sessions #2 and #3	
Casper-Stone Flow Phonation	Take a deep breath and say the number "one." As you say this number, let all your air out so that you run out of air speaking this number. Take a breath and continue counting to 10 in this way. Do not rush or you may get dizzy. If this happens, stop and rest until you recover. After each number, ask yourself if you ran out of air and if saying the number felt easy. Repeat this task, counting 2 numbers on each breath using the same technique.

continues

251

Table 6–7. *continued*

Treatment Task	Method
Easy Voice Onset During Single-Syllable Words	Take a breath and then say each of the following words using the same audible "h" sound as before, but use a staccato style of speaking to produce a shortened vowel and then the final speech sound. ("Heck," "Hook," "Hoop," "Hiss," "Hack," "Hope," "Hut," "Heat," "Hate")
Progression of Shortened Voicing Duration During Multisyllabic Words	As you say these words, try to keep the voiced part short and say the word as quickly as is comfortable. ("Hippy," "Henhouse," "Hamstring," "Heater," "Hockey," "Hoosier," "Halftime," "Hopper," "Haughty," "Hometown," "Happy," "Hokey")
Progress to "h"-loaded Phrases	Use the same shortened voicing pattern with these phrases. Insertion of pauses may also help impose shortened voicing on these. ("Heat the home," "He hissed at her," "Hope he heals," "Happy hens," "Help his hiccups," "He's a hero," "Hit with her hammer," "Hess was hateful")
Daily Phrase Activity	Each day, Ms X will practice saying her self-selected daily phrases using shortened voicing duration every time she says: "Hi! How are you?" "Come in the house, Daisy!"
An exercise log sheet and audio recording were provided to Ms X to use during her home practice	Instructed to practice these exercises 2-3 times daily
Session #4	
Easy Voice Onset During Single-Syllable Words	Take a breath and then say each of the following words using the same audible "h" sound as before, but use a staccato style of speaking to produce a shortened vowel and then the final speech sound. ("Heck," "Hook," "Hoop," "Hiss," "Hack," "Hope," "Hut," "Heat," "Hate")
Progression of Shortened Voicing Duration During 2-Syllable Words	As you say these words, try to keep the voiced part short and say the word as quickly as is comfortable. ("Hippy," "Henhouse," "Hamstring," "Heater," "Hockey," "Hoosier," "Halftime," "Hopper," "Haughty," "Hometown," "Happy," "Hokey")
Progress to "h-loaded" Phrases	Use the same shortened voicing pattern with these phrases. Insertion of pauses may also help impose shortened voicing on these. ("Heat the home," "He hissed at her," "Hope he heals," "Happy hens," "Help his hiccups," "He's a hero," "Hit with her hammer," "Hess was hateful")

Table 6–7. *continued*

Treatment Task	Method
Progress to Sentences Loaded With Voiceless Speech Sounds	Continue practicing speaking with shortened voicing duration and pause insertion using these sentences. ("He took the pepper." "She cooked fish." "Ted sipped turtle stew." "Can she speak today?" "Take this cake for Sue." "Teach puppies to sit." "Feed corn and seeds to chickens." "Throw ten touchdowns.")
Shortened Voicing Duration With Voiced Words	Practice using easy voice onset and shortened voicing duration on single-syllable words with all-voiced speech sounds. ("And," "Man," "Arm," "Egg," "Made," "Noon," "Mole," "Lean," "Gone")
Expand to 2-Syllable All-Voiced Words	Practice using easy voice onset and shortened voicing duration on 2-syllable all-voiced words. ("Many," "Narrow," "Melon," "Ladle," "Gallon," "Arrow," "Needle," "Borrow," "Believe," "Wonder," "Redeem")
Daily Phrase Activity	Practice using shortened voicing duration on 3 self-selected daily phrases. Ms X chose: "May I try the coffee?" "Can I water the flowers?"
Self-Monitor During 1 Conversation	During 1 conversation during the day, purposefully use the voicing strategies for 2 minutes and monitor your success.
An exercise log sheet and audio recording were provided to Ms X to use during her home practice	Instructed to practice these exercises twice daily
Sessions #5 and #6	
Easy Voice Onset Practice With 2-Syllable Words	As you say these words, try to keep the voiced part short and say the word as quickly as is comfortable. ("Hippy," "Henhouse," "Hamstring," "Heater," "Hockey," "Hoosier," "Halftime," "Hopper," "Haughty," "Hometown," "Happy," "Hokey")
Practice Shortened Voicing Duration 2-Syllable All-Voiced Words	Practice using easy voice onset and shortened voicing duration on 2-syllable all-voiced words ("Many," "Narrow," "Melon," "Ladle," "Gallon," "Arrow," "Needle," "Borrow," "Believe," "Wonder," "Redeem")
Shortened Voicing Duration During All-Voiced Phrases and Sentences	Practice using easy voice onset and shortened voicing on these phrases and sentences. Insertion of pauses may also help shorten voicing. ("My mom knew Mary." "Were you really there?" "Randy made millions." "Danny whines all day." "Larry arose early." "Lenny drained the oil." "Running many more." "leading the way." "Mining the moon.")

continues

Table 6–7. *continued*

Treatment Task	Method
Practice Skills in Sentences With Mixed Speech Sounds	Practice using easy voice onset and shortened voicing on these sentences. ("What is the date today?" "When should I bring this?" "What assignment should be presented to the class?" "Susie makes gourmet ice cream and frosting." "Can I bring a dessert to the party?" "The boat hit the iceberg and sank." "The dog paced to and fro panting." "I would love some chocolate chip cookies." "My voice is strong and clear.")
Self-Monitor During 2 Conversations	During two conversations during the day, purposefully use the voicing strategies for 2-5 minutes and monitor your success.
An exercise log sheet and audio recording were provided to Ms X to use during her home practice	Instructed to practice these exercises 2-3 times daily

Sessions #7 and #8

Treatment Task	Method
Review Speaking Using Voiceless-Loaded Sentences	Continue practicing speaking with shortened voicing duration and pause insertion using these sentences. ("He took the pepper." "She cooked fish." "Ted sipped turtle stew." "Can she speak today?" "Take this cake for Sue." "Teach puppies to sit." "Feed corn and seeds to chickens." "Throw 10 touchdowns.")
Practice Skills in Sentences With Mixed Speech Sounds	Practice using easy voice onset and shortened voicing on these sentences. ("What is the date today?" "When should I bring this?" "What assignment should be presented to the class?" "Susie makes gourmet ice cream and frosting." "Can I bring a dessert to the party?" "The boat hit the iceberg and sank." "The dog paced to and fro panting." "I would love some chocolate chip cookies." "My voice is strong and clear.")
Paragraph Reading	Practice reading aloud using reduced voicing duration and pause insertion. Use a standard passage, a paragraph Ms X selects from a book she is reading, or the newspaper. During initial practice, it may be important to mark phrases where she should stop to replenish her air supply. She should gradually become more independent in self-evaluating her accuracy.
Self-Monitor During Two 5-Minute Conversations	During 2 conversations during the day, purposefully use the voicing strategies for 5 minutes and monitor your success. These can include telephone conversations as well. The clinician may surprise Ms X with a phone call during the week to determine how well she is doing outside of the therapy room.
An exercise log sheet and audio recording were provided to Ms X to use during her home practice	Instructed to practice these exercises 2-3 times daily at home

Ms. Jones exhibited significantly reduced supraglottic squeeze associated with phonation compared to pretreatment. Further, during sustained phonation at comfortable and low pitches and during loud phonation, Ms. Jones successfully used a breathier phonation that resulted in the absence of enhanced adductory/abductory (ie, horizontal) oscillation of the vocal folds, as seen pretreatment.

Acoustic Measures. As shown in Table 6–5, Ms. Jones was measured with a more typical F0 during sustained phonation of /a/ with less noise in her voice (higher CPP value). Interestingly, Ms. Jones showed an increased pitch range even though this was not a focus of treatment, and articulation rate increased to 4.5 syllables per second, which nears the typical rate of 5 syllables per second.

Aerodynamic Measures. As shown in Table 6–5, average airflow fell to more typical levels and intraoral pressure also dropped slightly. This resulted in a higher laryngeal resistance due to the elevated measure of intraoral peak pressure relative to average airflow.

Patient Self-Assessment. Ms. Jones's scores on the VHI reduced significantly, although they remained elevated, suggestive of a mild to moderate voice impairment. As shown in Table 6–5, Ms. Jones's scores continued to be spread across all domains, with a slightly higher functional subscore compared to physical and emotional scores. A therapeutic effect requires a change in score of 18 points or greater. Thus, a total score change of 65 points indicates a significant improvement.

Summary and Concluding Remarks

Voice therapy focused on training Ms. Jones to improve utilization of her respiratory apparatus to speak with increased airflow or use of expiratory respiratory muscles rather than squeezing at the larynx during voicing. In addition, she was encouraged to speak using a staccato-like method to learn the sensation of reduced voicing duration. Insertion of pauses was also helpful. Progression from easy-onset speech stimuli to gradually more complex speaking contexts enabled Ms. Jones to transfer the strategies for reducing the perception of vocal tremor to conversation level. Posttreatment scores demonstrated significant clinical gains associated with reduced strain and improved respiratory drive during speaking as well as more typical articulatory rate and reduced perception of vocal tremor during connected speech. During her 3-month posttreatment follow-up session, Ms. Jones showed continued generalization of speaking strategies in a way that she reported aligned well with her typical speaking style. Interestingly, she also reported that daily vocal warm-ups using some of the speech treatment exercises helped her implement speaking strategies each day. Ms. Jones was discharged from treatment and recommended to return if her vocal tremor worsened or if she required additional support implementing speaking strategies.

 CASE STUDY 6.5

Multimodality Voice Therapy for an Adult Classical Singer With Vocal Tremor

Kristen Bond

Voice Evaluation

Case History

Chief Complaint. Vocal fatigue, phonation breaks, "wide" vibrato

I had the pleasure of seeing this patient for a comprehensive voice and upper airway evaluation. The physician diagnosed the patient with dysphonia and vocal tremor.

History of Voice Complaint. The patient (LL) is a 54-year-old cisgender female pursuing evaluation due to voice difficulty beginning gradually approximately 5 years ago. She reports no singular event at the onset of this problem. Her complaints include progressive

256 Voice Therapy: Clinical Case Studies

vocal fatigue during the course of the day, most notably during and immediately following singing; "wide" vibrato; and difficulty with sustained phonation, including reduced phrase length in singing, delayed voicing onsets, and loss of upper range. She also notes vocal inconsistency characterized by phonation breaks and registration breaks in speech. Her singing teacher advised the patient that these issues were related to "lack of breath support" and recommended additional home practice; however, she also advised the patient to pursue further evaluation with an ENT to rule out pathology. Two years ago, the patient pursued diagnosis with an otolaryngologist, who visualized mild edema and erythema generalized in the laryngeal area. The physician diagnosed her symptoms as the result of LPR and advised her to "take a break" from singing. LL complied with modified voice rest for several weeks, including cessation of all singing and limited daily voice use, and began use of omeprazole. Although she described mild improvement for the rare heartburn she used to experience, LL did not experience relief of symptoms from her original voice complaint. LL reports her primary goal is increased ease and control in her singing voice.

Voice Use. LL is an avocational classical soprano and served as a church cantor for 15 years, but she has reduced her vocal load from weekly services to an average of 5 services a year. She cited that this change is a result of prior recommendations for modified vocal rest and LPR, as well as continued decline in vocal quality. She works as a marketing consultant with moderate vocal demand, including weekly hour-long presentations and dinner meetings with clients. She also volunteers 2 days a week at an animal shelter, which requires conversation with staff and adopters in a noisy environment.

Medical History. LL received a diagnosis of intention tremor in her hands 2 years ago but prefers not to take propranolol to control her symptoms. She recently became more con-

cerned about her hand tremor, as her mother had this, as well as a "shaky" voice for much of her adult life. LL has noticed that social drinking results in improvement in her hand tremor and increased vocal ease. She also has a known history of environmental allergies with subsequent sinus congestion and postnasal drip. LL continues to take 40 mg of omeprazole daily and does not report common reflux symptoms. LL is a lifelong nonsmoker. She drinks 4 to 6 cups of water daily as well as 2 cups of decaffeinated tea.

> There are several important medical findings in this paragraph. Presence of a hand tremor, family history of tremor, and being alcohol responsive (ie, her voice improves with drinking alcohol) are signs that are consistent with essential voice tremor.

Auditory-Perceptual Evaluation

The CAPE-V[24] was administered. The patient was determined to have an overall CAPE-V score of 31/100, indicating a dysphonia of a moderate nature. Aberrant features identified in the voice included primary mild-moderate but variable strain, secondary tremor, and intermittent onset delays that worsen with prolonged speech. Pitch was within normal limits for age and gender. The patient's resonance was focused in the epilaryngeal region, with auditory qualities reflective of tongue tension. Respiration appeared to be primarily abdominal-thoracic. Frequent breath holding was observed prior to voicing onset.

Quality-of-Life Impairment

1. VHI-10[27]: 11/40 (threshold = 11)[28]
2. Voice Catastrophization Index (VCI)[50]: 29/52
3. The Vocal Fatigue Index (VFI)[74]:
   a. Vocal tiredness and avoidance of activities: 23/44 (threshold = 27)
   b. Pain: 1/20 (threshold = 7)

c. Rest: 6/12 (higher scores indicate greater symptom improvement with rest)

Laryngeal Palpation

The paralaryngeal musculature was palpated to assess the presence of laryngeal tension, which was rated on a 1 to 5 scale (1 = perceptually typical muscle tone and flexibility, 5 = maximal constriction and immobility).

1. 3/5 at the thyrohyoid space with mild pain reported bilaterally
2. 3/5 at the base of the tongue (just superior to the body of the hyoid) with mild pain
3. Raised laryngeal position, as assessed by palpation of hyoid
4. 3/5 restriction of laryngeal flexibility to the left; 4/5 restriction with movement to the right; pain reported bilaterally

Laryngeal Imaging

LL was examined using a distal chip nasoendoscope to assess soft palate closure, vocal fold amplitude, mucosal wave, phase closure, symmetry, periodicity, vertical level, symmetry, robustness of abductory and adductory motion, and supraglottic activity. An intermittent, low-amplitude, and low-frequency oscillation was observed at the base of the tongue and in the pharyngeal walls on sustained vowels (/i/), which corresponded with auditory perception of vocal tremor. Intermittent phonation breaks occurred in coordination with observed vocal fold oscillation and glottic underclosure.

Acoustic Analysis and Aerodynamic Assessment

All data were gathered utilizing the Pentax Medical Computerized Speech Laboratory with Multi-Dimensional Voice Program 6600, Analysis of Dysphonia in Speech (ADSV), real-time pitch analysis, and Phonatory Aerodynamic System (Pentax Medical, Montvale, NJ). Norms utilized represent

information from Awan et al (2016),[75] Patel et al (2018),[33] and Shao et al (2010).[76] A headset microphone (Audio-Technica ATM 73-a) was placed at a 45-degree angle at 2 cm from the mouth for data acquisition. Results of the assessment are presented in Table 6–8.

Stimulability Testing

Trial therapy was conducted with considerations for patient goals, as well as expected outcomes from behavioral modifications alone on vocal tremor. Given the patient-stated goals to reduce sensation of fatigue and to increase phrase length in singing, LL was trialed with several vocal "unloading" tasks with the understanding that these techniques may make the tremor initially more apparent to an outside listener.

> The author aptly points out that people with vocal tremor often use compensatory muscle tension to stabilize the vocal mechanism in an effort to make the vocal tremor less audible.

LL first performed lip trills to evaluate the perceptual effect of improved flow and reduced glottic press on sustained phonation. She described increased ease of production in both sustained modal phonation and glides throughout the phonatory range, and the sound of the lip vibration impeded the perception of tremor. She transitioned from lip trills to an orally resonant /u/ with cueing for lightly breathy onset in both modal phonation and inflection glides. While tremor was more apparent in single-phoneme productions, she again described a reduced level of effort to achieve sustained phonation. Carryover of breathy quality into segments from sacred songs resulted in moderately improved vocal flexibility and improved patient comfort.

The clinician performed circumlaryngeal massage, which targeted the tongue, thyrohyoid space, and lateral laryngeal flexibility.

Table 6–8. Pretreatment and Posttreatment Measurements: Acoustic and Aerodynamic

	% Jitter	% Shimmer	ATRI %	FTRI %	Fatr (Hz)	Fftr (Hz)	D2
Normative Data	0.483, SD 0.209	1.045, SD 0.040	0.417, SD 1.005	0.157, SD 0.25	1.106, SD 2.338	1.154, SD 1.46	1.575, SD 0.275
Pretreatment	0.98	2.143	3.312	2.487	4.12	3.18	2.875
Posttreatment	0.695	2.012	2.128	1.895	4.36	3.01	2.974

	Mean Flow Rate, Sustained Vowel (L/sec)	Subglottic Pressure (Psub) on Modal Sustained Vowel /a/ (cmH$_2$O)
Normative Data	0.11, SD 0.05	6.91 cmH$_2$O, SD 1.69
Pretreatment	0.09	8.98
Posttreatment	0.14	7.23

Following approximately 10 minutes of clinician-performed massage, the patient described an "open" sensation in speech and recognized further improved oral resonance.

Impressions

The patient presents with a moderate dysphonia characterized by strain and pitch oscillation with sustained phonation, diagnosed as vocal tremor with secondary MTD in com-

> When participating in the shared decision-making process, it is incumbent on the clinician to provide all treatment options. In this case, the clinician informed the patient of medical management options including botulinum toxin injections and propranolol. However, many patients choose not to use either of these treatments. Especially in singers, botulinum toxin injections can result in other secondary effects that make singing more difficult. This singer elected for more conservative management via voice therapy.

pensation. She describes improvement in perceptual effort with voicing after trial therapy and has enthusiasm for behavioral treatment.

Plan of Care

Treatment is recommended. The patient appears to be a good candidate for voice therapy considering the impact of voice on social demands and motivation to improve. Therapy will be conducted for 4 to 6 sessions of 45 to 60 minutes each, 4 times monthly. Reevaluation will occur after 90 days or with any change in status.

The long-term goal is to restore functional voice, including reducing vocal fatigue and perceptual effort, for daily occupational, social, and emotional needs. Long-term goals include improved perceptual vocal effort in speech and singing tasks, as well as further reduced laryngeal tension with use of circumlaryngeal massage. If, after vocal unloading, the patient feels that the tremor is more audible than she is comfortable with, she agreed to revisit trials for propranolol or botulinum toxin injection with the physician.

The patient's short-term goals include:

1. LL will reduce subglottic pressure through semi-occluded vocal tract postures to achieve increased vocal efficiency throughout her vocal range.
2. LL will use easy onsets to reduce glottic hyperfunction and resulting vocal fatigue.
3. LL will perform circumlaryngeal massage to achieve reduced paralaryngeal engagement to increase oral resonance and reduce phonatory effort.

Decision Making

LL's primary complaint is vocal strain characterized by significant supraglottic, glottic, and paralaryngeal hyperfunction. Because vocal tremor is involuntary, therapy is not intended to eliminate the presence of tremor, but to increase patient comfort by reducing compensatory behaviors. Trial therapy indicated patient stimulability for increased phrase length and perception of reduced effort, facilitated by increased flow and decreased hyperfunction. The perceptual similarity between the rate of LL's vocal tremor and classical singing vibrato, approximately 1.5 semitones, is comparable to the findings in previous studies examining the frequency magnitude of operatic singing vibrato.[77]

Intervention

Session #1. Short-term goal: Reduce subglottic pressure through use of semi-occluded vocal tract postures throughout the phonatory range. LL was first guided to raise awareness of the sensation of free airflow with trials for a variety of semi-occluded postures, including straw phonation in water, lip trills, and tongue trills. She described an "easier, open" sensation during lip trills in modal phonation. She achieved modal phonation and pitch glides with low perceptual effort using lip trills initially performed from A3 to D5. Tremor was initially difficult to discern due to her stabilizing moderate paralaryngeal engagement. Maximum phonation time and tonal consistency were gradually increased, with cueing for "even flow" throughout phonation, as the patient initially demonstrated a tendency to increase strain at range extremities. Clinician modeling to increase speed of range extension during trills, paired with movement (gentle arm swing), promoted reduced effort and increased range (glides achieved from F3 to A5).

Semi-occluded postures were transitioned to /u/, during which vocal tremor was more audible. The clinician counseled LL regarding the trade-off between reduced strain and increased perception of tremor in sustained phonation. Due to LL's stated priorities for greater vocal ease and mild severity of the tremor, she agreed to continue to pursue therapeutic intervention. Following clinician modeling for easy onset, she demonstrated easy-onset /u/, which was then contrasted with glottal onset in single phonemes and short phrases in modal registration. Perception of tremor was mildly reduced with easy onset, and LL independently described the sensation of increased forward resonance, noting a "buzz" in her mouth and forehead. (See Video 17 Contrasting Glottic Onset Types by Bond.)

Session #2. All short-term goals were addressed this session, including use of easy onsets and semi-occluded vocal tract postures to decrease glottic hyperfunction and resulting vocal fatigue, as well as use of circumlaryngeal massage to reduce paralaryngeal engagement. LL began by demonstrating easy onsets in single words and short phrases, followed by negative practice between glottic and breathy onset. The clinician observed significant strain in the patient's vocal quality and proceeded to laryngeal palpation to evaluate the presence of paralaryngeal muscular engagement. LL demonstrated significant tension at the thyrohyoid space (rated 5/5, with 5 = significantly altered muscular resistance to touch). The thyroid cartilage approximated the hyoid bone, and her larynx was significantly elevated. LL reported pain with light touch to each of these areas. The clinician performed circumlaryngeal massage to achieve improved thyrohyoid space with gentle downward sweeping motions along the length of the muscle, as well as a gentle lowering of the thyroid cartilage using light pressure on the superior edge, just lateral to the anterior notch. LL described an "open" feeling in her throat following this intervention, and she was then instructed in each technique to practice twice daily at home for approximately 10 minutes total per day.

Return to easy onsets at the phoneme and phrase level demonstrated improvement in perceptual vocal strain, with dual increase in oral resonance and perception of tremor. Easy onsets were scaffolded into oral reading with paragraphs loaded with initial vowels, with patient-reported increase in sensation of an "open voice." Additionally, the patient and clinician collected a list of phrases within the patient's current church music repertoire containing opportunities for easy onset, to be practiced daily in oral reading. The clinician instructed her to continue use of lip trills during her daily singing warm-up routine, as used in her first session.

Session #3. All short-term goals were addressed this session (use of easy onsets, semi-occluded vocal tract postures, and circumlaryngeal massage). LL initiated the session by demonstrating easy onsets as practiced in her functional phrases and oral reading homework, with guided negative practice to further establish kinesthetic awareness for "extremes" in sensation between full glottal onset and breathy onset. She then demonstrated lip trills and sustained /u/ in modal register and pitch glides across registers, as instructed previously, with evenness of flow maintained from her initial therapy session. She continued to show increased strain in upper range extension at the passaggio (G#4), leading to use of palpation for muscular ten-

sion. LL demonstrated tension at the thyrohyoid space (rated 3/5, showing improvement from the last therapy session) and mildly elevated laryngeal position. LL demonstrated circumlaryngeal massage techniques independently, as used in her home practice, including gentle, downward sweeping motions from the thyrohyoid space and a gentle lowering of the thyroid cartilage. The patient again described the sensation of tension relief and then demonstrated lip trills above G#4 with perceptually improved access to head-voice registration as well as patient-reported increase in phonatory ease. Audible tremor was increased with this release, but it was perceptually similar to vibrato, and the patient was pleased with the perceptual change from a "belt" quality to a classical voice approach to upper range with head-voice quality.

> The author skillfully illustrates how to work with the patient not to eliminate vocal tremor, which is not possible through voice therapy, but rather to help audibly connect the tremor to the patient's vibrato such that the listener does not recognize it as aberrant.

The patient then demonstrated scaleform tasks with easy-onset /u/ on scale degrees 1-3-5-3-1 from A3 to A5, with increased oral opening with vowels D5 and above, to reduce patient perception of vocal effort and to optimize acoustic parameters. LL carried over previously created easy-onset phrases into scaleform tasks (eg, "Alleluia") and performed throughout her phonatory range. These tasks were alternated with lip trills matching the same scaleform pattern to promote improved flow. The clinician provided her with written notation for tasks created during this session for home use.

Session #4. Easy onsets and semi-occluded postures were applied in this patient session. LL described improved vocal endurance and length of sustained phonation during home practice and during the week's church service. She initially performed lip trills using pitch glides throughout her range, followed by an /u/ glide with easy onset and increased flow. The patient transferred easy onsets and flow into a current performance piece she is preparing for her parish, with observed improvement in access to upper range, consistency of tonal quality, and increased phrase length (having stated, "I couldn't get through this phrase last month—now I think I could have kept going"). The presence of tremor mildly impacted the consistency of sudden registration shifts; however, it was perceptually similar to vibrato, and the patient implemented increased flow and was intermittently perceptible during generated conversation.

Therapy Outcomes

Auditory-Perceptual Evaluation and Patient Self-Assessment. The CAPE-V, VHI-10, VCI, and VFI were readministered to assess patient perception of treatment impact. LL's CAPE-V score was 25/100, exhibiting a continued mild impairment in vocal quality and reflecting reduction in strain (mild, intermittent). She scored 7/40 on the VHI-10 (score previously 11/40), 13/52 on the VCI (previously 29/52), and 12/44 on the Vocal Tiredness and Avoidance subscale of the VFI (previously 23/44).

Acoustic and Aerodynamic Assessment. Acoustic measures indicated a mild reduction in vocal noise, with little change to measurements of the amplitude of vocal tremor. Reduction in glottic hyperfunction resulted in increased mean flow rate and reduced subglottic pressure (see Table 6–8).

Summary and Concluding Remarks

LL presented with a mild essential voice tremor resulting in strain and vocal effort, particularly in sustained phonation. Considering her response to tension reduction through circumlaryngeal massage and improved vocal consistency through increased coordination of airflow on voicing, LL elected to undergo 4 therapy sessions to trial her response to these interventions for improved voice comfort rather than other treatment modalities such as the use of botulinum toxin injections or medications. LL experienced improvements in fatigue and in oral resonance across her conversational and singing voice using these techniques. Voice therapy focused on improving respiratory coordination to voicing onset to reduce hyperfunctional compensation at the level of the larynx. This was achieved with a progressive introduction of high-flow phonatory activities such as lip trills to carry over into semi-occluded postures with easy onsets. LL's exit scores indicated both patient-perceived improvement and instrumental measures showing improved voicing coordination.

 CASE STUDY 6.6

The SLP's Role in Deep Brain Stimulation for Vocal Tremor

Elizabeth DiRenzo

Voice Evaluation

Case History

Chief Complaint. Shaky voice, vocal fatigue

I had the pleasure of seeing this patient for a comprehensive voice and upper airway evaluation. The patient was referred to the SLP by neurology and neurosurgery. The patient was diagnosed with essential tremor of the head and neck with concern for onset of concurrent essential vocal tremor (EVT).

History of Voice Complaint. Patient RE is a 70-year-old cisgender male. The patient reports a 30-year history of head and neck tremor. He was formally diagnosed by a neurologist with essential tremor 25 years ago. Initially, the head tremor was not severe and did not impair his ability to function in any significant way. However, it has significantly worsened over time, particularly in the past 10 years. At times, he requires a neck brace to assist in holding his neck steady. He also reports that he must hold his chin to drink and rest his head on his hand to read. In addition, the patient reports a gradual onset of voice changes starting about 5 years ago that have also worsened over time. There was no specific inciting event. Current voice symptoms include increased vocal effort and vocal fatigue and an overall decline in voice quality. Voice reportedly sounds tremulous and shaky and worsens with generalized fatigue and during stressful situations. He often avoids talking on the phone. The patient has not received the services of an SLP for this problem. The patient does not have any additional relevant medical comorbidities and does not currently take any prescription medications. He has previously trialed several medications, including propranolol, primidone, and Klonopin, to treat his essential tremor without significant benefit in extremity tremor or voice. However, the patient does feel that alcohol helps reduce the severity of his tremor symptoms in both his head and voice. The patient was recently evaluated by neurology and neurosurgery and was felt to be a potential candidate for DBS therapy to treat his debilitating, medication-refractory essential tremor.

Voice Use. The patient retired 3 years ago from teaching middle school. The progression of the head tremor and voice changes influenced his decision to retire. The patient is still socially active. He regularly plays guitar with friends and surfs. He and his wife have a 25-year-old daughter. He will sometimes avoid speaking to friends and family because of his voice changes.

Laryngeal Imaging

Laryngeal videostroboscopy was performed in conjunction with laryngology. The evaluation was conducted transnasally with a flexible distal chip videolaryngoscope. There was mild periarytenoid and postcricoid edema and erythema. There was normal mobility of the arytenoids with full range of motion. The true vocal fold edges were smooth bilaterally. There were no mucosal lesions or masses seen. On stroboscopy, there was phase asymmetry with complete glottic closure on modal phonation. The mucosal wave was intact. There was mild supraglottal hyperfunction with primarily mediolateral compression.

Given the patient's history of essential tremor, specific information regarding the oscillatory movement of the muscles of the vocal tract and larynx was also collected. The vocal tract and larynx were viewed while breathing at rest and during sustained voicing of /i/ at a comfortable pitch and loudness. A validated scale, the Vocal Tremor Scoring System (VTSS), was used to grade the oscillatory movement of the muscles of the vocal tract and larynx.[44] Tremor severity was graded on a 0 to 3 scale where 0 = absent, 1 = mild, 2 = moderate, and 3 = severe. EVT was graded in the following anatomic sites: palate, base of tongue (BOT), pharyngeal walls (PW), larynx global (LG), supraglottis (SG), and true vocal folds (TVF). Results are presented in Table 6–9.

Quality-of-Life Impairment

The VHI-10 was administered.[27] The patient scored 20/40, with a score greater than 11 indicative of impairment.[28]

Auditory-Perceptual Assessment

The CAPE-V was administered.[24] The patient was determined to have an overall CAPE-V score of 47/100, indicating a dysphonia of a moderate nature. Aberrant perceptual features

Table 6–9. Vocal Tremor Scoring System (VTSS) Results

VTSS Rating					
Palate	BOT	PW	LG	SG	TVF
2	1	2	2	3	3

identified in the voice included primary shakiness and secondary strain. Overall vocal pitch and loudness were noted to be within normal limits. However, there were perceived rhythmic fluctuations in vocal pitch and loudness, most obviously during sustained vowel phonation. Fluctuations were perceived also during sentence production, but were less notable than on sustained vowels, particularly during voiceless-loaded sentences. Resonance was focused in the laryngeal region. Respiration was primarily abdominal.

Acoustic Assessment

All data were gathered using Computerized Speech Lab (CSL˜; Pentax Medical, Montvale, NJ) software and hardware in a sound-treated room. Instrumental Assessment of Vocal Function (IVAP) protocols[33] were utilized to collect a subset of acoustic measures using the Multidimensional Voice Profile (MDVP) and Analysis of Dysphonia in Speech and Voice (ADSV) software. To obtain voice samples, a head-worn, unidirectional microphone was placed over the patient's ears and at 6 cm from the patient's mouth. He was then asked to sustain the vowel /a/ at a comfortable pitch and loudness for approximately 5 seconds. A middle 2-second portion of the vowel was utilized for analysis. Results of the assessment are provided in Table 6–10. Normative data were obtained from studies by Xue and Deliyski (2001)[78] and Murton et al (2020).[79]

EVT is characterized by rhythmic modulations in F0 and intensity during sustained vowel phonation. Consequently, the Praat Speech Analysis program (University of Amsterdam) was also utilized to measure rate and magnitude, or extent, of F0 and intensity modulations.[55] The rate of F0 and intensity modulations in Hz was determined by counting the total number of cycles of modulation over 1 second. The total number of cycles was then averaged across two, 1-second intervals. The extent of F0 and intensity was determined by measuring the maximum and minimum F0 and intensity for each cycle of modulation across 2 seconds. The range of modulation was divided by the sum of the minimum and maximum values and then multiplied by 100 to obtain percent modulation. Results of the assessment are presented in Table 6–11.

Table 6–10. Acoustic Assessment Results

Sustained /a/ Assessment					
Average F0 (Hz)		SD F0 (Hz)		Jitter (%)	
Value	Norm	Value	Norm	Value	Norm
89.4	127.6 ± 29.18	3.2	3.12 ± 1.56	2.6	2.10 ± 1.56
Shimmer (dB)		NHR		CPP (dB)	
Value	Norm	Value	Norm	Value	Norm
0.5	0.49 ± 0.31	0.1	0.18 ± 0.08	10.20*	11.46

Normative data obtained from Xue SA, Deliyski D. Effects of aging on selected acoustic voice parameters: Preliminary normative data and educational implications. *Educ Gerontol.* 2001;27:159-163; Murton O, Hillman R, Mehta D. Cepstral peak prominence for clinical voice evaluation. *Am J Speech Lang Pathol.* 2020;29:1596-1607. *indicates abnormal value.

Table 6–11. F0 and Intensity EVT Modulation

Sustained /a/ Assessment			
F0 Modulation		Intensity Modulation	
Rate (Hz)	Extent (%)	Rate (Hz)	Extent (%)
4.5	5.6	4.5	33.8

Stimulability

The clinician targeted easy voice onset to facilitate reduced effort during voicing, anterior voice focus to improve resonance and projection, and increased articulation rate to reduce the duration of voicing segments and diminish overall perception of shakiness. The patient was mildly stimulable for improvement in voice symptoms. Specifically, he noted an increase in ease of phonation, but not a significant reduction in perception of EVT.

Impressions

The patient presents with a moderate-severe dysphonia secondary to EVT. Moderate to severe oscillations were observed in the palate, pharyngeal walls, larynx global, supraglottis, and true vocal folds. Acoustic analysis revealed reduced CPP. Typical EVT occurs at a rate of 4 to 8 Hz. Today, the patient's rate of F0 and intensity modulations was 4.5 Hz with greater extent of intensity modulation as compared to F0 modulation. Perceptually, the patient presents with a primarily shaky voice with some mild secondary strain. The patient is highly motivated to improve his voice quality.

Plan of Care

The patient is scheduled to undergo bilateral DBS of the ventral intermediate nucleus (Vim) to treat the debilitating and medication-refractory essential tremor of the head and neck. Vim stimulation immediately suppresses essential tremor symptoms. DBS of the Vim may also be beneficial for treating EVT. Consequently, the clinician plans to reassess the voice approximately 2 to 3 months following surgery. The clinician will also reevaluate further stimulability testing and recommendations for formal voice therapy at that time.

Decision Making

Essential tremor can affect the structures of the larynx and vocal tract. It is estimated that 25% of individuals with essential tremor have a co-occurring EVT. In EVT, oscillations of the muscles of the larynx and vocal tract result in alterations in vocal pitch and loudness. Perception of changes in pitch and loudness correlate with acoustic modulations of F0 and intensity, respectively. Patients with EVT experience reduced speech intelligibility and significant social embarrassment due to their tremulous voice. There are no curative treatments for EVT. In fact, EVT is considered one of the most difficult-to-treat voice disorders. EVT has been treated with injections of botulinum toxin to the thyroarytenoid muscle of the vocal folds. However, for this patient, oscillations were not isolated only to the vocal folds. Moderate to severe oscillations were present in other areas of the larynx and vocal tract including the palate, base of tongue, larynx globally, and supraglottis, thus likely reducing the effectiveness of this treatment for this patient. In addition, inconsistent improvements in EVT are observed with pharmacotherapy, including the classes of medications trialed by this patient. The patient also did not receive significant benefit from medications for either his head or voice tremor. There is some evidence that voice therapy can be beneficial for a subset of patients with EVT. This involves teaching the patient modified speech patterns to reduce the perception of EVT.[63] The patient was trialed with some of these strategies, and while he noted improvement in vocal ease, there were no significant perceptual improvements. This was likely due, in part, to the overall high severity of his EVT. However, since a full course of voice therapy was also not completed, it is difficult to determine the overall impact of behavioral treatment for this patient.

DBS is a nondestructive neurosurgical treatment for essential tremor and involves the placement and stimulation of electrodes into one or both sides of the basal ganglia of the brain. There is an emerging body of literature that DBS of the Vim is beneficial for treating EVT.[80–82] This includes a decrease in the perception of EVT but also objective reductions in the rate and extent of frequency and intensity modulations. However, stimulation-induced side effects, including dysarthria, are also common. Specific deleterious speech effects may include reduced voicing and imprecise oral articulation during the production of consonants and vowels.[83] Consequently, speech production following DBS should be monitored. Given the patient had elected to undergo DBS to treat his head and neck tremor, the clinician elected to defer a formal trial of voice therapy and instead reassess voice following DBS surgery. Postoperative outcomes and treatment efficacy also rely on other factors, including postoperative DBS programming. The programming process takes more than 1 visit over a period of weeks or months to ensure optimal stimulation settings and symptom relief. Consequently, the clinician elected to wait until after programming to reassess the voice. In addition, the treatment team wanted to monitor for any DBS-induced dysarthria. When making decisions for these patients, it is important to acknowledge that, unlike essential tremor, DBS is currently not a standard of care for EVT. The primary purpose of DBS for patients with EVT is to treat tremor of the extremities, not voice. As a result, EVT reduction is not the primary focus when choosing chronic implant positions of DBS electrodes and during programming. It is currently unknown whether specific electrode locations and programming parameters optimize EVT outcomes.

Intervention

The patient underwent awake, computer robot-assisted image-guided placement of DBS electrodes into the thalamic nucleus bilaterally by a frameless approach, with intraoperative electrophysiology and fluoroscopy in conjunction with neurosurgery and neurology. DBS programming sessions were completed with neurology following surgery at approximately 2, 4, and 10 weeks. Voice was reassessed 12 weeks following surgery. The patient states that he has recovered well from surgery without complications. In terms of his symptoms, he reports that his head and neck tremor is nearly eliminated. He also notes the shakiness in the voice has dramatically improved. Specifically, he is no longer limiting his voice use or avoiding specific communicative situations (eg, telephone calls). Comprehensive voice assessment was repeated to assess for improvements in EVT. Results are as follows.

Laryngeal Imaging

Repeat laryngeal videostroboscopy was completed. The VTSS revealed reductions in the severity of oscillations at all evaluated sites; specifically, there were mild oscillations in the pharyngeal walls and no detectable oscillations in the palate, BOT, LG, SG, and TVF (Table 6–12).

Quality-of-Life Impairment

The VHI-10 score was 5/40 (threshold = 11). This is a 15-point reduction from the initial assessment.

266 Voice Therapy: Clinical Case Studies

Table 6–12. VTSS Results Post-DBS Surgery

VTSS Rating					
Palate	BOT	PW	LG	SG	TVF
0 (–2)	0 (–1)	1 (–1)	0 (–2)	0 (–3)	0 (–3)

Parentheses indicate +/– changes from initial assessment

Auditory-Perceptual Assessment

The patient was determined to have an overall CAPE-V score of 5/100, indicating a dysphonia of a mild nature. This is a 42-point reduction from the initial assessment. The perceptual feature of shakiness was substantially reduced from the initial evaluation, with minimal perceived rhythmic fluctuations in vocal pitch and loudness during sustained vowel phonation. No detectable fluctuations were appreciated during sentence production. There was minimal perceivable strain. Resonance was forward focused.

Acoustic Assessment

Acoustic assessment using MDVP and ADSV software revealed reductions in SD F0, jitter, and shimmer. However, these values were within normal range at initial assessment for the aged male voice. CPP increased and no longer meets a pathologic threshold (Table 6–13). EVT was still detected acoustically. However, there was a substantial reduction in the rate and extent of F0 and intensity modulations (Table 6–14).

Impressions

The patient presents with a mild dysphonia secondary to EVT. Overall, substantial improvements in multiple parameters of EVT are appreciated following DBS surgery. Specifically, only mild oscillations were observed in the pharyngeal walls. CPP is now within normal range. Although EVT could still be detected acoustically, the rate and extent of F0 and intensity modulations were also reduced.

Only very mild shakiness was perceived during sustained vowel phonation. No significant vocal handicap was reported. Informal observations of speech did not reveal evidence of dysarthria, including reduced voicing or imprecise articulation. The patient is extremely pleased with the improvements in his symptoms and reports that his voice is "normal." The clinician determined that no further voice therapy is needed at this time. Of note, the long-term efficacy of DBS for tremor may decrease over time secondary to patient-developed stimulation tolerances. Consequently, the clinician recommends voice reassessment in 6 to 9 months or sooner if voice symptoms worsen.

Summary and Concluding Remarks

For patients with essential limb tremor not responsive to medication, surgical therapies are standard of care and can abolish severe tremor. DBS is a nondestructive neurosurgical treatment for essential limb tremor. There is emerging evidence that DBS may also be beneficial for treating EVT. In current standards of practice, treating EVT is not the primary goal of DBS surgery. In this patient, the primary purpose of DBS was to treat medication-refractory limb tremor; therefore, EVT was not considered when chronic implant position for the deep brain stimulating electrode was chosen. However, DBS was beneficial for treating EVT in this patient. The optimal target for EVT might be slightly different from the target for limb tremor. It is also important to remem-

Table 6–13. Acoustic Assessment Post-DBS Surgery

Sustained /a/ Assessment					
Average F0 (Hz)		SD F0 (Hz)		Jitter (%)	
Value	Norm	Value	Norm	Value	Norm
91.6 (±2.2)	127.6 ± 29.18	1.3 (−1.9)	3.12 ± 1.56	0.8 (−1.8)	2.10 ± 1.56
Shimmer (dB)		NHR		CPP (dB)	
Value	Norm	Value	Norm	Value	Norm
0.2 (−0.3)	0.49 ± 0.31	0.1 (0)	0.18 ± 0.08	14.0 (±3.8)	11.46

Parentheses indicate +/− changes from initial assessment

Table 6–14. F0 and Intensity EVT Modulation Post-DBS Surgery

Sustained /a/ Assessment			
F0 Modulation		Intensity Modulation	
Rate (Hz)	Extent (%)	Rate (Hz)	Extent (%)
3 (−1.5)	1.1 (−4.5)	3 (−1.5)	4.3 (−29.5)

Parentheses indicate +/− changes from initial assessment

ber that there are reports of adverse speech effects with DBS implantation. Stimulation-induced dysarthria is a potential side effect of DBS treatment. Consequently, speech should be monitored postoperatively in these patients. Finally, it is of note that EVT was reduced but not eliminated following DBS treatment. This patient was pleased with his progress and did not elect to pursue postoperative voice therapy. However, this highlights that many patients may be candidates for postoperative voice therapy to maximize voice outcomes following DBS surgery. Patients should be considered for voice therapy following DBS if there is a need to further diminish perception of EVT and improve ease of phonation.

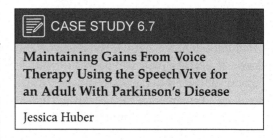

CASE STUDY 6.7

Maintaining Gains From Voice Therapy Using the SpeechVive for an Adult With Parkinson's Disease

Jessica Huber

Voice Evaluation

Case History

Chief Complaint. Reduced loudness, weak/breathy voice, disfluencies, difficulty being understood

Patient SM was referred for a comprehensive voice and upper airway evaluation by his otolaryngologist. The patient was diagnosed with dysphonia associated with hypokinetic dysarthria and Parkinson's disease.

History of Voice Complaint. Patient SM is a 68-year-old cisgender man who was diagnosed 1.5 years ago with Parkinson's disease (PD). His first symptoms of the disease were voice related and included reduced loudness and breathiness. The onset of his voice symptoms was about 2 years before diagnosis, and the process in receiving a diagnosis was difficult. The patient retired 6 months ago from his job as a sales manager for an agricultural equipment company. His voice issues significantly interfered with his ability to continue to meet the requirements of his job. Changes to motor control and cognition resulted in SM surrendering his license to drive. Current voice symptoms include reduced loudness, increased vocal effort, breathiness, and monotonicity. He reports no pain in the laryngeal area or neck and no choking or difficulty swallowing. The patient saw an SLP when he was diagnosed and underwent a course of speech treatment using the Lee Silverman Voice Treatment Program (LSVT-LOUD).[84] The patient and spouse both reported that the patient did well with LSVT-LOUD in the treatment room with the therapist but struggled to carry the louder voice over into everyday communication environments, including at his job. He continues to complete the LSVT-LOUD exercises several days a week. The patient reports no medical comorbidities. He takes pramipexole 3 times per day and amantadine twice a day to control his Parkinson's disease symptoms. He reports no change to his voice or communication with these medications.

Voice Use. The patient reports that voice use is rather minimal, especially during the day when his wife is at work. During the day, he is usually at home since his Parkinson's disease has impaired his ability to drive. When his wife returns home from work, they chat during the evening. He sees family and friends occasionally over the weekends. His wife reports that he initiates conversations less often and responds to questions with less information than he used to. The patient reports that his communication is frustrating since he often has to repeat what he says.

Laryngeal Imaging

The otolaryngologist performed laryngeal videostroboscopy transorally with a rigid videolaryngoscope. No lesions were present. Full abduction and adduction of vocal folds was present, but moderately reduced glottal closure was noted, consistent with vocal fold bowing often present in PD. Moderate supraglottal squeezing in the anterior-posterior dimension was present, but no false fold hyperfunction.

Vocal Effort, Fatigue, and Pain

The patient reports that his voice tires when he is socializing on the weekends. He does not notice any fatigue on weeknights when conversing with just his wife. Talking in loud environments is very difficult and tiring. He reports feeling like he has to "push" his voice to produce audible speech.

Quality-of-Life Impairment

The Communicative Participation Item Bank–Brief[85] was administered to determine effects of the voice issues on his communicative participation. Both the patient and his wife completed the form due to well-established impairments in self-perception of vocal loudness associated with PD.[86] He reported some difficulty in general, with a standard score of 52.7/71, especially when trying to get a turn in a conversation, saying something quickly, and speaking to people he does not know. His wife reported more significant difficulty in participation for SM, with a standard score of 41.10/71.

Auditory-Perceptual Assessment

The CAPE-V[24] was administered. The patient was determined to have an overall CAPE-V score of 31/100, indicating moderate dysphonia. Aberrant perceptual features identified in the voice included breathiness (49/100), strain (19/100), high pitch (21/100), and low loudness (48/100), with loudness decay present. Moderate dysprosody and mild hypernasality were also observed. Respiration was primarily abdominal-thoracic. Breath holding was not observed. The patient took preparatory inhalations prior to utterances most of the time. Articulation was mildly impaired, rate was slightly fast with short rushes of speech present, and mild disfluencies were present. The Sentence Intelligibility Test[87] was administered. The patient was rated 82% intelligible at the sentence level in quiet.

Acoustic and Aerodynamic Assessment

All data were gathered utilizing Glottal Enterprises equipment with custom Matlab software for measurements. Aerodynamic protocols were those established within the Stathopoulos laboratory.[17] Briefly, these protocols include holding the mask securely against the patient's face and checking the pressure (pitot) tube for any blockages (ie, from spit). Further, adequate lip seal and velopharyngeal closure were ensured for pressure measurements. The patient produced 3 strings of 7 syllables of /pa/ and repeated a short sentence ("Buy Pop or Pop a Papa") 3 times. The patient was instructed to complete these slowly, connecting the vowels and consonants as much as possible. He was able to complete the speech tasks adequately. However, due to weak lip seal and hypernasality, accurate estimates of subglottal pressure could not be obtained. A headset microphone was placed at a 45-degree angle at 6 inches from the mouth to acquire acoustic data (see Table 6–15 for results). Normative data were obtained from Matheron et al (2017),[17] Huber and Darling (2011),[88] Rojas et al (2020),[89] Enright et al (1994),[90] and McClaran et al (1995).[91]

Respiratory Assessment

Breath locations were identified visually as the patient spoke, using protocols developed in the Huber laboratory.[92] Pauses over 150 ms were identified on a spectrogram and the number of pauses that coincided with a breath were counted (Figure 6–1). Maximum expiratory pressure was assessed using an inspiratory/expiratory respiratory pressure meter with nose clips. Vital capacity was obtained using a digital spirometer and nose clips.

Stimulability

The patient was stimulable for increased loudness using external cues, including targeting 78 dB on a sound pressure level meter and speaking in noise. However, the patient did not maintain increased loudness with internal cues (ie, talk at twice your comfortable loudness). The patient increased sound pressure level by 3 dB in conversation during a 1-session trial with the SpeechVive device (Figure 6–2). (See Video 18 Calibrating the SpeechVive by Huber.)

Cognitive Assessment

Cognition was assessed using the Cognitive-Linguistic Quick Test.[93] The patient's composite score was 3.4, indicating mild cognitive impairment. He scored in the moderately impaired range for memory and the mildly impaired range for language.

Impressions

SM demonstrated a mild-moderate impairment in speech production that was characterized by moderate breathiness, reduced loudness, and dysprosody. Acoustic and aerodynamic results corroborated the auditory-perceptual findings. Sound pressure level was low. Aerodynamic results indicated reduced vocal fold closure and poor vocal fold valving. Respiratory results indicated low maximum expiratory pressure, short utterances, and a lack of pauses for emphasis (most pauses were to breathe). Mildly reduced communicative participation was reported, more so by the patient's wife than by the patient himself. The patient was stimulable for increased loudness when elicited using external cues. Cognition was found to be mildly impaired, with a moderate impairment in memory.

Voice Therapy: Clinical Case Studies

Table 6–15. Acoustic and Aerodynamic Assessment Results

Measurement	Task	Patient Value	Normative Value Mean (SD)	Abnormal?
Sound Pressure Level (SPL)	Monologue	74.8 dB	78 dB (0.82)	Slightly low
Utterance Length	Monologue	8.2 syllables	13.2 syllables (1.01)	Low
Speech Rate	Monologue	4.46 syllables/sec	3.90 syllables/sec (0.019)	High
Fundamental Frequency	Vowel in syllable train	123.36 Hz	123.04 Hz (8.02)	WNL
Maximum Flow Declination Rate	Vowel in syllable train	44.81 L/sec/sec	354.5 L/sec/sec (62.16)	Very low
Open Quotient	Vowel in syllable train	0.779	0.640 (0.036)	High
Peak-to-Peak Airflow	Vowel in syllable train	0.068 L/sec	0.257 L/sec (0.045)	Very low
Minimum Airflow	Vowel in syllable train	0.106 L/sec	0.005 L/sec (0.380)	Slightly high
Percent of Breath Pauses	Monologue	97%	N/A	Likely high
Maximum Expiratory Pressure	N/A	83 cmH$_2$O	188 cmH$_2$O	Very low
Vital Capacity	Slow vital capacity	4.03 L	4.16 L (0.679)	WNL

dB = decibels; Hz = hertz; L/sec = liters per second; L/sec/sec = liters per second per second; cmH$_2$O = centimeters of water

In this case, the author documents reduced vocal fold closure and poor vocal fold valving per aerodynamic testing as well as a glottal gap seen on videostroboscopy. Below, Huber recommends voice therapy following the injection augmentation, which highlights the importance of both complete glottal closure (targeted with injection augmentation) and adequate respiratory drive (targeted in the voice therapy) to optimize overall voice and speech communication.

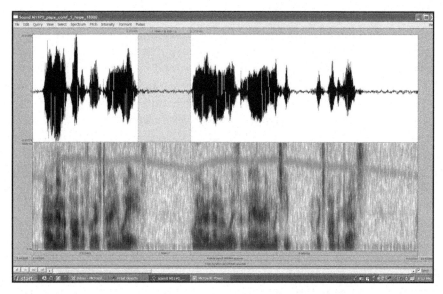

FIGURE 6–1. Spectrographic display of a pause over 150 ms in length.

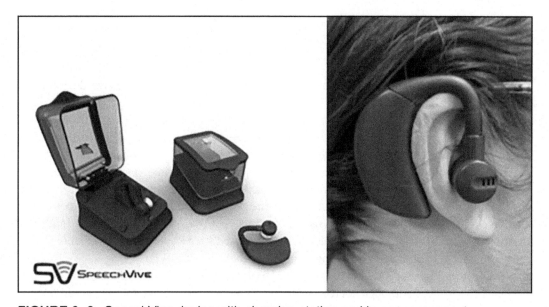

FIGURE 6–2. SpeechVive device with charging station and in-ear component.

Plan of Care

The patient will return to the otolaryngologist who recommended a trial vocal fold injection to increase vocal fold closure before starting behavioral voice treatment. He will be seen for 2 treatment sessions (45 minutes each) per week for 6 weeks. Daily homework will be assigned. Improvements in loudness, voice quality, and communicative participation will be the foci of treatment.

Long-Term and Short-Term Goals:

1. SM will improve voice production and respiratory support for speech.

a. SM will wear the SpeechVive device daily during communicative environments and will speak with the device on for at least 30 minutes per day.
b. SM will increase sound pressure level to 78 dB during conversation with the SpeechVive device on, without any further cueing.
c. SM will utilize the PhoRTE® program to increase vocal loudness and vocal endurance with normal prosodic features. (For more information on PhoRTE®, see Case Study 5.2 by Ziegler and Hapner: Phonation Resistance Training Exercises [PhoRTE®] to Treat an Adult With Presbyphonia.)
d. SM will increase expiratory muscle strength so maximum expiratory pressure is over 100 cmH₂O.
2. SM will increase communicative participation.
a. SM will answer the phone over 50% of the time at home.
b. SM will increase his initiation of conversations by 15%.

Decision Making

Since the patient had already been treated with LSVT-LOUD without successful carryover, treatment was designed to use alternative treatment approaches. Given his moderate difficulty with memory, the SpeechVive device was recommended for the patient. Due to the strong respiratory component of the patient's symptoms, the EMST-150 from Aspire Products was recommended for the patient. Although not relevant to voice, memory and executive function skills were addressed during treatment in addition to the treatment described below. When possible, cognitive skills were practiced with the SpeechVive device in place and using improved voice techniques, consistent with progress in PhoRTE®.

Intervention

The otolaryngologist administered a bilateral vocal fold injection augmentation using an injectible that lasts 3 to 4 months. After the injection, voice quality was improved and breathiness was reduced but still present. Sound pressure level (loudness) did not improve following the injection. Post injection voice therapy was initiated.

Short-Term Goal #1. *SM will wear the SpeechVive device daily during communicative environments and will speak with the device on for at least 30 minutes per day.* SM and his wife were taught how to care for and wear the SpeechVive device. He was instructed to wear the device in quiet communicative environments daily and to speak with it on every day, either in conversation or while reading aloud from clinician-provided reading passages. At the start of treatment, the patient read aloud for 15 minutes per day and, across the first 3 weeks, worked up to reading aloud 30 minutes per day.

Short-Term Goal #2. *SM will increase sound pressure level to 78 dB during conversation with the SpeechVive device on, without any further cueing.* The SpeechVive device plays noise in one ear when the patient speaks. The device was set to sense the patient's voice and the noise output was set to elicit a 3-dB increase in sound pressure level during reading. Device settings were checked every week in therapy, increasing the intensity of speech elicited until the target of 78 dB was reached. This ensured consistent workload for the patient and increased his SPL in small increments (1 dB) to reach the 78-dB goal. (See Video 18 Calibrating the SpeechVive by Huber.)

Short-Term Goal #3. *SM will utilize the PhoRTE® program to increase vocal loudness and vocal endurance with normal prosodic features.* The patient completed the PhoRTE® program[54] during therapy and at home while wearing the SpeechVive device. He practiced all 5 of the exercises prescribed in the PhoRTE® program during each session: sustained "ah," glides using an "ah," functional phrases in stronger voice at higher and lower pitch, and conversing in strong voice. The SLP used cueing to encourage the patient, as well as self-perceptual activities to help him rate his voice quality, pitch change, and vocal loudness. She gave him immediate and consistent feedback early on, fading to intermittent feedback over the first 4 weeks. In the last 2 weeks, SM was primarily providing his own feedback with small corrections from the SLP.

Short-Term Goal #4. *SM will increase expiratory muscle strength so maximum expiratory pressure is over 100 cmH_2O.* The EMST-150 from Aspire Products was used to achieve this goal. The EMST device was set to 75% of maximum expiratory pressure. The SLP instructed the patient to perform exercises in an upright, seated position and to wear nose clips during exercises. She told him to breathe in as much as possible before blowing into the device. He blew for 3 seconds after the valve of the device opened each time. The patient completed 25 expiratory breaths (in sets of 5) 1 day per week during therapy and 4 days per week at home. Maximum expiratory pressure was checked each week, and the device was reset to ensure that overload of the muscles was maintained at 75% of maximum expiratory pressure.

Short-Term Goal #5. *SM will answer the phone over 50% of the time at home.* The patient logged each call he answered. In treatment sessions, the clinician and patient discussed barriers or concerns to increasing his use of the phone and brainstormed solutions. SM started with a goal of answering the phone 10% of the time and slowly increased this goal every week.

Short-Term Goal #6. *SM will increase his initiation of conversations by 15%.* To start with, SM logged the times he initiated conversations in the first week, with the help of his wife. During therapy, the clinician and patient discussed barriers he faced in initiating conversations and brainstormed solutions for both familiar and unfamiliar conversational partners. He tracked initiations, with assistance from his wife, each week. This was the toughest goal for SM. He started by initiating 2 conversations with familiar partners in week

1 and slowly built on successes to increase the number of initiations. He moved to initiating conversations with unfamiliar partners in week 5.

Session Plan (Two Sessions per Week)

1. Measure SPL in conversation and reset settings on SpeechVive, if necessary (session #1 each week)
2. Review EMST completion logs and revise settings on EMST-150, if necessary (session #2 each week)
3. Practice PhoRTE® exercises with Speech-Vive device on
4. Review communication participation goals, identify successes and barriers, and discuss methods to overcome barriers (while wearing the SpeechVive device)
5. Review homework assignments and answer questions from patient and his wife

Posttherapy Outcomes and Conclusions

The patient was dismissed from treatment after 6 weeks and was asked to come back for a reassessment in 6 months.

SM was compliant with wearing the SpeechVive device. On average, he wore it 6 days per week and spoke for 65 minutes per day on the device. SM's sound pressure level was maintained at 78 dB during conversation by the end of treatment when he was wearing the SpeechVive device. Without the device, his sound pressure level was 76 dB on average during a monologue. It was recommended that he continue to wear the device daily.

SM was compliant with his home program, completing all exercises (EMST and PhoRTE®) 4 days per week on average. After 6 weeks of treatment, SM's loudness and breathiness were improved. Post-treatment, breathiness and hypophonia were rated as mild. Speech intelligibility increased to 88%. Dysprosody was slightly improved. It was recommended that the patient continue to practice PhoRTE® exercises 3 to 5 times per week.

Maximum expiratory pressure increased to 95 cmH$_2$O. The clinician recommended that he continue to use the device 5 days per week, with quarter-turn increases when he finds that the device feels easier.

SM was compliant with answering the phone at home, more so when his wife was at work. He was compliant with tracking his initiations and logging barriers and concerns for the treatment sessions. By the end of treatment, he was initiating 20% more often than pretreatment. Before treatment was terminated, the clinician and patient developed 3 additional communication participation goals that were salient to SM. She recommended that he continue to work to improve his communicative participation.

Conflict of Interest Statement

Huber is the inventor of the SpeechVive device. She owns shares in SpeechVive, Inc., the company that manufactures and sells the device. Huber also serves on the medical advisory board for Rock Steady Boxing.

References

1. Ludlow CL, Adler CH, Berke GS, et al. Research priorities in spasmodic dysphonia. *Otolaryngol Head Neck Surg.* 2008;139(4): 495-505. doi:10.1016/j.otohns.2008.05.624
2. Simonyan K, Barkmeier-Kraemer J, Blitzer A, et al. Laryngeal dystonia: Multidisciplinary update on terminology, pathophysiology, and research priorities. *Neurology.* 2021;96(21):989-1001. doi:10.1212/WNL.00 00000000011922
3. Blitzer A, Brin MF, Simonyan K, Ozelius LJ, Frucht SJ. Phenomenology, genetics, and CNS network abnormalities in laryngeal dystonia: A 30-year experience. *Laryngoscope.* 2018;128(suppl 1):S1-S9. doi:10.1002/lary.27003
4. Shoffel-Havakuk H, Marks KL, Morton M, Johns MM III, Hapner ER. Validation of the

OMNI vocal effort scale in the treatment of adductor spasmodic dysphonia. *Laryngoscope.* Published online October 12, 2018. doi:10.1002/lary.27430
5. Merati AL, Heman-Ackah YD, Abaza M, Altman KW, Sulica L, Belamowicz S. Common movement disorders affecting the larynx: A report from the neurolaryngology committee of the AAO-HNS. *Otolaryngol Head Neck Surg.* 2005;133(5):654-665. doi:10.10 16/j.otohns.2005.05.003
6. Ludlow CL, Domangue R, Sharma D, et al. Consensus-based attributes for identifying patients with spasmodic dysphonia and other voice disorders. *JAMA Otolaryngol Head Neck Surg.* 2018;144(8):657-665. doi:10.1001/jamaoto.2018.0644
7. Yiu Y, Baylor CR, Bamer AM, et al. Validation of the Communicative Participation Item Bank as an outcome measure for spasmodic dysphonia. *Laryngoscope.* 2021; 131(4):859-864. doi:10.1002/lary.28897
8. Hoffman MR, Jiang JJ, Rieves AL, McElveen KAB, Ford CN. Differentiating between adductor and abductor spasmodic dysphonia using airflow interruption. *Laryngoscope.* 2009;119(9):1851-1855. doi:10.1002/lary.20 572
9. Sapienza CM, Walton S, Murry T. Adductor spasmodic dysphonia and muscular tension dysphonia: Acoustic analysis of sustained phonation and reading. *J Voice.* 2000;14(4): 502-520. doi:10.1016/S0892-1997(00)800 08-9
10. Marks KL, Díaz Cádiz ME, Toles LE, et al. Automated creak differentiates adductor laryngeal dystonia and muscle tension dysphonia. *Laryngoscope.* 2023;133(10):2687-2694. doi:10.1002/lary.30588
11. Colton R, Casper J, Leonard R. *Understanding Voice Problems: A Physiological Perspective for Diagnosis and Treatment.* Lippincott Williams & Wilkins; 2006.
12. Torrecillas V, Dwenger K, Barkmeier-Kraemer JM. Classification of vocal tremor using updated consensus-based tremor classification criteria. *Laryngoscope Investig Otolaryngol.* 2021;6(2):261-276. doi:10.1002/lio2.544
13. Sherer TB, Chowdhury S, Peabody K, Brooks DW. Overcoming obstacles in Parkinson's

disease. *Mov Disord.* 2012;27(13):1606-1611. doi:10.1002/mds.25260

14. Broadfoot CK, Abur D, Hoffmeister JD, Stepp CE, Ciucci MR. Research-based updates in swallowing and communication dysfunction in Parkinson disease: Implications for evaluation and management. *Perspect ASHA Spec Interest Groups.* 2019;4(5):825-841. doi: 10.1044/2019_pers-sig3-2019-0001

15. Schapira A, Chaudhuri K, Jenner P. Nonmotor features of Parkinson disease. *Nat Rev Neurosci.* 2017;18(7):435-450.

16. Mu L, Chen J, Sobotka S, et al. Alpha-synuclein pathology in sensory nerve terminals of the upper aerodigestive tract of Parkinson's disease patients. *Dysphagia.* 2015;30(4):404-417. doi:10.1007/s00455-015-9612-7

17. Matheron D, Stathopoulos ET, Huber JE, Sussman JE. Laryngeal aerodynamics in healthy older adults and adults with Parkinson's disease. *J Speech Lang Hear Res.* 2017;60(3):507-524. doi:10.1044/2016_JSLHR-S-14-0314

18. Duffy J. *Motor Speech Disorders: Substrates, Differential Diagnosis, and Management.* e-Book. Elsevier Health Sciences; 2019.

19. Ramig LO, Sapir S, Countryman S, et al. Intensive voice treatment (LSVT®) for patients with Parkinson's disease: A 2 year follow up. *J Neurol Neurosurg Psychiatry.* 2001;71(4):493-498. doi:10.1136/jnnp.71.4.493

20. Pu T, Huang M, Kong X, et al. Lee Silverman Voice Treatment to improve speech in Parkinson's disease: A systemic review and meta-analysis. *Parkinsons Dis.* 2021;2021. doi:10.1155/2021/3366870

21. Watts CR. A retrospective study of long-term treatment outcomes for reduced vocal intensity in hypokinetic dysarthria throat disorders. *BMC Ear Nose Throat Disord.* 2016; 16(1):1-7. doi:10.1186/s12901-016-0022-8

22. McLaney E, Morassaei S, Hughes L, Davies R, Campbell M, Di Prospero L. A framework for interprofessional team collaboration in a hospital setting: Advancing team competencies and behaviours. *Healthc Manag Forum.* 2022;35(2):112-117. doi:10.1177/084047042 11063584

23. Gutierrez D, Simpson CB, Hapner ER. Exploring models of interdisciplinary voice

care. Poster presented at: *The Fall Voice Conference.* October 6-8, 2022, San Francisco.

24. Kempster GB, Gerratt BR, Abbott KV, Barkmeier-Kraemer J, Hillman RE. Consensus auditory-perceptual evaluation of voice: Development of a standardized clinical protocol. *Am J Speech Lang Pathol.* 2009;18(2): 124-132. doi:10.1044/1058-0360(2008/08-0017)

25. Daraei P, Villari CR, Rubin AD, et al. The role of laryngoscopy in the diagnosis of spasmodic dysphonia. *JAMA Otolaryngol Head Neck Surg.* 2014;140(3):228-232. doi:10.1001/jamaoto.2013.6450

26. Poburka BJ, Patel RR, Bless DM. Voice-Vibratory Assessment With Laryngeal Imaging (VALI) form: Reliability of rating stroboscopy and high-speed videoendoscopy. *J Voice.* 2017;31(4):513.e1-513.e14. doi:10.1016/j.jvoice.2016.12.003

27. Rosen CA, Lee AS, Osborne J, Zullo T, Murry T. Development and validation of the Voice Handicap Index-10. *Laryngoscope.* 2004;114(9 I):1549-1556. doi:10.1097/0000 5537-200409000-00009

28. Arffa RE, Krishna P, Gartner-Schmidt J, Rosen CA. Normative values for the Voice Handicap Index-10. *J Voice.* 2012;26(4):462-465. doi:10.1016/j.jvoice.2011.04.006

29. Shembel AC, Rosen CA, Zullo TG, Gartner-Schmidt JL. Development and validation of the cough severity index: A severity index for chronic cough related to the upper airway. *Laryngoscope.* 2013;123(8):1931-1936. doi:10.1002/lary.23916

30. Gartner-Schmidt JL, Shembel AC, Zullo TG, Rosen CA. Development and validation of the Dyspnea Index (DI): A severity index for upper airway-related dyspnea. *J Voice.* 2014;28(6):775-782. doi:10.1016/j.jvoice.2013.12.017

31. Castro ME, Sund LT, Hoffman MR, Hapner ER. The Voice Problem Impact Scales (VPIS). *J Voice.* 2024;38(3):666-673. doi:10.1016/j.jvoice.2021.11.011

32. Barkmeier JM, Case J. Differential diagnosis of adductor-type spasmodic dysphonia, vocal tremor, and muscle tension dysphonia. *Curr Opin Otolaryngol Head Neck Surg.* 2000;8(3):174-179.

33. Patel R, Awan S, Barkmeier-Kraemer J, et al. Recommended protocols for instrumental assessment of voice: American Speech-Language-Hearing Association expert panel to develop a protocol for instrumental assessment of vocal function. *Am J Speech Lang Pathol.* 2018;27(3):887-905.

34. Evatt M, Freeman A, Factor S. Adult-onset dystonia. *Handb Clin Neurol.* 2011;100:481-511.

35. Martino D, Liuzzi D, Macerollo A, Aniello MS, Livrea P, Defazio G. The phenomenology of the geste antagoniste in primary blepharospasm and cervical dystonia. *Mov Disord.* 2010;25(4):407-412. doi:10.1002/mds.23011

36. Battistella G, Simonyan K. Clinical implications of dystonia as a neural network disorder. In: Shaikh A, Sadnicka A, eds. *Basic and Translational Applications of the Network Theory for Dystonia in Advances in Neurobiology.* Springer; 2023:223-240.

37. Kaye R, Blitzer A. Chemodenervation of the larynx. *Toxins (Basel).* 2017;9(11):1-16. doi:10.3390/toxins9110356

38. Simpson CB, Lee CT, Hatcher JL, Michalek J. Botulinum toxin treatment of false vocal folds in adductor spasmodic dysphonia: Functional outcomes. *Laryngoscope.* 2016;126(1):118-121. doi:10.1002/lary.25515

39. Justicz N, Hapner ER, Josephs JS, Boone BC, Jinnah HA, Johns MM. Comparative effectiveness of propranolol and botulinum for the treatment of essential voice tremor. *Laryngoscope.* 2016;126(1):113-117. doi:10.1002/lary.25485

40. Mendelsohn AH, Berke GS. Surgery or botulinum toxin for adductor spasmodic dysphonia: A comparative study. *Ann Otol Rhinol Laryngol.* 2012;121(4):231-238. doi:10.1177/000348941212100408

41. Murry T, Woodson GE. Combined-modality treatment of adductor spasmodic dysphonia with botulinum toxin and voice therapy. *J Voice.* 1995;9(4):460-465. doi:10.1016/S0892-1997(05)80211-5

42. Creighton F, Hapner E, Klein A, Rosen A, Jinnah H, Johns M. Diagnostic delays in spasmodic dysphonia: A call for clinician

education. *J Voice.* 2015;29(5):592-594. doi:10.1016/j.jvoice.2013.10.022

43. Kirke DN, Battistella G, Kumar V, et al. Neural correlates of dystonic tremor: A multimodal study of voice tremor in spasmodic dysphonia. *Brain Imaging Behav.* 2017;11(1):166-175. doi:10.1007/s11682-016-9513-x

44. Bové M, Daamen N, Rosen C, Wang CC, Sulica L, Gartner-Schmidt J. Development and validation of the Vocal Tremor Scoring System. *Laryngoscope.* 2006;116(9):1662-1667. doi:10.1097/01.mlg.0000233255.57425.36

45. Jacobson E. *Progressive Relaxation.* 2nd ed. University of Chicago Press

46. Roy N, Ford CN, Bless DM. Muscle tension dysphonia and spasmodic dysphonia: The role of manual laryngeal tension reduction in diagnosis and management. *Ann Otol Rhinol Laryngol.* 1996;105(11):851-856. doi:10.1177/000348949610501102

47. Stemple JC, Weiler E, Whitehead W, Komray R. Electromyographic biofeedback training with patients exhibiting a hyperfunctional voice disorder. *Laryngoscope.* 1980;90(3):471-476. doi:10.1002/lary.5540900314

48. Wang F, Yiu EM. Is surface electromyography (sEMG) a useful tool in identifying muscle tension dysphonia? An integrative review of the current evidence. *J Voice.* 2024;38(3):800.e1-800.e12. doi:10.1016/j.jvoice.2021.10.006

49. Stemple J, Roy N, Klaben B. *Clinical Voice Pathology: Theory and Management.* 6th ed. Plural Publishing; 2018.

50. Shoffel-Havakuk H, Chau S, Hapner ER, Pethan M, Johns MM. Development and validation of the Voice Catastrophization Index. *J Voice.* 2019;33(2):232-238. doi:10.1016/j.jvoice.2017.09.026

51. Leung JS, Rosenbaum A, Holmberg J, et al. Improved vocal quality and decreased vocal effort after botulinum toxin treatment for laryngeal dystonia. *Auris Nasus Larynx.* 2024;51(1):106-112. doi:10.1016/j.anl.2023.06.004

52. Ziegler A, Verdolini Abbott K, Johns M, Klein A, Hapner ER. Preliminary data on two voice therapy interventions in the

treatment of presbyphonia. *Laryngoscope.* 2014;124(8):1869-1876. doi:10.1002/lary.24548

53. Barkmeier-Kraemer J. Updates on vocal tremor and its management. *Perspect Voice Voice Disord.* 2012;22(3):97-103. doi:10.1044/vvd22.3.97

54. Belsky MA, Shelly S, Rothenberger SD, et al. Phonation resistance training exercises (PhoRTE) with and without expiratory muscle strength training (EMST) for patients with presbyphonia: A noninferiority randomized clinical trial. *J Voice.* 2023;37(3):398-409. doi:10.1016/j.jvoice.2021.02.015

55. Lederle A, Barkmeier-Kraemer J, Finnegan E. Perception of vocal tremor during sustained phonation compared with sentence context. *J Voice.* 2012;26(5):668.e1-668.e9. doi:10.1016/j.jvoice.2011.11.001

56. Leeper HA, Jones E. Frequency and intensity effects upon temporal and aerodynamic aspects of vocal fold diadochokinesis. *Percept Mot Skills.* 1991;73(3 pt 1):880-882. doi:10.2466/pms.1991.73.3.880

57. Louzada T, Beraldinelle R, Berretin-Felix G, Brasolotto AG. Oral and vocal fold diadochokinesis in dysphonic women. *J Appl Oral Sci.* 2011;19(6):567-572. doi:10.1590/S1678-77572011000600005

58. Awan SN, Roy N, Jetté ME, Meltzner GS, Hillman RE. Quantifying dysphonia severity using a spectral/cepstral-based acoustic index: Comparisons with auditory-perceptual judgements from the CAPE-V. *Clin Linguist Phon.* 2010;24(9):742-758. doi:10.3109/02699206.2010.492446

59. Heman-Ackah YD, Sataloff RT, Laureyns G, et al. Quantifying the cepstral peak prominence, a measure of dysphonia. *J Voice.* 2014;28(6):783-788. doi:10.1016/j.jvoice.2014.05.005

60. Gaskill CS, Awan JA, Watts CR, Awan SN. Acoustic and perceptual classification of within-sample normal, intermittently dysphonic, and consistently dysphonic voice types. *J Voice.* 2017;31(2):218-228. doi:10.1016/j.jvoice.2016.04.016

61. Hwa Chen S. Sex differences in frequency and intensity in reading and voice range profiles for Taiwanese adult speakers. *Folia Phoniatr Logop.* 2006;59(1):1-9. doi:10.1159/000096545

62. Lundy DS, Roy S, Xue JW, Casiano RR, Jassir D. Spastic/spasmodic vs. tremulous vocal quality: Motor speech profile analysis. *J Voice.* 2004;18(1):146-152. doi:10.1016/j.jvoice.2003.12.001

63. Barkmeier-Kraemer J, Lato A, Wiley K. Development of a speech treatment program for a client with essential vocal tremor. *Semin Speech Lang.* 2011;32(1):43-57.

64. Smitheran JR, Hixon TJ. A clinical method for estimating laryngeal airway resistance during vowel production. *J Speech Hear Disord.* 1981;46(2):138-147.

65. Leeper H, Graves D. Consistency of laryngeal airway resistance in adult women. *J Commun Disord.* 1984;17(3):153-163.

66. Jacobson BH, Johnson A, Grywalski C, et al. The Voice Handicap Index (VHI): Development and validation. *Am J Speech Lang Pathol.* 1997;6(3):66-69. doi:10.1044/1058-0360.0603.66

67. Louis E, Gerbin M. Voice handicap in essential tremor: A comparison with normal controls and Parkinson's disease. *Tremor Other Hyperkinet Mov.* 2013;3. doi: 10.7916/D8KD1WN3

68. Barkmeier-Kraemer J. Hiding vocal tremor. In: Behrman A, Haskell J, eds. *Exercises for Voice Therapy.* 2nd ed. Plural Publishing; 2013:196-199.

69. Barkmeier-Kraemer J. Evaluation and treatment of vocal tremor. In: Maryn Y, De Bodt M, eds. *Neurolaryngologie (StEMINARIES 2015-2016).* Vlaamse Vereniging voor Logopedisten; 2016:12-25.

70. Bhatia KP, Bain P, Bajaj N, et al. Consensus statement on the classification of tremors from the task force on tremor of the International Parkinson and Movement Disorder Society. *Mov Disord.* 2018;33(1):75-87. doi:10.1002/mds.27121

71. Barkmeier-Kraemer JM. Isolated voice tremor: A clinical variant of essential tremor or a distinct clinical phenotype? *Tremor Other Hyperkinet Mov.* 2020;10:1-8. doi:10.7916/tohm.v0.738

72. Twohig A, Finnegan E. The effect of vowel duration on tremor severity for patients with vocal tremor. [Undergraduate thesis] Iowa City, Iowa: *Department of Speech Pathology and Audiology, University of Iowa*; 2008.

73. Khoury S, Randall D. Treatment of essential vocal tremor: A scoping review of evidence-based therapeutic modalities. *J Voice*. 2024;38(4):922-930. doi: 10.1016/j.jvoice.2021.12.009

74. Nanjundeswaran C, Jacobson BH, Gartner-Schmidt J, Verdolini Abbott K. Vocal Fatigue Index (VFI): Development and validation. *J Voice*. 2015;29(4):433-440. doi:10.1016/j.jvoice.2014.09.012

75. Awan SN, Roy N, Zhang D, Cohen SM. Validation of the Cepstral Spectral Index of Dysphonia (CSID) as a screening tool for voice disorders: Development of clinical cutoff scores. *J Voice*. 2016;30(2):130-144. doi:10.1016/j.jvoice.2015.04.009

76. Shao J, MacCallum JK, Zhang Y, Sprecher A, Jiang JJ. Acoustic analysis of the tremulous voice: Assessing the utility of the correlation dimension and perturbation parameters. *J Commun Disord*. 2010;43(1):35-44. doi:10.1016/j.jcomdis.2009.09.001

77. Lester-Smith RA, Story BH. The effects of physiological adjustments on the perceptual and acoustical characteristics of vibrato as a model of vocal tremor. *J Acoust Soc Am*. 2016;140(5):3827-3833. doi:10.1121/1.4967454

78. Xue SA, Deliyski D. Effects of aging on selected acoustic voice parameters: Preliminary normative data and educational implications. *Educ Gerontol*. 2001;27(2):159-168. doi:10.1080/03601270151075561

79. Murton O, Hillman R, Mehta D. Cepstral peak prominence values for clinical voice evaluation. *Am J Speech Lang Pathol*. 2020;29(3):1596-1607. doi:10.1044/2020_AJSLP-20-00001

80. Ruckart KW, Moya-Mendez ME, Nagatsuka M, Barry JL, Siddiqui MS, Madden LL. Comprehensive evaluation of voice-specific outcomes in patients with essential tremor before and after deep brain stimulation. *J Voice*. 2022;36(6):838-846. doi:10.1016/j.jvoice.2020.09.013

81. Erickson-DiRenzo E, Kuijper FM, Barbosa DAN, et al. Multiparametric laryngeal assessment of the effect of thalamic deep brain stimulation on essential vocal tremor. *Park Relat Disord*. 2020;81:106-112. doi:10.1016/j.parkreldis.2020.10.026

82. Erickson-DiRenzo E, Sung CK, Ho AL, Halpern CH. Intraoperative evaluation of essential vocal tremor in deep brain stimulation surgery. *Am J Speech Lang Pathol*. 2020; 29(2):851-863. doi:10.1044/2019_AJSLP-19-00079

83. Mücke D, Hermes A, Roettger TB, et al. The effects of thalamic deep brain stimulation on speech dynamics in patients with essential tremor: An articulographic study. *PLoS One*. 2018;13(1):e0191359. doi:10.1371/journal.pone.0191359

84. Ramig L, Halpern A, Spielman J, Fox C, Freeman K. Speech treatment in Parkinson's disease: Randomized controlled trial (RCT). *Mov Disord*. 2018;33(11):1777-1791. doi:10.1002/mds.27460

85. Baylor C, Yorkston K, Eadie T, Kim J, Chung H, Amtmann D. The communicative participation item bank (CPIB): Item bank calibration and development of a disorder-generic short form. *J Speech Lang Hear Res*. 2013;56(4):1190-1208. doi:10.1044/1092-4388(2012/12-0140)

86. Ho AK, Bradshaw JL, Iansek R. Volume perception in Parkinsonian speech. *Mov Disord*. 2000;15(6):1125-1131. doi:10.1002/1531-8257(200011)15:6<1125::AID-MDS1010>3.0.CO;2-R

87. Yorkston K, Beukelman D, Tice R. The Sentence Intelligibility Test. 1996. Lincoln, NE: Tice Technologies.

88. Huber JE, Darling M. Effect of Parkinson's disease on the production of structured and unstructured speaking tasks: Respiratory physiologic and linguistic considerations. *J Speech Lang Hear Res*. 2011;54(1):33-46. doi:10.1044/1092-4388(2010/09-0184)

89. Rojas S, Kefalianos E, Vogel A. How does our voice change as we age? A systematic review and meta-analysis of acoustic and perceptual voice data from healthy adults over 50 years of age. *J Speech Lang Hear Res*. 2020;63(2):533-551.

90. Enright PL, Kronmal RA, Manolio TA, Schenker MB HR. Respiratory muscle strength in the elderly. Correlates and reference values. Cardiovascular Health Study Research Group. *Am J Respir Crit Care Med.* 1994;149(2):430-438.

91. McClaran SR, Babcock MA, Pegelow DF, Reddan WG, Dempsey JA. Longitudinal effects of aging on lung function at rest and exercise in healthy active fit elderly adults. *J Appl Physiol.* 1995;78(5):1957-1968. doi:10.1152/jappl.1995.78.5.1957

92. Sevitz JS, Kiefer BR, Huber JE, Troche MS. Obtaining objective clinical measures during telehealth evaluations of dysarthria. *Am J Speech Lang Pathol.* 2021;30(2):503-516. doi:10.1044/2020_AJSLP-20-00243

93. Helm-Estabrooks N. *Cognitive-Linguistic Quick Test.* 2001.

7

Upper Airway

Introduction: Refractory Chronic Cough

Laurie Slovarp

Chronic cough (CC), defined as a cough lasting 8 weeks or more, impacts approximately 10% of adults worldwide.[1] The most common causes of CC are asthma, eosinophilic airway disease, rhinosinus conditions (sometimes referred to as upper airway cough syndrome), and gastroesophageal reflux disease (GERD); however, up to 20% of patients do not respond to medical treatment for these conditions.[2,3] The nomenclature for this condition varies widely throughout the literature, including idiopathic CC, refractory CC (RCC), unexplained CC, difficult-to-treat cough, and neurogenic cough. Some sources delineate RCC from unexplained CC and idiopathic CC.[4] These sources describe RCC as a cough where a known medical etiology has been determined (eg, sinusitis) but medical treatment for the condition has not resolved the cough, and unexplained or idiopathic CC as a cough where no medical etiology can be determined. For simplicity, the term "RCC" is used in this chapter to describe any patient with a CC that has not responded to guideline-based medical management.

The impact of RCC on mental health and quality of life is significant. RCC can cause disruption of daily activities such as talking, socializing, working, eating, and sleeping,[5,6] contributing to clinical depression in an estimated 50% of patients.[7] Approximately 60% of women report urinary incontinence.[8] Behavioral treatment provided by a properly trained speech-language pathologist (SLP) has proven efficacy, typically requires only 2 to 4 sessions, and comes with zero negative side effects.[9,10] While there is no evidence-based systematic approach that indicates when SLP treatment should be considered, medical evaluation should always precede consideration of behavioral treatment.

The nomenclature for SLP treatment for RCC also varies widely in the literature, including physiotherapy, speech, and language therapy intervention (PSALTI),[11] behavioral cough therapy,[12] speech pathology treatment (SPT),[13] cough control therapy,[9] cough suppression therapy,[14] and behavioral cough suppression therapy (BCST).[10,15] In this chapter, the term "BCST" will be used to highlight it as a behavioral treatment with an emphasis on volitional cough suppression.

Blager et al (1988)[16] initially described SLP treatment for RCC, drawing upon techniques utilized for hyperfunctional voice disorders and incorporating aspects of psychotherapy. During that period, the underlying mechanisms and cause of the cough were not yet understood, leading to the conclusion that it was a conversion disorder. Fortunately, significant advances have been made in understanding and treating RCC. A wealth of evidence now indicates hypersensitivity of the cough reflex as the underlying pathophysiology responsible for RCC.[4,17,18] The exact mechanisms responsible for this hypersensitivity, however, have not been fully elucidated. The prevailing theory is that inflammation resulting from an identifiable precipitating condition, such as upper respiratory infection, sinusitis, or GERD, is the initial cause of hypersensitivity. Once hypersensitivity sets in, the cough is then perpetuated by the cough itself, likely in part due to persistent inflammation as a result of phonotrauma. In other words, coughing begets inflammation, which begets more coughing, which begets more inflammation, and so on. The *use-it-or-lose-it* principle of neuroplasticity is also likely a factor. The more one coughs in response to an urge to cough (UTC), the more the neural mechanism causing the UTC is strengthened. This condition is now commonly termed "cough hypersensitivity syndrome (CHS)" and is thought to be a distinct clinical entity.[19]

Evidence suggests multiple areas within the nervous system as potential sites for hypersensitization.[4] Studies have implicated peripheral processes such as increased expression of sensory receptors expressed on airway vagal C-fibers contributing to increased excitability, and the role of endogenous adenosine triphosphate (ATP), thought to be released during inflammation, as a signaling molecule sensitizing vagal afferent neurons. These findings have led to several clinical trials in search of a pharmaceutical solution in the form of peripheral receptor antagonists; however, the clinical benefit of these medications has been marginal.

Brain imaging research underscores the crucial role of central processes in RCC. Functional MRI studies have shown heightened activity in midbrain structures involved in processing of cough stimuli.[20,21] Moe et al[22] contrasted activity in multiple brain areas in RCC patients and matched healthy counterparts focusing on differences in neural activity when cough stimulation is adjusted so that both groups experience similar UTC sensation (ie, a lower dose for RCC patients). In this scenario, RCC patients exhibited less neural activity in the medullary brainstem regions where airway afferents terminate, greater activity in the midbrain, and comparable activity in the primary sensory cortex. This data challenges the hypothesis that hypersensitivity is primarily due to heightened peripheral afferent signaling, suggesting instead that low-level sensory input is amplified at the level of the midbrain. Other studies show decreased activity in the dorsomedial prefrontal and anterior midcingulate cortices—areas known to be involved in cough suppression.[20] Moreover, Namgung et al,[23] using brain MRI, found differences in frontal lobe areas known to be involved in bottom-up sensory processing and top-down attentional control, and these findings were associated with heightened cough severity and psychological and social impacts. Collectively, these data provide strong mechanistic support for BCST which, as a behavioral therapy, targets central processes. For SLPs treating RCC, possessing a fundamental understanding of these underlying mechanisms is crucial. This knowledge serves multiple purposes, including informing the rationale behind BCST and enabling SLPs to effectively explain the disorder and its treatment to patients. Such clarity enhances the likelihood of patient adherence to the recommended therapy.

The ultimate goals of BCST are to (1) improve cough control and (2) reduce cough sensitivity by reducing laryngeal irritation and inflammation and strengthening cough suppression neural pathways. These goals are targeted by improving laryngeal hygiene (eg, improving hydration, reducing phonotrauma) and suppressing cough. For patients **without** chronic pulmonary disease, BCST is intended to be a restorative treatment. In other words, the goal is not to make a patient excellent at suppressing cough, but rather to change cough sensitivity so that cough suppression is no longer needed. While we do not anticipate BCST to have a similar restorative effect on individuals **with** chronic pulmonary disease (eg, chronic obstructive pulmonary disease, interstitial lung disease), due to other factors contributing to their chronic cough, these patients still exhibit a component of CHS, which often contributes to dry coughing bouts.[24] Consequently, BCST may be beneficial in these cases for improving cough control. Anecdotal evidence indicates patients with pulmonary disease can typically discern between a dry cough and a productive cough. Since suppressing a productive cough is not recommended, it is crucial to clearly explain to patients with pulmonary disease that they should only suppress dry cough, not productive cough.

Although a fully standardized BCST program has not been described, most sources outline BCST as comprising 4 main components: (1) education, (2) cough suppression techniques, (3) laryngeal hygiene, and (4) psychoeducational counseling.[11,25] Conceptually speaking, the first 3 components are relatively straightforward; however, the fourth component may appear somewhat ambiguous. It can be beneficial to view the fourth component as *self-efficacy*, as its primary objective is to instill in the patient a sense of empowerment, encouraging them to believe that they can take control of their cough and effect a change in their condition. This is a crucial component of the treatment as BCST will only work if the patient consistently adheres to the treatment.

Education is the first step toward achieving self-efficacy. Most patients with RCC have already seen several practitioners without benefit and are likely reluctant to go to an SLP, given they don't have a "speech" disorder. Subsequently, the SLP should educate the patient during the first session and should include a clear and knowledgeable explanation of CHS as the cause of the cough as well as a clear rationale for BCST. Regarding cough suppression, the SLP's job is to explain the purpose of cough suppression, instruct the patient in various cough suppression strategies, and encourage the patient to figure out what works for them. Cough suppression strategies may include breathing techniques, laryngeal relaxation, and sensory replacement strategies (eg, hard swallowing or the Masako maneuver). During breathing techniques, the laryngeal and respiratory musculature are engaged in functional tasks in opposition to their action during coughing (eg, prolonged exhale rather than abrupt, high-velocity exhale). Relaxation strategies help to reduce heightened laryngeal muscle tension experienced with cough. Motor replacement strategies provide a competing sensorimotor stimulus to overcome urge to cough in the larynx. It's important the patient understands the treatment is not in the cough suppression techniques or strategies, but rather in suppressing cough when an urge to cough is present. In this regard, patients should be told they are free to try anything they like (other than anything that numbs the throat, such as a menthol cough lozenge) to find out what works for them.

Adherence to treatment is paramount. The therapy will not yield results if the patient only suppresses their cough when coughing is inconvenient or when cough suppression is most convenient. A few consecutive days of dedicated effort is often sufficient to observe a noticeable difference. It is beneficial to explain this to patients so they can plan and allocate time accordingly. It is important to emphasize that 100% success in suppressing cough is not expected or necessary, particularly initially, but attempting to suppress cough consistently is necessary. Patients should make an earnest attempt to suppress their cough every time they feel a UTC and try to interrupt coughing if complete prevention is not possible.

Suppression efforts should continue, even if there is breakthrough coughing, until the UTC has fully dissipated, which may take several minutes. They should also be informed the UTC will likely temporarily intensify before diminishing. It is crucial to convey that this temporary increase does not imply that the strategy is exacerbating the condition. Employing the analogy of a mosquito bite can be helpful—just like resisting the urge to scratch, the itch often worsens before it ultimately subsides.

BCST typically requires no more than 4 sessions and has no reported negative side effects. Studies have shown it improves quality of life and reduces cough sensitivity, frequency, and severity.[11,15,26,27]

In one randomized controlled trial (RCT) 88% of participants with RCC who received BCST reported clinically relevant improvements compared to 14% on placebo.[26] In a single cohort study involving 164 patients from over 15 separate clinics, 70% achieved a clinically meaningful improvement and 58% reported they were quite to completely satisfied with their cough status following BCST.[15]

Case Studies

 CASE STUDY 7.1

Behavioral Cough Suppression Therapy (BCST) for an Adult With Chronic Refractory Cough

Lisa Zughni

Evaluation

Case History

History of the Problem. Patient DW is a 43-year-old cisgender female referred by pulmonology for a comprehensive voice and upper airway evaluation due to a chief complaint of chronic refractory cough for over 5 years. Although she could not recall a clear inciting event at the time of onset, she believes she may have had an upper respiratory infection, which eventually resolved, but cough persisted. She describes 2 different "types" of cough: (1) a single dry cough and/or throat clear that occurs frequently throughout the day, as well as (2) episodic coughing "attacks" that can last up to several minutes at a time. During these coughing attacks, she reports difficulty with inhalation, with occasional stridor. Coughing attacks are severe to the point of gagging and occasional urinary incontinence. Triggers for cough include exertion, cold air, dust, smoke, strong scents (eg, cleaning products, dryer sheets), voice use, and swallowing particulate foods (eg, nuts, granola). She notices a cough if she uses her voice extensively or tries to project her voice. She reports that she doesn't cough if she is not moving, talking, or eating. Her cough occurs mostly during the day, but she has had infrequent nocturnal coughing episodes that wake her up at night. She describes having a momentary "warning sign" for her cough, which is a tickle in the middle of her throat. She uses her inhaler when she has coughing episodes but is unsure if this is helpful or not. Sips of water can help interrupt coughing episodes if she catches it early enough. She feels like she also clears her throat/coughs frequently throughout the day due to the feeling of excess mucus in her throat, though her cough is nonproductive. Apart from her coughing episodes, she denies dyspnea. She eats a general diet with thin liquids and denies any signs or symptoms of aspiration or pharyngeal residue; however, she does endorse consistent cough with particulate foods, which she now avoids (eg, nuts, granola). Her weight has been stable, and she denies any recent pneumonia. Although voice is not her chief concern, she does describe her voice as more "gravelly" and "froggy" than it used to be. She has not seen an SLP previously.

Medical History. Patient DW has undergone a thorough workup for chronic cough to date. She has seen a pulmonologist for evaluation, including chest x-ray, pulmonary function tests, bronchoscopy, and methacholine challenge. Although nothing definitively revealed the cause of the cough, she reports being diagnosed with "borderline asthma" and was prescribed an albuterol inhaler. She has seen an outside general otolaryngologist who performed laryngoscopy, which she reports showed "signs of silent reflux" (there was no access to this report). The otolaryngologist prescribed 20 mg of omeprazole daily. She reports no change in her cough despite taking omeprazole consistently for over 8 weeks. She has also seen an allergist and underwent allergy testing, which did not reveal the cause of cough.

Social History. Patient DW is married with 2 young children and works in human resources as a manager for a medium-sized company. She has moderate voice demands, including extensive Zoom meetings and phone calls. She reports that her coworkers have commented on her cough and are "used to" disruptive coughing during calls and meetings. She does not smoke, drinks 2 cups of coffee per day and about 32 ounces of water per day, and reports minimal alcohol intake.

Quality-of-Life Assessment

Patient DW was provided with 5 patient-based questionnaires to complete during her initial visit including the Voice Handicap Index–10 (VHI-10), Reflux Symptom Index (RSI), Eating Assessment Tool–10 (EAT-10), Dyspnea Index (DI), and Cough Severity Index (CSI).[28–32] Scores are depicted in Table 7–1.

Auditory-Perceptual Assessment

The Consensus Auditory-Perceptual Evaluation of Voice (CAPE-V) protocol was used to rate Patient DW's voice quality.[33] Ratings were based on sustaining the vowels /a/ and /i/, reading of sentences, and conversational speech. The following ratings refer to a visual analog scale of 100 mm. The patient presented

Table 7–1. Patient-Reported Outcome Measures and Scores

Patient-Reported Outcome Measure	Score
Voice Handicap Index–10 (VHI-10)	2/40
Eating Assessment Tool–10 (EAT-10)	4/40
Reflux Symptom Index (RSI)	26/40
Dyspnea Index (DI)	9/40
Cough Severity Index (CSI)	34/40

with mild dysphonia (14 mm) consistently characterized by mild roughness (13 mm) and mild-moderate strain (22 mm). Loudness was mildly increased (8 mm) and pitch was rated mildly decreased (12 mm). Decreased coordination of respiration and phonation was noted during conversation with breath-holding patterns as well as posterior tone focus and intermittent glottal fry.

Laryngeal Imaging

Laryngeal Videostroboscopy. In conjunction with the laryngologist, the SLP completed laryngeal videostroboscopy with a transnasal distal chip endoscope. During the examination protocol, the patient demonstrated normal vocal fold mobility. The vocal folds were very mildly erythematous and edematous, but no discrete lesions were noted. Glottic closure was largely complete with a small posterior glottic gap. Vibratory parameters were largely normal, with periodic vibration and normal mucosal wave but with mild phase asymmetry. There was moderate sphincteric phonatory hyperfunction noted with connected speech tasks during videostroboscopy.

Flexible Endoscopic Evaluation of Swallowing (FEES). Due to patient reports of cough triggered by certain foods, a subsequent swallowing evaluation was conducted during laryngoscopy. The Murray Secretion Scale score was 0 and no excessive mucus was noted within the larynx or pharynx.[34] Bilateral pharyngeal squeeze was observed with high-pitched /i/ and velopharyngeal closure was adequate. With thin liquids and solids trials, there was timely swallow initiation, complete whiteout, no evidence of penetration/aspiration, and no retention of bolus within the pharynx. There was no coughing during the FEES exam. Oropharyngeal swallow function was reassuring.

Stimulability

During the evaluation, DW experienced a coughing episode triggered by voice use while providing the case history. This provided an excellent opportunity to trial cough reduction strategies to assess stimulability to behavioral intervention. The SLP instructed her in a brief version of relaxed throat breathing to interrupt the acute cough episode, including exhalation on /ʃ/ and nasal inhalation with cues for shoulder release. Patient DW was able to interrupt her cough after about 15 seconds of moderate clinician cueing and demonstration. Once she gained control of her cough, she started to talk again, which led to immediate resumption of cough. With minimal cueing, she was able to interrupt the cough almost immediately and regain control of her breathing. She was then instructed not to talk but to hum gently instead. She was cued to sigh on a hum and say "mmhmm" before talking. She was able to resume providing her clinical history without inducing cough again.

Clinical Impressions

Overall, Patient DW's symptoms and evaluation results were consistent with chronic refractory cough due to laryngeal hypersensitivity as well as mild muscle tension dysphonia (MTD) contributing to patient's cough. The team explained that the etiology of her chronic cough was unclear but thought to be either neurogenic in nature following her possible URI and/or chronic exposure to noxious irritants.[35,36] Options for intervention were presented to the patient by the multidisciplinary team with primary recommendation for BCST with an SLP. Pending the results of cough suppression therapy, the use of neuromodulators or superior laryngeal nerve blocks may also be considered in the future.[37,38] The SLP reviewed the results of the evaluation with the patient, as well as the theory behind laryngeal hypersensitivity and the BCST approach to reduce laryngeal responsiveness.

Plan of Care

The team recommended that the patient complete a course of BCST with an SLP for 3 to 4 sessions over 60 days, scheduled once every 2 weeks. Patient DW preferred to participate in therapy via telehealth. The general goals of cough suppression therapy typically include (1) education, (2) laryngeal hygiene, (3) implementation of cough reduction strategies to prevent or interrupt inappropriate laryngeal motor response (cough/throat clear) in the presence or absence of triggers, and (4) psychoeducational counseling.[39]

Specific goals outlined for DW during the course of intervention were to:

1. Demonstrate understanding of chronic refractory cough and describe a theoretical framework to understand laryngeal hypersensitivity
2. Identify and minimize potential laryngeal irritants/triggers for cough
3. Utilize relaxed throat breathing to prevent or interrupt coughing episodes
4. Independently utilize cough/throat clear reduction strategies to reduce inappropriate motor reactions (ie, throat clears) in the presence or absence of triggers
5. Utilize target voice techniques to produce a more efficient voice without vocal strain to reduce cough triggered by voice use

Decision Making

Patient DW was considered an excellent candidate for BCST due to her ability to identify clear triggers and warning signs for cough, her excellent stimulability during initial evaluation, and her high level of motivation. It is common for patients with chronic refractory cough to be skeptical of a behavioral therapy approach, particularly after extensive workup with multiple medical specialists. Patients are often confused about the role of an SLP in cough management, and a high level of clinician knowledge and explanation may be needed to get "buy-in" from the patient. If possible, stimulability testing using cough suppression strategies at the initial visit can be crucial in demonstrating the efficacy of behavioral cough intervention. Although DW was initially skeptical of an SLP as part of her care team, she was highly motivated and felt confident in this approach by the end of the visit. Although the cause of DW's cough may not be clear, the team felt confident that DW could successfully participate in a behavioral cough reduction approach using principles of motor relearning to reduce the learned laryngeal motor response and promote overall laryngeal desensitization.

> Zughni mentions using principles of motor relearning to reduce the laryngeal motor response. It is well established that principles of motor learning form the basis of much of voice therapy due to the need to adapt motor behaviors. Motor learning includes principles of practice and feedback that have demonstrated success in giving the patient tools to change their aberrant motor response and regain control of behaviors believed to cause cough.

Intervention

Goal #1

DW will demonstrate understanding of chronic refractory cough and describe a theoretical framework to understand laryngeal hypersensitivity.

Rationale and Intervention. Education is a crucial aspect of behavioral intervention for chronic refractory cough. It is important for the patient to understand the normal cough reflex response and abnormal laryngeal hypersensitivity so they can reframe their thinking about their cough and emphasize voluntary control of the laryngeal response to innocuous triggers. The explanation of typical symptoms and triggers common with laryngeal hypersensitivity often encourages patient buy-in and reassurance that this is an appropriate plan of care for their particular problem. The clinician should discuss the goals of cough suppression therapy and the treatment approach, including education/counseling, laryngeal hygiene such as identifying and reducing triggers, direct cough suppression techniques and, in DW's case, voice therapy. The overarching goal of therapy is to break the cycle of laryngeal responsiveness (cough response) despite the urge to cough by utilizing cough suppression techniques (similar to suppressing the urge to scratch a mosquito bite). With time, this can lead to overall laryngeal desensitization and decreased laryngeal hypersensitivity.[36,39,40] DW quickly demonstrated understanding of this theoretical framework and the goals of therapy, which further increased her motivation to participate. This goal was largely addressed in the first therapy session, though education was woven throughout the course of therapy.

Goal #2

Identify and minimize potential laryngeal irritants/triggers for cough.

Rationale and Intervention. This is another important aspect of cough suppression therapy and includes overall laryngeal hygiene as well as personalized identification of triggers. For DW's case, identified triggers for cough included exertion, cold air, dust, smoke, strong scents, voice use, and swallowing particulate foods. DW had excellent self-awareness and identification of triggers; however, for some patients, it is necessary to explore triggers more and possibly utilize a checklist to increase awareness.[39,40] She also reported infrequent nocturnal episodes that wake her up at night, which may suggest reflux as a possible contributor to cough. The medical team recommended that she continue omeprazole during BCST to control acid reflux as a potential trigger contributing to cough. It is important to recognize comorbidities and to work with the medical team to treat any potential triggers or contributors to laryngeal hypersensitivity.[41]

The clinician recommended that DW limit caffeine intake, increase water intake, avoid smoke, and utilize a headset when speaking on Zoom calls or phone calls to reduce possible vocal strain.[42] The clinician also discussed the importance of taking voice breaks throughout the day as needed. This goal was largely addressed in the first therapy session, though, as self-awareness increases, additional irritants and triggers may be identified throughout the course of therapy.

> The author points out an important point for the treating clinician. Patients often lack self-awareness of triggers and precough sensations when they enter therapy. Once patients develop an internal locus of control and become aware of trigger sensations to reduce coughing, they may realize that there are additional triggers for their cough and/or additional precough sensations. The clinician is guided to iteratively check with their patients about cough discoveries between sessions.

Goal #3

DW will utilize relaxed throat breathing to prevent or interrupt coughing episodes.

Rationale and Intervention. Relaxed throat breathing techniques are a hallmark of behavioral intervention for patients with chronic cough. The goal of relaxed throat breathing is to focus on expiration rather than inspiration, transfer any airway resistance from the larynx to the oral cavity, and encourage an overall more relaxed laryn-

geal posture.[36,39] Relaxed throat breathing was initially instructed at rest in the absence of triggers during the first therapy session. (See Video 20 Relaxed Throat Breathing by Slovarp.) Although DW responded best during the evaluation with exhalation on /ʃ/, this technique was modified during therapy sessions to a more traditional quick-release breathing technique including pursed lip exhalation with gentle nasal inhalation. This led to the same "open throat" feeling for DW and was less conspicuous in everyday use. The SLP instructed her to begin with pursed lip exhalation to create resistance to airflow. After 4 to 5 seconds, she would gently inhale through her nose for 1 to 2 seconds without holding her breath. She was cued for abdominal breathing and shoulder release to reduce laryngeal tension. Once she was able to demonstrate this technique independently in the absence of triggers, known triggers were introduced including mild scents, physical activity, and particulate foods during the second and third therapy sessions. The SLP instructed DW to begin relaxed throat breathing prior to the introduction of triggers and to continue with the breathing technique despite the presence of triggers. Her successes and limitations with the techniques depending on the trigger and situation were discussed to create a personalized plan for DW. She noted the most success using quick-release breathing techniques in combination with sips of water. With sips of water trials, she was instructed to swallow with her chin slightly tucked and then exhale with pursed lips, and to continue the breathing technique until the tickle in her throat diminished. She continued these desensitization trials independently, which improved her confidence and voluntary control of the cough response. By her third session, DW reported more confidence and success using the techniques. She was able to consistently swallow problem foods without any urge to cough and had reduced the overall frequency, duration, and severity of her coughing episodes in the presence of triggers using the above techniques. DW was able to independently prevent coughing in the presence of triggers with 85% accuracy during her third therapy session. In the one desensitization trial that she was not able to prevent, she was able to successfully interrupt the cough within 3 seconds using cough suppression techniques.

Goal #4

The patient will independently utilize cough/throat clear reduction strategies to reduce inappropriate motor reactions (ie, throat clears) in the presence or absence of triggers. (See Video 19 Throat Clearing Reduction Strategies by Zughni.)

Rationale and Intervention. Patient DW's frequent throat clears throughout the day were approached separately from her cough episodes. The SLP taught DW strategies to replace or suppress throat clearing, including (1) sips of water, (2) humming, and (3) relaxed throat breathing.[39] DW was encouraged to take a sip of water using an effortful swallow with her chin tucked at the first urge to clear her throat. This posture reduces entrance to the airway and effortful swallow increases pharyngeal contraction, which may lead to increased sensory input during the swallow. The SLP also instructed DW in gentle humming using a barely adducted laryngeal posture to focus on anterior oral vibrations rather than vocal strain.[43] Last, the previously instructed relaxed throat breathing promotes a more relaxed and open laryngeal posture and helps suppress throat clearing. These strategies were taught during the first therapy session and DW responded best to a combination of these strategies. She felt that a sip of water followed by relaxed throat breathing was the most effective for her. If she needed to speak while still feeling a tickle in her throat, she hummed or said "mmhmm" to shift the focus from her throat to the front of her face while voicing. The SLP instructed her to suppress or even delay her throat clear response using these techniques with the goal of reducing the over-

all frequency of throat clearing throughout the day. With time, this reduction in frequency of laryngeal response is thought to lead to lower laryngeal hypersensitivity.[36,39,40] It's important to set realistic expectations for patients that the urge to cough or throat clear will not go away immediately—it takes conscious effort and time to reduce laryngeal reactivity prior to feeling a reduction in the urge to clear their throat. By DW's third session, she felt that she had reduced her throat clearing frequency by about 50%. The clinician noted a 75% reduction in frequency of throat clearing during the therapy session compared to the first therapy session.

Goal #5

The patient will utilize target voice techniques to use a more efficient voice without vocal strain to reduce cough triggered by voice use.

Rationale and Intervention. Although the voice was not a complaint for DW, it needed to be addressed as a main trigger for her cough. The goal was to improve efficiency of voice use in everyday conversation to decrease phonatory hyperfunction as a potential cause of her cough. The first step was increasing DW's self-awareness of vocal strain. This started in the first therapy session during instruction of gentle humming as a throat clear reduction strategy. With voice exploration using principles of resonant voice therapy (RVT), DW was eventually able to sense anterior oral vibrations within her lips while producing an easy voice with /m/ (many cases use RVT techniques for therapy. Case Study 3.7 by Orbelo, Li, and Verdolini Abbott discusses a systematic approach to resonant voice therapy, Lessac-Madsen Resonant Voice Therapy LMRVT). She utilized negative practice to increase her awareness of vocal strain triggering her cough. She was able to reproduce a tickle in her throat while using negative practice (which DW labeled as her "old" voice compared to her target "easy" voice). This clearly illuminated the impact vocal strain had on

DW's cough. During the second therapy session, she quickly advanced to conversational voice use by using principles of Conversation Training Therapy (see Case Study 3.1 by Gartner-Schmidt and Gillespie on Conversation Training Therapy).[44] For DW, the goal of voice therapy wasn't to produce a "perfect" voice, as this was not her chief complaint. Rather, the goal was to reduce strain and posterior tone focus, as this was considered the trigger for her cough. She was able to use her "easy" voice with attention to crisp, clear articulation and the mouthfeel of certain consonants as well as negative practice to solidify her control of the target voice during conversation. If she started to feel a tickle in her throat while talking, she could easily "recalibrate" with "mmhmm" or humming and maintain the target voice using these techniques. By the end of the third session, DW was able to maintain her target voice in conversation with 80% accuracy for at least 10 minutes at a time, requiring minimal clinician cueing and independent brief recalibration with dedicated humming.

Therapy Outcome

Patient DW underwent 3 sessions of cough suppression therapy over 6 weeks. She messaged the clinician to cancel her last session of cough suppression therapy, as she reported significant improvement at that time. She felt like she was "at least 80% better" overall and continuing to make progress. She mentioned that her coworkers had even commented on her lack of cough/throat clearing during meetings. She felt that she was able to voluntarily control both the frequency and severity of her cough and reported less mental effort to reduce laryngeal response. Although her cough wasn't 100% resolved at this point, she was very happy with her progress and felt confident that she had the tools at her disposal to practice independently and continue to make progress on her own. She was discharged from formal therapy.

During her follow-up appointment with the laryngologist, 3 months following the original evaluation and 6 weeks following the end of therapy, she demonstrated continued improvement as evidenced by the change in her patient-reported outcome measures (Table 7–2). As such, she was not interested in further medical or surgical interventions for cough. DW was encouraged to reach out in the future with any questions or concerns or for a refresher session of BCST as needed. Like many patients with chronic refractory cough, BCST was a crucial and effective treatment option for DW, and SLPs should consider themselves an integral part of the care team for this patient population.

Table 7–2. Posttherapy Patient-Reported Outcome Measures and Scores

Patient-Reported Outcome Measure	Score
Voice Handicap Index–10 (VHI-10)	0/40
Eating Assessment Tool–10 (EAT-10)	1/40
Reflux Symptom Index (RSI)	6/40
Dyspnea Index (DI)	3/40
Cough Severity Index (CSI)	6/40

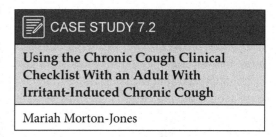

CASE STUDY 7.2

Using the Chronic Cough Clinical Checklist With an Adult With Irritant-Induced Chronic Cough

Mariah Morton-Jones

Voice Evaluation

Chief Complaint. Cough. This patient was seen in person at the multidisciplinary clinic for a comprehensive upper airway evaluation. She was seen by the laryngologist and SLP on the same day and was diagnosed with irritant-induced chronic refractory cough.

Case History

Patient KM is a 41-year-old cisgender female that reports a 2-year history of cough. The cough originally began after a common cold, which occurred shortly after starting her new job as a quality control inspector for an automobile plant that makes parts for major car companies. The cough was initially productive, producing a thick yellowish, greenish mucus. Additional symptoms included sneezing, nasal congestion, and a scratchy throat. She took over-the-counter cold medicine, which reportedly cleared up the majority of her symptoms, including the stuffy nose, sneezing, and thick mucus; however, the cough symptoms persisted and the cough became a dry cough as other symptoms resolved. On the day of the evaluation, she reported that the cough was present initially when she was at her desk and when entering the manufacturing area of the plant, where car parts are being assembled. She reported that she is able to suppress the cough when at her desk but that the coughing episodes occur throughout the entire day and last for nearly 1 minute. She endorsed a tickle feeling in her throat prior to coughing. Her job requires her to walk through the manufacturing area of the car plant, which contains a significant amount of dust, debris, chemicals, noise, and cold air. She also noticed the cough worsened when attempting to have conversations with coworkers in the car plant, a noisy environment.

The patient reports no medical comorbidities and denied a smoking history, dyspnea, and dysphagia.

KM was first seen by her primary care provider and given an inhaler without benefit and was subsequently seen by an allergist and reported that the results were unremarkable. KM lived in a rural community and visited the ear, nose, and throat doctor (ENT) in the neighboring county. The ENT prescribed her gabapentin, which reportedly improved symptoms for 3 months; however, she was unsure of the dosage. After 3 months, the medication stopped working and started causing drowsiness. As time progressed, she would avoid talking with family members after returning home from work because of persistent cough lasting for several hours after leaving her job. KM underwent a gastrointestinal (GI) evaluation and had been taking omeprazole for mild GERD symptoms for many years, with no change in cough symptoms. She previously benefited from Flonase, but reported it was no longer effective since starting her new position as a quality control inspector. After discontinuing use of the gabapentin, KM was seen by a local pulmonologist and underwent PFT, all of which was unremarkable. The pulmonologist then referred KM to the specialized cough clinic within the multidisciplinary voice center in her state, which is nearly 3 hours away from her rural community.

Given that the patient's cough triggers were potentially related to her rural home environment and work environment in the automobile industry,[45,46] there was suspicion for exposure to specific irritants not as common in urban and metropolitan areas. The Irritant-Induced Occupational Exposures Chronic Cough Clinical Checklist[47] was used to assess for exposure to such triggers. Identifying environmental and occupational triggers can be crucial for laryngeal desensitization and may assist in supporting cough suppression strategies.[48]

The Chronic Cough Clinical Checklist is a comprehensive list of nearly 220 documented cough irritants categorized by general environmental exposures and occupational exposures. Use of the checklist is beneficial to ensure a comprehensive cough assessment is completed, especially for patients such as KM with a complex work environment exposing her to numerous extrinsic and intrinsic agents that may be less obvious or well known, especially to early-career clinicians with emerging expertise and experience with treating cough. It may also assist patients in providing a more accurate and comprehensive history if they

292 Voice Therapy: Clinical Case Studies

have never been asked or thought about their cough as irritant induced.

The SLP asked the patient to review the checklist and to determine if any of the listed irritants were possible triggers. With such prompting, KM was able to identify that dust (road dust), debris, oil mist and straight cutting oil exposure, and vehicle exhaust were triggers for her cough (Figure 7–1).[48]

Laryngeal Imaging

Laryngeal videostroboscopy performed transnasally with a flexible distal chip videolaryngoscope revealed postcricoid edema. However, no supraglottal, hypopharyngeal, or vocal fold masses or lesions were present. Bilateral vocal fold adduction and abduction were fully intact with complete glottal closure. Mucosal wave, amplitude of lateral excursion, and periodicity were intact bilaterally. No supraglottic hyperfunction was present.

Vocal Effort, Fatigue, and Pain

The OMNI Vocal Effort Scale (OMNI-VES)[49] was completed. The patient rated vocal effort on a 0 to 10 scale where 0 = "extremely easy" to produce voice and 10 = "extremely hard" to produce voice. The patient reported that vocal effort was 0/10 during the evaluation and 2/10 at worst, occurring at the end of the day, attributed solely to the amount of coughing that occurred during the day.

Patient-Reported Quality-of-Life Impairment

1. VHI-10: 0 (threshold = 11)[28,50]
2. DI: 0 (threshold = 4)[31]
3. CSI: 26 (threshold = 5)[32]
4. Glottal Function Index: 0 (threshold = 5)[51]
5. EAT-10: 0 (threshold = 3)[30]

Auditory-Perceptual Assessment

The CAPE-V[33] was administered. The patient was determined to have an overall CAPE-V score of 15/100, indicating a dysphonia of a mild nature. Aberrant perceptual features identified in the voice included mild roughness. Overall vocal loudness was noted to be within normal limits (WNL). Pitch of the voice was WNL for age and gender as well as com-

---

General Exposures
  Smoke/smoking/tobacco use
    ☑ Second-hand tobacco smoke (e.g. cigarettes)

  Fumes/perfumes/scents/odors/fragrance
    ☑ Car exhaust

Occupational Exposures
  Dust/debris
    ☑ Road dust

  Oil exposure
    ☑ Oil mist

    ☑ Straight cutting oils

FIGURE 7–1. Patient KM's cough trigger inventory.

fortable according to the patient report. Resonance was forward focused. Respiration was primarily abdominal-thoracic.

Manual Palpation Assessment

Muscle tension was assessed following a 1-minute coughing episode that occurred during the evaluation and was rated on a 0 to 5 scale where 0 = "no tension" and 5 = "most tension." Results indicated:

1. 2/5 tension at the thyrohyoid space without report of pain
2. 0/5 tension at the base of tongue (BOT)/suprahyoid region without report of pain
3. 2/5 restriction of lateralization of thyroid cartilage bilaterally

Acoustic and Aerodynamic Assessment

Acoustic and aerodynamic assessment measures were not obtained, given the lack of voice complaints and only mild auditory-perceptual dysphonia (15/100 on the CAPE-V), as well as the recent unremarkable PFT completed by the outside pulmonologist. Results revealed vital capacity, forced vital capacity, and inspiratory flows were WNL, indicating no concerns for pulmonary restriction or lung disease underlying the cough.

Impressions

Following the comprehensive evaluation, it appeared the patient presented with an irritant-induced RCC that began after starting a job at a new automobile manufacturing plant, impacting all aspects of her life. The patient's verbalized eagerness, motivation, and attentiveness to resolve her cough symptoms were strong indicators that may assist with her success in behavioral management.

Decision Making and Plan of Care

Given that allergy, GI, and pulmonology testing were unremarkable, and that subsequent prescribed medications and inhalers were used with no improvement, KM's symptoms were determined to be related to chronic refractory cough. The treatment options were discussed, specifically the benefits of behavioral cough suppression and respiratory retraining therapy.[52] The efficacy of BCST via teletherapy was discussed given that the patient lives in a rural area nearly 3 hours from the clinic.[53] Following some additional counseling from the SLP and laryngologist, KM decided that she would begin BCST via teletherapy. Therapy was recommended for a total duration of 2 months, with an anticipated 3 to 5 sessions of 45 minutes each, occurring once every 2 weeks.

> Telehealth access exponentially expanded out of necessity during the COVID-19 pandemic in 2020. Studies have demonstrated that certain therapies delivered via telehealth can be just as effective as when delivered in person. Here, the author quotes a study from 2022, and an even more recent scoping review in 2024 demonstrated that BCST provided via telehealth is effective.[54]

Goals:

1. Provide psychoeducational counseling to the patient on irritant-induced chronic cough and describe the theoretical framework to better understand laryngeal hypersensitivity.
2. The patient will increase awareness of irritant cough triggers by logging specific situations, times, and days when the cough is most severe with assistance from the Occupational Exposures on the Chronic Cough Clinical Checklist.
3. The patient will increase hydration and implement the trained breathing strategies and cough suppression techniques when she feels the tickle sensation to replace the coughing behavior and reduce laryngeal irritation.

Intervention: Behavioral Cough Suppression Therapy (BCST)

Session #1

Goal #1. *Provide psychoeducational counseling to the patient on irritant-induced RCC and describe the theoretical framework to better understand the laryngeal hypersensitivity.*

Health beliefs, learning, and expectations from BCST may influence upper airway sensory responses.[55] Therefore, behavioral management began with psychoeducational counseling in which the SLP not only explained irritant-induced chronic refractory cough and laryngeal hypersensitivity, but also listened to the patient's health beliefs and goals for behavioral intervention.

The SLP provided education on irritant-induced chronic refractory cough as well as the objectives and benefits of BCST. They discussed, through use of visual aids, that there are many receptors on the outer epithelial layer of the upper airway. Such receptors send signals to the brain to elicit cough when harmful stimuli are present, such as smoke, fumes, food, or liquid.[56,57] The SLP explained that this type of cough is beneficial and serves as a protective mechanism for the larynx. The clinician also explained that persistent cough may perpetuate hypersensitivity, causing overstimulation and leading to continued cough when not needed or in the presence of minimal amounts of an irritant that are typically tolerable. Through thorough discussion, counseling, and education, the SLP worked with the patient to understand that, at this point, behavioral modifications to suppress the cough are possible, not harmful, and necessary to reduce laryngeal hypersensitivity and persistent disruptive cough. KM and the clinician discussed that various breathing strategies and suppression techniques would be introduced to replace the behavior. KM demonstrated understanding that, given her extensive workup with the allergist, GI, and pulmonologist, she did not have a condition causing the cough that could be treated with medication. KM expressed eagerness to continue the therapeutic process. Although this patient demonstrated buy-in during the evaluation and initial session, some patients may need additional counseling or education.

Goal #2. *The patient will increase awareness of irritant cough triggers by logging specific situations, times, and days when the cough is most severe with assistance from the Occupational Exposures on the Chronic Cough Clinical Checklist.*

The remainder of the first session was spent in discussion revisiting the occupational exposures of the Chronic Cough Clinical Checklist initially filled out during the evaluation. The clinician asked KM to check if there were any additional triggers she noticed since the evaluation. The clinician also encouraged the patient to take the checklist with her, mark any other triggers she discovered, and log daily situations, times, or days when the cough occurred in relation to the marked triggers. KM determined that keeping a log in the Notes application of her iPhone was easiest and decided she would email her log and notes to the clinician at the beginning of each session.

BCST progressed to discussing feasible ways to avoid certain locations at her place of employment where the identified irritants were in abundance. Given that secondhand smoke was an identified trigger, KM and the clinician determined that she could use a different entrance into the building to avoid the designated smoking area for employees.

> Initially, it is often wise to encourage patients to avoid situations where cough triggers are known, as the author recommends in this case. As therapy advances, gradual reexposure to these situations can be trialed.

Goal #3. *The patient will increase hydration and implement the trained breathing strate-*

gies and cough suppression techniques when she feels the tickle sensation to replace the coughing behavior and reduce laryngeal irritation.

Relaxed throat breathing strategies were first trained to promote maximal abduction of the vocal folds (maximal activation of the posterior cricoarytenoid muscle) and to prevent forceful adduction of the vocal folds that occurs with coughing. KM was trained in sniff inhalation with either 1 or 2 sniffs to promote maximal abduction, followed by exhalation via fricative consonants (/s/ or /ʃ/) or pursed lips. The clinician cued the patient to think of an "open throat" while practicing the trained breathing strategy several times. By the conclusion of the first session, KM demonstrated preventing the cough twice with the breathing technique. The SLP encouraged the patient to practice the trained breathing techniques regularly throughout her day as well as when she knows she will be entering an area of the automobile plant where the irritants are present. The SLP also addressed the importance of sipping water regularly throughout her day and specifically when she feels the urge to cough. (See Video 20 Relaxed Throat Breathing by Slovarp.)

Session #2

Goal #2. *The patient will increase awareness of irritant cough triggers by logging specific situations, times, and days when the cough is most severe with assistance from the Occupational Exposures on the Chronic Cough Clinical Checklist.*

KM reported that the office's break room shares a wall with the outside designated smoking area for employees and if she sat at the table next to the wall, her cough symptoms worsened. Getting through her lunch and 15-minute breaks without coughing was challenging. It was discussed that KM would try sitting on the opposite side of the break room during lunchtime and breaks.

Goal #3. *The patient will increase hydration and implement the trained breathing strate-*

gies and cough suppression techniques when she feels the tickle sensation to replace the coughing behavior and reduce laryngeal irritation.

The clinician encouraged the patient to be as diligent as possible during the session by using the hard sip of water, dry swallow, or trained breathing strategy when she felt the urge to cough. KM was then trained in an additional relaxed throat breathing strategy in which she exhaled through a straw. It was important to practice all options for exhalation during the session and give KM the agency and autonomy to select which breathing technique was most comfortable. KM was observed to intermittently use a significant amount of upper extremity and shoulder movement with inhalation, suggestive of laryngeal tension and possible shallow breathing with the trained technique. KM was cued to reduce her effort with inhalation and was reminded that the sniffs alone will provide maximum vocal fold opening. Given that BCST was occurring via teletherapy, the SLP cued KM to watch her shoulder movement in the video as she practiced the breathing. She was then able to complete multiple repetitions with visual cues and minimal clinician cueing. KM then reported that 2 sniffs following exhalation through the straw was most relaxing. She was encouraged to use this technique when possible, keeping a straw at her desk for practice.

Session #3

Goal #2. *The patient will increase awareness of irritant cough triggers by logging specific situations, times, and days when the cough is most severe with assistance from the Occupational Exposures on the Chronic Cough Clinical Checklist.*

At the start of the third session, KM reported that entering a different door alleviated the cough in the morning because she was able to avoid the smoking area. KM also reported that it was helpful to sit near the opposite wall of the break room and take regular sips of water. The clinician encouraged her

296 Voice Therapy: Clinical Case Studies

to continue to use these strategies to reduce irritant exposure.

Goal #3. *The patient will increase hydration and implement the trained breathing strategies and cough suppression techniques when she feels the tickle sensation to replace the coughing behavior and reduce laryngeal irritation.*

Exhalation through the straw was advanced to straw phonation as a semi-occluded vocal tract exercise. (See Video 28 Straw Phonation in Water Hierarchy by Codino.) The SLP educated the patient on how to achieve respiratory phonatory coordination. Initially, KM found phonation through the straw challenging, suggestive of possible breath-holding behaviors and laryngeal tension. The clinician cued KM to place her hand in front of the straw to feel the gentle airflow on her hand and encouraged her to maintain such airflow through phonation. KM was then able to complete short periods of sustained phonation with greater ease and focus on an "open throat" posture. KM and the clinician discussed that the ability to have a straw with her at all times would pose a challenge during her workday, but that practice at her desk was possible. KM was encouraged to determine 1 additional form of exhalation to use when the straw was not available. She noted that the /s/ exhalation was also comfortable and was encouraged to use such breathing techniques.

Given that she was unable to avoid the manufacturing area of the car plant due to her work as a quality control inspector, the SLP encouraged KM to wear her mask in those areas and to implement her breathing techniques with 2 sniffs and fricative exhalation. The SLP also introduced the use of nonmedicated and nonmenthol lozenges she could suck on regularly throughout the day, even when in the manufacturing plant.

Session #4

This session was scheduled nearly 1 month out to ensure maintenance of trained strategies and reduced cough symptoms.

Goal #2. *The patient will increase awareness of irritant cough triggers by logging specific situations, times, and days when the cough is most severe with assistance from the Occupational Exposures on the Chronic Cough Clinical Checklist.*

The clinician revisited the Chronic Cough Clinical Checklist that KM initially filled out during the evaluation and first session. KM was able to note which triggers were no longer an issue and which triggers she was able to manage with trained strategies. It was critical during the final session that the patient was able to verbalize and demonstrate independently which techniques and strategies she implemented to reduce exposure and avoid laryngeal irritation. The clinical checklist was beneficial as an outcome measure, visually demonstrating to the patient and clinician previously identified irritants and an opportunity to discuss if exposure to the known irritants is no longer triggering due to reduced hypersensitivity of the upper airway.

Goal #3. *The patient will increase hydration and implement the trained breathing strategies and cough suppression techniques when she feels the tickle sensation to replace the coughing behavior and reduce laryngeal irritation.*

By the final session, the clinician noted that the patient was able to suppress and prevent the cough by either performing breathing techniques, taking a sip of water, or wearing her mask in areas with significant debris. KM reported her cough symptoms had reduced by 85%.

Treatment Results and Summary

KM successfully moved through the described therapy in 4 sessions. Throughout the progression of the therapeutic process, KM also implemented the breathing techniques, increased her water intake regularly throughout her day, began sucking on nonmedicated lozenges, and inhaled steam in the evenings. Through her dedicated home practice, by the final visit,

KM reported that use of the breathing techniques or lozenges in conjunction with wearing her mask in manufacturing areas reduced her cough by nearly 95%, which for KM was a success. The laryngeal hypersensitivity decreased significantly and KM reported that the occasional times she would walk by the designated smoking area no longer triggered a cough response.

BCST was successful in reducing KM's irritant-induced cough. Given the patient's complex environmental and occupational exposures, use of the Chronic Cough Clinical Checklist during the evaluation to identify irritants and in the final therapy session as an outcome measure to assess progress was beneficial for both KM and the SLP.

CASE STUDY 7.3

Behavioral Cough Suppression Therapy for an Adult With Underlying Respiratory Disease

Laurie Slovarp

Evaluation

Chief Complaint. This patient was referred by her pulmonologist, who diagnosed her with restrictive and obstructive lung disease and chronic cough.

History of Upper Airway Complaint

Patient DS is a 73-year-old cisgender woman who was referred by her pulmonologist for chronic cough. DS reported her cough started over 30 years ago with no apparent cause except that she recalled having "laryngitis" for about a week prior to the onset of the cough. She had been to multiple specialists for numerous tests and treatments for her cough, including chest CT scan, videostroboscopy, PFT, bronchoscopy, allergy testing, and a modified barium swallow study. She was eventually diagnosed with mixed restrictive and obstructive lung disease. Her pulmonary records indicated her lung disease was fairly well managed, yet her cough had persisted. Prior treatments for her cough included reflux medications, various nasal sprays, saline nasal rinses, several different inhalers, codeine, Tessalon Perles, and gabapentin. Codeine relieved her cough but was not a long-term solution due to dependency risk and side effects. She did not tolerate the side effects of gabapentin.

> Restrictive lung diseases are those that make it difficult to expand the lungs, resulting in reduced lung volume. Pulmonary fibrosis is an example of a restrictive lung disease. Other examples include interstitial lung disease and sarcoidosis. Obstructive lung diseases are those that make it difficult to exhale all the air out of the lungs. Emphysema, chronic bronchitis, chronic obstructive pulmonary disease (COPD), and asthma are all examples of obstructive lung diseases.

She stated her cough was productive approximately 50% of the time (worse in the morning), producing thick, sticky mucus that she would either expectorate or swallow. The rest of her coughs were dry and often led to severe bouts, sometimes to the point of gagging. She usually experienced an urge to cough (UTC) in her throat before the dry coughs, which she described as a tickle or itch. She occasionally produced mucus at the end of a coughing bout but it was not as thick or sticky as the morning coughing. She reported the dry coughing bouts occurred daily and were the most impactful to her quality of life as they frequently disrupted conversation, caused urinary incontinence, and prevented her from attending many social events such as church, yoga class, and the theater. She reported her cough was often triggered by strong fragrances such as perfumes or scented soaps, the smell of smoke, cold air, and talking or laughing. She

Voice Therapy: Clinical Case Studies

also stated if she used a Q-tip in her left ear, it caused coughing.

> The ear-cough reflex is also known as Arnold's nerve cough reflex and is more prevalent in individuals with chronic cough than those without chronic cough.[58] It occurs when manipulation of the outer ear, as in using a Q-tip, stimulates the auricular branch of the vagus nerve.

DS's medical history included obstructive sleep apnea (adequately managed with continuous positive airway pressure [CPAP]) and GERD. She did not experience heartburn as long as she took her reflux medication (20 mg pantoprazole before breakfast and dinner). She was very adherent with the medication. She also reported occasional dysphonia and exertional dyspnea. She stated that it was usually more difficult to breathe in than out during her dyspnea and that her breathing was noisy. She denied symptoms of postnasal drip or dysphagia.

Laryngeal Hygiene. >64 ounces of water daily, 1 cup of coffee every morning, 40 pack-year, meaning they have smoked on average 1 pack (20 cigarettes) per day for 40 years, history of smoking until quitting 16 years prior; no history of alcohol or recreational drug use; no remarkable phonotraumatic behaviors other than coughing

Laryngeal Imaging

Laryngeal videostroboscopy was performed transorally with a rigid laryngoscope.

Salient Examination Findings. No supraglottal, hypopharyngeal, or laryngeal masses; full abduction and adduction of both vocal folds; complete glottal closure; mild vocal fold edema and erythema; copious sticky, lightly colored thick mucus throughout the larynx; mucosal wave and amplitude appeared slightly reduced, but this was difficult to assess

fully due to presence of the mucus; other stroboscopic parameters appeared grossly WNL.

Patient-Reported Outcome Measures

1. **Leicester Cough Questionnaire (LCQ)**[59]: A validated survey of cough whereby patients rate 19 items from "never" to "always" regarding their perception of cough-related quality-of-life impact. Lower scores indicate greater impact on quality of life. A score of 17/21 or higher is considered WNL.
   - Physical score: 3.88
   - Psychological score: 4.00
   - Social score: 3.41
   - Total score: 11.29 (indicative of significant negative impact of cough on quality of life)
2. **VHI-10**[28]: 14/40 (threshold = 11)[50]

Auditory-Perceptual Assessment

The CAPE-V[33] was administered with an overall score of 17/100, indicating mild dysphonia. Aberrant perceptual features identified in the voice included primary roughness (15/100) during conversation and primary strain (15/100) during sustained phonation.

Sustained Phonation. 8 seconds due to interruption from cough; strained quality

Observational/Perceptual Speaking Assessment

Respiratory and speech patterns were assessed while the patient read the Rainbow Passage. Aberrant features included thoracic breathing pattern with intermittent breath holding and consistently audible inhalation (moderate severity).

Laryngeal Palpation

The patient reported mild tenderness in the left hyoid cornu. Laryngeal lateralization was slightly reduced. Moderate suprahyoid muscular tension was present.

Urge-to-Cough (UTC) Assessment

The patient rates 0 ("no urge") to 10 ("very, very strong urge")[18] after a 15-second exposure to smells/odors from household items (eg, laundry soap) and completing vocal and respiratory tasks. The UTC Assessment is an unvalidated assessment; however, anecdotal evidence indicates it is a useful tool if any of the tasks elicit coughing, as it suggests cough hypersensitivity. Since the assessment is not validated, and because symptoms of cough hypersensitivity vary widely across patients, it should never be used as a sole basis for diagnosing cough hypersensitivity. It can be helpful for testing stimulability to cough suppression, challenging the patient in cough suppression in future sessions, and assessing treatment progress (Table 7–3).

Acoustic and Aerodynamic Assessment

Aerodynamic assessment equipment was not available. Acoustic assessment was not completed because it was not deemed necessary for determining a treatment plan or for assessing progress in this patient, whose dysphonia was mild and not a primary complaint.

> Note that there are differences of opinion regarding assessment for cough among several of the authors. Several have indicated that a full voice evaluation was conducted since voicing/talking were triggers for cough. In this case, the author reports it was not necessary to complete the instrumental acoustic and aerodynamic assessment as it would not change the treatment. The American Speech-Language-Hearing Association (ASHA) practice portal indicates there are no standard guidelines for evaluation or treatment, only recommendations. The clinician is guided to use good clinical judgement in choosing evaluation methods and to have sound rationale for what to include or not include in their assessments. The clinician is also guided to review the article titled *Recommended Protocols for Instrumental Assessment of Voice: American Speech-Language-Hearing Association Expert Panel to Develop a Protocol for Instrumental Assessment of Vocal Function* by Patel et al (2018).[60]

Table 7–3. Urge to Cough (UTC) Assessment Results

Stimulant	*UTC Score*	*Cough Count*
Baseline	0	0
Chlorine Bleach	2	1
Perfume	4	4
Dry Laundry Soap	3	1
Gasping Breathe In ×2	2	1
Sustained Phonation	1	0
Reading the Rainbow Passage	3	3
Sustained Phonation	2	2
Projecting Voice	1	0

Stimulability

After instruction in relaxed throat breathing for cough suppression (the author calls this *cough-control breathing* when describing it to the patient for face validity purposes), DS was able to fully suppress her cough when exposed to the smell of bleach and laundry soap. (See Video 20 Relaxed Throat Breathing by Slovarp.) She was able to limit coughing to 1 cough when exposed to perfume. She was also given brief instruction in relaxed phonation, which she practiced during sustained phonation. This consisted simply of cueing her to relax and to let her air out rather than push it out. Within a minute or so of practicing, she was able to sustain phonation for over 15 seconds with less strain in her voice and no coughing. She was also instructed in quiet breathing while breathing through her mouth. Although she struggled to make her breathing completely silent, she was able to greatly reduce the sound of her breathing. After practicing quiet breathing through her mouth, the SLP encouraged her to try it through her nose and to focus on feeling slight air turbulence at the nares. Focusing on the feel of airflow distal to the larynx tends to help keep the vocal tract open and relaxed so that airflow is maximized. This can be helpful during nasal breathing when it is more difficult to hear glottal constriction. DS commented she had never noticed how loud or tight her breathing was even at rest. She also commented that taking in a deep breath through her mouth without noise felt less irritating in her throat and less likely to lead to a UTC.

Impressions

DS's symptoms suggested CHS as the cause for her dry coughing bouts.[18] The primary indicators of CHS included (1) dry coughing bouts preceded by UTC in the throat that can be severe enough to cause gagging; (2) UTC and cough elicited by exposure to fragrances, cold air, and phonation; and (3) cough elicited with stimulation of the left ear canal. This is known as Arnold's nerve cough reflex and is also a sign of hypersensitivity of the vagus nerve and consistent with a diagnosis of CHS.[61] Although DS was diagnosed with restrictive and obstructive lung disease, which certainly contributed to her cough, cough hypersensitivity commonly co-occurs with inflammatory lung conditions, and was likely making her cough worse.[24,62] Although full recovery of the cough was not expected given her pulmonary condition, BCST was expected to help minimize cough hypersensitivity and maximize cough control.

DS also had mild dysphonia characterized by a mildly rough and strained voice quality. Mild vocal fold edema and erythema were observed on videostroboscopy, which were suspected to be due to persistent phonotrauma from the cough. The edema was likely the cause of the roughness in her voice but the strain in her voice suggested a component of MTD. Her response to stimulability for relaxed phonation indicated her coughing triggered by talking was likely due to the MTD.

DS also presented with intermittent exertional dyspnea characterized by more difficulty breathing in than out and noisy breathing. This suggested a possible component of inducible laryngeal obstruction (ILO). Audible inhalation was observed consistently throughout the session, even at rest, indicating her glottis was likely slightly constricted at all, or nearly all, times. This meant that her vocal folds were frequently in the line of airflow, which was likely contributing to dehydration of the vocal folds and exacerbation of laryngeal irritation.

Readiness and Prognosis

DS's distress over her persistent cough and its detrimental effects on her quality of life indicated she was ready for therapy. The results of the stimulability testing were encouraging, pointing to a favorable prognosis for reducing her dry cough. It is important to note that the primary objective of the treatment was not to address her productive cough directly; however, by diminishing overall cough frequency, it was anticipated that the reduction in laryngeal irritation and inflammation would decrease her productive cough episodes.

Plan of Care

BCST[9] with inclusion of resonant voice principles for up to 5 sessions was recommended.

Long-Term Goals:

1. The patient will score at least 15 on the LCQ from a baseline of 11.29.
2. The patient will be able to attend at least 2 social events (eg, church, yoga class, a movie) without having to leave the room because of her cough.
3. The patient will experience 0 severe coughing bouts for at least 5 days in a row.
4. The patient will score no more than 11 on the VHI-10 from a baseline of 14.

Short-Term Goals:

1. The patient will explain CHS and the rationale for BCST with no more than minimal assistance.
2. The patient will be able to fully suppress dry cough in at least 50% of opportunities.
3. The patient will be able to minimize dry cough severity in at least 80% of opportunities where she is not able to fully prevent her cough.
4. The patient will use quiet breathing at least 80% of the time throughout each therapy session with no more than minimal cues.
5. The patient will be able to read the Rainbow Passage without UTC or cough.

Decision Making

Several factors influenced clinical decision making and prognosis in this case. Since suppressing a productive cough is contraindicated, the therapy plan focused strictly on the dry cough and included education about how to discriminate dry from productive cough. Fortunately, this was not difficult for her since her dry cough was nearly always preceded by a UTC in the throat. She was instructed to pay close attention to this feeling and implement a cough suppression strategy at the slightest increase in UTC. Since she presented with a strained voice that elicited coughing during sustained phonation, the plan included instruction in resonant voice. The therapy plan also included respiratory retraining to address glottic constriction and reduce audible inhalation, which was suspected to be contributing to laryngeal irritation. Breathing with the vocal folds in a slightly closed position can be very drying and exacerbate irritation so it was important to address this. Additionally, performing cough-control breathing techniques with a constricted glottis had the potential to worsen laryngeal irritation and trigger UTC, which would likely worsen the cough rather than be helpful. The patient had a pulmonary condition that contributed to her cough. This influenced 2 factors:

1. **Prognosis.** Since BCST is not expected to treat a chronic pulmonary disease, full resolution of her cough was not expected. However, given that she was stimulable for cough suppression in the initial visit, and that her primary complaint was about dry coughing bouts, her prognosis for improvement was excellent. A conservative LCQ score of 15 was set as the long-term goal, due to her pulmonary disease, rather than the normal threshold of approximately 17.
2. **Treatment Planning.** Since suppressing a productive cough is contraindicated, it was important to focus strictly on the dry cough and include education about how to discriminate dry from productive cough.

302   Voice Therapy: Clinical Case Studies

Intervention

Goal #1

Goal #1. *The patient will explain CHS and the rationale for BCST with no more than minimal assistance.*

This goal was addressed during the initial assessment session via verbal education and a written handout. Verbal education went something like, "*Your symptoms suggest you have a condition called cough hypersensitivity syndrome (CHS), which is the likely cause of your dry cough. We all have a cough reflex. The sensitivity of that reflex varies a bit from patient to patient, but it shouldn't be triggered by harmless things like the faint smell of a perfume, cold air, or talking. These are clear indications of cough hypersensitivity. Researchers can measure individuals' cough reflex sensitivity by exposing them to a cough stimulant, such as capsaicin, which is what is in pepper spray. Capsaicin will make every person cough at a certain dose. Researchers have found that people with cough hypersensitivity cough at lower capsaicin doses compared to those without a chronic cough. Research has also revealed that changes in the nervous system are the cause of the cough hypersensitivity. There are sensory nerves in our throat that protect your airway. These nerves send signals to the brain when activated, telling your brain you need to cough to protect your airway. There are small molecules on these nerves, which are the key players in activating the nerve. These molecules have been measured in research with biopsy studies, and people with CHS have more of them than those without CHS. Other research has also found differences in the brains of people with CHS. Specifically, an area of the brain responsible for cough suppression is less active in individuals with CHS compared to healthy individuals. The goal of BCST is to help you learn to suppress your dry cough. When you suppress the cough over time, your nervous system changes by reducing the hypersensitivity. In your case, we know you have a chronic pulmonary disease which, unfortunately, will always*

be a driving force to some degree of hypersensitivity; however, if you can suppress your dry cough with reasonable success, we anticipate you'll achieve some reduction in sensitivity and you'll improve control of your cough, which will reduce the impact it is having on your life."

Goals #2 and #3

Goal #2. *The patient will be able to fully suppress dry cough in at least 50% of opportunities.* **Goal #3.** *The patient will be able to minimize dry cough severity in at least 80% of opportunities where she is not fully suppressing her cough.*

These goals were targeted in tandem. Table 7–4 outlines cough suppression strategies. The clinician taught the first strategy to the patient during the evaluation session. The clinician recommended that DS practice 10 cycles of relaxed throat breathing 4 to 5 times each day, when not feeling a UTC, to create muscle memory and improve automaticity of the technique. (See Video 20 Relaxed Throat Breathing by Slovarp.) The SLP taught the other strategies in the first treatment session and emphasized the importance of finding what strategies work the best for DS. She also emphasized that what matters is suppressing a cough when feeling a UTC. In this regard, DS was free to modify each strategy or try other things to suppress her cough. (See Video 21 Box Breathing by Slovarp.)

Goal #4

Goal #4. *The patient will use quiet breathing at least 80% of the time throughout each therapy session with no more than minimal cues.*

This goal was targeted briefly during the evaluation session and then again during session #2. The patient was educated on how vocal fold position influences airflow sound. The clinician modeled stridor and an audible inhalation without stridor and asked her to imitate each. She was able to do these easily. She was informed of what her body was doing to make the two different breath sounds. She

Table 7–4. Cough Suppression Strategies

Name	Description	Tips
Relaxed-Throat Breathing	Quick inhale through nose followed by a long exhale through pursed lips, a coffee straw, or while saying "ssssss"	• If the patient tends to breath hold or constrict at the larynx, cue them to focus on hearing lots of air turbulence at the exit (ie, the lips, end of the straw, or loud "sss"). This helps ensure the larynx is open. • Some people do best if they push air out forcefully. Others do better if they simply let the air out. • If a quick sniff in causes cough, slow it down. • Adding a swallow once in a while before or after the exhale can be helpful.
Box Breathing	3-4 count in through nose, 3-4 count breath hold, swallow, 3-4 count exhale	Breath in should be through the nose; exhale can be through the nose or mouth.
Relaxation	• Release neck and shoulder tension. • Abdominal breathing	This should be targeted during breathing techniques if needed.
Swallow Strategies	1. Sipping water 2. Effortful swallow 3. Masako (swallow with tongue between teeth) HINT: The idea is to create a competing sensation in the throat to override the UTC. The Masako helps because it usually results in the greatest sensation.	• Some patients prefer small sips. Others find gulping water more effective. • Effortful swallow can be done with or without a Valsalva. Pressing the hands forcefully together during the swallow can also be helpful.
Distraction	• Suck on a nonmedicated lozenge or sugar-free candy, sip water, chew gum or ice chips. • Blow on a tissue when doing relaxed-throat breathing and focus on making the tissue fly. This also helps reduce laryngeal constriction.	

was then instructed to take a silent breath in through the mouth. Although her breath-in was not completely silent, it was much quieter. She was informed that her breath-in was quieter because the vocal folds opened wider, which led to less air turbulence. The clinician emphasized that she didn't have to know what she was doing differently with her laryngeal muscles to breathe quietly. She simply needed to think her breath-in should be quiet and her brain would take care of the rest. She was then instructed to contrast some loud breaths in with quiet breaths in and to pay attention to the feel and to the ease of airflow with each. After this, she stated that she felt less irritation in her throat with quiet breaths and that the air flowed in much easier.

Goal #5

Goal #5. *The patient will be able to read the Rainbow Passage without UTC or cough.*

This goal was targeted during sessions #2 and #3. Treatment started with education about how the voice works (with emphasis on importance of relaxed laryngeal muscles) and instruction in resonant voice techniques including general neck and shoulder relaxation, strategies to promote unrestricted airflow during phonation, and mask-of-face humming followed by chanting and gradual reduction of the chanting to normal prosody during automatic speech tasks, then reading aloud, and finally conversation.

The clinician asked the following questions at each treatment session:

- What percentage of the time did you try to suppress your dry cough?
- What strategies did you try and what did you like best?
- What percentage of the time were you able to fully prevent the cough?
- Of those you were not able to fully prevent, what percentage were you able to minimize?
- Has the frequency of feeling a UTC decreased overall?

She also asked DS to demonstrate the techniques. The SLP only gave further instruction to improve accuracy if the technique was not helpful. If DS performed a technique different from was instructed, but reported it was working well to suppress the cough, the technique was not modified.

> The author highlights a critical concept here regarding technique accuracy. The purpose of cough replacement strategies is not to be good at the technique, but to use the technique to successfully prevent or abort a cough. Thus, the technique was not modified if it was successful, even if it differed from the way it was originally taught.

Posttreatment Outcomes

At the first treatment session, DS had greatly improved, and she was delighted with the results. She reported she was usually able to tell the difference between her productive and dry cough and she was able to fully suppress her dry cough 60% to 70% of the time. She was able to minimize the severity of at least 90% of coughs she was not able to fully prevent and had only had 2 minor coughing bouts since the first session. She also noticed a reduction in how strong and how often she felt the UTC. By session #3, she was able to suppress close to 90% of her dry coughs and she had not had any coughing bouts since session #2. She was also able to hold a 5-minute conversation with no remarkable strain in the voice and no coughing. Her progress on long-term goals was as follows:

1. **The patient will score at least 15 on the LCQ from a baseline of 11.29.** GOAL MET. Her LCQ score at session #3 was 19.7, indicating her cough was no longer negatively impacting her quality of life. (Normal threshold for the LCQ is 17.05 in individuals without chronic cough.[6])

2. **The patient will be able to attend at least 2 social events (eg, church, yoga class, a movie) without having to leave the room because of her cough.** GOAL MET. DS stated she had attended 1 movie and church and she didn't need to get up during either to deal with her cough.
3. **The patient will experience 0 severe coughing bouts for at least 5 days in a row.** GOAL MET.
4. **The patient will score no more than 11 on the VHI-10 from a baseline of 14.** GOAL MET. DS scored 9 on the VHI-10 at session #3.

 CASE STUDY 7.4

Interprofessional Use of SLN Injection and BCST for an Adult With Chronic Refractory Cough

Edie R. Hapner and C. Blake Simpson

Evaluation

Chief Complaint. Chronic refractory cough, episodic dyspnea, and voice change

I had the pleasure of seeing this patient for a comprehensive voice and upper airway evaluation as part of the SLP/laryngologist interprofessional assessment. The patient was diagnosed with chronic refractory cough and associated changes in voice.

History of the Complaint

Patient CC is a 53-year-old cisgender woman who reports an 8-month history of chronic cough after contracting SARS-CoV-2 (COVID-19). Cough currently occurs in ballistic episodes more than 10 times per day, sometimes resulting in secondary voice changes with shortness of breath and occasional stridor. Her cough is preceded by a tickling or dry sensation on the right side of her throat. Coughing can be so violent that she has occasional urinary incontinence and vomiting. Talking and exposure to strong fragrances or smoke exacerbate her symptoms. She often feels like she is "drowning in phlegm," but the cough is dry and she is only able to expectorate a small amount of mucus.

The patient was not hospitalized with SARS-CoV-2, but she reports experiencing severe upper respiratory symptoms with ballistic coughing for more than 2 weeks. She was treated with Paxlovid and her URI symptoms waned, but the cough persisted. She was subsequently treated by her general practitioner (GP) for the cough, who prescribed an antibiotic, inhaled glucocorticosteroid inhaler (fluticasone), and rescue inhaler (Ventolin). She reported little cough relief from the inhalers and antibiotics. Following, she was placed on an oral steroid dose pack and noted a reduction in the severity of the cough while on the medications. However, about 2 days after finishing the steroid dose pack, ballistic coughing returned. Her GP then referred her to a community otolaryngologist who placed her on a proton pump inhibitor (PPI) (omeprazole) BID for suspected laryngopharyngeal reflux (LPR) as the cause of cough. Despite all previous treatments, she continued to experience ballistic coughing episodes at least 10 times per day. The community otolaryngologist referred Patient CC to a pulmonologist to determine if pulmonary disease or long COVID could be precipitating the cough. Pulmonary function testing (PFT) was completed with no evidence of obstructive or restrictive lung disease, and the rescue inhaler and steroid inhaler were therefore discontinued. However, PFT did indicate a blunted flow volume loop (Figure 7–2) that might represent an extrathoracic obstruction such as ILO, which could be associated with her episodic shortness of breath and stridor.

Patient CC reports the cough has taken a toll on her occupational and social life. She works as an HR counselor for a large urban hospital and must participate in orientation sessions for approximately 30 new employees

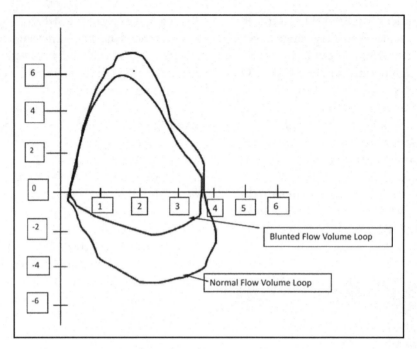

FIGURE 7–2. Blunted flow volume loop.

once monthly, regularly counsel employees face to face, and conduct meetings both virtually and in person each week. She reports that chronic coughing during and since the COVID-19 pandemic can often "clear a room" during an attack, and she has to explain that her cough is not contagious, something she described as frustrating and exhausting.

> For patients with suspected ILO or EILO, PFT with a flow volume loop provides important information. A flow volume loop is a pictorial representation of the inhale-exhale-inhale cycle, and a normal flow volume loop has a representative egg-like shape. When there is a restriction in the inhalation cycle due to extrathoracic obstruction, such as in ILO or EILO, the loop will take on a blunted or cut-off inhalation, usually seen in the repeat inhalation. In these cases, the shape of the flow volume loop will be more pyramidal than egg-like, as seen in Figure 7–2.

Patient CC notes chronic vocal roughness that is exacerbated on the days she has to conduct orientation meetings. She has foregone social events, singing in the church choir, and talking on the telephone due to coughing and voice changes, and this makes her feel disconnected and isolated.

Laryngeal Imaging

Laryngeal endoscopy was performed transnasally with a flexible distal chip videolaryngoscope because CC's case history amplified concerns for a postviral motion asymmetry or ILO that cannot be effectively assessed with rigid laryngoscopy. Laryngeal endoscopy was performed to assess motion during rest breathing and speech, while exposed to cough triggers, and during speech tasks. Videostroboscopy was used to assess glottal closure and vocal fold pliability that cannot be assessed with the use of constant light imaging. Salient examination findings during constant halogen light indicated normal-appearing laryngeal structures with normal-appearing mucosa and little to no mucus; full abduction and adduction; no evidence of paradoxical adduction on inspiration; and no supraglottal or hypopharyngeal masses. Utilizing the Voice Assessment for Laryngeal Imaging (VALI)[63] to assess stroboscopic findings at modal pitch (190-198 Hz for this patient), results indicate:

1. Glottal closure: Elongated posterior gap
2. Amplitude of lateral excursion: Normal at 30% bilaterally
3. Mucosal wave: Normal at 40% of the superior surface of the folds bilaterally
4. Vertical level: On plane
5. Nonvibrating portion: None present
6. Supraglottic activity: Minimal but clearly present anterior-posterior compression
7. Free edge contour: Normal/straight
8. Phase closure: Nearly equivalent with occasions of increased open phase
9. Phase symmetry: 20% of the time asymmetry noted
10. Regularity: 90% of examination regular

Vocal Effort, Fatigue, and Pain

The patient rated her vocal effort using the OMNI-VES[49] where 0 = "extremely easy" to produce voice and 10 = "extremely hard" to produce voice. The patient reported that vocal effort was 6/10 during the evaluation and 10/10 at worst, occurring on days when she was required to do significant talking.

Measures of Patient-Reported Quality-of-Life Impairment

1. VHI-10[28]: 32/40 (threshold = 11)[50]
2. CSI[32]: 35/40 (threshold = 3)
3. DI[31]: 20/40 (threshold = 3)
4. LCQ[59,64]
   a. Total score: 79/133 (threshold = 17.68)
   b. Physical domain: 25/56 (threshold = 5.36)
   c. Psychological domain: 27/49 (threshold = 5.81)
   d. Social domain: 27/27 (threshold = 6.06)

5. Voice Problem Impact Scales (VPIS)[65]
   a. Work life/daily activities: 6/7
   b. Social life: 7/7
   c. Home: 4/7
   d. Overall: 5.7

Auditory-Perceptual Assessment

The CAPE-V[33] was administered and the patient received an overall score of 36/100, indicating a dysphonia of a moderate nature. Aberrant perceptual features identified in the voice included primary strain and secondary roughness. Overall vocal loudness was noted to be WNL. Pitch of the voice was WNL for age and gender but with occasional drop of pitch and loss of airflow at the ends of breath groups during conversational speech. Resonance was focused in the laryngeal region. Respiration was primarily abdominal-thoracic. There was consistent breath holding with poor coordination of airflow with phonation.

Manual Palpation Assessment

Manual palpation indicated pain over the thyrohyoid region on the right with the stimulus to cough during palpation of that space. Muscle tension was assessed and rated on a 0 to 5 scale where 0 = "no tension" and 5 = "most tension" with the following results:

1. 4/5 tension at the thyrohyoid space with report of pain; cough induced by palpation on the right side. Patient endorsed that was where she felt the source of the cough.
2. 3/5 tension at the base of tongue (BOT)/ suprahyoid region without report of pain
3. 4/5 laryngeal height as assessed by palpation of the hyoid
4. 4//5 restriction of lateralization of thyroid cartilage bilaterally

Acoustic and Aerodynamic Assessment

All data were gathered utilizing the Pentax Medical Computerized Speech Laboratory with Multi-Dimensional Voice Program 6600,

Analysis of Dysphonia in Speech (ADSV), Real-Time Pitch Analysis, and Phonatory Aerodynamic System. Norms utilized represent information from Recommendations for the Instrumental Assessment of Voice[60] using an omnidirectional headset microphone (Shure SM 48) and Extech Sound Level Meter was placed at a 45-degree angle at 2 cm from the mouth for data acquisition.[66] Results of the assessment are detailed in Tables 7–5 and 7–6.

Stimulability and Commitment/Confidence
The patient was stimulable for reducing pain and tension in the perilaryngeal musculature with short-duration manual palpation of the thyrohyoid space and reducing continuous, uncontrolled coughing with use of *rescue breathing* or positive expiratory pressure (PEP) breathing, which is a normal inhalation and exhalation against a resistance that provides back pressure to the airways to keep them open.

Table 7–5. Acoustic Assessment Results

	Rainbow Passage	Sustained Vowel	Norms	X Indicates Abnormal
Mean F0 (Hz)	189 Hz	206 Hz	M 121-163 Hz F 200-266 Hz	
SD (Hz)	27.89 Hz	N/A	<29.1 Hz	
Physiological Pitch Range (Hz)	150-550 Hz		M 190-550 Hz F 130-750 Hz	X (a functional result of secondary MTD)

Sustained Vowel /a/	Results	Norms	X Indicates Abnormal
CPP (dB)	7.321 dB	F 10.74, M 13.03	
CPP SD (dB)	4 dB	F 2.37, M 0.75	
L/H Spectral Ratio (dB)	25 dB	F 32.99, M 38.12	
L/H Spectral Ratio SD (dB)	3 dB	F 1.05, M 1.31	
Mean CPP F0 (Hz)	200 Hz	F 210.37, M 110.89	
CPP F0 SD (Hz)	9 Hz	F 10.74, M 0.75	
CSID	36	F 4.43, M 3.58	X

Table 7–6. Aerodynamic Assessment Results

	Results	X Indicates Abnormal
Vital Capacity (L) (expiratory volume)	2.64 L	
MFR (L/sec): Vowel (mean airflow during voicing)	0.21 L/sec	X (likely a result of the elongated posterior glottal gap and air loss)
MFR (L/sec): Rainbow Passage	0.17 L/sec	
Duration (sec)	33 sec	
Breaths (#)	4	
Psub (cmH$_2$O)	6.59 cmH$_2$O	

To use PEP or rescue breathing, the patient was asked to inhale through the nose and complete a slow, sustained exhalation through pursed lips with a voiceless fricative like /s/, /f/, or /ʃ/.

Utilizing the ruler exercise[67] (Figure 7–3) to assess readiness for change, the patient indicated that gaining control of her cough was of the utmost importance to her at a rating of 10/10 and that her confidence to complete the treatments suggested to gain this control was 9/10.

Impressions

The patient presents with chronic refractory neurogenic cough as a result of CHS likely from a postviral vagal neuropathy with secondary MTD and episodic ILO.

Plan of Care

The laryngologist and SLP discussed the multi-specialty protocol used to treat chronic refractory neurogenic cough/CHS with the patient. This includes use of superior laryngeal nerve (SLN) steroid injection[38] immediately followed by BCST.[9]

Prognosis is good for improved cough suppression, reduction of MTD symptoms, and elimination of episodic ILO based on stimulability testing, evidence for the use of SLN injections reducing the urge to cough

(UTC) by 80% to 100% in most patients,[68] and the evidence that BCST reduces cough frequency by 74% to 100% in most patients.[9] Additionally, Patient CC had confidence in her care providers and in her ability to adhere to the recommended treatment. Most importantly, however, eliminating her cough and returning to her pre-illness lifestyle was of the utmost importance to her.

Patient CC underwent a right SLN block on the day of her assessment in the interprofessional clinic and was instructed to return in 1 week to begin BCST. Therapy will be conducted once weekly in 45-minute sessions per Voice Center protocol, and the patient will return to the laryngologist/SLP interprofessional clinic in 6 weeks to determine need for additional SLN injections and any further BCST.

Long-Term Goals. The patient will regain the ability to participate in her high vocal load at work, attend social events, and return to singing through elimination or significant reduction of the episodic cough, dyspnea with stridor, and dysphonia.

Short-Term Goals:

1. The patient will reduce the urge to cough by 80% or greater as measured by self-report.

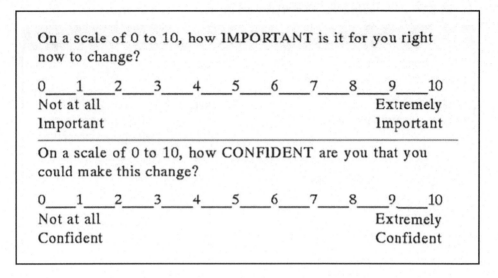

FIGURE 7–3. Ruler exercise. *Source*: From Behrman A, Haskell J, eds. *Exercises for Voice Therapy*. 3rd ed. Plural Publishing; 2020:1-289. Copyright © 2020 Plural Publishing, Inc. All rights reserved.

2. The patient will increase the ability to control the cough by 80% as measured by self-report.
3. The patient will improve the ability to identify the onset of stridor and dyspnea and reduce the severity of the episode and frequency of episodes to once weekly or less per self-report.
4. The patient will improve vocal endurance by reducing vocal effort, thereby reducing daily fatigue after mandatory talking at work or in social situations.

Decision Making

The decision to use a multimodality approach to chronic cough treatment at the Voice Center resulted from observation that patients receiving only SLN injection without committing to BCST returned for 8+ repeated SLN injections.[69] Patients with ballistic cough who received a single SLN injection and engaged in BCST often came to their first therapy session saying that they were *better than before the injection, but not all the way better*. Starting BCST with someone who has already experienced improvement in their ability to control a cough as a result of the SLN injection may improve the trajectory of therapy.

The underlying theory regarding use of SLN injections in those with chronic cough is that the SLN is implicated in the development of chronic neuropathic cough. The SLN provides sensation to the larynx including pain, touch, and temperature.[37] As a result of postviral neural damage to the internal branch of the SLN, a state of laryngeal hypersensitivity causes the larynx to overreact to stimulation. The injection, consisting of a long-acting anesthetic and a steroid (1-2 mL of 1:1 triamcinolone 40 mg and 1% lidocaine with 1:200,000 epinephrine) is theorized to disrupt the cough-signaling pathway, thereby reducing the urge to cough.[38]

BCST is also hypothesized to disrupt the laryngeal hypersensitivity that leads to cough. The progression of therapy and therapeutic tasks presented here are derived from a well-established body of literature that suggests the 4 elements of BCST are education, vocal hygiene training, cough suppression, and psychoeducational counseling.[70]

Voice Therapy Intervention

The patient received a right-sided SLN injection at the initial office visit and was guided to spend the next week improving overall hydration through (1) utilizing a portable steam inhaler at least 3 times a day, (2) using glycerin-based lozenges to soothe the throat rather than menthol-based cough drops (with patient education that neither of these actually touch the vocal folds, but rather are used to soothe the throat only), and (3) maintaining adequate systemic hydration through drinking water and reducing drying products such as caffeine and alcohol. The clinician reminded Patient CC to use rescue breathing and gave her a handout with written instructions for various ways to exhale against resistance (eg, voiceless fricative, through a straw with or without water). Therapy was scheduled for 1 week later. (For examples of exhaling against resistance, see Figures 7–4 and 7–5 as well as Video 21 Box Breathing by Slovarp, Video 24 Cup Phonation by Castro, and Video 28 Straw Phonation in Water Hierarchy by Codino.)

At each of the 4 therapy sessions scheduled 1 week apart, the patient was asked a series of questions in Table 7–7, completed the LCQ and CSI, and was asked, "What percent better is your cough?" This information was garnered as outcome measures and was presented to the patient in graphic form to open discussion about the trajectory of her recovery. This allowed the patient to fully appreciate her role in her own recovery and her progress (or setbacks) and to explore the whys.

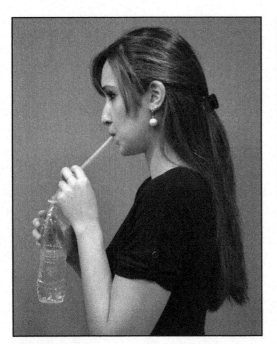

FIGURE 7–4. Cup bubbles. *Source:* From Behrman A, Haskell J, eds. *Exercises for Voice Therapy*. 3rd ed. Plural Publishing; 2020:1-289. Copyright © 2020 Plural Publishing, Inc. All rights reserved.

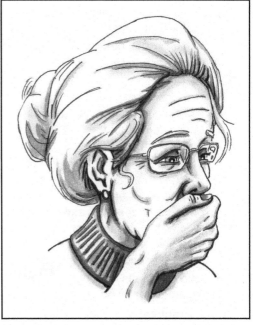

FIGURE 7–5. Hand-over-mouth. *Source:* From Behrman A, Haskell J, eds. *Exercises for Voice Therapy*. 3rd ed. Plural Publishing; 2020:1-289. Copyright © 2020 Plural Publishing, Inc. All rights reserved.

Table 7–7. Intervention

Therapy Protocol	Specific Patient Response
Session #1	• **Outcomes:** Patient reported 70% better
• **Outcome Measures:**	• **Indirect Therapy:** Reviewed status of improved systemic and surface hydration; patient reported she used steaming 3-4 times per day the past week
○ What percent better are you since the SLN injection?	
○ Complete LCQ and CSI to document post-SLN, pretherapy status	• **Direct Therapy:**
• **Indirect Therapy:**	○ Patient reported she had 1 episode a day but that she was able to stop the episode without coughing with the use of rescue breathing. Said she uses /ʃ/ on exhalation generally.
○ Provide education on the biological function of cough and the difference when cough is nonproductive/neurogenic	
○ Review status of improved systemic and surface hydration	○ Practiced multiple methods of cough replacements, but patient believes that use of the "sip of water-swallow" and eventually just a hard swallow will work best.
• **Direct Therapy:**	
○ Review the use of rescue breathing and PEP breathing	
a. Document the number of dyspneic episodes with or without stridor that occurred the prior week	
b. Did rescue breathing reduce the severity or eliminate the episodes of dyspnea?	
○ Introduce cough replacement behaviors	
c. Discuss the idea that cough is a vicious cycle, and the goal is to disrupt the cycle and identify the sensations associated with the UTC	
d. Discuss that the goal is to respond differently every time one feels the "tickle" and use a different, less traumatic response to the "tickle" or other sensation	
○ Practice methods of cough replacements	
• **Home Practice:** Continue tracking episodes of dyspnea, voice change, and cough	

Table 7–7. *continued*

Therapy Protocol	Specific Patient Response

Session #2: One Week Later
• **Outcome Measures:**
   ○ Document percent better
• **Direct Therapy:**
   ○ Introduce semi-occluded vocal tract strategies to maintain a relaxed laryngeal posture and as a recalibration method.
     a. Cup bubbles (see Figure 7–4)
     b. Cup bubbles to straw phonation
     c. Straw phonation to transfer /w/ words to /ʍ/
   ○ Begin to transfer to conversation using patient awareness of change in voice and to return to any level of this task as a recalibrator during 10-minute conversational practice
• **Home Practice:** Continue journaling. Use recalibrator straw in 5- to 10-minute conversational practice sessions with people and environment the patient feels comfortable with.
	• **Outcomes:** Reported symptoms are 80% better. Patient reported:
	   ○ Able to talk on the phone 3 times the past week for up to 15 minutes each call without coughing
	   ○ Reported she has advanced to using only an effortful swallow when she felt the "tickle. Noted she felt dyspneic only 3 times during the week and started rescue breathing in these instances and was able to stop the episode all 3 times.
	• **Direct Therapy:** Recalibrated with cueing to use the straw successfully 70% of the time

Session #3: One Week Later
• **Outcome Measures:**
   ○ Document percent improved
• **Direct Therapy:**
   ○ Introduce hand over mouth as another semi-occluded therapy task option that easily transfers to a conversational setting (see Figure 7–5)
   ○ Practice transfer to conversation using patient awareness of voice changes or tension
• **Home Practice:** Continue journaling. Use hand-over-mouth recalibrator in both spontaneous and 5- to 10-minute conversational practice sessions with comfortable people and environment.
	• **Outcomes:** Patient reported symptoms are 85%-90% better. Patient reported:
	   ○ She was able to conduct most meetings at work the past week for up to 30 minutes of talk time without coughing or voice change
	   ○ Not feeling the throat tickle as often
	   ○ Dyspneic only once, while getting into an elevator with a man with lots of cologne. She started rescue breathing and got off the elevator at the next floor, and this stopped the episode
	• **Direct Therapy:**
	   ○ Practiced using the straw as a recalibrator and said it was useful but wondered if there was something less noticeable she could use in conversation
	   ○ Hand over mouth was successful at avoiding UTC 75% of the time

continues

314 Voice Therapy: Clinical Case Studies

Table 7–7. *continued*

Therapy Protocol	Specific Patient Response

Session #4: One Week Later
 	
• **Outcome Measures:**
  ○ Document percent improved
  ○ Document episodes of dyspnea or voice change this past week
 	
• **Direct Therapy:**
  ○ Introduce cough triggers from evaluation in a safe and controlled environment, emphasizing the importance of using trusted and successful techniques to reduce UTC
  ○ Spend time assuring the patient
  ○ Start with triggers less likely to produce cough and progress to more likely triggers, supporting the patient to utilize acquired tools to stop or reduce the response and dyspnea
	• **Outcomes:** Reported symptoms are 90%-95% better.
	  ○ No episodes of dyspnea or voice change in past week
	  ○ Able to go to church and sing in the congregation without coughing
	  ○ Went out to dinner with 2 friends in a minimally noisy restaurant without coughing
	
	• **Direct Therapy:**
	  ○ Introduced triggers that she had reported made her cough during the voice evaluation. The clinician intentionally spent time assuring the patient she was in a safe environment if she did experience any problems with breathing or uncontrolled cough.
	  ○ Reviewed the tools she was able to use to stop the episode by reviewing her trajectory chart of improvements in the PROMs and her activities. Started with those less likely to trigger and progressed to those more likely to trigger, supporting the patient to utilize her tools to stop or reduce the response.
	  ○ Utilized conversation with progressive exposures of alcohol hand wash to disinfectant cleaning wipes of the therapy table, air freshener in the room, to finally perfume.
	  ○ Each time the patient was instructed to keep talking and to indicate by pointing to a scale of 0-10 (0 = no problems and 10 indicates profound problems) placed on the table in front of her regarding how much tension, vocal effort, urge to cough, and dyspnea she was experiencing.
	  ○ The patient was told to determine when she needed to use her tools and decided her tool progression would be hand over mouth if she felt vocal effort or voice change starting; rescue breathing with any dyspnea; and sip of water swallow if UTC. Throughout the exposures, she started using the tools between 3-4 on the scale and did not need to discontinue talking

Table 7–7. *continued*

Therapy Protocol	Specific Patient Response
Session #4 *continued*	at any time. Following this task that took approximately 30 minutes of the session, the patient and clinician walked outside the building to the area designated as the smoking area. The patient was encouraged to continue talking and use tools as needed. During the smoke exposure, the patient noted increased difficulty to continue talking without stopping or to do rescue breathing, and the task was aborted after about 3 minutes of exposure. Once the patient left the smoking area, her breathing returned to normal.
• **Return Visit With Physician:** 2 weeks later, 6 weeks after initial appointment. Patient is offered repeat SLN injection at this appointment.	The patient noted to the physician that she felt 95% better and felt she was able to control most situational triggers. She was offered a second SLN block and chose to see if she could continue her progress to eliminate her dyspnea, cough, and dysphonia without an additional block. The patient and clinician determined she did not need consistent therapy appointments at this time and a telehealth follow up was scheduled in 3 weeks to confirm that she continues to progress toward resolution.

Summary and Concluding Remarks

Chronic cough, especially that with a neurogenic origin, presents a challenge to the clinician. In this case, the patient had been coughing for more than 8 months. She had seen multiple medical practitioners and had been told that her cough was because of multiple diagnoses and that the onset of her problems was from a virus that, during the pandemic of 2020 to 2022, was cloaked in misinformation, fear of dying, and frank examples of people diagnosed with long COVID who were not recovering fully. The practitioner should not be surprised if patients are leery of being offered yet another treatment that perhaps, once again, may not work. Using the ruler exercise is a simple method to assess where patients stand on their self-efficacy for participating in their care and to emphasize the importance of addressing what can be multiple issues with chronic cough (ie, dyspnea, ILO, dysphonia). This patient had done her research and knew that the laryngologist had successfully developed the use of an SLN injection and that the Voice Center was known for its multispecialty approach to chronic cough. This undoubtedly improved her confidence in the practitioners and the treatment recommendations.

CASE STUDY 7.5

Interprofessional Use of Neuromodulators and BCST for an Adult With Chronic Refractory Cough

Juliana Litts and Daniel Fink

Evaluation

Chief Complaint. Chronic cough for over 10 years

We had the pleasure of evaluating this patient in our interdisciplinary clinic with a fellowship-trained laryngologist and a voice and upper-airway-specialized SLP. The patient was referred by a private practice otolaryngologist in the community.

History of Cough Complaint

The patient (DT) is a 52-year-old cisgender female with a history of more than 10 years of coughing. Her cough was precipitated by an upper respiratory infection and has been chronic since that time. She complains of a nonproductive cough triggered in her throat, including the sensation of a tickle in the throat and what she describes as "mucus buildup" in the throat. She notes her tickle sensation and cough are worse when she is exposed to cold air and when she walks into air-conditioned rooms. She also notes a sensation of mucus that triggers a cough and tends to be worse with prolonged phonation. She is a public speaker and reports high voice demand. She describes her cough as short episodes of 3 to 4 coughs that can occur throughout the day. She very rarely has long coughing jags, but when she does, they can last 45 to 60 seconds. She never coughs when she is sleeping at night. She has never smoked. Her previous ENT physician started her on a trial of low-dose gabapentin, which improved her symptoms by about 40% to 50%. At the time of her initial visit, she was taking 100 mg of gabapentin in the morning and 200 mg of gabapentin at night as prescribed. She has no sinonasal complaints. She previously had heartburn symptoms multiple times per week, but this has resolved since she started taking a daily H2 blocker prescribed by her primary care physician. Her cough did not change after starting her H2 blocker. She is not taking any angiotensin-converting enzymes (ACE) inhibitors, specifically lisinopril, which is known to have cough as a side effect. ACE inhibitors are used to relax blood vessels and lower blood pressure.

Previous Workups in Other Specialties. DT had full workups in several other specialties. She had a negative allergy workup, a normal pulmonary function study, and a normal chest x-ray.

Previously Trialed Therapies. DT had no change in her cough despite being prescribed many different trials of medications over the years including allergy medications, steroid inhalers, reflux management, Tessalon Perles, and guaifenesin. She was temporarily on oral steroids due to an unrelated infection and found that her cough resolved only while she was on the steroids.

Other Related Symptoms and History. DT reports no significant symptoms of dyspnea or dysphagia. She notes mild hoarseness when she does a lot of talking, but this is not significantly limiting to her. She had no previous surgeries in her head, neck, or chest, and she has never been intubated for longer than 24 hours. She does have obstructive sleep apnea (OSA), which is successfully treated with CPAP. She has no other significant medical problems.

Laryngeal Imaging and Auditory-Perceptual Analysis

A 70-degree rigid laryngeal videostroboscopy exam was performed, and perceptual analysis of voice was completed by a voice-specialized SLP using CAPE-V[33] scoring (0-100 scale of severity) with findings detailed in Table 7–8.

Objective acoustic and aerodynamic analysis was not completed for this patient as

Table 7–8. Results of Laryngeal Imaging Examination and Clinician's Perceptual Assessment

Assessment Parameter	Findings
Hypopharynx	No pooling of secretions at base of tongue and pyriform sinuses, no mucosal lesions, pharyngeal wall motion intact
Larynx	R TVF: full abduction and adduction, no masses, no atrophy
	L TVF: full abduction and adduction, no masses, no atrophy
Stroboscopy	Closure: normal/complete
	Amplitude: normal bilaterally
	Mucosal wave: mildly reduced bilaterally
	Periodicity: normal
	Phase symmetry: symmetric
Auditory-Perceptual Assessment: CAPE-V	Overall severity: 32/100
	Roughness: 22/100
	Breathiness: 5/100
	Strain: 28/100
	Asthenia: 0/100

she was seen for her initial visit at a satellite clinic where there is no equipment to perform this type of analysis.

Impression

The laryngologist and SLP discussed the patient history and physical exam together. They concluded DT presented with chronic cough most likely related to laryngeal hypersensitivity that has been exacerbated by her high voice use that is mildly inefficient.

Plan of Care

Multidisciplinary evaluation and discussion led to a two-pronged treatment plan, including titrating up on the dose of gabapentin DT was taking to maximize therapeutic benefit and working on behavioral management of her cough symptoms by engaging in BCST with an

SLP. The recommended duration of BCST is typically 2 to 3 therapy sessions that are 2 to 3 weeks apart. Goals for BCST target increasing patient knowledge about chronic cough, improving patient awareness of sensations that trigger cough behaviors, providing substitute behaviors to interrupt the cough response, and decreasing underlying laryngeal hypersensitivity that is contributing to the presenting chronic cough symptoms.

Decision Making

Chronic cough is a challenging problem to treat, as it can have several underlying etiologies, including allergies, pulmonary disease, sinus disease, reflux, and laryngeal hypersensitivity. It is important to rule out other possible etiologies of cough before diagnosing laryngeal hypersensitivity. Detailed case histories

318   Voice Therapy: Clinical Case Studies

are critical to make this determination. Important questions to ask include:

1. Where do you feel the cough triggered? Cough triggered in the throat is much less likely to be related to pulmonary issues.
2. What triggers the cough? Cough triggered during or after eating can indicate dysphagia or acid reflux. Cough triggered with nasal congestion can indicate sinonasal disease.
3. Is the cough dry or productive? Productive coughs have an underlying cause that is not related to laryngeal hypersensitivity.
4. Does your cough wake you from sleep at night? Cough that can be behaviorally managed typically does not wake the patient from sleep at night.
5. What kinds of medications have you tried and what were the outcomes? This can help rule in or rule out contributory factors. For example, if inhaled steroids lessen the cough, cough-variant asthma or eosinophilic bronchitis should be considered and the patient sent to pulmonology.

It should also be considered that cough is often multifactorial, making it critical to ensure other cough etiologies are ruled out and/or treated before starting behavioral management. BCST can be completed alone or in conjunction with medical management with no significant difference in efficacy.[71] In this case, the decision to continue treatment with gabapentin and add BCST was determined because DT was already taking gabapentin with good results on a very low dose. Of note, neuromodulator medication can have significant side effects, especially as dosing increases, and this should be considered when choosing this treatment option.

Intervention

Medical Intervention

On initial evaluation, the patient was taking 300 mg of gabapentin total per day and receiving a modest benefit without side effects. The laryngologist recommended the patient increase by 300 mg every 3 days to a maximum dose of 600 mg 3 times daily (total 1800 mg) or until the cough was approximately 80% improved. This is based on the dosing in the randomized, double-blinded, placebo-controlled trial, which showed a significant improvement in cough-specific quality of life, cough severity, and cough frequency compared with placebo.[72] Had the patient been medication naïve, the clinicians might have also considered pregabalin or amitriptyline. Pregabalin is in the same family as gabapentin (gabapentinoids) and works similarly by blocking a subset of central voltage-gated calcium channels.[4] These medications are used to attempt to treat cough as either a peripheral or central neuropathic disorder.

Pregabalin in conjunction with BCST has been shown to reduce cough as measured by the LCQ compared with placebo and BCST.[71] This effect was maintained after discontinuation of therapy, unlike gabapentin in the above-noted trial.

Amitriptyline, a tricyclic antidepressant, is commonly used, again to treat what is felt to be, at least in part, a neuropathy. Jeyakumar et al demonstrated amitriptyline 10 mg nightly over 10 days to be more effective than guaifenesin in reducing cough.[73] Ryan and Cohen found that over 2 to 3 years, 67% of patients reported over 50% improvement in cough symptoms on amitriptyline.[74] While studies indicate benefit with such medications, up to one-third of patients on these medications will experience side effects that impair their ability to use the medication, including blurry vision, confusion, dry mouth, headache, memory loss, nausea or vomiting, and sedation or drowsiness, and patients should be warned about this, particularly with higher dosages.[75]

Behavioral Intervention

Behavioral therapy was initiated approximately 3 weeks after starting to titrate the patient's gabapentin dose. DT was taking 300 mg of gabapentin in the morning and 900 mg of gabapentin at night. Her cough was about 75% better overall. BCST has been shown to be effective for 87% of patients in reducing chronic cough symptoms. The typical duration of therapy is 1 to 4 sessions and contains 4 major components of therapy that were used for DT's therapy.[9] DT's therapy consisted of two 45-minute sessions, including all 4 of these components in each session.

Education

This component involves explanation of the cough mechanisms in the setting of laryngeal hypersensitivity where cough is triggered by nontussive or low levels of tussive stimuli in the absence of a physiological need to cough. For DT, this was most likely initiated by some postviral neuropathy related to her upper respiratory infection from more than 10 years ago. It is important to explain that although the urge to cough is real, there is no physiological benefit to cough (in this case), and the repeated coughing behavior without need can contribute to laryngeal hypersensitivity. It is important to reinforce the capacity of the brain to develop voluntary control over these cough behaviors, similar to any other mechanical behaviors such as the urge to scratch a poison ivy rash.

Cough Suppression Strategies

Cough suppression strategies include behavior substitution, breathing control, and laryngeal reposturing techniques to release laryngeal constriction and prevent or interrupt cough episodes. It is important that the patient understands that these strategies are not intended to immediately eliminate the sensation that triggers the urge to cough. The point is to control the behavioral response, which allows the body to desensitize, implement new behaviors, and learn to appropriately ignore nontussive or low-tussive stimuli.

1. **Behavior substitution strategies** include using a hard or effortful swallow (dry or with a sip of liquid) to avoid the cough behavior. It is important to emphasize to the patient that the hard swallow is not intended to take away the urge to cough. To help with patient buy-in to this very simple behavior substitution, the clinician should clearly explain why this will help suppress a cough by using the following script or something similar: *"We use the hard swallow technique for 3 reasons. (1) A swallow is intended to clear out anything that is in your throat that is not supposed to be there. As your swallowing function is fine and you can eat and drink whatever you want, we know that your swallow will clear out any excess mucus or anything that is stuck in your throat. (2) If there is any area of mucosal dryness or irritation in the throat, the swallow provides a mucus bath for all of the lining inside your throat. It can soothe this area of irritation that could be caused by some dryness. (3) The hard swallow also gives your body an opportunity to stop and reassess the sensory information that is coming from your throat. It gives you a moment to decide if you really need to cough or if you really just want to cough. A 'need to cough' situation is if you have a piece of pancake stuck in your throat and you cannot breathe or if you take a bite of a powdered sugar doughnut and breathe in some of the powdered sugar. A 'want to cough' situation is basically everything else. Once you realize that this urge to cough is really a representation*

320   Voice Therapy: Clinical Case Studies

of you wanting to cough but not needing to cough, then we can start using some other breathing techniques to help control this urge to cough."

2. **Breathing control strategies** focus on using exhalation to prevent breath holding. After the patient does the hard swallow, she can slowly exhale to maintain control of her breathing and not allow any buildup of pressure in her lungs. After a slow exhale, instruct the patient to use a short, completely silent inhale of air through the nose. The silence of the inhale prevents high velocity of large volumes of air moving through the pharynx while it is irritated. Imagery of collecting air in the nasopharynx and then sending it back out through pursed lips on the exhale can offer a sensory distraction that keeps the brain from perseverating on the urge to cough that is coming from the throat. DT practiced feeling the difference in laryngeal irritation when using a diaphragmatic breathing technique versus feeling the sensation of air collecting in the back of the nose. Breathing control strategies can also be used to interrupt a cough once it has started. This technique involves trying to shape the cough, which is a spastic and uncontrolled exhalation, into a smooth and forceful breath out through pursed lips. Similar to the previous breathing technique described, the breath in happens through the nose and is completely silent and controlled. It is also important that this breath in through the nose is short, as we want to limit the volume and velocity of air traveling through the irritated larynx. Instruct the patient to use this breath cycle until the cough has subsided and the breathing is back under control. It is important to remind the patient not to use the breathing techniques for longer than

necessary and to return to a more normal breathing pattern as soon as possible, as it can cause lightheadedness. Most patients are able to control a triggered cough after about 2 or 3 of those breath cycles with some practice. This significantly reduces both the amount of time the patient will stay in a coughing jag and the irritation input to the larynx.

3. **Laryngeal reposturing** can use resonant voice strategies and basic training gestures to help alter sensation and reduce laryngeal constriction. Some patients will present with cough symptoms and endorse a sensation of throat tightness. Basic training gestures such as lip trills, tongue trills, or tongue out trills are great exercises that the patient can implement into their daily life, which will encourage a reduction in laryngeal tension (see Case Study 3.7 by Orbelo, Li, and Verdolini Abbott on LMRVT for basic training gestures). It is reasonable to suggest to the patient that they implement these exercises for 5 to 10 seconds as needed throughout the day. The patient can select a life event that reminds them to do these exercises, such as every time they stop at a stoplight or a stop sign while driving, every time they walk into the kitchen to get something, or every time they send an email or finish a phone call. For some patients, these exercises will be irritative and trigger a cough. Allow the patient to decide which exercises make their throat feel better and less irritated.

Reducing Laryngeal Irritation

Reducing laryngeal irritation is achieved by reducing exposure to cough-triggering irritants by avoiding smell and cold air triggers, improving hydration, reducing phonotraumatic behaviors such as excessive yelling, and improving overall voicing efficiency. Controlled exposure to irritants and practic-

> In cases of laryngeal hypersensitivity, there can be significant variability among patients regarding what tasks provide relief and what tasks exacerbate irritation. Sometimes, tasks that are designed to provide relief, such as a semi-occluded vocal tract exercise, can paradoxically contribute to a sensation of irritation. The authors here acknowledge that some exercises will not work for some patients and that multiple tasks should be trialed to allow the patient to select which ones feel effective.

ing cough-avoidant strategies can be helpful to use in therapy to improve behavior control over the cough mechanism. If the patient presents with a strong cough response to odors, have the patient make a list of odors that cause irritation and may trigger a cough. The patient should rank this list from least triggering to most triggering. Instruct the patient to find something that has low irritation. This could be a mild spice or some unscented deodorant. The patient can open the product and set it on the table in front of them while using their strategies to control their cough response. If this does not trigger a response, have the patient move the odor closer to their nose for a single sniff of the product and then have them move it away from their face. Continue to have the patient use their cough suppression strategies to manage the cough behavior. Continue working up the hierarchy toward more irritative products as the patient improves in their skills of controlling their cough. This will encourage the patient in their own success and demonstrate to them the effectiveness of these cough suppression strategies.

Psychoeducational Counseling

Psychoeducational counseling addresses motivation, enables adherence to therapy, and facilitates appropriate beliefs about the patient's condition and the role of behavioral

therapy. It is important for the patient to take ownership and control of their cough and to recognize that symptomatic improvement relies heavily on their commitment to change their behavior. This can be done at the end of the session while you are reviewing strategies and giving patients their homework tasks. Assure the patient that the expectation is not to stop all of their coughs. The initial goal for the patient is for them to stop a minimum of 1 out of 10 coughs. This can mean preventing a cough from happening completely or it can mean stopping a longer coughing jag significantly earlier than it would have stopped if not using their techniques. Encourage the patient to aim for more than 10% improvement every day but reinforce that if they can be 10% better every day, the cough can be resolved or mostly resolved in about 4 to 6 weeks. Use this time to remind the patient that behavior change is hard, and it is okay for them to have times where they are not perfect in their therapy tasks.

Posttreatment Reflection

DT had an excellent symptomatic response to the combination of neuromodulator and behavioral treatments for her cough. After the first session, she understood and embraced her role as the primary source for change in her symptoms. She went home with her homework tasks of using a hard swallow and her breathing techniques to stop her coughs. She was extremely compliant with her homework tasks, and at her second therapy session 2 weeks later, she reported a 60% improvement in her symptoms using her strategies. At the second session, DT discussed that she found it difficult to remember to use her cough suppression strategies when she was in work meetings, and the clinician discussed some strategies to set reminders in her phone before the start of meetings. DT was instructed to follow up with an update in the patient portal if her symptoms did not completely resolve before her follow-up with the laryngologist. She returned for a follow-up appointment with her laryngologist as recommended about 3 months after her initial evaluation. At that time, she was having no complaints with her cough. The clinician recommended she start to slowly wean off the gabapentin to see if she could control her cough symptoms without the medication. She was reminded to continue to use her cough suppression strategies while titrating off her medication to maintain her symptom resolution. DT was instructed to contact the laryngologist if her cough symptoms returned as she was weaning off the gabapentin, as she might need to be on a low dose to maintain resolution of symptoms. DT was able to wean completely off the gabapentin and stay symptom free.

> While this may seem far-fetched to one who has not worked with many chronic cough patients, the idea that someone could be coughing for 10 years and then find resolution with the use of systematic medication trials of higher-dosed medical therapy and the use of BCST is not uncommon for those seeing many of these patients. It reminds the clinician that duration of cough should not be a deterrent to attempting treatment.

Introduction: Inducible Laryngeal Obstruction (ILO)

Mary J. Sandage

Inducible laryngeal obstruction (ILO) is a disorder of the upper airway that is characterized by episodes of partial to complete adduction of the vocal folds during inhalation. These breathing "attacks" can occur while one is awake, asleep, sedentary, or active. The clinical presentation is marked by difficulty inhaling and the perception of throat tightness, with or without stridor. It can start suddenly or gradually and does not respond to rescue asthma medications. Frequently misdiagnosed as asthma, most individuals will have many months or years pass from their first breathing attack to proper diagnosis. While not a disorder of communication, it is an upper airway disorder amenable to SLP treatment.

Historically, physicians used the term *vocal cord dysfunction* for this condition; however, a European Respiratory Society consensus now prefers *inducible laryngeal obstruction* (ILO).[76] SLPs specializing in this disorder adopted this term in lieu of the prior term of *paradoxical vocal fold motion* (PVFM). When this condition occurs during exercise, the term *exercise-induced laryngeal obstruction* (EILO) is used.[77] Historically, other terms have been used, several of which indicate a specific underlying etiology, as described below.

The etiology for this upper airway disorder can vary and generally falls into one of the following groups: irritant induced, exercise induced, psychogenic causes, or neurologic causes.[78] ILO/EILO/PVFM can occur in males and females and has been identified in ages ranging from infancy to the eighth decade of life. The prevalence of this disorder is not well understood. A 5% to 8% prevalence is described in adolescents and over 20% for elite athletes and combat soldiers.[77] The clinical presentation can range from occasional, brief experiences of throat narrowing and difficulty inhaling to temporary loss of consciousness. ILO mimics other upper airway conditions and may also co-occur with other upper airway conditions such as asthma, angioedema, and panic attack. Sandage et al (2023) give a comprehensive account of common and rare mimics of this clinical entity and provide a clinical worksheet to aid in the differential diagnosis.[79]

Prior to referral for SLP services, it is critical for patients to have a pulmonary assessment to definitively rule asthma in or out. An endoscopic evaluation to rule out extrathoracic obstruction and supraglottic tissue collapse during exertion is also necessary, considering conditions such as bilateral vocal fold paralysis, obstructive vocal process granuloma, recurrent respiratory papillomatosis, or unresolved laryngomalacia, all of which may compromise the airway without affecting voice quality. Many individuals with ILO have concurrent medical conditions, such as panic attacks or asthma, the latter of which can co-occur in 40% to 60% of patients. Success of behavioral intervention is enhanced when a complete medical assessment is obtained and all ILO mimics are considered.

Irritant-induced ILO typically develops after repeated exposure or a single bout of overwhelming exposure to environmental agents that trigger a protective response in the upper airway. These irritants may be intrinsic, such as LPR, or extrinsic, such as fumes, fragrances, or smoke. Given the biological role of the larynx as a lower airway protector, ILO is considered a defensive posture of the larynx that occurs after a threshold of tolerance to the irritant is surpassed. In Case Study 7.7, Rammage discusses her theory of ILO as a central sensitivity syndrome through a case illustration of ILO that developed secondary to chemical exposure. Recent work in the area of laryngeal chemosensation suggests that even a trivial amount of the irritant may, over time, be enough to trigger an upper airway response.[80] Once the trigger is identified, limiting exposure will be a component of treatment. For an example of irritant-induced ILO in the work setting, see Case Study 7.6 by Maira describing how odor exposure developed into ILO.

Individuals with ILO typically see many different medical specialists (ie, pulmonologists and allergists) without resolution of the breathing attacks. Successful treatment is best achieved via concurrent medical management of triggers (eg, LPR and allergies), lim-

ited exposure to environmental triggers, and SLP therapy. For more challenging clinical presentations, such as the individual with an overwhelming single chemical exposure that triggered the initial event, referral for counseling may be warranted. Psychogenic causes for ILO are rare. Similar to spasmodic dysphonia, initial accounts of ILO attributed the origin to psychogenic pathology without consideration of the far more prevalent irritant-induced etiology. Overemphasis on psychogenic etiology may undermine timely, effective medical and behavioral interventions required for rapid recovery of symptoms.

Respiratory laryngeal dystonia, the neurologic variant of inspiratory stridor observed through the life span, is distinct from the time-limited, episodic nature of ILO, presenting as persistent difficulty inhaling while awake with resolution of symptoms while sleeping.[81] The etiologies include brainstem compression, cortical or upper motor neuron injury, nuclear or lower motor neuron injury, or movement disorder.[82] The clinical presentation is distinct from irritant-induced and psychogenic etiologies in that the neurologic variant presents as difficulty inhaling all day during waking hours—it is not characterized as rather short, time-limited breathing events that resolve after a time and then recur later in the same day. A rarer presentation of a neurally mediated laryngeal adduction during inspiration is diaphragmatic flutter.[81] Neurologic variants will require medical intervention (tracheotomy, pharmacotherapy, or surgery) and patients with suspected neurologic etiology should be referred immediately for medical assessment before initiating SLP therapy, which will have little to no benefit.

The primary goals of the initial patient interview are to identify the likely etiology and triggers of the breathing attacks if they were not clearly identified prior to referral. Careful case history will also elucidate if other upper airway disorders are co-occurring. Have the client explain in detail the exact nature of the breathing events without asking leading questions. Discerning the exact nature of the individual's breathing difficulty is important for development of an individualized treatment plan.

- Do you have trouble inhaling, exhaling, or both? (If the answer is only exhaling, asthma is more likely; if the answer is both inhaling and exhaling, then extrathoracic obstruction should be ruled out.)
- Do you make a noise when it happens? Can you imitate the noise?
- Do you feel tightness anywhere when these breathing events happen? In your chest, throat, or both?
- What typically triggers an event?
- How often do these breathing events happen?
- How long do they last? (If the events last all day long and only remit with sleeping, then a neurologic etiology should be ruled out.)
- Do you do anything for them? What works? What doesn't?
- Do you use an inhaler? Does the inhaler work? How long does it take to work?
- Have you ever passed out?
- Have you ever been to the emergency room or been hospitalized for these breathing events?

The primary goal of medical and behavioral intervention is complete resolution of the ILO/EILO/PVFM events. The breathing recovery method trained may be similar among individuals;[83] however, the details and timing of the intervention will be client specific. The breathing recovery therapy has 3 basic components, the third one being the rescue breathing technique: (1) body awareness training via a progressive tightening-relaxing activity, (2) training lower abdominal/rib cage expansion during inhalation, and (3) rapid,

deep nasal sniff or oral straw-sip inhalation followed by complete exhalation using a front sibilant or fricative sound (eg, /s/, /f/). All 3 steps should be practiced while asymptomatic so that the client can easily implement step 3 when a breathing attack is imminent. The rescue breathing technique should be started before the breathing attack occurs so that it can be avoided completely. Success of this method hinges on careful client interview to discern the first physiologic signal that a breathing attack is imminent, with rapid employment of step 3 before experiencing any air hunger.

Athletes represent a special subpopulation because, in general, EILO events occur at a rather predictable time and the unique features of each sport will require specific adaptations. The timing for medications and meals should be adapted for the athlete to have optimal LPR control. For example, instead of taking reflux medications as commonly prescribed, the athlete may need to take medication an hour before the first training session of the day. Type and timing of preworkout meals may need to be altered to reduce additional reflux symptoms during training. Finally, the athlete will need to train the breathing recovery exercises regime in a sport-specific manner rather than while sedentary. Sport-specific training, done in conjunction with the coach and athletic trainer, can forge a path to complete recovery from the EILO events. The Olin Exercise-Induced Laryngeal Obstruction Biphasic Inhalation (EILOBI) breathing techniques have been developed specifically for athletes.[84] This chapter includes cases of EILO authored by Sandage and Nauman (Cases 7.8 and 7.9), describing their assessment, treatment specifics, and clinical outcomes.

Published outcomes for treatment efficacy in this population are limited but supportive of the efficacy of SLP intervention in as few as 2 therapy sessions using a telepractice model[85] and a median of 3 in-person treatment sessions.[86]

CASE STUDY 7.6

Long-Term Management of PVFM in an Adult Following an Environmental Fume Exposure

Carissa Maira

Evaluation

History of the Upper Airway Complaint

I had the pleasure of evaluating LC at the request of otolaryngologist Dr X. LC is a 49-year-old cisgender female with a 6-month history of chronic cough, dysphonia, and episodic dyspnea (described as a "choking feeling"). She reported onset of symptoms following an accidental exposure at her place of work. She noted that one Monday morning, she was the first to arrive at her office building. Upon opening the door and taking the first step into the building, she began coughing uncontrollably. She ran out of the building but could not stop coughing for several hours. She later found out that the floors in the office had been refinished over the weekend, and she had inhaled polyurethane fumes. Symptoms at onset were frequent bouts of coughing, constant throat pain, shortness of breath, and severe dysphonia. Symptoms have improved with pulmonology intervention with use of Singulair, Flovent, and Ventolin for the past 3 months for diagnosed reactive airway disease. Workup included positive methacholine challenge and normal chest x-ray. Dr X prescribed omeprazole to manage LPR and gabapentin for sensory neuropathic cough 4 weeks prior. LC reports consistent adherence to all the above medications since they were prescribed.

Despite medical management, the patient reports persistent mild but chronic voice changes. At rest, there is no dyspnea, but she reports multiple daily episodes of dyspnea, described as a choking sensation and feeling as though she cannot take in a full breath. These episodes are typically precipitated by strong odors (such as cleaning agents), smoke, perfume, fumes, dust, or moderate activity (eg, taking her dog for a walk or climbing stairs). Spicy or strongly flavored foods often induce a "choking" sensation. Rarely (once per week or less), symptoms occur without any inciting stimulus, usually when she is under increased stress at work. The albuterol inhaler (Ventolin) does not stop the episode, but her episodes improve with relaxed breathing and being still. During episodes, she reports that her voice changes from her baseline mild hoarseness to a whisper with only occasional airy, squeaky sounds produced. That voice change lasts for several hours up to several days.

Medical history is remarkable for difficulty sleeping: Her PCP prescribed Soma and Xanax as needed for sleep. She had no formal psychiatric diagnosis.

Social History. LC did not use tobacco, and rarely drank alcohol. She noted increased stress after her brother was in a severe motor vehicle accident (approximately a year before her exposure), in which he sustained a spinal cord injury resulting in paraplegia. Patient LC lives with her dog. She is still working in the building where the exposure occurred as a personal assistant but is in the process of applying for long-term disability and filing a lawsuit against the office building landlord for their role in the exposure.

Laryngeal Imaging

Preliminary training in "rescue breathing strategies" (described below) was performed prior to videostroboscopic examination. Laryngeal videostroboscopy was completed with a transnasal distal chip endoscope. During the examination, the patient demonstrated normal arytenoid mobility and no fatigability; however, the arytenoids were slightly adducted during rest breathing. The vocal fold edges were smooth. There was mild evidence of

326 Voice Therapy: Clinical Case Studies

phonotrauma with an increased number of visible blood vessels on the superior surface. Glottic closure was complete with a pressed phonation pattern (increased closed quotient and reduced amplitude of lateral excursion). Mucosal wave was intact bilaterally. Vibration was periodic. There was supraglottic hyperfunction, both mild ventricular compression and anterior position of the arytenoids, consistent with MTD.

Auditory-Perceptual Evaluation, Visual Evaluation, and Manual Palpation

The CAPE-V[33] was utilized to assess overall severity of voice quality and to quantify aberrant perceptual features identified in the voice.[87] The overall score was 35/100, indicating moderate vocal quality deficits. Aberrant perceptual features identified in the voice included breathiness and strain. Overall vocal intensity was reduced, and overall vocal pitch was normal. Resonance was laryngeal/pharyngeal in quality. During respiration, there was only upper thoracic and clavicular motion. There was minimal to no excursion of the lower thoracic ribs or abdomen during inhalation or exhalation. The patient spoke in short phrases with shallow, audible breaths between phrases. Her rate of speech was perceptually increased. On palpation, there was a narrow thyrohyoid space and palpable base of tongue tension.

Aerodynamic Measures

The Pentax Medical (Montvale, NJ) Phonatory Aerodynamic System (PAS) model #6600 was utilized to acquire and analyze aerodynamic measures. Results indicated normal vital capacity of 2.91 L. Mean expiratory flow rate was normal on sustained vowels at 0.09 L/sec but reduced in running speech at 0.05 L/sec, consistent with the findings of mild MTD. The patient was unable to shout for a measure of maximal loudness. A minimal increase in vocal loudness was produced with strain and roughness. Loudness range was 62 to 80 dB SPL.

Acoustic Measures

Acoustic measures were obtained utilizing the Pentax Medical (Montvale, NJ) Computerized Speech Lab (CSL) with ADSV™, Multi-Dimensional Voice Program (MDVP™), and Real-Time Pitch™. A headset microphone was placed at a 45-degree angle at 2 cm from the mouth for data acquisition. Results are detailed in Table 7–9.

These findings indicated normal mean F0 in speech and normal SD of F0 (a measure of overall speech prosody). Pitch and loudness control and flexibility were reduced, with a decreased upper and lower F0 range and a voice break in the midrange. Cepstral Peak Prominence (CPP) was slightly reduced, consistent with the perceptual assessment of breathiness and strain. Cepstral Spectral Index

Table 7–9. Acoustic Assessment Results

Speaking Fundamental Frequency (SF0)	205 Hz
Standard Deviation of SF0	22 Hz
Physiological Pitch Range	172-583 Hz
Fundamental Frequency on Sustained Vowels	212 Hz
Cepstral Peak Prominence (CPP) /a/	9.573 dB
Cepstral/Spectral Index of Dysphonia (CSID™)	39

of Dysphonia (CSID) was consistent with the perceptual CAPE-V score, indicating moderate dysphonia.

Trial Therapy/Stimulability

The patient was trained in 2 rescue breathing strategies: pursed-lip breathing[88] and sniff/hiss.[78,89] Pursed-lip breathing is performed by puckering the lips as though drinking through a straw and maintaining this position during inhalation and exhalation. The patient controls the degree of resistance by controlling the aperture of the lips. In the sniff/hiss strategy, the patient is cued to exhale on the sound /s/ until nearly out of air, then relax and allow a passive recoil breath in through the nose. LC appeared stimulable to both strategies during preexamination trials. During LC's videostroboscopic exam, the clinician guided her through 3 productions of each strategy with the endoscope in place. Both pursed-lip posture and sniff/hiss resulted in full abduction of the arytenoids. The clinician recorded and reviewed this with her at the end of the examination. Seeing the effect of the strategies on increasing the size of her airway was reinforcing for LC. She said, "Oh, wow, it really does give me more room to breathe when I do those exercises!"

> Biofeedback with the use of laryngeal endoscopy and cueing of relaxed throat breathing, resulting in reduction or elimination of hyperadducted vocal fold postures, has been demonstrated in multiple studies and most recently in LeBlanc et al (2021).[90]

Impression

Overall, evaluation results were consistent with episodes of PVFM or ILO exacerbated by underlying reactive airway disease and LPR. The patient had also developed maladaptive compensatory mild-moderate MTD, with reports of severe episodes of aphonia (not observed during evaluation). LC presents as an excellent candidate for voice and respiratory retraining therapy. The clinician reviewed the results of the evaluation with the patient, particularly the effectiveness of both the sniff/hiss and pursed-lip breathing strategies to maintain an open glottis. The clinician asked her to practice these strategies 5 times daily and to use them (along with her albuterol inhaler) for relief when the "choking" sensation occurs, as well as to use them instead of coughing to reduce phonotrauma.[39]

Plan of Care

It is anticipated that 6 sessions over 90 days will be required to resolve the patient's complaints.

Long-Term Goal. The patient will engage in normal activities of daily living without dyspnea.

Short-Term Goals:

1. The patient will demonstrate abdominal (versus habitual clavicular) breathing with 80% accuracy during rest breathing in a seated position.
2. The patient will demonstrate rescue breathing strategies (pursed-lip breathing and/or sniff/hiss) with 80% accuracy during rest breathing in a seated position.
3. The patient will speak with a resonant voice at the phrase level with 80% accuracy as judged by clinician perception.

Decision Making

The complexities of LC's case included underlying pulmonary disease with a positive methacholine challenge (indicating mechanical breathing difficulties that required medical intervention) as well as possible secondary gains with a pending lawsuit. However, she was stimulable to trial therapy: Based on laryngeal imaging findings, she could achieve a more open airway with both pursed-lip breathing and sniff/hiss. These were promising "rescue breathing" replacement strategies to break

328 Voice Therapy: Clinical Case Studies

cycles of PVFM as well as alternatives to cough to reduce her phonotrauma. The voice change was also complicated; there were signs of phonotrauma, and she was coughing frequently, so managing that physical aspect made sense. Additionally, she had reported episodes of complete voice loss. It is possible that those were repeated hemorrhages, but it seemed more likely to be episodic severe MTD. The only way to know for sure would be to scope her again during an episode of voice loss, and it would be easier to achieve that while she was engaged in therapy.

> There is always a possibility of working with patients who are pursuing legal intervention or workers' compensation when the cause of their problem is believed to result from a workplace incident. This should not be a factor in determining the candidacy of a patient for therapy, and in this case, the clinician points to all the reasons to take this patient into therapy to address her upper airway/breathing and voice concerns. If the clinician is concerned about the impact of a pending case in their therapy, they are guided to talk with risk management, a department in most medical centers that can best guide the clinician.

In addition to the rescue breathing strategies, it was important to address her chronic moderate dysphonia, muscular tension, and shallow breathing. LC was not aware of her breathing patterns and didn't notice her breath until it was at a crisis level. LC reported environmental stress and lacked a strong support system. The clinician considered the value of encouraging LC to engage with a counselor or psychologist to help manage these aspects of her disordered breathing but also wanted to offer her immediate help. The clinician decided to start by working on developing mindfulness/awareness of breathing

and encouraging abdominal respiration and relaxed throat breathing to build awareness of baseline tension and promote a more relaxed laryngeal posture.[91]

> In this case, the author is referencing the possibility that this episodic loss of voice is more muscular in nature and may represent a significant secondary MTD due to episodic breathing problems changing the balance of the muscles used in producing voice. (Review Case Studies 4.1, 4.2, and 4.3 for guidance on therapy tools to use in addressing MTD.) Further into this case, the author notes that during an episode of aphonia, a repeat laryngeal imaging was conducted and there was no evidence for hemorrhage, so MTD was hypothesized as the cause of the aphonia.

Due to observations of high thoracic/clavicular breathing and the link between intercostal muscle tension and anxiety symptoms, progressive relaxation exercises were incorporated in the plan of care, which would also increase mindfulness of tension throughout the body.[92] To address her MTD, use of Vocal Function Exercises (VFEs)[93] was planned to balance the subsystems of respiration, phonation, and resonance. However, since VFEs do not address running speech, and given the videostroboscopy findings of pressed phonation and supraglottic hyperfunction, the clinician also used RVT[43] in speech and introduced conversation to train LC to utilize a barely adducted glottal configuration during speech.

Intervention

Session #1: In Person, Two Hours

When LC returned for her first voice therapy session, she was aphonic and only able to communicate in a whisper. She had walked into a store that was selling scented candles and had a long coughing bout and immediate voice change. She did not attempt to use the alternative behaviors trained in the evaluation because she felt the issue was in her chest, not her throat. Because of the abrupt voice change after coughing, brief transoral videostroboscopy was implemented, and there was no vocal fold hemorrhage. During the course of that examination, it was observed that with her tongue protruded and the endoscope pressing on the tongue slightly, the voice cleared to a normal quality. The laryngologist confirmed acute MTD exacerbation leading to aphonia. The remainder of the first therapy visit was devoted to regaining voicing: LC was asked to protrude her tongue and hold it with gauze (as during the transoral videostroboscopy). (See Video 30 Tongue Stretches by Schneider.) Meanwhile, the clinician applied gentle pressure at the base of tongue at the midline under the chin, at the point of demarcation between the mandible and the soft tissue of the floor of the mouth (anterior belly of the digastric muscle and mylohyoid). The clinician then asked the patient to keep that area completely relaxed while saying "Don't work here at all" and while phonating /m/. It took 20 minutes for clear voice to be consistently established on /m/ (10 consecutive accurate repetitions). Then, the clinician was able to remove the tactile feedback while LC continued with successful productions. After consistent voice was established and maintained without clinician cues for 10 consecutive accurate repetitions, LC was able to release the gauze from her tongue (producing 10 more accurate repetitions of /m/), then allow her tongue to rest inside her mouth for 10 accurate repetitions of /m/. The biggest hurdle in generalization to speech was the transition from /m/ to /m/ + vowel. After several tries with the clinician coaching, "Don't let ANYTHING change; just open your mouth," the patient was successful in producing /ma/, then /mi/, /mo/, and so on. Once voicing was firmly established on /m/ + vowel sounds for at least 10 consecutive repetitions, the patient was guided to produce negative practice for a single sound (returning to

her aphonic presentation from the beginning of the session), then to return immediately to the rehearsed target voice. Once she was able to consistently perform this activity, she advanced to the same pattern (10 target repetitions, 1 "wrong on purpose," 10 target repetitions) on /m/-initial words, phrases laden with /m/, and sentences with varied phonemes not laden with nasals. Negative practice for stimuli longer than 1 syllable was only for the first word of the stimulus with immediate return to target voice. After an hour of drill, the patient was able to produce conversation at a slow rate of speech with intense concentration, slowly increasing the rate of speech as she became more confident. The entire process from walking in the door with aphonia to normal voice took 2 hours, including laryngeal examination. The clinician left the patient to practice independently for a portion of the generalization practice while attending to another patient. As the patient left the session, the clinician gave her a "voice recovery" handout that included step-by-step instructions beginning with "Stick out your tongue and hold it with a piece of gauze" and outlining each step she had just completed, up through spontaneous speech.

Session #2: In Person, One Hour

LC came back 1 week later with a return to her baseline moderate dysphonia. At this point, the clinician was able to resume the original plan of care. The session goals were to introduce progressive relaxation and VFEs as well as to reinforce the rescue breathing strategies trained at the initial evaluation. The session began with a quick check-in, where LC revealed that she had maintained voicing for the past week for the most part. There was one episode of voice loss, but she was able to use the voice recovery handout from session #1 independently to regain her voice. Practice then moved on to mindfulness via progressive relaxation. LC was guided to focus on one part of the body at a time, first contracting muscles and creating tension, then releasing fully. In this manner, she was able to relax the muscles in her forehead, cheeks, jaw, tongue, shoulders, throat, chest, and abdomen. The clinician emphasized focusing without judgment on the sensation of tension versus relaxation in the throat, in the abdomen, and in the movement of breath, noticing how tension in the abdomen changed the depth and flow of breath. Through this practice, LC recognized an easier flow of breath when she relaxed her abdomen and a higher locus of breath (chest) when she tightened her abdomen. That relaxed abdominal breathing was then applied to sound during modified VFEs. LC was trained to produce a modified kazoo buzz sound by gently approximating her lips and phonating an /o/ vowel (a never-ending "w" as though about to say the word "whoa" but forgetting to open the mouth). LC continued to monitor her expiratory airflow to avoid breath holding. She placed her finger in front of her lips to ensure continuous and consistent airflow. She performed ascending-descending glides and sustained phonation exercises with the modified kazoo buzz sound. Finally, rescue breathing sniff/hiss and pursed-lip breathing exercises were retrained and practiced, utilizing them organically any time the urge to cough arose during the session. At this stage, LC did not recall the rescue breathing strategies independently until she began to cough and the clinician cued her to use a replacement strategy. For homework, the clinician asked her to complete progressive relaxation, rescue breathing techniques (5 sets of 5 breaths of either technique), and VFEs twice daily using a recording made during her session, as well as to utilize the breathing techniques to prevent or stop coughing. (See Video 5 Vocal Function Exercises by Stemple.)

Session #3: In Person, 45 Minutes
LC returned in 1 week with baseline moderate dysphonia and reported no further episodes of aphonia. She practiced modified VFEs

once daily and a few repetitions of the rescue breathing. She was still coughing but was able to use either the sniff/hiss or pursed-lip breathing strategy to reduce the duration of her coughing episodes, and the cough was no longer progressing to PVFM/dyspnea. Session goals were to advance progressive relaxation, reinforce VFEs, reinforce and increase independence with rescue breathing strategies, and introduce modified RVT. First, to deactivate lingering tension, LC performed self-guided circumlaryngeal massage. The clinician then guided LC through an advanced version of progressive relaxation where she tightened her entire body for a few seconds, then released. The clinician guided her through releasing the muscles in her forehead, cheeks, jaw, tongue, shoulders, throat, chest, and abdomen without first having to contract them. She performed VFEs with increased accuracy of abdominal respiration and consistency of phonation as well as slightly increased range of motion (ROM) as measured through F0 range. When she began to cough during a treatment session, she required strong clinician cues to use her replacement strategy. She resisted this treatment, but ultimately, with a lot of encouragement, was able to prevent a cough episode using the sniff/hiss technique. At this point, she finally "bought in" to this aspect of the therapy and more consistently attempted to use the replacement strategies. The clinician then turned the attention to voicing. Using the mindful sensation she had developed during progressive relaxation and VFEs as a guide, as well as the work in session #1 focusing on producing voice near the front of her mouth, the clinician and LC engaged principles of RVT. Specifically, the clinician guided LC to feel the difference between her habit of mild-moderate muscle tension and a completely relaxed voice with sensation on /m/ in the mouth, lips, and front of her face. She worked at the sound level (/m/ and "m-hm") throughout this session in the same format as session #1 (10 repetitions in target voice, 1 in habit voice [negative practice], 10 in target voice) and was able to progress to /m/-initial words and nasal-laden phrases. For homework, the clinician asked her to practice advanced progressive relaxation, rescue breathing techniques, VFEs, and resonant voice phrases twice daily using the recording made during her session. LC expressed motivation to utilize the breathing techniques to prevent or stop coughing but did not think she could practice twice daily due to time commitments. With discussion of lifestyle, she realized she could practice in the car and in the shower. Neither of those times permitted the use of paper handouts, but she could practice with the session recording while in the car and, in the shower, she could make up words with "m" and "n."

Session #4: In Person, 45 Minutes
LC returned in 1 week with persistent moderate dysphonia. She reported inconsistent success using the rescue breathing techniques to prevent coughing episodes. She had practiced either VFEs or RVT for a few minutes once daily and never consistently practiced the breathing exercises. At this point, the clinician and LC discussed her goals and how she might best meet them. LC was tearful and concerned that her medical record reflected that she was trying her best. The clinician and patient developed a plan to create a very fast (2-minute) practice routine she could memorize and perform multiple times during the day, which she felt she could commit to during her upcoming vacation. First, LC was trained to perform a quick scan-and-release progressive relaxation in just a few seconds by silently thinking about relaxing the key areas: face, throat, shoulders, chest, belly. The modified VFE program was condensed to only 2 repetitions of maximal sustained phonation and 1 ascending-descending glide. RVT techniques were advanced from nasal-laden phrases to conversation with "m-hm" or extended /m/ thrown in periodically so that she could practice RVT covertly. After establishing awareness and successful production of the target voice, negative practice was again used (10 seconds in habit voice) to give LC the mastery experience of "fixing" her own voice in running speech. Her conversational speech continued to lapse into laryngeal tone focus during conversation, but she demonstrated the ability to return to target resonant voice with carrier "m-hm" as soon as she became aware of the change. At this point, that awareness was driven by the clinician pointing out the change; LC was not yet independently aware when her voice drifted back to habit voice. Homework was to perform the quick scan-and-release progressive relaxation in just a few seconds, 1 rescue breath (either strategy), reduced VFEs, and 1 minute of spontaneous speech with resonant voice followed by 10 seconds of habit voice and immediate return to resonant voice.

Session #5: In Person, 45 Minutes
LC returned 4 weeks later, having taken a 2-week vacation and then needing time to catch up at work. She reported that when she returned from vacation, her voice was completely clear and effortless, and she had not had an episode of cough or PVFM during her entire vacation. When returning to the scene of her initial exposure at her office as well as the stresses of work, she felt her throat tighten and she once again began to struggle with maintaining attention to producing a target voice. She recognized the interplay between her underlying anxiety and her waxing and waning symptoms but was not open to seeking professional guidance for the anxiety. She was concerned about a formal psychiatric diagnosis being made because she thought it could undermine her lawsuit. The session was spent reinforcing all activities from previous sessions: deactivation of tension via gentle pressure on the base of tongue muscles externally, progressive relaxation, modified VFEs, forward focus/resonant voice in conversation, and rescue breathing exercises. She was

consistently successful during the session and expressed confidence in her ability to continue independent practice. The patient and clinician agreed she was ready to discharge from direct therapy to independent practice at this point, with the understanding that external factors and underlying stress/anxiety would likely result in variable degrees of success with the techniques outside the therapy room.

Session #6: In Person, 45 Minutes

LC returned 3 months later, reporting a debilitating relapse in her cough, for which her doctors recommended she not work for 4 weeks. The trigger for the relapse on that occasion was walking past a person smoking on the street during a work trip to New York. Her voice was very low in pitch and strained. Her breathing pattern was high and shallow. Both improved with retraining in low abdominal breathing and return to twice-daily VFEs as well as attention to forward focus/resonant voice. This same pattern occurred several times over the next year. LC would experience improvement to near-normal, then would experience a recurrence, including a significant voice change. She returned for a truncated course of voice therapy (1-2 "refresher" sessions) each time it occurred. During one of these visits, she and the clinician had a lengthy discussion about stress management. LC concluded that talking with a trained counselor would be beneficial. She did ultimately see a counselor for several sessions and learned techniques to better manage her anxiety. She also became independent in resolving the voice changes that occurred after relapses by independently implementing therapy techniques and viewing home practice videos created during her therapy sessions. Her pulmonologist would not permit controlled desensitization challenges with odor provocations. However, after repeated training, LC became adept at automatically implementing breathing strategies to avoid PVFM episodes when entering areas with odors or smoke. She continued to have flare-ups of reactive airway disease when ill with upper respiratory infections. Coughing and PVFM episodes due to odors became less frequent over time, and her ability to manage them increased to a completely independent level. Her stress level reduced significantly after she obtained long-term disability status and when the lawsuit was settled in her favor, removing her from the trauma of revisiting the site of her original exposure and allowing her to find occupation in a lower-stress field.

Summary

When patients experience a significant exposure to laryngeal irritants, there can be long-lasting symptoms, and voice therapy may involve an initial more consistent and intensive phase followed by sporadic visits during relapses over a long duration. In this case, LC required a coordinated treatment approach including medications through pulmonology, voice and respiratory retraining therapy, and professional counseling. Relapses were frequent while the patient dealt with the stressors of work and sued the landlord of her office building. She consistently demonstrated gains during therapy sessions, but her success outside the therapy room was limited by the recurring trauma of revisiting the site of her original exposure as well as the stress of her occupation. Despite this, she progressed toward independence in applying therapy techniques. The use of audio recordings and videos with supplemental handouts was particularly helpful to reinforce strategies during periods of relapse, which were sometimes weeks or months apart. Although she has become adept at managing her PVFM and MTD, 4 years after the initial exposure, she still is unable to tolerate being in a room with strong odors for extended periods. However, she is no longer afraid to walk down the street or past a perfume counter, and she has not lost her voice in over 2 years. Perhaps more importantly, if she were to lose her voice, she knows how to fix it herself.

CASE STUDY 7.7

Treating Irritable Larynx in an Adult Within the Framework of Central Sensitivity Syndrome

Linda Rammage

Evaluation

History of the Upper Airway Problem

Over the previous 18 months, DD had experienced progressive difficulty with voice quality, breathing, and swallowing. She became aware of the first symptom: progressively "squeaky," effortful voice during the day, when she started working in a department store, adjacent to the perfume department. Several weeks later, her breathing also was affected when she was in the store. She described a wheezing sensation in her throat and effort in her chest when she was trying to breathe in, which worsened the longer she spoke, as did her dysphonia. A few months later, DD began to experience difficulty swallowing. She described increasing effort to swallow solid food and a feeling of panic when preparing to go on her lunch breaks. She typically took her break with a longtime friend, who regularly expressed great concern about DD's symptoms and proposed that she might have throat cancer from her husband's secondhand smoke or from the chemicals coming from the perfume department that seemed to aggravate DD's symptoms. DD asked her manager for a transfer to another department, and he complied. She was transferred to a clothing section and initially felt relieved until she noticed a peculiar scent as she opened some new garment packages. These odors triggered the same throat symptoms: increased dysphonia followed by difficulty breathing in. Her doctor recommended that she go on medical leave. As her symptoms persisted, her concern about cancer increased, despite a clear chest x-ray and an otolaryngologist's exam of "negative findings." She was sleeping poorly and waking frequently, gasping for breath. DD contracted COVID-19 several months prior to our consultation, and she suffered ongoing chronic coughing spells triggered by talking and certain odors, as well as globus and stuffy nose. She often woke up coughing and breathing through her mouth.

Medical History. DD had undergone abdominal surgery and sustained back injuries during a motor vehicle accident. Her mother died of colon cancer. She reported that she currently suffered from or had previously experienced the following problems: anxiety; (presumed) asthma; arthritis; breathing problem; fatigue; chronic coughing and choking; depressed mood; heartburn; hoarseness; irritable bowel; lump in throat sensation; multiple chemical sensitivity (MCS); neck or back injury; postnasal drip (PND); severe snoring; swallowing problem; and chronic throat clearing. DD had been moderately overweight all her life, but she had gained an additional 25 pounds while on medical leave. She did not eat regular meals during the day but enjoyed a large meal in the evening. She drank 8 cups of water daily. She was a lifelong abstainer from alcohol and tobacco and did not drink caffeine. DD's family doctor had initially treated her for "asthma" by prescribing antianxiety medication and steroid inhalers to reduce her "asthma" attacks based on symptoms of difficulty breathing in and coughing, particularly in the presence of certain odors and cold temperatures. No airborne allergies were identified. Consultation with a respiratory specialist yielded results inconsistent with asthma.

Psychosocial History. DD was 54 and married with 3 adult children, one of whom still lived at home. Her husband was a heavy smoker, but had recently limited smoking to outdoors. She stated she was happily married, but worried about her husband's health. DD had enjoyed her job in sales. Quitting her job had negative economic and emotional impacts. DD stated that her husband's business was experiencing some slowdowns,

334   Voice Therapy: Clinical Case Studies

which increased the financial burden on the family.

Patient Self-Assessment

DD completed the Voice-Related Quality of Life (V-RQOL).[94] Scores were: social-emotional domain: 15/16; physical functioning domain: 22/24; total raw score: 37, indicating significant negative impact on voice-related quality of life.

Evaluation Procedures

DD underwent evaluation of her problem with an interprofessional team composed of a laryngologist, SLP, and psychiatrist. The psychiatrist on the voice care team obtained a comprehensive psychosocial history, helped DD manage psychological factors, and advised on and prescribed optimal use of neuropsychotropic medications.

Interprofessional Team History

The voice care team identified physiological and emotional factors that likely contributed to the development of irritable larynx syndrome (ILS) and/or acted as symptom triggers. Among the potential predisposing factors:

- **Abdominal Tension.** DD's history of multiple abdominal surgery and lower back injury may have contributed to the tendency to hold her abdominal muscles in a "splinting" behavior to inhibit painful abdominal muscle stretching on inspiration. She was aware of tension in her abdomen and back when she recalled her mother's fight with colon cancer. These reactions could act as "tone modulators," making her more susceptible to reacting to ILS triggers.[35]
- **Gastroesophageal Reflux.** DD identified chronic heartburn, globus pharyngeus, sensation of postnasal drip, chronic throat clearing, and choking when supine. All are common symptoms of LPR. These symptoms increased as she became more sedentary, went to bed immediately after

meals, and gained weight. More intense coughing, particularly at night, may have exacerbated her reflux since coughing is associated with heightened abdominal pressure. Her nasal obstruction onset with COVID-19 symptoms resulted in a dominance of oral breathing, which often serves as a cough trigger and can exacerbate adductor laryngospasm (AL).

- **Psychological Factors.** DD's preoccupation with the possibility she had cancer caused growing anxiety and was fueled by the unabated throat and breathing symptoms. It was evident that DD was burdened by unexpressed fear that she would inherit her mother's colon cancer given her history of abdominal problems, or alternatively that her long-term exposure to her husband's secondhand smoke might have induced cancer, as was inadvertently reinforced by her work friend. Furthermore, it was clear that DD had developed anticipatory anxiety about her throat, specifically her difficulty breathing in certain environments. Her anxiety may have been borne of previous inconclusive or inadequately explained diagnoses of "borderline asthma" and "multiple chemical sensitivities," particularly as she was cautioned against exposing herself to environmental agents and had already been exposed to triggering irritants for prolonged periods. A symbolic olfactory association also may have existed during the onset of symptoms. On reflection and discussion with the psychiatrist, DD stated that she had never appreciated perfumes since she was a child because a relative whom she distrusted and feared always wore strong perfume when she visited.
- **Central Sensitivity Syndrome (CSS).** DD had been suffering from several symptoms that led to diagnosis of multiple Central Sensitivity Syndrome (CSS). If ILS represents a CSS, DD may have been predisposed to neuroplastic changes that affect

the sensory-motor system, with other physiological and psychological factors contributing the laryngopharyngeal focus for symptom formation.[35,48]

> The clinician is guided to reflect on the discussion earlier in this chapter of a centrally mediated CHS that likely represents a subtype of CSS. Here, CSS is implicated in the cause of irritable larynx and laryngeal adductory breathing spasms. It has been said that CSS is an umbrella term for a variety of centrally mediated hyperresponsive somatic problems, and there is quite a fascinating body of literature that spans many medical specialties.

Body Alignment and Use

Visual observation and manual techniques revealed spinal lordosis, head retraction, and jaw jutting posture in sitting position. Effortful swallowing and AL were both triggered by jaw jutting posture. DD's scapulae were moderately adducted and tender. Her head was held rigidly on her neck and suboccipital muscles were very tender to palpation. Circumferential palpation of DD's abdomen and lumbar spine regions revealed minimal palpable displacement on inhalation during speech and at rest in upright positions.[95]

Oral Breathing

DD reported she had been mouth breathing frequently due to chronic nasal congestion. Oral breathing offers lower airway resistance in the upper airway and provides none of the filtering, warming, and humidifying functions of nasal breathing, so it introduces an external irritant to the laryngeal region and may invoke laryngeal "valving" or coughing to filter the inspiratory air.

Paralaryngeal Muscle Evaluation

Using the 0 to 3 Likert scale grading criteria, the clinician manually evaluated 4 paralaryngeal muscle groups at rest and during vocal activities.[96] Suprahyoid, thyrohyoid, and cricothyroid muscles all were maximally tight (score 3) and her cricoid cartilage was displaced anteriorly. Lateral laryngeal mobility was limited, suggesting cricopharyngeus muscle hypertonicity.

Acoustic and Auditory-Perceptual Evaluation

Mean F0 during speech was 278 Hz (above normative range); speaking F0 range was 270 to 314 Hz (above normative range); and physiologic F0 range, produced during glissando productions on "oo-siren" and phonation with simultaneous lip trilling, was 125 to 857 Hz (normal range). Dynamic intensity range was 42 dB (normal range). CPP values were outside the normal range.[97] DD's CAPE-V score of 35/100 indicated her speaking voice was characterized by consistent moderate strain and breathiness but normal voice quality during laughter and spontaneous vocal responses such as "um-hm." Phrasing was intermittently affected by shortness of breath. Intermittent voiced inspiration was noted.

Laryngeal Imaging

Laryngeal imaging using a transnasal fiberoptic scope initially elicited an AL response to the sensory stimulus; adductory laryngospasm and voiced inspiratory stridor were viewed and recorded. Muscle misuse patterns observed in the laryngopharynx included larynx elevation for speech and pitch ascension, elongated vocal fold posture during speech, and absence of vocal fold shortening during pitch descent. During evaluation of vocal fold vibratory patterns with stroboscopic light, notable features included reduced amplitude of vibration bilaterally, incomplete closure during high-pitched phonation, and reduced mucosal wave bilaterally. Several signs of reflux were noted, including erythema in the posterior glottis, edematous arytenoid and interarytenoid regions, and pseudosulci inferior to the vocal fold margins.

It is a common practice to rule out GERD and LPR as triggers for ILS. Often, physicians use a positive response to a diagnostic trial of PPIs as a means to rule in or out LPR and GERD. However, there remains controversy regarding the laryngeal signs of GERD and/or LPR. The reader is guided to critically read the literature on the evidence of laryngeal signs of reflux.[98]

Trial of Therapy Techniques (Stimulability)

Therapy trials were initiated during the laryngeal examination, using recordings and real-time transnasal fiber-optic laryngeal imaging for visual feedback as facilitation exercises were introduced. Using a nasal breathing focus beginning with sniffing, DD was able to reverse her AL symptoms while watching the video monitor. Vibratory amplitude, mucosal wave, and closure patterns were normalized when techniques were introduced to improve coordination between speech breathing and phonation in modal register. Spontaneous utterances "m-hm" and "Hm!" allowed her to initiate phonation in her natural modal register area, around 180 Hz, and a pulsing voiced fricative production on /z/ allowed her to sustain normal phonation. "Z-pulses" are elicited by modeling a sustained /z/ while producing a rhythmic F0 and intensity pulse at a typical speaking rate.[99]

Decision Making

The voice care team and DD employed a client-centered model to define dominance of potential factors contributing to her symptoms. The client-centered ALERT Model was introduced to help DD understand the potential presence and dominance (size) of Anatomical, Lifestyle, Emotional, Reflux, and Technique factors and their potential interactions.[100] DD sketched her ALERT profile based on her understanding and beliefs. Since all components were important, they were assigned equivalent sizes

(Figure 7–6). Discussions around dominance and negative impact of symptoms led to decisions about hierarchy of the treatment program components.

Rehabilitation Approach

A multifactorial and interprofessional approach to treatment addressed the anatomical, lifestyle, and emotional factors contributing to DD's ILS symptoms.[48] This treatment plan is based on dominance and hierarchy of symptoms. Our interprofessional team therefore uses the term "level" rather than "long-term goal."

Level 1

Minimize sensory stimuli acting as internal (eg, reflux) and external (eg, odors) triggers, identify triggers, and maximize reflux management/compliance.

Goal #1. *DD will demonstrate an understanding and acceptance of ILS as CSS.* Using video recordings and references, the voice care team reassured DD that she did *not* have laryngeal cancer and that the symptoms she suffered can be explained by ILS.

Rationale. DD needed to understand the concept of ILS as a central nervous system (CNS) hypersensitivity syndrome to maximize treatment compliance and reduce emotional factors. CSS and CHS can both be considered CNS sensory disorders.

Goal #2. *Minimize sensory reflux stimuli that trigger AL, dysphonia, chronic cough, and globus.* The physician prescribed a PPI BID. DD and her daughter viewed a client education tool on LPR.[101] The otolaryngologist initiated treatment to manage DD's nasal congestion to minimize oral breathing, which aggravated her symptoms. DD's husband participated in discussions about symptom triggers, DD's anxiety about his health, and eliminating airborne irritants including secondhand smoke.

Rationale. DD's medical history suggested that reflux played a major role in predisposing her to laryngeal muscle spasm and

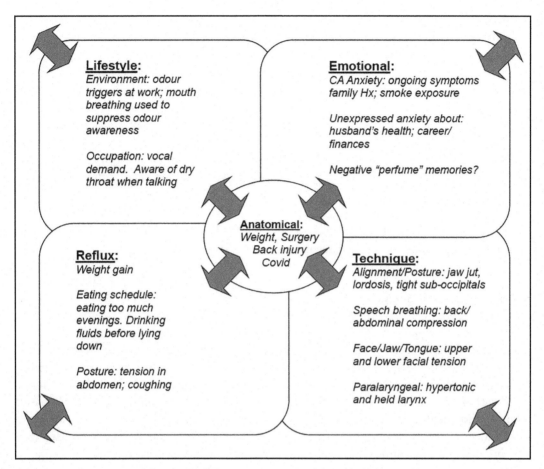

FIGURE 7–6. DD's ALERT profile.

coughing, which had increased since she gained weight. LPR may have also contributed to oral breathing as an airway irritant. Her husband needed to understand the potential trigger of secondhand smoke.

Level 2

Reprogram the habituated motor response: Desensitize and use principles of motor re-learning.

Goal #3. *DD will learn about maladaptive motor responses causing ILS symptoms.* Psychotherapy was offered to help make DD aware of the role that unexpressed negative emotions play in hyperkinetic muscle activity and of how olfactory stimuli can trigger ILS symptoms. The psychiatrist helped DD recognize how her fears about her health and olfactory memories, and sensory stimuli from reflux or airborne irritants, became inappropriately associated to cause abnormal muscle responses to normal sensory stimuli and how the pain sensation was reinforced through fear of what it might represent. This information was shared with the SLP so the professionals could apply common language and concepts in their interventions. The SLP and psychiatrist introduced physical activity and relaxation to assist DD in recognizing sensations associated with muscle tension and relaxation, as well as the emotional effects of physical activity.

Rationale. Understanding the complex physiological connection between sensory, emotional, and motor systems is essential to successful motor learning outcomes. Since endorphins are among the most powerful chemical treatments for negative affect, a regular physical fitness regime has the potential to minimize the dose and number of pharmacotherapies required.

> The clinician is guided to consider interprofessional collaboration with a variety of professionals. In this case, the author was able to seamlessly collaborate with a mental health professional. This collaboration improved communication and likely the care and positive outcome for this patient.

Voice Therapy. Simultaneous with psychotherapy and physical fitness programs, weekly speech-language pathology sessions were offered for 2 months (8 sessions) to help DD learn to extinguish maladaptive motor responses and learn more appropriate functional patterns for breathing and speech. DD's husband and daughter were asked to participate in formal therapy sessions to learn about ILS, provide support, and help with home practice and carryover. The most distressing symptoms of AL and chronic coughing were targeted first in therapy to empower DD with skills for immediate relief.

Goal #4. *DD will change her breathing pattern focus.* "Back breathing" was introduced: With head dropped forward and spine flexed, DD was instructed to notice which parts of her back moved during breathing. Once able to identify movements in her back, she was asked to continue attending to the sensation of back breathing in upright positions and to note how back breathing also facilitated natural abdominal breathing.[99]

Rationale. Ergonomic position changes minimized tension in the upper torso, helped release abdominal splinting, and served as a distraction from attending to the typical negative feedback of chest tension and effort that DD associated with inspiration. It eliminated DD's confusion about abdominal breathing, since "relaxed abdominal breathing" training had been previously unsuccessful.

Goal #5. *DD will learn to prevent and abort AL and coughing reactions.* Having already demonstrated appropriate inspiratory vocal fold posture during sniffing, DD was instructed to draw air slowly through the nose "filter" while her head and arms were dropped forward gently so she could identify areas of her back that were expanding to pull the air inward. The concept of nasal "circle" breathing was introduced to provide imagery that retains an abducted vocal fold position during the rest breathing cycle. DD would use the circle nasal breathing activity throughout her day to visualize the open airway and feel natural back movements. She would use nasal breathing to enjoy pleasant odors and imagine smelling a favorite food to pair positive olfactory activity with appropriate breathing patterns. She would use a combination of circle nasal/back breathing and successive water swallows through a straw to abort cough episodes. (See Video 21 Box Breathing by Slovarp, similar to circle breathing described here.)

Rationale. The sniffing/nasal breathing focus works on the same principle as "pursed lips breathing,"[102] by introducing a restriction in the upper airway that forces a compensatory reaction to abduct the vocal folds maximally. By imagining she was smelling something pleasurable, DD was able to pair olfactory sensations with appropriate breathing sensations. Circle breathing through the nose facilitates abducted vocal fold posture throughout the breathing cycle. In addition to breathing techniques, successive water swallows were introduced to initiate natural vertical movements of the larynx, thus reducing the posterior grip on the larynx from the cricopharyngeus muscle. Use of a straw for successive water swallows controls the amount of water in each swallow and maintains a neutral and safe swallowing position of the head and neck so the passage of fluid is not perceived as an airway threat that triggers ILS symptoms.

Goal #6. *DD will improve body posture and reduce specific muscle misuses in the abdomen, head, face, and neck.* Appropriate alignment and training in awareness of "tense" versus "neutral" muscles was paired with selective manual therapy to optimize function in neck, face, laryngeal, and pharyngeal muscles that had been chronically hypertonic.[99]

Rationale. Normalizing posture alignment is essential to restoring natural breathing patterns and neutralizing laryngeal suspension systems. Negative practice allows individuals to contrast voluntary isometric muscle activity with "release of muscle contraction" and provides a concrete sensory reference when hypertonicity has become the "normal" state and sensory feedback from muscle spindles has been reduced or altered.

Goal #7. *DD will learn how to consistently initiate and sustain voice in modal register with minimal muscle misuse in laryngeal suspension muscles.* Voice onset techniques that were successful during diagnostic therapy were applied. Coordinated voice onset (CVO) activities allow patients to experience natural abdominal muscle activity and resonance sensations simultaneously with easy voice onset. Two CVO activities were explored: (1) CVO on "spontaneous" utterances "um-hum" /mhm/ (vocal sound for "Yes") and "Hm!" (vocal sound for "That's interesting!") and (2) "Z-pulses," which provide feedback on the voiced fricative about continuous airflow and simulate speech inflections in a continuous phonation segment.[99,103] DD's response to these techniques was evaluated to determine which she could apply most immediately and effectively to speech. She chose CVO ("Hm!"/"m-hm") to cue her modal register, since she had noticed normal voice during this type of utterance in the past and was immediately able to apply it to short responses, such as "Sure," "Hi," and "OK."

A hierarchical approach was used to transfer the CVO sensations to speech within the first therapy session: serial speech ("HmMonday; HmTuesday . . . "); memorized passages; carrier phrases ("HmI'm going to the market to buy some _____"); and conversational speech. Subsequently, DD used "Z-pulses" and "V-pulses" to transfer CVO rapidly to speech phrases. Negative practice was used to enhance motor learning: The clinician asked DD to produce her "weak, high voice," then to use therapy cues to optimize her voice.

Rationale. Hypertonicity in laryngeal suspension muscles, most notably suprahyoid muscles, was noted during DD's attempts to initiate speech. Spontaneous voice-onset activities such as CVO tend to elicit natural modal register phonation with appropriate vocal fold adduction associated with low phonation threshold pressures, and CVO allowed DD to feel normal abdominal muscle activity and extinguish extraneous muscle activity. Voiced fricative productions use the principle of semi-occluded vocal tract to optimize vocal fold closure while providing resonance feedback. Pulsing engages the natural prosody and simulates stressed syllable productions in speech.[99]

Goal #8. *DD will learn to incorporate her therapy strategies to prevent inappropriate laryngeal motor reactions in the presence of triggers.* The clinician introduced a desensitization program in later stages of the therapy to allow DD to incorporate her management strategies when exposed to odors that previously triggered ILS symptoms. DD applied circle nasal breathing to situations she had previously found challenging, setting her own schedule and hierarchy, starting with scheduled exposures in the clinic and in her home.

Rationale. The desensitization program allowed DD to learn to extinguish the maladaptive responses to normal sensory stimuli and gave her the control and confidence to return to previously problematic environments, including her workplace.

340 Voice Therapy: Clinical Case Studies

Level 3

Capitalize on neural plasticity to reprogram the CNS.

Goal #9. *DD will work with the medical team to explore use of neuropsychotropic medication.* In consultation with DD, her general practitioner and the laryngologist, the psychiatrist took responsibility for determining which, if any, prescription medications, such as selective serotonin reuptake inhibitors, combined serotonin and norepinephrine reuptake inhibitors, tricyclic antidepressants, or a centrally active antispasmolytic drug might assist DD in reducing ILS symptoms. DD decided to defer medications based on her rapid improvement with therapy.

Rationale. Some patients with ILS and other CSS symptoms benefit from centrally active prescription medications. The neurons involved in the sensory-motor disorder of ILS and other types of CSS use chemicals to communicate with each other, and altering the communication reduces symptoms.

Treatment Outcomes: Three-Month Posttreatment Initiation

Symptom Abatement. DD reported that she was swallowing more easily, coughing less, and breathing and sleeping better within 3 weeks of reflux therapy. She had lost 5 pounds. DD recognized a significant reduction in her general body pain and fatigue. V-RQOL scores at 3 months were: social-emotional domain: 9/16; physical functioning domain: 11/24; and total raw score: 20/50, indicating a reduction in negative symptom impact on quality of life compared to her previous score of 37/50.

General Posture and Laryngeal and Paralaryngeal Muscle Use. Progressive improvement in body alignment and laryngeal postures were noted. DD monitored tension in her neck, face, jaw, tongue, and suprahyoid muscles several times daily and used appropriate strategies to release tension sites.

Laryngeal Imaging. Laryngeal imaging with the transnasal scope confirmed lowered larynx during phonation; modal register phonation; and normal vocal fold closure pattern, vocal fold vibratory amplitude, and mucosal wave bilaterally. DD experienced adductory spasm when the flexible scope was inserted but controlled the symptoms using circle nasal breathing and performing her "body meditation." The laryngeal exam revealed reduced erythema and edema in the larynx.

Acoustic and Perceptual-Acoustic Evaluation. DD's CPP values were WNL. DD's speaking voice was predominantly clear and produced in the modal register, with a mean F0 of 185 Hz. When she spoke of issues that caused anxiety, such as returning to work and financial pressures, she tended to revert to her "squeaky voice." She recognized the voice change and, with the assistance of the SLP, was able to recover clear modal register phonation.

Summary and Concluding Remarks

ILS is presented as a central sensitivity syndrome and as a hyperkinetic/hypertonic response in the laryngopharynx to normal stimuli. Since neural plasticity can cause long-term changes in muscle use patterns through a variety of mechanisms at the peripheral and central nervous system levels, treatment typically needs to be directed toward reprogramming subconscious movement patterns. An interprofessional approach is often helpful in determining the complex interactions between symptom formation and sensory triggers and planning the most effective treatment.

The rapid abatement of DD's ILS symptoms can be attributed largely to her motivation to improve her health and return to a normal lifestyle. An intelligent and insightful woman, she was able to recognize and evaluate her physical and emotional responses to various situations and employ appropriate techniques to reduce or extinguish inappropriate muscle responses to symptom triggers. The interprofessional team provided consistent messages about the causes and appropriate treatments for her symptoms. Although it was almost a year after her first visit to the voice clinic that she claimed to be "symptom free," DD accepted the gradual improvement as a predictable response and gave herself due credit for the amount of time and effort she contributed to the changes she made.

 CASE STUDY 7.8

Behavioral Management for Exercise-Induced Laryngeal Obstruction (EILO) in a Collegiate Swimmer

Mary J. Sandage

Evaluation

Chief Complaint. Difficulty breathing while swimming

Patient II, an 18-year-old cisgender female college student on a swim scholarship, was referred by her pulmonologist and sports medicine physician for an assessment to rule out probable EILO.

History of Breathing Concern

The patient attended the initial speech-language pathology evaluation by herself and served as the sole reporter for her behavioral and medical history. She described some confusion about the referral to an SLP, as she did not believe that she had any difficulty with her speech. It was explained that the evaluating SLP specialized in upper airway breathing disorders in athletes and worked closely with pulmonologists, allergists, and sports medicine physicians. The patient described a successful high school swimming career with subsequent recruitment to an excellent collegiate swim program. During high school, she competed in the 200- and 400-meter freestyle; however, during her first season of collegiate swimming, her coach changed her training and competition to the 200-meter freestyle. She described intermittent breathing problems during swimming for about 3 years with a diagnosis of asthma 2 years prior to her referral to the Voice & Upper Airway Clinic. The sports medicine physician for the swim team referred the patient for a pulmonology assessment to definitively rule asthma in or out. The pulmonology assessment consisted of a negative methacholine challenge, negative chest x-ray, and spirometry with a flat inspiratory flow volume loop that was consistent with extrathoracic obstruction *during inhalation*. When the pulmonologist ruled out asthma, they suspected EILO and referred the patient for assessment and treatment. When prompted about difficulty inhaling, exhaling, or both when breathing events occurred, the patient described primary difficulty with inhaling and no trouble exhaling. She denied making any noise, stridor, or wheezing when the breathing events happened; however, she described throat tightness and some tightness in her upper torso. When asked to describe a typical breathing event in detail, she indicated that the breathing difficulty generally occurred during timed trials in practice and in competition when she was swimming the 200-meter freestyle. She reported that the first 100 meters of the race went well; however, she noticed more difficulty breathing during the last 100 meters. She related that she wasn't able to get enough air in fast enough and, as a result, her times were slower than those that she typically achieved in practice. She reported that at first, this happened occasionally; however, by the time of the evaluation, it was occurring every time she was being timed in practice and in every competitive race. The patient initially thought she was experiencing asthma attacks that were not getting less frequent with the rescue inhaler, having been diagnosed with asthma 2 years prior by her pediatrician. The patient indicated that when a breathing event occurred, she would take her rescue inhaler as soon as she got out of the pool and her breathing seemed better within a couple of minutes. She indicated that the only thing that really made the breathing problem better was to stop swimming and take her rescue inhaler. Breathing difficulties had slowly worsened over the course of the season and, at the time of the evaluation, she described breathing trouble every time she was being timed or in competition. The patient denied breathing difficulty with any other exercise activities or activities of daily living. She also denied any difficulty breathing at night.

When asked about her typical swimming style and breathing strategy when free of breathing events, she described training in a competition pool with 50-meter lanes. She reported that she takes a breath about 2 swim strokes before a turn and then again when she resurfaces after a turn. She also indicated that her coach didn't care how many strokes she put between each breath as long as she continued to improve her times. Her coach encouraged her to try to avoid taking a breath during the last 50 meters of the race. This latter direction was new, per client report, and she described feeling a lot of pressure to achieve this benchmark. When asked specifically about her exhaling strategy while swimming, the patient reported that she generally held her breath and then let it out as fast as she could before turning her head to take another breath.

> The author does a nice job here of specifying questions specific to swimming breathing that can impact feelings of dyspnea and additional breathing burdens. Each sport at this elite level has its own unique breathing rhythm, and it is incumbent on the treating clinician to learn more about the physical and respiratory demands of the patient's preferred sport. This can be done through direct consultation with trainers and coaches in the sport in addition to querying the patient about their specific breathing patterns and concerns.

The patient described her first year on a collegiate swim team as challenging and stressful and described anxiety about losing her scholarship if her breathing problem was not resolved quickly. She indicated setting high personal goals for herself, both academically and athletically, with the ultimate goal to make the US Olympic swim team.

The patient's medical history is remarkable for diagnosed allergies to pollen, mold, and dust mites, the primary symptoms of which included nasal congestion and sneezing. The patient denied other chronic medical conditions and surgical history. She indicated that she did not smoke or drink alcohol. When asked about symptoms of LPR, she indicated that she experienced a persistent globus sensation and often cleared her throat secondary to a perception of phlegm in her throat. She attributed the throat irritation to her history of allergies. She described some nausea and acidy burps before and during swim meets, for which she took over-the-counter antacids. The patient reported that she took birth control pills and, when her allergies were bothering her, over-the-counter allergy medication. Albuterol, a rescue inhaler, had been prescribed for her to take when she experienced asthma attacks, and she reported that the inhaler didn't help her breathing problem. When asked about her eating habits, the patient indicated that she frequently eats a high-protein snack before practice (eg, peanut butter sandwich), and she also typically snacks before bed. She described drinking about 4 to 5 carbonated beverages per day as well as sports drinks during and after practice. Socially, the patient reported that she didn't have much of a social life due to swim team practices both before and after classes; however, she indicated that she had close friends on the swim team. She also described missing her family, who lived about 11 hours away from her university.

Auditory-Perceptual Evaluation of Voice Quality

Using both informal and formal methods, the evaluating clinician judged the patient's voice quality. During conversation, the evaluating SLP did not note any voice disturbances. The CAPE-V[33] was used as a formal voice quality assessment and found no discernible dysphonia.

Laryngeal Imaging

The structure and function of the patient's upper airway were assessed using a flexible nasal endoscope, which was carefully advanced along the floor of the patient's nostril after application of topical nasal anesthetic. The flexible endoscope was advanced through the nasopharynx and the tip of the endoscope was positioned with a complete view of the laryngeal structure during resting breathing and breathing maneuvers. The patient's larynx was observed during several cycles of rest breathing to allow the patient to get used to the endoscope and to observe the behavior of the upper airway during unstressed rest breathing. Frequent "twitching" of the arytenoid cartilages during resting breathing was observed, with a patent airway during both inspiration and expiration. The tissue of the membranous vocal folds appeared smooth but somewhat edematous bilaterally, characterized by infraglottic edema bilaterally, which was observed during maximum abduction. Additionally, posterior laryngeal edema and interarytenoid tissue changes were observed, consistent with clinical signs for LPR. When the patient was asked to quickly take a maximum inhalation then exhale quickly and completely through the mouth, the patient was observed to narrow the vocal folds about 50% to 60% of the width of the glottis during inhalation. Given that the referring pulmonologist had ruled out asthma (asthma is a contraindication for panting, which can trigger an asthma attack), the patient was asked to pant, during which the arytenoid cartilages were also observed to "twitch." At this point in the endoscopic assessment, the patient was asked to view the screen and was oriented to the anatomical structures of her larynx. When asked to imitate what a breathing attack felt like, the patient produced near-complete vocal fold adduction with no production of stridor but obvious glottal narrowing. The patient was able to match the perception of throat tightness with the image of glottal narrowing. The patient was then asked to sniff in quickly and deeply through her nose and then exhale out of her mouth, observing her larynx rapidly lower and widely abduct during the sniff and then remain open during exhalation. Finally, the patient was asked to sip air in through a narrow mouth opening, as if sipping through a straw, with subsequent wide abduction of the glottis during inspiration. For purposes of visual feedback with the endoscope still in place and to strengthen the subsequent training of the breathing recovery exercises, the patient was asked to imitate what a breathing attack felt like and then perform the sip inhale on the following breath to simulate application of the breathing recovery method. The dynamic endoscopic laryngeal assessment was reviewed with an otolaryngologist, who concurred with the observation of clinical signs of LPR and ruled out other laryngeal obstruction or disease.

> It is a common practice to rule out GERD and LPR as triggers for EILO. Often, physicians consider patient-reported symptoms of acid reflux and use a diagnostic trial of PPIs to rule in or out LPR and GERD. However, controversy remains regarding the laryngeal signs of GERD and/or LPR. The reader is guided to critically read the literature on the evidence of laryngeal signs of reflux.[98]

Impressions

The patient's pulmonary and otolaryngology assessments ruled out medical diagnoses that are part of the differential diagnosis for EILO (eg, pulmonary disease [including asthma], subglottic stenosis, bilateral vocal fold paralysis, laryngeal mass lesion, unresolved laryngomalacia).[79] Key medical assessment information supporting the diagnosis of EILO included the negative methacholine challenge and the flow-volume loop showing a truncated inspiratory loop only with no expiratory obstruction. Additionally, the account that her breathing difficulties resolved only a couple of minutes after taking her rescue inhaler signaled that her difficulty was not asthma—the rescue inhaler would not have worked that quickly per the pulmonologist report. The medical information in combination with the patient's description and imitation of the breathing "attacks," as well as the information gleaned from the dynamic endoscopic assessment, supported the diagnosis of EILO and indicated it would be safe to proceed with counseling and treatment.

Plan of Care

The treatment program designed for Patient II consisted of the following: counsel the patient about the differences between asthma and EILO and offer a theoretical framework to understand why these breathing attacks may have occurred; counsel her regarding dietary and behavioral changes that may improve symptoms of LPR; train breathing recovery exercises adapted for swimming; and implement step-by-step application of the recovery exercises to swimming, with the ultimate goal of total elimination of the breathing attacks.

Decision Making

Many patients who carry the diagnosis of asthma and then are suddenly told that they never had asthma in the first place are reluctant to drop the asthma mantle. Detailed descriptions of the physiological differences between the two diagnoses, differences between triggers and, finally, differences in treatment approaches are important components to include. Counseling also can help patients understand that the breathing attack is not their fault and that they have control over the difficulty—a critical shift from external to internal locus of control. For this patient, stress may have played a role, but it was clear that there was a probable physiologic trigger from

undertreated LPR. Understanding the role of LPR as a trigger helped focus the patient on a systemic approach to recovery. Given that the patient described symptoms of LPR and that the endoscopic assessment indicated clinical signs of the same, counseling Patient II about behavioral and dietary changes to reduce LPR was appropriate. Elite athletes who follow a rigorous training regime require adapted LPR counseling tailored to their sport. With all other obstructive conditions ruled out, counseling regarding the condition completed, and medical/behavioral management of LPR initiated, it was safe to train a breathing recovery program with a measure of confidence that the breathing strategies would be successful in remediating Patient II's breathing difficulties in the pool. The breathing recovery program typically used by the evaluating clinician included 3 basic steps: (1) body awareness, (2) establishment of lower torso/belly breathing, and (3) training of a quick, deep nasal sniff followed by complete exhale through the mouth.[83] Step 2 of the program, establishment of lower torso/belly breathing, was not appropriate for the patient to use in the pool. Most swimmers are coached to maintain a "streamlined" position in the pool, which translates to a perfectly straight spine with limited chest and abdominal excursion during inhalation. The goal of the streamlined position is to create a body silhouette whereby the shoulders cut through the water first with little or no drag created by chest or abdominal excursion. To train belly breathing with a swimmer might slow her down instead of speeding her up in the pool. Additionally, counseling the patient to pursue a physical profile that was in direct disagreement with her coach's training may have undermined the SLP's ability to successfully engage the coach in the generalization process. The application of the recovery exercise to elite sport required a structured step-by-step approach to support the athlete in generalizing to the pool what was relatively easy to do while sitting in a chair in the therapy room or at home. The cardiopulmonary requirements of swimming the 200-meter freestyle far exceeded those required for the therapy room. Finally, the specificity requirement for training a new physical skill required that the exercises be generalized to a pool environment while employing the freestyle stroke.

Intervention

Goal #1

Goal #1. *Counsel the patient about the differential diagnosis of EILO and describe a theoretical framework to understand the physiologic triggers for the events.*

Visual feedback was provided during the endoscopic assessment, empowering her to see that she had at least 2 strategies for getting her throat open during inhalation, either via a deep, quick nasal sniff or during a sip inhale through her lips, allowing her to match the physical perception of throat tightness with narrowed vocal folds and demonstrating how the sniff or sip inhale would open her vocal folds. Taking time to describe EILO and how it is different from asthma, identifying her triggers for it, and providing visual feedback helped the patient overcome her initial confusion about the role of the SLP and build her self-efficacy for successful use of the breathing recovery method.

Goal #2

Goal #2. *The patient will make dietary and behavioral changes to reduce the symptoms of LPR.*

The clinician reviewed foods that exacerbate reflux and asked the patient to avoid the following foods until her breathing attacks were well controlled: chocolate, nuts/peanut butter, carbonated and acidic drinks, fried food, onions, spicy foods, and high-fat foods. Because of her high calorie needs, the patient was asked to refrain from high-fat foods only prior to practice and bedtime. The patient's physician prescribed medication for LPR, and

medication delivery was timed to get maximum coverage while swimming.

Goal #3

Goal #3. *Train a breathing recovery program with special adaptations for the elite swimmer.*

Step 1, training body awareness, was appropriate for this patient without much adaptation. The progressive awareness tasks, a combination of progressive relaxation and mindfulness, were trained, and the patient was directed to complete the exercise at least twice daily when not at swim practice. The third goal of the breathing recovery program (the quick, deep nasal sniff in, followed by the slow, complete exhale) required significant adaptation for this patient. Patient II competes at the middle distance 200-meter freestyle, a stroke that requires her face to be in the water most of the time while taking as few breaths as possible for the fastest time. Given that she described nasal congestion as a symptom of her intermittent allergies, it was more appropriate to train the quick "straw" sip method of inhalation. The patient was trained to purse her lips as if sipping through a straw, draw air in quickly and completely, and then follow the inhalation with a complete exhalation out of her mouth. Complete exhalation during practice breathing while out of the pool was critical to avoid hyperventilation and the sensation of lightheadedness. During swimming, the patient described that after taking a breath, she held it and then rapidly exhaled just before taking another breath. The tension in her throat from this breath-holding habit may have contributed to extraneous neck tension and laryngeal adduction; therefore, she was asked to stop holding her breath and exhale over a period of time leading up to her next breath to allow for greater inhalation. This last direction was discussed with the patient's coach, and he concurred that this change should translate into improved swim performance and more optimal streamlined position. The clinician asked Patient II to perform an appropriate repeat demonstration of the exercises trained during the initial evaluation and to focus on the sensation in her throat to discern when it felt tight and when it felt open. The SLP also asked her to avoid breath holding between the inhalation and the exhalation.

Goal #4

Goal #4. *The patient will apply the recovery exercises in the pool, gradually working up to race speed, timed trials and, finally, competition.*

The generalization program started in the pool given the marked differences for breathing in a horizontal position in water. Using a lane away from the swim team, she was instructed to swim slowly, incorporating the recovery exercise with her stroke. Time was spent at this stage while she learned to coordinate the extended exhale before the head turn and straw sip for inhalation. She quickly adapted to the inhalation pattern but had more difficulty stopping the breath holding, a long-standing practice of hers. Given that the straw-sip inhalation would not provide enough oxygen for a middle-distance elite swimmer, she was directed to reserve the straw-sip inhalation for the point in the race right before she would typically experience throat tightness. Because she knew the distance in the race at which the breathing attack typically occurred, she could start the recovery exercise before this and completely avoid the attack. After 2 poolside therapy sessions, a baseline of success was established with the new breathing strategies, and the patient's coach and trainer completed the remainder of the generalization.

> In this case, the author has access to the pool to train and observe the patient during her chosen sport of swimming. Not all clinicians have this type of access, so it becomes necessary to work with trainers, coaches, and perhaps colleagues who have pool access to practice carryover of newly learned skills and address episodes of dyspnea.

Intervention Outcomes

Patient II received 3 sessions of therapy over the course of 1 month and attended 1 follow-up session a month after discharge from treatment. At the final clinic visit, approximately 8 weeks after her initial diagnosis, Patient II reported that she no longer experienced any breathing difficulty when competing at the 200-meter freestyle. She also described that she was gradually able to avoid the throat tightness completely and had recently started swimming successfully without the straw-sip inhalation. She was most excited to report she had steadily improved her race time. Her disposition during the clinic visit was optimistic, and she no longer reported anxiety about keeping her athletic scholarship.

The outcome of therapy was attributed to the patient's high level of motivation and compliance with the combination of behavioral and medical management for LPR as well as the breathing training. Vital aspects of the behavioral management program included cultivation of an internal locus of control for the EILO events and high efficacy expectations for the breathing recovery method, 2 critical components for therapy success. The support of the patient's family and the coaching staff were also key contributors to her rapid recovery.

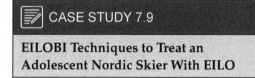

CASE STUDY 7.9

EILOBI Techniques to Treat an Adolescent Nordic Skier With EILO

Emily A. Nauman

Evaluation

Patient NN received a standard assessment for EILO,[79] including history of present illness, review of other diagnostics from other medical specialties, auditory-perceptual assessment, patient-reported outcome measures, and laryngeal imaging.

History of Present Illness

Patient NN is a 16-year-old cisgender female high school varsity athlete competing in Nordic skiing, cross-country, and lacrosse. Patient NN was referred by her pulmonologist for a speech-language pathology evaluation and continuous laryngoscopy during exercise (CLE) that confirmed EILO, formerly known as exercise-induced vocal cord dysfunction (EI-VCD) or paradoxical vocal fold motion (EI-PVFM).[104] Patient NN presented to the speech pathology evaluation with her mother, who also provided background history.

Onset of NN's symptoms began after a SARS-CoV-2 infection and another viral illness for which she was treated with antibiotics due to a working diagnosis of pneumonia/bronchitis. Following recovery from the illnesses, NN's chief complaint was episodic breathing difficulty while Nordic skiing and running. She had no difficulty with breathing during exercise before this time and no medical comorbidities. She denied common signs and symptoms of reflux, dysphagia, allergies, and nasal drainage. She had not received speech-language pathology services for this problem in the past. Prior therapeutic trials included albuterol; however, NN reported it was not beneficial in alleviating or preventing breathing symptoms during exercise.

Patient NN characterized the episodic dyspnea events as a gradual increase in difficulty on inhalation with associated throat tightness and stridorous breathing on inhalation as exercise became more strenuous and intense. She reported the breathing problem was worse in competitions than in practices. She noted higher altitude and cold weather (below 20 degrees Fahrenheit) exacerbated breathing symptoms while exercising. She had noted episodes of presyncope (the feeling you are about to faint) during severe dyspneic events but denied full syncope. Patient NN denied simultaneous chest pain and audible wheeze on exhalation during breathing problem events. She denied muscular weakness and pallor. She reported no throat clearing, coughing, or dysphonia during events, but did endorse dysphonia and occasional persistent throat tightness following episodes.

Patient NN noted that the breathing problem occurred in about 100% of exercise events and that dyspnea symptoms typically began within 5 minutes of beginning to exercise. Typical severity rating was a 6, on a 1 to 10 scale (with 10 representing "severe"). Patient NN reported that, if she stopped exercise to rest, it would usually take her about 45 seconds to 1 minute to recover. Reinitiating exercise resulted in dyspnea at the same severity or worse as the initial episode. Outside of exercise, episodic dyspnea events could be triggered by ascending stairs and occasionally during stressful situations.

Prior Diagnostics

Patient NN was seen for a pulmonary evaluation prior to the speech pathology evaluation. She completed a chest x-ray that was WNL. Pulmonary function tests revealed forced expiratory volume in the 1st second of exhalation (FEV1) of 106% with 7% improvement with albuterol. NN's pulmonary evaluation ruled out other medical diagnoses that are essential for the differential diagnosis of EILO (eg, subglottic stenosis, bilateral vocal fold paralysis, laryngomalacia).

> Several authors in this chapter highlight the importance of ruling out several pulmonary and cardiac diseases or disorders prior to hypothesizing that the problem is ILO or EILO. Full otolaryngology and pulmonology workup are important prior to treating ILO/EILO. If the patient has not received these workups, it is important that the SLP refer for them prior to treatment. In the case of EILO, a cardiology referral may be warranted as well, as shortness of breath and cough are also cardinal signs of possible cardiac abnormalities.

348 Voice Therapy: Clinical Case Studies

Auditory-Perceptual Evaluation

Patient NN's vocal quality was assessed using both informal and formal methods. During conversation, the SLP perceived mild-moderate dysphonia. Using the CAPE-V[33] parameters, the patient's voice was evaluated while reading aloud the 6 sentences of the CAPE-V protocol and sustaining /a/ and /i/ vowels. The SLPs rated NN's voice as 27/100 in overall severity on a scale of 0 (no dysphonia) to 100 (severe dysphonia).

Patient-Reported Outcome Measures

1. Exercise-Induced Laryngeal Obstruction Dyspnea Index (EILODI): 26/48 (score of 6 is considered a minimal clinically important difference)[105]
2. DI: 31/40 (score above 10 is considered abnormal)[31]

Review of Recent Laryngeal Imaging

The patient had completed a CLE 1 month prior to speech-language pathology evaluation.[106,107] Results of examination and video from CLE were reviewed with the patient and her mother. CLE revealed normal glottic and supraglottic anatomy; normal, symmetrical vocal fold adduction and abduction at rest; and moderate inappropriate inspiratory glottic adduction and mild inspiratory arytenoid prolapse during high-intensity exercise. Cardiopulmonary exercise tolerance test and CLE

CLE provides a definitive look at the larynx during increasing demands of exercise and during the patient's perceived increase in shortness of breath (SOB). The reader is advised to review the literature on CLE as well as the benefits and feasibility of CLE. There are several methods of continuously examining the larynx during exercise, and the reader is guided to examine the level of evidence each provides toward the hypothesis that EILO is the cause of the exercise-induced dyspnea.

---

test data revealed moderate upper airway obstruction without bronchoconstriction.

Impressions

Patient NN's clinical signs and symptoms were consistent with that of EILO. Pulmonary testing ruled out the presence of asthma, and an EILO diagnosis was confirmed using the gold standard of CLE. Given the confirmed EILO diagnosis combined with the patient's high level of motivation for treatment and strong family support, Patient NN was an excellent candidate for respiratory retraining therapy with an SLP.

Plan of Care

Speech-language pathology treatment was recommended and NN initiated treatment on the same day as her speech-language pathology evaluation. The patient was recommended to complete 3 60-minute follow-up sessions, completing 1 session every 1 to 2 weeks. Her goals for therapy included:

Short-Term Goal #1. NN will name up to 3 common signs and symptoms associated with EILO diagnosis following education given minimal assistance.

Short-Term Goal #2. NN will implement respiratory retraining techniques utilizing diaphragmatic support given limited to minimal clinician cueing across 2 sessions.

Short-Term Goal #3. NN will implement the EILOBI breathing technique within 20 to 30 minutes of exercising (eg, walking, running, stationary bike) given limited to minimal clinician cueing and will report an EILO symptoms severity rating of 3 or less (0 = "no EILO symptoms"; 10 = "severe EILO symptoms") across 2 sessions.

Short-Term Goal #4. NN will implement sport-specific modifications to the EILOBI breathing technique given limited to minimal clinician cueing across 2 sessions

Long-Term Goal. NN will independently implement respiratory retraining techniques within her preferred format of exercising (eg, running, Nordic skiing) to manage and/or prevent EILO symptoms as measured by patient report.

Decision Making

Patient NN was an excellent candidate for behavioral therapy. She expressed high motivation for improving EILO symptoms and had a strong support system from her family and her Nordic skiing coaches. Possible barriers to treatment included NN's stress management as it related to her need to perform at a high level within athletics and school. The treatment approach designed for Patient NN consisted of thorough education about the EILO condition; instruction on specific respiratory retraining techniques that NN would apply during skiing and running for EILO symptom control; and practice of implementation of breathing techniques during exercise to improve patient accuracy and independence. The goals of therapy were targeted to first improve the patient's management of EILO symptoms during exercise, with the ultimate goal of prevention of EILO symptoms all together.

The speech-language pathology evaluation contained assessment, education about the EILO condition, and initial instruction and practice of specific respiratory retraining techniques. Due to the patient's participation in high levels of exertion, the SLP instructed the patient on the Olin EILOBI technique, as these respiratory retraining techniques have a high level of perceived clinical effectiveness in high-performance athletes.[84]

The Olin EILOBI breathing technique is a biphasic inspiratory respiratory retraining technique involving a transition from high resistance to low resistance that forcibly abducts the vocal folds on inspiration. There are 3 variants for the EILOBI breathing technique: tooth variant, lip variant, and tongue variant. The tooth variant was used for Patient NN, as it provided the most optimal vocal fold opening as seen on endoscopy. The biphasic breathing maneuver has 2 parts:

- **Part 1 (High Resistance Phase).** The patient's lower lip is placed in front of the upper teeth. The patient inhales via the mouth in this position to create a high inspiratory resistance. Inhalation in this phase lasts for about 1 second before transition to part 2.
- **Part 2 (Low Resistance Phase).** The patient then drops the lower lip and the jaw abruptly, continuing to inhale via the mouth. Inhalation in this phase involves incorporation of lower rib excursion on inhalation to gain efficiency and fullness of breath on inspiration.

The biphasic breath is then completed on a 4-cycle breath pattern. The patient is instructed to complete a deliberate or slightly longer exhalation, which precedes the biphasic inhalation. The biphasic inhalation is then completed with a comfortable or typical exhalation. The patient then completes 3 normal breaths in between each biphasic breath (Figure 7–7).

Intervention

Evaluation Day

Goals Addressed During Initial Instruction on Evaluation Day:

Short-Term Goal #1. NN will name up to 3 common signs and symptoms associated with EILO diagnosis following education given minimal assistance. (Goal #1 met by the end of the session.)

Short-Term Goal #2. NN will implement respiratory retraining techniques utilizing diaphragmatic support given limited to minimal clinician cueing across 2 sessions. (Goal #2 in progress.)

Patients need to have a firm understanding of what is normal as it relates to the larynx and breathing to better understand what is abnormal in the context of EILO. Teaching the patient about common signs and symptoms

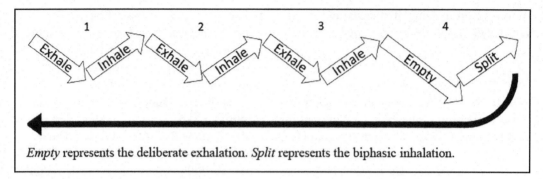

FIGURE 7–7. 4-cycle breath pattern.

of EILO and describing how these clinical symptoms differ from other breathing problems, such as asthma, can help the patient appropriately identify the possible source of the breathing problem in the moment of breathing difficulty. This can also assist the patient in early symptom identification, and therefore early symptom management, to prevent a severe breathing problem event from occurring.

Many patients who receive an EILO diagnosis have gone through many breathing evaluations, only to be told all respiratory functions appear normal. Taking careful time to review the results of laryngeal imaging/CLE is extremely helpful that can validate that the patient does, in fact, have a real reason to be breathless during exercise. In this case, after the SLP reviewed the CLE images with Patient NN, she stated: "It's so nice to know that I'm not crazy, and that there is a reason why I'm having such a hard time breathing."

While the etiology of EILO is still yet to be discovered, describing a possible theoretical framework founded in the physiologic functions of the larynx for why the condition might have developed can be empowering to the patient. In NN's case, she had 2 significant upper respiratory infections that resulted in an increase in phonotraumatic behaviors such as coughing. This laryngeal trauma led to subsequent laryngeal irritation and hypothesized laryngeal hypersensitivity. Understanding the physiologic role of the larynx as it relates to 2 back-to-back upper respiratory illnesses helped validate to the patient that the breathing problem was not her fault.

Patient NN was provided instruction on the EILOBI breathing technique at the initial evaluation.[84] When thinking about behavioral therapy, SLPs use specific respiratory retraining techniques and provide step-by-step directions on how to accurately complete a breathing technique or strategy. It is also important to consider the principles of motor learning and incorporate repeated opportunities for practice to promote good skill acquisition and the retention and implementation of the skill without much mental thought. The initial targets of therapy in this case were focused on improving the mechanics of the EILOBI technique and on completing high-volume practice.

Using visual aids and clinician demonstration, NN first practiced the technique at rest, sitting in a chair in the clinic room. The Olin EILOBI breathing technique consists of a 4-cycle breath pattern in which patients learn to take a biphasic inhalation on every fourth breath (see Figure 7–7). (See Video 22 Tooth Variant EILOBI Breathing Technique by Nauman.) Most patients are unfamiliar with counting or pacing breath patterns; therefore, a focus of the initial instruction on this technique was to have the patient become more comfortable with planning the biphasic inhalation and practicing the 4-cycle breath pattern. Practice of the technique was first done at rest and then was advanced to walking on the treadmill. Once the 4-cycle breath pattern appeared more fluid, specific step-by-step instruction was provided to the patient regarding the biphasic inhalation. Patient NN was instructed to focus on a single aspect of the biphasic inhalation given clinician prompting and shaping until the overall accuracy of the mechanics of the EILOBI technique improved during exercise.

While difficulty with breathing during exercise was the primary reason for NN to seek out therapy, NN had discussed in the detailed case history interview that stressful situations could also trigger her breathing symptoms. The literature outlines several different behavioral health areas in treating EILO. Many authors in research have noticed personality features that stand out in a prototypical patient with EILO: a type A perfectionist who is competitive and has unreasonably challenging self-standards. In a recent review completed by Røksund and colleagues (2017), the authors describe that most patients with EILO exhibited an appropriate behavioral response to severe respiratory distress.[108]

At the end of the initial session, the SLP educated the patient regarding stress as a common trigger for breathing symptoms. This led to NN expressing feelings of unmanaged stress due to the high demand of upcoming Nordic races on top of schoolwork and an open dialogue about the recommendation of seeking out a mental health provider to assist in stress management.

To help the patient attain the long-term goal of being able to independently manage and/or prevent EILO symptoms, the SLP gave Patient NN a home exercise program including independent practice of employing the EILOBI respiratory retraining technique at low levels of exertion (eg, walking around the house/neighborhood) and during recovery periods at Nordic practice.

Speech-Language Pathology
Follow-Up Session #1

Goals Addressed During Follow-Up Session #1:

Short-Term Goal #2. NN will implement respiratory retraining techniques utilizing diaphragmatic support given limited to minimal clinician cueing across 2 sessions. (Goal #2 met by the end of the session.)

Short-Term Goal #3. NN will implement the EILOBI breathing technique within 20 to 30 minutes of exercising (eg, walking, running, stationary bike) given limited to minimal clinician cueing and will report an EILO symptoms severity rating of 3 or less (0 = "no EILO symptoms"; 10 = "severe EILO symptoms") across 2 sessions. (Goal #3 in progress.)

Short-Term Goal #4. NN will implement sport-specific modifications to the EILOBI breathing technique given limited to minimal clinician cueing across 2 sessions. (Goal #4 in progress.)

NN returned for her first follow-up session expressing good compliance with practicing the technique while skiing; however, she noted some difficulty with maintaining good accuracy with increased levels of exertion or when she felt fatigued. Follow-up session #1 then targeted accuracy of mechanics at faster speed intervals. Patient practiced the EILOBI breath during jogging and running intervals with the clinician cueing for specific improvements she could make to the EILOBI breath. By the end of follow-up session #1, NN's accuracy of technique had significantly improved, and she reported improved EILO symptom control at higher running levels. The patient's home exercise program was then increased to implementing the EILOBI breathing technique during all high levels of exertion and full Nordic practices.

Speech-Language Pathology Session #2

Goals Addressed During Follow-Up Session #2:

Short-Term Goal #3. NN will implement the EILOBI breathing technique within 20 to 30 minutes of exercising (eg, walking, running, stationary bike) given limited to minimal clinician cueing and will report an EILO symptoms severity rating of 3 or less (0 = "no EILO symptoms"; 10 = "severe EILO symptoms") across 2 sessions. (Goal #3 in progress.)

Short-Term Goal #4. NN will implement sport-specific modifications to the EILOBI breathing technique given limited to minimal clinician cueing across 2 sessions. (Goal #4 in progress.)

Due to NN's improving accuracy of respiratory retraining technique, follow-up session #2 was targeted at simulating a Nordic ski track and practicing modifications of EILOBI technique for racing. The patient completed running intervals on treadmill rolling hills (up to incline 8.5) as Nordic ski tracks often contain hills at varying degrees. While it is not possible to fully recreate skiing within the clinic setting, modifications such as adding incline and varying speeds (eg, increasing speed on the "downhill") can simulate the exertional level that could be expected within a Nordic ski route. Additionally, it is common for patients to have difficulty completing the 4-cycle breath pattern while racing as there are many other areas of focus that patients need to attend to.

> Many clinics have gym equipment available to allow training of breathing techniques during exercise. Breathing patterns vary across different types of physical activity, and it is important to explore methods of practicing the specific exercise causing the dyspneic episodes and practice during that exercise. This can be difficult, and often the clinician does not have a pool or football field or basketball court available. Explore other options, including referring to a colleague who does have those resources, working with the athletic trainer and patient to see if they are amenable to the clinician attending a practice or using the facilities for therapy or, as in this case, finding methods to simulate the exercise task, intensity, and breathing required.

Patient NN was instructed to practice intermittently taking 1 aspect of the EILOBI breath (eg, empty phase into the biphasic inhale) without the 4-cycle breath pattern. At first, the clinician told the patient when to take the breath to help NN get used to monitoring for EILO symptoms during in-between biphasic breaths. After this, the patient then independently completed the biphasic inhale as she felt like she needed it throughout the simulated "ski route." Across exertional activity within the clinic setting, the patient reported EILO symptoms severity decreased any time she took a tooth-variant EILOBI breath. Patient NN also was beginning to independently monitor and self-correct when the mechanics of the EILOBI technique were imprecise.

Patient NN noted at the end of follow-up session #2 that this coming weekend's competition would determine if her Nordic team would go to the state championship. NN also reported that she had started working with a mental health provider with regard to her stress management, and while there was a lot riding on this up-and-coming race, she was feeling more confident that her breathing problem would be better controlled due to the combination of speech-language pathology treatment and counseling. Patient NN's home exercise program was then advanced to implementing the EILOBI breathing technique using sport-specific modifications (eg, taking EILOBI split breath as needed) at Nordic practices and during her next race.

Speech-Language Pathology Session #3
Goals Addressed During Follow-Up Session #3:

Short-Term Goal #3. NN will implement the EILOBI breathing technique within 20 to 30 minutes of exercising (eg, walking, running, stationary bike) given limited to minimal clinician cueing and will report an EILO symptoms severity rating of 3 or less (0 = "no EILO symptoms"; 10 = "severe EILO symptoms") across 2 sessions. (Goal #3 met by the end of the session.)

Short-Term Goal #4. NN will implement sport-specific modifications to the EILOBI breathing technique given limited to minimal clinician cueing across 2 sessions. (Goal #4 met by the end of the session.)

Patient NN returned for a third follow-up session noting that, unfortunately, her Nordic team had lost the competition, but that her breathing was well managed throughout the entirety of the race. She noted lacrosse season was starting in addition to an intensive cardio training involving a significant amount of running for off-season Nordic skiing. She reported using the tooth-variant EILOBI breathing technique while running and when playing lacrosse, but she was having difficulty implementing it due to the presence of a mouth guard.

The clinician taught her how to modify the EILOBI technique when the mouth guard was in place, and NN practiced the modifications while walking, jogging, and running on the treadmill. These modifications included instruction by the SLP to practice implementing a lower jaw position (eg, yawning jaw position) when transitioning from part 1 to part 2 of the biphasic inhale to allow for increased

airflow while the mouth guard was present. NN was also instructed regarding the lip-variant EILOBI technique. This variant can be a helpful modification when mouth guards are in place as it takes away the high resistance phase from placing the lower lip against the upper teeth and instead creates the high resistance phase using both upper and lower lip occlusion. NN noted a sensation of less forcefulness compared to using the tooth-variant EILOBI, but found it was easier to get air in when the mouth guard was present.

Posttreatment Outcomes

Long-Term Goal. NN will independently implement respiratory retraining techniques within her preferred form of exercising (eg, running, Nordic skiing) to manage and/or prevent EILO symptoms as measured by patient report. (Long-term goal met.)

After completing 3 follow-up sessions of therapy, the patient then completed a phone check-in with the SLP 1 month after her last visit. NN reported the breathing problem was still present during exercise; however, she had avoided being subbed out of lacrosse games due to lack of EILO symptom control. She also noted excellent control over EILO symptoms despite exercising intensely for her off-season cardio training. NN expressed optimism for her next Nordic season and excitement that her breathing felt controlled.

Although the patient's EILO symptoms were still present during exercise at the time of discharge, the patient was independently and successfully managing symptoms. She was able to employ respiratory retraining techniques in high-stress situations with overall good symptom improvement across a variety of athletic settings. The patient's success in therapy was attributed to her high motivation and compliance as well as to the support of her family, coaches, and mental health counselor.

References

1. Song WJ, Chang YS, Faruqi S, et al. The global epidemiology of chronic cough in adults: A systematic review and meta-analysis. *Eur Respir J.* 2015;45(5):1479-1481. doi:10.1183/09031936.00218714

2. Irwin RS, French CL, Chang AB, et al. Classification of cough as a symptom in adults and management algorithms: CHEST guideline and expert panel report. *Chest.* 2018; 153(1):196-209. doi:10.1016/j.chest.2017 .10.016

3. Kang SY, Song WJ, Won HK, et al. Cough persistence in adults with chronic cough: A 4-year retrospective cohort study. *Allergol Int.* 2020;69(4):588-593. doi:10.1016/j .alit.2020.03.012

4. Mazzone SB, McGarvey L. Mechanisms and rationale for targeted therapies in refractory and unexplained chronic cough. *Clin Pharmacol Ther.* 2021;109(3):619-636. doi:10.1002/cpt.2003

5. French C, Crawford S, Bova C, Iriwn RS. Change in psychologic, physiologic, and situational factors in adults after treatment of chronic cough. *Chest.* 2017;152(3):547-562

6. Chamberlain SAF, Garrod R, Douiri A, et al. The impact of chronic cough: A cross-sectional European survey. *Lung.* 2015; 193(3):401-408. doi:10.1007/s00408-015-9701-2

7. Dicpinigaitis P, Tso R, Banauch G. Prevalence of depressive symptoms among patients with chronic cough. *Chest.* 2006;130(6):1839-1843.

8. Dicpinigaitis PV. Prevalence of stress urinary incontinence in women presenting for evaluation of chronic cough. *ERJ Open Res.* 2021;7(1):00012-02021. doi:10.1183/23120 541.00012-2021

9. Vertigan AE, Haines J, Slovarp L. An update on speech pathology management of chronic refractory cough. *J Allergy Clin Immunol Pract.* 2019;7(6):1756-1761. doi: 10.1016/j.jaip.2019.03.030

10. Slovarp L, Loomis BK, Glaspey A. Assessing referral and practice patterns of patients with chronic cough referred for behavioral cough suppression therapy. *Chron Respir Dis.* 2018;15(3):296-305. doi:10.1177/1479 972318755722

11. Chamberlain Mitchell SAF, Garrod R, Clark L, et al. Physiotherapy, and speech and language therapy intervention for patients with refractory chronic cough: A multicentre randomised control trial. *Thorax.* 2017;72(2):129-136. doi:10.1136/ thoraxjnl-2016-208843

12. Wright ML, Sundar KM, Herrick JS, Barkmeier-Kraemer JM. Long-term treatment outcomes after behavioral speech therapy for chronic refractory cough. *Lung.* 2021; 199(5):517-525. doi:10.1007/s00408-021-00481-3

13. Vertigan AE, Kapela SL, Ryan NM, Birring SS, McElduff P, Gibson PG. Pregabalin and speech pathology combination therapy for refractory chronic cough a randomized controlled trial. *Chest.* 2016;149(3):639-648. doi:10.1378/chest.15-1271

14. Chamberlain S, Garrod R, Birring SS. Cough suppression therapy: Does it work? *Pulm Pharmacol Ther.* 2013;26(5):524-527. doi:10.1016/j.pupt.2013.03.012

15. Slovarp LJ, Jetté ME, Gillespie AI, Reynolds JE, Barkmeier-Kraemer JM. Evaluation and management outcomes and burdens in patients with refractory chronic cough referred for behavioral cough suppression therapy. *Lung.* 2021;199(3):263-271. doi:10.1007/s00408-021-00442-w

16. Blager FB, Gay ML, Wood RP. Voice therapy techniques adapted to treatment of habit cough: A pilot study. *J Commun Disord.* 1988;21(5):393-400. doi:10.1016/0021-9924(88)90024-x

17. Morice AH, Millqvist E, Bieksiene K, et al. ERS guidelines on the diagnosis and treatment of chronic cough in adults and children. *Eur Respir J.* 2020;55(1):1901136. doi:10.1183/13993003.01136-2019

18. Chung KF. Approach to chronic cough: The neuropathic basis for cough hypersensitivity syndrome. *J Thorac Dis.* 2014; 6(suppl 7):S699-S707. doi:10.3978/j.issn.20 72-1439.2014.08.41

19. Chung KF, McGarvey L, Mazzone S. Chronic cough and cough hypersensitivity syndrome. *Lancet Respir Med.* 2016;4(12): 934-935. doi:10.1016/S2213-2600(16)30 373-3

20. Ando A, Smallwood D, McMahon M, Irving L, Mazzone SB, Farrell MJ. Neural correlates of cough hypersensitivity in humans: Evidence for central sensitisation and dysfunctional inhibitory control. *Thorax.* 2016;71(4):323-329. doi:10.1136/ thoraxjnl-2015-207425

21. Mazzone SB, Cole LJ, Ando A, Egan GF, Farrell MJ. Investigation of the neural control of cough and cough suppression in humans using functional brain imaging. *J Neurosci.* 2011;31(8):2948-2958. doi:10 .1523/JNEUROSCI.4597-10.2011

22. Moe AAK, Singh N, Dimmock M, et al. Brainstem processing of cough sensory inputs in chronic cough hypersensitivity. *eBioMedicine.* 2024;100:104976. doi:10.1016/j.ebiom.2024.104976

23. Namgung E, Song W-J, Kim Y-H, An J, Cho YS, Kang D-W. Structural and functional correlates of higher cortical brain regions in chronic refractory cough. *Chest.* 2022;162(4):851-860. doi:10.1016/j.chest .2022.04.141

24. Doherty MJ, Mister R, Pearson MG, Calverley PMA. Capsaicin responsiveness and cough in asthma and chronic obstructive pulmonary disease. *Thorax.* 2000;55(8): 643-649. doi:10.1136/thorax.55.8.643

25. Vertigan A, Gibson P. *Speech Pathology Management of Chronic Refractory Cough and Related Disorders.* Compton Publishing; 2016.

26. Vertigan AE, Theodoros DG, Gibson PG, Winkworth AL. Efficacy of speech pathology management for chronic cough: A randomised placebo controlled trial of treatment efficacy. *Thorax.* 2006;61(12):1065-1069. doi:10.1136/thx.2006.064337

27. Ryan NM, Vertigan AE, Bone S, Gibson PG. Cough reflex sensitivity improves with speech language pathology management of refractory chronic cough. *Cough.* 2010;6(1):1-8. doi:10.1186/1745-9974-6-5

28. Rosen CA, Lee AS, Osborne J, Zullo T, Murry T. Development and validation of the Voice Handicap Index-10. *Laryngoscope.* 2004;114(9 I):1549-1556. doi:10.10 97/00005537-200409000-00009

29. Belafsky PC, Postma GN, Koufman JA. Validity and reliability of the Reflux Symptom Index (RSI). *J Voice.* 2002;16(2):274-277. doi:10.1016/S0892-1997(02)00097-8

30. Belafsky P, Mouadeb D, Rees C, et al. Validity and reliability of the Eating Assessment Tool (EAT-10). *Ann Otol Rhinol Laryngol.* 2008;117(12):919-924. doi:10.1177/ 000348940811701210

31. Gartner-Schmidt JL, Shembel AC, Zullo TG, Rosen CA. Development and validation of the Dyspnea Index (DI): A severity index for upper airway-related dyspnea. *J Voice.* 2014;28(6):775-782. doi:10.1016/j .jvoice.2013.12.017

32. Shembel AC, Rosen CA, Zullo TG, Gartner-Schmidt JL. Development and validation of the Cough Severity Index: A severity index for chronic cough related to the upper airway. *Laryngoscope.* 2013;123(8):1931-1936. doi:10.1002/lary.23916

33. Kempster GB, Gerratt BR, Abbott KV, Barkmeier-Kraemer J, Hillman RE. Consensus Auditory-Perceptual Evaluation of Voice: Development of a standardized clinical protocol. *Am J Speech Lang Pathol.* 2009;18(2):124-132. doi:10.1044/1058-03 60(2008/08-0017)

34. Pluschinski P, Zaretsky E, Stöver T, Murray J, Sader R, Hey C. Validation of the secretion severity rating scale. *Eur Arch Otorhinolaryngol.* 2016;273(10):3215-3218. doi:10 .1007/s00405-016-4073-7

35. Morrison M, Rammage L, Emami AJ. The irritable larynx syndrome. *J Voice.* 1999; 13(3):447-455. doi:10.1016/S0892-1997(99) 80049-6

36. Gibson PG, Vertigan AE. Management of chronic refractory cough. *BMJ.* 2015;351. doi:10.1136/bmj.h5590

37. Altman KW, Noordzij JP, Rosen CA, Cohen S, Sulica L. Neurogenic cough. *Laryngoscope.* 2015;125:1675-1681. doi:10.1002/ lary.25186

38. Simpson CB, Tibbetts KM, Loochtan MJ, Dominguez LM. Treatment of chronic neurogenic cough with in-office superior laryngeal nerve block. *Laryngoscope*. 2018; 128(8):1898-1903. doi:10.1002/lary.27201

39. Vertigan AE, Theodoros DG, Winkworth AL, Gibson PG. Chronic cough: A tutorial for speech-language pathologists. *J Med Speech Lang Pathol*. 2007;15(3):189-206.

40. Shembel AC, Sandage MJ, Verdolini Abbott K. Episodic laryngeal breathing disorders: Literature review and proposal of preliminary theoretical framework. *J Voice*. 2017;31(1):125.e7-125.e16. doi:10.1016/j.jvoice.2015.11.027

41. Soni RS, Ebersole B, Jamal N. Treatment of chronic cough: Single-institution experience utilizing behavioral therapy. *Otolaryngol Head Neck Surg (United States)*. 2017; 156(1):103-108. doi:10.1177/01945998166 75299

42. Tomassi NE, Castro ME, Timmons Sund L, Díaz-Cádiz ME, Buckley DP, Stepp CE. Effects of sidetone amplification on vocal function during telecommunication. *J Voice*. 2021;37(4):553-560. doi:10.1016/j.jvoice.2021.03.027

43. Verdolini K, Druker DG, Palmer PM, Samawi H. Laryngeal adduction in resonant voice. *J Voice*. 1998;12(3):315-327. doi:10.1016/S0892-1997(98)80021-0

44. Gartner-Schmidt J, Gherson S, Hapner ER, et al. The development of conversation training therapy: A concept paper. *J Voice*. 2016;30(5):563-573. doi:10.1016/j.jvoice.2015.06.007

45. Ameille J, Wild P, Choudat D, et al. Respiratory symptoms, ventilatory impairment, and bronchial reactivity in oil mist-exposed automobile workers. *Am J Ind Med*. 1995; 27(2):247-256. doi:10.1002/ajim.4700270 209

46. Denton E, Hoy R. Occupational aspects of irritable larynx syndrome. *Curr Opin Allergy Clin Immunol*. 2020;20(2):90-95. doi:10.1097/ACI.0000000000000619

47. Sandage MJ, Ostwalt ES, Allison LH, Cutchin GM, Morton ME, Odom SC. Irritant-induced chronic cough triggers: A scoping review and clinical checklist. *Am J Speech Lang Pathol*. 2021;30(3):1261-1291. doi:10.1044/2021_AJSLP-20-00362

48. Morrison M, Rammage L. The irritable larynx syndrome as a central sensitivity syndrome. *Can J Speech Lang Pathol Audiol*. 2010;34(4):282-289.

49. Shoffel-Havakuk H, Marks KL, Morton M, Johns MM III, Hapner ER. Validation of the OMNI vocal effort scale in the treatment of adductor spasmodic dysphonia. *Laryngoscope*. Published online October 12, 2018. doi:10.1002/lary.27430

50. Arffa RE, Krishna P, Gartner-Schmidt J, Rosen CA. Normative values for the Voice Handicap Index-10. *J Voice*. 2012;26(4):462-465. doi:10.1016/j.jvoice.2011.04.006

51. Bach K, Belafsky P, Wasylik K, Postma G, Koufman J. Validity and reliability of the Glottal Function Index. *Arch Otolaryngol Head Neck Surg*. 2005;131:961-964. doi:10.1016/j.jvoice.2024.04.004

52. Gibson PG, Vertigan AE. Speech pathology for chronic cough: A new approach. *Pulm Pharmacol Ther*. 2009;22(2):159-162. doi:10.1016/j.pupt.2008.11.005

53. Sundholm N, Shelly S, Wright ML, Reynolds J, Slovarp L, Gillespie AI. Effect of behavioral cough suppression therapy delivered via telehealth. *J Voice*. Published online December 20, 2022. doi:10.1016/j.jvoice.2022.11.015

54. Pommer A, Sarmento A, Singer A, Loewen H, Torres-Castro R, Sanchez-Ramirez DC. Virtual assessment and management of chronic cough: A scoping review. *Digit Heal*. 2024;10. doi:10.1177/20552076241239239

55. Novaleski CK, Mainland JD, Hegland KW, Aleksandruk MM, Dalton PH. Characterization of ethyl butyrate–induced cough before and after breath control techniques in healthy adults. *Am J Speech Lang Pathol*. 2023;32(2):675-687. doi:10.1044/2022_AJ SLP-22-00233

56. Driessen AK, McGovern AE, Narula M, et al. Central mechanisms of airway sensation and cough hypersensitivity. *Pulm Pharmacol Ther*. 2017;47:9-15. doi:10.1016/j.pupt .2017.01.010

57. Mazzone SB. An overview of the sensory receptors regulating cough. *Cough*. 2005; 1(1):1-9. doi:10.1186/1745-9974-1-2

58. Dicpinigaitis PV, Kantar A, Enilari O, Paravati F. Prevalence of Arnold nerve reflex in adults and children with chronic cough. *Chest*. 2018;153(3):675-679. doi:10.1016/j.chest.2017.11.019

59. Birring SS, Prudon B, Carr AJ, Singh SJ, Morgan L, Pavord ID. Development of a symptom specific health status measure for patients with chronic cough: Leicester Cough Questionnaire (LCQ). *Thorax*. 2003; 58(4):339-343. doi:10.1136/thorax.58.4.339

60. Patel RR, Awan SN, Barkmeier-Kraemer J, et al. Recommended protocols for instrumental assessment of voice: ASHA expert panel to develop a protocol for instrumental assessment of vocal function. *Am J Speech Lang Pathol*. 2018;27(3):887-905.

61. Mai Y, Zhan C, Zhang S, et al. Arnold nerve reflex: Vagal hypersensitivity in chronic cough with various causes. *Chest*. 2020; 158(1):264-271. doi:10.1016/j.chest.2019.11.041

62. McCallion P, De Soyza A. Cough and bronchiectasis. *Pulm Pharmacol Ther*. 2017; 47:77-83. doi:10.1016/j.pupt.2017.04.010

63. Poburka BJ, Patel RR, Bless DM. Voice-Vibratory Assessment With Laryngeal Imaging (VALI) form: Reliability of rating stroboscopy and high-speed videoendoscopy. *J Voice*. 2017;31(4):513.e1-513.e14. doi:10.1016/j.jvoice.2016.12.003

64. Reynolds JE, Jetté ME, Wright ML, Sundar KM, Gillespie AI, Slovarp LJ. Normative values for the Leicester Cough Questionnaire in healthy individuals. *Ann Otol Rhinol Laryngol*. 2023;132(6):705-708. doi:10.1177/00034894221112517

65. Castro ME, Sund LT, Hoffman MR, Hapner ER. The Voice Problem Impact Scales (VPIS). *J Voice*. 2024;38(3):666-673. doi:10.1016/j.jvoice.2021.11.011

66. Titze IR. Toward standards in acoustic analysis of voice. *J Voice*. 1994;8(1):1-7. doi:10.1016/S0892-1997(05)80313-3

67. Hapner ER. The ruler exercise. In: Behrman A, Haskell J, eds. *Exercises for Voice Therapy*. Plural Publishing; 2020:27-29

68. Duffy JR, Litts JK, Fink DS. Superior laryngeal nerve block for treatment of neurogenic cough. *Laryngoscope*. 2021;131(10): E2676-E2680. doi:10.1002/lary.29585

69. Shaha M, Hoffman MR, Hapner ER, Simpson CB. Membranous vocal fold lesions in patients with chronic cough: A case series. *J Voice*. 2023:1-7. doi:10.1016/j.jvoice.2023.02.006

70. Vertigan AE. The larynx as a target for treatment in chronic refractory cough. *Curr Otorhinolaryngol Rep*. 2019;7:129-136.

71. Vertigan AE, Kapela SL, Ryan NM, Birring SS, McElduff P, Gibson PG. Pregabalin and speech pathology combination therapy for refractory chronic cough: A randomized controlled trial. *Chest*. 2016;149(3):639-648. doi:10.1378/chest.15-1271

72. Ryan N, Birring S, Gibson P. Gabapentin for refractory chronic cough: A randomized, double-blind, placebo-controlled trial. *Lancet*. 2012;380:1583-1589.

73. Jeyakumar A, Brickman TM, Haben M. Effectiveness of amitriptyline versus cough suppressants in the treatment of chronic cough resulting from postviral vagal neuropathy. *Laryngoscope*. 2006;116(12):2108-2112. doi:10.1097/01.mlg.0000244377.60334.e3

74. Ryan MA, Cohen SM. Long-term follow-up of amitriptyline treatment for idiopathic cough. *Laryngoscope*. 2016;126(12):2758-2763. doi:10.1002/lary.25978

75. Cohen S, Misono S. Use of specific neuromodulators in the treatment of chronic, idiopathic cough: A systematic review. *Otolaryngol Head Neck Surg*. 2013;148(3):374-382. doi: 10.1177/0194599812471817

76. Halvorsen T, Walsted ES, Bucca C, et al. Inducible laryngeal obstruction: An official joint European Respiratory Society and European Laryngological Society statement. *Eur Respir J*. 2017;50(3). doi:10.1183/13993003.02221-2016

77. Clemm HH, Olin JT, McIntosh C, et al. Exercise-induced laryngeal obstruction (EILO) in athletes: A narrative review by a subgroup of the IOC consensus on "acute respiratory illness in the athlete." *Br J Sports*

Med. 2022;56(11):622-629. doi:10.1136/bjsports-2021-104704

78. Mathers-Schmidt BA. Paradoxical vocal fold motion: A tutorial on a complex disorder and the speech-language pathologist's role. *Am J Speech Lang Pathol.* 2001;10(2):111-125. doi:10.1044/1058-0360(2001/012)

79. Sandage MJ, Milstein CF, Nauman E. Inducible laryngeal obstruction differential diagnosis in adolescents and adults: A tutorial. *Am J Speech Lang Pathol.* 2023;32(1):1-17. doi:10.1044/2022_AJSLP-22-00187

80. Song WJ, Chung KF. Exploring the clinical relevance of cough hypersensitivity syndrome. *Expert Rev Respir Med.* 2020;14(3):275-284. doi:10.1080/17476348.2020.1713102

81. Sandage MJ, Billingsley CP, Hatcher JL, Petty B, Olin JT. When inspiratory stridor is not paradoxical vocal fold motion/inducible laryngeal obstruction: A case study of diaphragm flutter. *Perspect ASHA Spec Interest Groups.* 2021;6(3):596-600. doi:10.1044/2021_persp-21-00039

82. Maschka DA, Bauman NM, McCray PB, Hoffman HT, Karnell MP, Smith RJH. A classification scheme for paradoxical vocal cord motion. *Laryngoscope.* 1997;107(11):1429-1435. doi:10.1097/00005537-199711000-00002

83. Sandage M, Zelazny S. Paradoxical vocal fold motion in children and adolescents. *Lang Speech Hear Serv Sch.* 2004;35:353-362.

84. Johnston KL, Bradford H, Hodges H, Moore CM, Nauman E, Olin JT. The Olin EILOBI breathing techniques: Description and initial case series of novel respiratory retraining strategies for athletes with exercise-induced laryngeal obstruction. *J Voice.* 2018;32(6):698-704. doi:10.1016/j.jvoice.2017.08.020

85. Towey MP. Speech therapy telepractice for vocal cord dysfunction (VCD): Mainecare (Medicaid) cost savings. *Int J Telerehabil.* 2012;4(1):37-40. doi:10.5195/ijt.2012.6095

86. Drake K, Palmer AD, Schindler JS, Tilles SA. Functional outcomes after behavioral treatment of paradoxical vocal fold motion in adults. *Folia Phoniatr Logop.* 2018;69(4):154-168. doi:10.1159/000484716

87. Zraick RI, Kempster GB, Connor NP, et al. Establishing validity of the Consensus Auditory-Perceptual Evaluation of Voice (CAPE-V). *Am J Speech Lang Pathol.* 2011;20(1):14-22. doi:10.1044/1058-0360(2010/09-0105)

88. Breslin EH. The pattern of respiratory muscle recruitment during pursed-lip breathing. *Chest.* 1992;101(1):75-78.

89. Murry T, Tabaee A, Aviv JE. Respiratory retraining of refractory cough and laryngopharyngeal reflux in patients with paradoxical vocal fold movement disorder. *Laryngoscope.* 2004;114(8):1341-1345. doi:10.1097/00005537-200408000-00005

90. LeBlanc RA, Aalto D, Jeffery CC. Visual biofeedback for paradoxical vocal fold motion (PVFM). *J Otolaryngol Head Neck Surg.* 2021;50(1):1-6. doi:10.1186/s40463-021-00495-0

91. Brugman SM, Newman K. Vocal cord dysfunction. *Med Sci Updat (National Jewish Cent Immunol Respir Med).* 1993;11:1-5.

92. Ritz T, Meuret AE, Bhaskara L, Petersen S. Respiratory muscle tension as symptom generator in individuals with high anxiety sensitivity. *Psychosom Med.* 2013;75(2):187-195. doi:10.1097/PSY.0b013e31827d1072

93. Stemple JC, Lee L, D'Amico B, Pickup B. Efficacy of Vocal Function Exercises as a method of improving voice production. *J Voice.* 1994;8(3):271-278. doi:10.1016/S0892-1997(05)80299-1

94. Hogikyan ND, Sethuraman G. Validation of an instrument to measure voice-related quality of life (V-RQOL). *J Voice.* 1999;13(4):557-569. doi:10.1016/S0892-1997(99)80010-1

95. Lieberman J. Principles and techniques of manual therapy: Application in the management of dysphonia. In: Harris T, Harris S, Rubin J, Howard D, eds. *The Voice Clinical Handbook.* Whurr; 1998:91-138.

96. Angsuwarangsee T, Morrison M. Extrinsic laryngeal muscular tension in patients with voice disorders. *J Voice.* 2002;16(3):333-343.

97. Murton O, Hillman R, Mehta D. Cepstral peak prominence values for clinical voice

evaluation. *Am J Speech Lang Pathol.* 2020; 29(3):1596-1607. doi:10.1044/2020_AJSLP-20-00001

98. Qadeer MA, Swoger J, Milstein C, et al. Correlation between symptoms and laryngeal signs in laryngopharyngeal reflux. *Laryngoscope.* 2005;115(11):1947-1952. doi:10.1097/01.mlg.0000176547.90094.ac

99. Rammage L. *Vocalizing with Ease.* 3rd ed.; 2023. Osterreuche Akademie der Wissenschaften

100. Rammage L, Shoja SMM. Muscle misuse disorders of the larynx. In: Wackym P, Snow J, eds. *Ballenger's Otorhinolaryngology: Head and Neck Surgery.* 18th ed. ; 2016. People's Medical Publishing House.

101. Rammage L. But doctor, I don't have heartburn! https://www.youtube.com/watch?v=cX24JfEfxTE

102. Blager F. Breathing exercises for cough: Pursed lips breath. National Jewish Medical and Research Center.

103. Rammage L. Approaches to voice therapy: Speech Language and Audiology Canada. Webcast available at: https://www.sac-oac .ca/event-education/approaches-to-voice-therapy-2015/

104. Christensen PM, Heimdal JH, Christopher KL, et al. ERS/ELS/ACCP 2013 international consensus conference nomenclature on inducible laryngeal obstructions. *Eur Respir Rev.* 2015;24(137):445-450. doi:10 .1183/16000617.00006513

105. Olin JT, Shaffer M, Nauman E, et al. Development and validation of the Exercise-Induced Laryngeal Obstruction Dyspnea Index (EILODI). *J Allergy Clin Immunol.* 2022;149(4):1437-1444. doi:10.1016/j.jaci .2021.09.027

106. Heimdal J-H, Roksund OD, Halvorsen T, Skadberg BT, Olofsson J. Continuous laryngoscopy exercise test: A method for visualizing laryngeal dysfunction during exercise. *Laryngoscope.* 2009;116(1):52-57.

107. Olin JT, Clary MS, Fan EM, Johnston KL, Strand M, Christopher KL. Continuous laryngoscopy quantitates laryngeal behaviour in exercise and recovery. *Eur Respir J.* 2016;48(4):1192-1200.

108. Røksund OD, Heimdal J, Clemm H, Vollsæter M, Halvorsen T. Exercise inducible laryngeal obstruction: Diagnostics and management. *Paediatr Respir Rev.* 2017;21: 86-94. doi:10.1016/j.prrv.2016.07.003

8

Performance Voice

Introduction

Marina Gilman

The human voice is capable of producing an amazing variety of sounds. Some are pleasing to the ear and others less so, depending on individual tastes and auditory sensibilities. Common to all vocal expressions ranging from laughing, crying, yelling, to screaming, and to all musical styles from classical to heavy metal, is the potential to produce all of these sounds while maintaining optimal laryngeal function.

Vocal demands encompass the basic ability to communicate and interact with family and colleagues, to be heard over noise or just to be heard, and to use the voice as a finely tuned instrument that responds easily, freely, and flexibly with a consistent and varied sound palate.

This chapter focuses on the management of avocational as well as professional singers, who must maintain a refined, flexible vocal instrument to function at a consistently proficient level and to use that same instrument, their voice, for daily communication.

It is the role of the voice clinician to facilitate the rehabilitation or restoration of vocal function based on the patient's specific vocal needs. For vocal rehabilitation to be effective,

it is very important that clinicians understand the anatomy and physiology of the vocal tract, respiration, resonance, and phonation not only abstractly, but also somatically within the postural dynamics of the whole body. A key to successful treatment outcomes is understanding how the presenting symptoms relate to the diagnosis as well as to the functional demands of the patient—in other words, knowing where or how the voice breaks down and considering the patient's culture (vocal, professional, and personal), body dynamics, and personality. Therapy goals, treatment plans, and therapeutic exercises are based equally on the history of the complaint, the medical diagnosis from the referring physician, the instrumental acoustic and aerodynamic evaluations, the audio-perceptual evaluations, and the vocal capabilities as they relate to the patient's professional and personal needs. This is especially true when dealing with the complexity of performers' lives and performance demands.

Voice clinicians do not necessarily have expertise in the specific vocal demands encountered by their patients. Knowledge of the patient's culture, lifestyle, rehearsal, and studio demands is useful, but key to successful rehabilitative treatment is taking a thorough history, ie, knowing what questions to ask regarding lifestyle, vocal demands, and training—not just how much but also what was taught. By truly listening to and watching the patient's body dynamics, the clinician can learn the nature of their patients' unique challenges and facilitate solutions.

When patients, especially seasoned professionals, present with vocal problems, it is very important to validate the patients' knowledge of their own voice. This is especially true with patients whose vocal demands extend to the extreme, as in shouting, screaming, or vocally aggressive contemporary genres. It is incumbent on the clinician to focus on balancing the vocal systems, helping the patient find more efficient ways to produce the necessary sounds, providing them with therapeutic strategies, and encouraging the patient to discover within themselves new pathways to accomplish their vocal goals. Our role is to rehabilitate the whole voice, with singing being only one aspect.

Many voice clinicians are hesitant to treat patients who are singers at any level, especially high-level professional singers. On the other hand, clinicians generally don't hesitate to treat a patient who may be a high-level actor or preacher because they feel they understand the "speaking voice." In fact, the clinician may well not understand the specific vocal demands and profession-specific "instrument tuning" needed by someone in the broadcast industry or a stage actor any more than they do a high-level rap singer. How systems interact changes depending on the task, whether yelling at a football game, singing opera over a large Wagnerian orchestra, or filling a theater with a stage whisper. However, voice clinicians do understand how the presenting pathology can disrupt the normal vibratory characteristics of the vocal folds and vocal mechanisms. They appreciate that the disruption in function might be more apparent in certain vocal expressions than others. For example, certain parts of the range may be significantly more dysphonic than others, or perhaps the issue occurs not when speaking at a normal pitch and loudness but with any change in modality such as singing, change in dynamics, or using a "stage voice."

Voice clinicians are trained to rehabilitate the voice in all its functions, including singing. In fact, many of the exercises used clinically originated in the singing studio. These tasks have effectively balanced the systems in the context of voice habilitation training and continue to do so in the context of rehabilitation.[1,2]

Speech pathologists don't coach repertoire; however, sections of repertoire can be used as a therapeutic tool in the same way standard sentences or phonemically loaded words are used clinically. In other words, the voice clinician can, and in many cases should, incorporate singing into therapy as a remediation strategy as long as it relates to the rehabilitation of laryngeal function.

Over the past few decades, as the field of voice has grown, an increasing number of speech-language pathologists (SLPs) working with patients with voice disorders have singing backgrounds or have dual degrees. The terms "singing voice specialist" and more recently "vocologist" are often used by both singing teachers as well as SLPs with additional degrees in voice even though their respective training and qualifications are very different. The terms are ill defined and used by some to designate expertise in working with elite singers. It is important to keep in mind that the SLP is certified and licensed medically to treat patients with voice disorders for purposes of rehabilitation, while the role of the singing teacher or coach is one of vocal enhancement or habilitation. Singing teachers and coaches can and should become part of the multidisciplinary voice team where appropriate.

Two issues often arise with respect to referral to a specialty clinician, vocal coach, or singing teacher. First, a referral should be made to a specialty clinician when the limits of the treating clinician's knowledge have been reached and when the treating laryngologist concurs that continuing therapy is appropriate. Second, when the patient is completing therapy and generalization of skills to repertoire may be appropriate, the patient should be referred to a vocal coach or singing teacher. As stated previously, sections of repertoire can be used as facilitating exercises; however, coaching of repertoire is out of the scope of clinical practice for the SLP, even if the clinician is also a singing teacher. Professional organizations such as the National Association of Teachers of Singing, the Voice and Speech Trainers Association, and the Pan-American Vocology Association are good sources of references for voice coaches and teachers.

Recent developments in neuroplasticity and changes in our understanding of the body/mind/brain relationship are introducing new elements to the therapeutic toolbox of voice clinicians. Motor learning theory and principles of exercise science are influencing therapy protocols.[3-5] Somatic methods and practices such as myofascial release, the Alexander Technique, the Feldenkrais® Method, yoga, and mindfulness have been found effective in voice rehabilitation.[6-9] Clinicians can and should embrace these "new tools" in their therapy toolkit. However, it is important to understand that many of these somatic and meditation/mindful practices also require special training. This is especially true of the manual therapies such as myofascial release or the hands-on elements of the Feldenkrais Method and Alexander Technique. If the clinician is not sufficiently trained in the specific modality, they should refer the patient to a qualified practitioner. It is always incumbent on the clinician to recognize the source of their therapeutic strategies and techniques and be clear with the patient and in their documentation as to what specifically was done as well as its source. Respecting the boundaries of one's training and knowledge as well as the legal scope of practice for the clinician will facilitate rather than hamper the patient's access to appropriate interventions.

This chapter contains 9 case studies exploring the specific occupational voice demands of a variety of styles. Eugenia Castro and Megan Urbano describe the case of a voice-over artist, Marina Gilman shares the road to vocal health for a praise and worship leader, and Maurice Goodwin explores the challenges of a high school music teacher. The case of a jazz singer by night and a teacher by day worked up in the interprofessional clinic with a laryngologist and speech pathologist is presented by Sarah Schneider and Mark Courey. Patricia Doyle and Starr Cookman present a case of a 9-year-old with nodules. Readers will learn about different genres of singing as explored by Jenny Muckala, who presents a case of a performing country singer with voice concerns. Wendy LeBorgne describes working with a traveling musical theater singer/actor, while Deb Phyland and Juliana Codino share the challenges faced by actors and aging performers, respectively.

Case Studies

 CASE STUDY 8.1

Multimodality Voice Therapy for an Adult Voice Actor/Singer With a Translucent Polypoid Lesion

M. Eugenia Castro and Megan Urbano

Voice Evaluation

Chief Complaint. Voice cracks during high-pitched character voices, discomfort with voicing, and vocal fatigue after performing extreme voices for her job as a voice actor

History of Present Illness. The patient was evaluated in an interprofessional clinic with a voice-specialized SLP and fellowship-trained laryngologist. The patient was diagnosed with dysphonia secondary to a left vocal fold translucent polyp by the laryngologist.

364 Voice Therapy: Clinical Case Studies

Case History

History of Voice Complaint. The patient, Operatic Ogre (OO), is a 33-year-old cisgender woman with a sudden onset of voice problems lasting 3 weeks at the time of the evaluation. She reports that the onset of symptoms was associated with a sudden voice crack when yelling for a voice recording. Afterward, she noted voice cracks in her upper singing and speaking range and difficulty singing softly in the high range. She reports she could avoid voice cracks but only when singing loudly.

During the initial diagnostic appointment, laryngeal imaging indicated significant edema. The clinician prescribed the patient a week of steroids accompanied by complete voice rest. At her follow-up, there was noted overall improvement in vocal fold edema at the lesion site; however, a small left vocal fold translucent polyp remained. A surgical approach was deemed unnecessary, and the patient was recommended to do a course of voice therapy. OO reported completing a self-imposed modified voice rest routine for a couple of weeks prior to evaluation without significant improvement in vocal fatigue and laryngeal tightness, which she attributed to being overly preoccupied about her voice. Her modal speaking voice was unaffected. Notably, she had experienced voice problems with similar symptoms 2 years prior. At that time, a videostroboscopy exam showed mild vocal fold inflammation without lesions. OO had not received the services of an SLP for her voice problems in the past. She currently has no complaints of dysphagia, dyspnea, or reflux symptoms.

Voice Use. OO is a professional voice-over actor (mainly working on video games) with prior experience as a classical soprano. She currently primarily performs classical musical theater and classical baroque. Her most frequent work involves conversational speech in modal register, but she sometimes voices an ogre, a well-known role of hers. This vocal style requires more demanding voice effects such as grunting and yelling. Doing these more vocally demanding tasks made her symptoms worse. She was also concerned that her voice cracked in the highest segment of her range and sometimes during high-pitched character voices (eg, cartoon princesses). The patient reports she currently does not have an established warm-up or cool-down routine. Her voice symptoms often worsen during conventions, when she is required to perform samples of her voice-over work and to engage in networking and meet and greets in noisy environments, such as booths in convention spaces.

Laryngeal Imaging

Laryngeal videostroboscopy was performed transorally with a rigid videolaryngoscope. Salient examination findings included no supraglottal or hypopharyngeal masses, full abduction and adduction of both vocal folds, and complete glottal closure. There was a decreased mucosal wave noted on the left true vocal fold with a small, translucent polypoid lesion in the striking zone, mid vocal fold free edge.

Patient-Reported Outcome Measures

The OMNI Vocal Effort Scale[10] was completed. The patient rated vocal effort on a 0 to 10 scale where 0 = "extremely easy" to produce voice and 10 = "extremely hard" to produce voice. The patient reported that vocal effort was 0/10 during the evaluation and 6/10 at worst, occurring at the end of the day.

Quality-of-Life Impairment:

1. Voice Handicap Index–10 (VHI-10)[11]: 13/40 (threshold = 11)[12]
2. Voice Catastrophization Index[13]: 17/52
3. Voice Problem Impact Scales (VPIS)[14]: On four 1 to 7 scales with equal-appearing intervals and end anchors where 1 = "not at all affected" and 7 = "profoundly affected," the patient self-scored the following:

a. Impact on work life or daily activities: 7/7
b. Impact on social life: 2/7
c. Impact on home life: 1/7
d. Overall impact: 5/7

After a collaborative review of VPIS answers, OO explained she was most impacted by her voice problems in her work life due to high-intensity vocal requirements. Her social life was affected because she began avoiding certain interactions to conserve her voice. However, she stated she could "push through" and continue on if absolutely needed, worsening her symptoms.

Auditory-Perceptual Assessment

The Consensus Auditory-Perceptual Evaluation of Voice (CAPE-V)[15] was administered. The patient had an overall score of 12/100, indicating a dysphonia of a mild nature. Aberrant perceptual features identified in the voice include primary roughness. Overall, vocal intensity was noted to be within normal limits. Pitch of the voice was within normal limits for age, gender, and stature. Resonance was focused in the oral region. Respiration appeared to be primarily abdominal-thoracic.

Extended range phonation was assessed from D3 to C6 (on the keyboard) in thyroarytenoid (TA)- and cricothyroid (CT)-dominant productions. Voice instability and breaks were noted in transitions from TA to CT dominance and occurred around E5 through A5. Epilaryngeal resonance was noted secondary to extraneous paralaryngeal muscle tension, particularly in CT dominance, which improved with change from /a/ to straw phonation productions.

Manual Palpation Assessment

Muscle tension was assessed and rated on a 0 to 5 scale where 0 = "no tension" and 5 = "most tension." Results indicated elevated hyoid position and reduced flexibility, 3/5 tension at the base of tongue, 5/5 during phonation, 3/5

tension at the lateral suprahyoid muscles, 4/5 tension at the thyrohyoid space, and reduced laryngeal flexibility.

Acoustic and Aerodynamic Assessment

OO demonstrated values slightly below normative data for F0 standard deviation when reading the Rainbow Passage and mean F0 in sustained phonation. Values were slightly above normative data for extended range and vital capacity, as expected in trained professional singers. She also demonstrated slightly elevated mean dB SPL in reading aloud as well as in conversational speech (Table 8–1). Of note, objective data collected must be interpreted with the consideration that normative data is not usually reported specifically for the professional voice user population. Professionally trained voice users may have greater control over their vocal apparatus and, as such, may conceal certain subtle symptoms in casual conversation.[16] Normative values and ranges are derived from Goy et al (2013), Siupsinskiene and Lycke (2011), Sanchez et al (2014), Buckley et al (2023), Zraick et al (2012), and Lewandowski et al (2018).[17-22]

Stimulability

Stimulability testing was conducted. The patient demonstrated decreases in voice breaks, reduced effort, and improved forward resonance when utilizing straw phonation in water.

Impressions

The patient presents with a mild dysphonia that limits communication and participation in all aspects of life, with particular negative impact on vocal tasks required for work.

Plan of Care

Voice therapy was recommended and considered medically necessary. The patient appeared to be a good candidate for therapy. Positive prognostic indicators included the patient's favorable response to stimulability testing and

Table 8–1. Complete Acoustic and Aerodynamic Assessment Chart

Normative ranges calculated for a cisgender female between the ages of 18 and 64. RB = Rainbow Passage, SP = sustained phonation, SD = standard deviation, CNV = conversation, MFR = mean airflow during voicing

Pitch: Frequency (Hz)	Results	Normative Range*	Outside Norms
Mean F0 (RP)	191.39	183-234	
SD F0 (RP)	26.76	34-57	✓
Mean F0 (CNV)	180.28		
Sustained Phonation (Hz)			
Mean F0 (SP)	192.02	213-293	✓
Max F0 (SP)	852	363-683	✓
Min F0 (SP)	159	117.7	✓
Range (in octaves)	2.42	1.85-3.05	
Vocal Intensity: Loudness (dB)			
Mean SPL (RB)	77.29	62-83	✓
Mean SPL (CNV)	82.79		
Mean SPL (SP)	85.45	68.9-80.2	✓
Voice Quality (dB): Analysis of Dysphonia in Speech and Voice (ADSV)			
CPP (SP)	13.43	<12.07** SD 1.99	
CPP (RP)	6.56	<7.40** SD 1.18	

Phonatory Aerodynamic System (PAS)	Results	Normative Data***	1SD	Outside Norms
Vital Capacity (L) (expiratory volume)	3.87	2.87 SD 0.69	✓	
MFR (L/sec): Vowel	0.188	0.13 SD 0.06		
MFR (L/sec): RP First 4 sentences	0.163	0.15 SD 0.05		
Duration (sec)	21	20.95 SD 2.06		
Breaths (#)	3	4.38 SD 1.44		

Table 8–1. *continued*

Phonatory Aerodynamic System (PAS)	Results		Normative Data***	1SD	Outside Norms
Psub (cmH$_2$O) (mean peak air pressure)	6.08	SD	5.4 1.37		
PTP (cmH$_2$O): Quietest Modal (mean peak air pressure)	2.25				
Laryngeal Resistance (cmH$_2$O/L/sec) (aerodynamic resistance)	50	SD	68.2 52.08		

*Goy et al (2013); Siupsinskiene & Lycke (2011); Sanchez et al (2014). Ranges indicate between 10th-90th percentile **Buckley et al (2023) ***F 18-39; Zraick et al (2012); Lewandowski et al (2018).

her expressed commitment to a behavioral therapy approach. The clinician explained the treatment options during the evaluation session, and the patient elected to begin therapy. Therapy was then planned to be conducted for 4 to 6 sessions of 45 to 60 minutes each. Sessions were conducted twice monthly for a total of 2 to 3 months.

The patient's long-term goal was to restore functional use of voice for daily occupational, social, and emotional needs. Short-term goals (STGs) were set to attempt changes in vocal function through the following strategies:

1. Use indirect strategies to improve vocal health and wellness by establishing a routine for hydration, warm-ups, resets, and cool-downs as well as to manage vocal load.
2. Improve glottal configuration to reduce vocal fatigue and effort using semi-occluded vocal tract (SOVT) exercises across an extended frequency range.[23]
3. Using Resonant Voice Therapy (RVT)[24] tenets, increase voicing efficiency and respiratory phonatory coordination across speech patterns used for extreme vocal effects and character voices.

This treatment plan was developed with the patient collaboratively, and she expressed agreement and an understanding of the clinician's recommendations.

Decision Making

Considering the intricacies of the patient's profession as well as a smaller lesion size and morphology, surgery was not recommended in favor of a conservative approach. Clinical hypothesis by the SLP and the laryngologist was that the lesion could be reduced with a behavioral intervention approach. Although the patient presented with an overall mild dysphonia, her voice symptoms significantly impacted her ability to work. Barriers to change included the patient's apprehension toward approaching casting directors and agents to advocate for her own vocal health. Goals were written to provide a well-rounded approach to improve overall vocal health and wellness to support a long-lasting career as a voice actor. An eclectic approach to voice therapy was implemented, including a combination of indirect and direct therapy with physiologic approaches. Indirect strategies included a patient-centered approach, incorporating thorough education of anatomy and physiology of vocal production, exploring meaningful

368 Voice Therapy: Clinical Case Studies

rationales for therapeutic techniques, and creating a vocal health and wellness program. Regarding physiologic approaches, SOVT exercises were implemented to optimize glottal configurations and potentially enhance reduction in phonotrauma.[23] RVT[24] tenets and elements from the Estill Voice Model[25] were used in a modified approach to target increased endurance and sustainable phonation patterns for extreme vocal effects and character voices. Therapy was delivered via telemedicine for easier access to care due to the patient's long commute to the clinic.[26]

Intervention

Session #1

Short-Term Goal #1. *Use indirect strategies to improve vocal health and wellness by establishing a routine for hydration, warm-ups, resets, and cool-downs as well as to manage vocal load.*

   Short-Term Goal #2. *Improve glottal configuration to reduce vocal fatigue and effort using semi-occluded vocal tract (SOVT) exercises across an extended frequency range.*[23]

   The first session focused predominantly on addressing both short-term goals #1 and #2. The clinician conducted a thorough discussion on vocal health and wellness strategies, first addressing systemic and topical forms of hydration.[27] OO reported that, when she moved to Los Angeles 5 years ago, she immediately noticed symptoms of dry throat and increased "clicking sounds," a term in voice acting for noticeable smacking of the tongue and lips on recording associated with dry mouth. The clinician advised OO to sip liquids throughout the day to improve overall hydration and use a nebulized isotonic saline solution prior, during, and after recording sessions as needed to improve topical hydration.[28] Finally, the clinician recommended using glycerin-based lozenges to stimulate saliva production and reduce dry mouth during recording sessions.

   In describing the intricacies of voice acting, OO reported that sessions are typically booked for 4 hours. The number of breaks given can vary based on the company and sound booth director. The clinician discussed education on vocal dose and budgeting to provide meaningful rationale for how different voices can cause faster onset of vocal fatigue.[29] While OO felt she could perform a full session with a high-pitched cartoon character voice with ease, the monster voice sessions were not only vocally fatiguing, but were also creating increased anxiety. OO worried the character voices would worsen phonotrauma, resulting in a negative impact on her singing voice. The clinician incorporated active listening and a collaborative approach to find solutions for these challenges. The consensus was for OO to present information via handouts addressing vocal health recommendations to her agent.

   To improve voicing efficiency and glottal configuration, SOVT exercises (ie, straw phonation in water) were introduced to create a warm-up routine. Initial practice sets included descending glides on the musical pattern 5-4-3-2-1 across physiological modal range. Beginning an exercise routine on a descending scale promotes laryngeal relaxation and can be used as a vocal reset when feelings of tension arise. Next, 3-5-1 and 1-5-1-5-1 gliding patterns were used to gradually ascend into the patient's higher ranges. The patient initially demonstrated increased airflow in her higher range, which was balanced to find forward resonance via vibrations at the lips and visual feedback from the bubbles created by blowing into the straw placed in water. Voice cracks in the high range decreased gradually as the patient gained proficiency with the task. (See Video 28 Straw Phonation in Water Hierarchy by Codino for an example of cup bubbles.)

Session #2

Short-Term Goal #3. *Using Resonant Voice Therapy (RVT)*[24] *tenets, increase voicing efficiency and respiratory phonatory coordination across speech patterns used for extreme vocal effects and character voices.*

During the second session, short-term goal #3 was addressed and SOVT exercises were reviewed. OO demonstrated improved respiratory/phonatory coordination throughout her frequency range. She had also independently included more complex phonatory patterns from her opera background, such as octave vocalises, to advance practice. Neck stretches were used to reduce strap muscle engagement and perception of vocal strain.

> A *vocalise* generally refers to a vocal task sung on vowels or consonant-vowel syllables to warm up the voice or practice a certain vocal requirement in a song. The pitch pattern of a vocalise is typically repeated in an ascending and descending pattern across the frequency range.

To continue building the patient's confidence in vocal growth, the high-pitched character voices were first targeted, as these voices were easier to maintain than the ogre and monster voices. During trials, OO demonstrated breath-holding patterns and exacerbated strap muscle engagement. OO was led through an exercise using /njæ/ sounds on a 3-2-1 musical pattern and implementing the /n/ and liquid glide /j/ to target the feel of oral and nasal resonance mix, also known as *twang*.[30] The clinician advanced trials to incorporate words, phrases, and full sentences using the initial /njæ/ sound as an anchor. OO said she had never felt such ease with her character voices in that part of her range! (See Video 23 Twang for Sustainable Character Voices by Urbano.)

Session #3
OO reported she had spoken to her agent and casting directors at her current job, arranging 2 weekly 2-hour video game recording sessions, reducing her vocal load. They graciously accepted her advocacy for improved vocal budgeting. At this time, OO started using a personal, portable nebulizer prior to, during, and after voice acting sessions and in her day-to-day life. She noted her voice felt "moisturized," lending ease to phonation.

Tenets of RVT and SOVT exercises previously established were applied to target comfortable and sustainable phonation in her yelling character voice as a precursor to targeting her ogre voice. Education was provided in safe belting technique and vocal effects such as growl and yelling.

> *Belting* is a musical theater style technique that uses the chest voice to produce a powerful sound.

The clinician used videostroboscopy examples of healthy vocal folds, demonstrating vocal effects via supraglottic rattle and shaping as aids to facilitate learning via a shared screen during telemedicine appointments. The previously introduced *twang* technique was used to optimize glottal posture with high belting/yelling vocal effects. The clinician guided OO in trials with /njæ/ on a descending pattern 5-4-3-2-1 across her physiological frequency range, but this time used her character voices, incorporating belting (increased TA dominance) and yelling (increased vocal intensity). Initially, she reported increased effort at the level of the throat when using her character voices versus her regular singing voice. Prompts to emulate a kitten's cry ("meow") were implemented to enhance aryepiglottic narrowing as described in the Estill Voice Model.[25] An "open throat" hand expression was also added as a facilitator to promote a simultaneous open and relaxed throat for kinesthetic and visual feedback.[25] This resulted in successful trials with reported effortless phonation.

Practice was advanced to incorporate cup phonation[31] as a facilitator to introduce trials with her ogre voices and growl effects. Trials were completed using sustained phonation with ease on a humming /m/ sound

370 Voice Therapy: Clinical Case Studies

and gradually "turning on" her growl effects to achieve her characteristic ogre voice. Cup phonation was added as a *safety net*, a means to optimize glottal postures and promote feelings of an open throat throughout explorations of extreme vocal effects. She was cued to maintain a tight seal around the mouth with the cup and maintain a target of low vocal effort. (See Video 24 Cup Phonation by Castro.) When adding growl, OO was guided to focus on feeling rattling somewhere in the resonating vocal cavity structures, above an imaginary line traced at the level of her chin. These facilitators prompted the production of growl by squeezing aryepiglottic folds versus straining at the level of the glottis, securing increased airflow during voicing.[32,33] The task was advanced to consonant-vowel-consonant combinations, words, and short phrases with and without the cup. Phrases were practiced with special attention to reduced vocal effort and then advanced to using lines from her prior ogre-voice roles. Contrasting practice was incorporated to facilitate greater vocal awareness. OO differentiated "uncomfortable" versus "comfortable" phonation and switched between them on command.

Session #4

At this point, OO felt she was making consistent progress toward her goals. However, she continued to experience vocal fatigue when attending video game or anime conventions (a Japanese style of cartooning), during which she would sit at a booth for meet and greets, participate in panel discussions, and spend a large part of the day with friends and other voice actors. As a well-known voice actress, she was expected to attend events throughout the year and historically regularly experienced voice loss afterward. The clinician and patient reviewed vocal health and wellness goals and implemented use of a microphone/speaker system at her booth to decrease the need to project.

A modified Conversation Training Therapy (CTT)[34] approach was introduced to spe-

cifically address ease with vocal projection. Using conversation with the clinician and cues of clear speech as the main stimuli, OO was guided to feel as if she had a "consonant salad" in her mouth while keeping the focus on crisp consonants as opposed to on her throat. (See Video 1 Mapping Speech Sound Sensations by Gartner-Schmidt.) Background noise was incorporated during practice trials to emulate a convention setting.

Session #5

OO returned for her last therapy session after attending an important convention. She reported she successfully implemented strategies learned during the therapeutic process. Her routine included using CTT in conversational speech, using a speaker/microphone in her booth, being mindful of vocal budgeting, taking a vocal nap before networking or social dinners, doing gentle SOVT exercises, and nebulizing at night before bed. As a result, she stated enthusiastically that this was the first convention she attended in a long time after which she hadn't lost her voice.

Given her improvements, the clinician and patient discussed readiness for discharge and collaboratively developed a maintenance program for OO to continue working toward her goals independently.

Posttreatment Outcome Measures

Measures for posttreatment and discharge decisions were patient led. Objective measures were not collected since OO's last session was conducted via telemedicine. A global rating of change scale[35] was administered to evaluate positive change posttreatment. On a 1 to 10 scale with equal appearing intervals and end anchors where 1 = "no change" and 10 = "considerable improvement," the patient self-reported an 8/10, which was considered significant improvement. She also self-reported a 90% improvement on a percentage of improvement scale (0%-100% improvement) when comparing pre- and posttreatment. She reported meeting all voice demands required for daily occupational, social, and emotional needs.

Clinician Reflections on Outcome

The patient benefited from an eclectic, holistic therapy approach that gave her the tools and autonomy to become a voice detective herself, identifying vocal problems and finding appropriate solutions. Due to her multifaceted vocal requirements, it was necessary to address the voice as a whole instrument, targeting her speaking, singing, and character voices. Following therapy, OO felt confident she could experiment freely with her voice with no symptoms, but she also had the security to bring her voice back to baseline if needed. This case seemed daunting at first due to the need to address unconventional and contrasting forms of vocal production; however, the clinicians incorporated several therapeutic approaches with individualized modifications, always supported by evidence-based practice.

 CASE STUDY 8.2

Onsite Voice Therapy for an Adult Theater Actor With Vocal Injury During Preparation and Performance

Debra Phyland

The following case gives the reader the privilege of learning about working in a medical system outside the US, in this case Australia, a country that has a robust speech-language pathology presence. The reader is encouraged to review the assessment and treatment tools that may be unfamiliar.

Voice Evaluation

Primary Complaint. Recent change in voice quality, reduced vocal stamina for performance requirements, longer than usual warm-up times, and decreased access to vocal dynamics meeting all voice demands required for daily occupational, social, and emotional needs.

This professional actor, a 26-year-old nonbinary individual assigned female at birth, was seen for an urgent comprehensive voice evaluation by our voice team (laryngologist and speech pathologist) following direct referral from the company manager of a touring professional theater production.

History of Voice Complaint

The patient reported a gradual 2-week onset of mild decline in vocal stamina and quality during play rehearsals/preview period, now with persistent mild dysphonia and mild odynophonia on sustained voicing, at 1 month following the onset of symptoms.

LF noted no obvious sentinel moment around the onset of the voice problem but had noticed increasing throat discomfort and huskiness within the first week of the rehearsal period during a scene that required shouting (1 month ago). They described their voice as usually clear but stated that it had now become mildly breathy, unreliable, and "coarse" with a slight lowering of their speaking voice pitch and reduction in pitch range, as well as a tendency to deteriorate with use. They also reported that they had taken a prednisone tablet (a prescription oral steroid) given to them by a friend for the opening night to try to fix their voice and that this had improved the "huskiness" but only temporarily—the quality again declined when they performed 2 shows the following day. Since then, their voice continues to fatigue and they are concerned by the increased vocal effort, slight pain with speaking, and occasional "cracking" on lines.

Medical and Vocal History. LF has been taking daily low-dose sertraline (25 mg) for anxiety and a contraceptive pill, both for several years, but takes no other prescribed medication. They reported very occasional reflux symptoms, which they manage with diet control, behavioral measures (≥2 hours before lying down after evening meal), and occasional use of dual-action Gaviscon™ (sodium alginate, bicarbonate, and calcium carbonate)

372 Voice Therapy: Clinical Case Studies

prior to bed. They reported to be in excellent health and have no other comorbidities.

LF reported no prior significant voice concerns, other than short-term common cold-related changes. Five years ago while at drama school, they consulted an ear, nose, and throat (ENT) specialist for a routine voice check-up and were told there were no abnormalities detected. Of note, on the first day of rehearsals in their current role, LF was also seen by the theater company's resident speech pathologist for a perceptual voice screen as per the occupational health program protocol and was deemed to be vocally healthy.

Voice Training and Prior Acting Experience. LF performed in amateur theater as a nonsinging actor throughout their teen years and received a bachelor of fine arts in acting 4 years ago from a well-recognized drama school. Since graduating, they have worked as a part-time waiter and sporadically as an actor for TV commercials and as a minor role or extra in several miniseries. They have also undertaken further acting classes with a focus on film and TV but no additional voice classes.

Current Vocal Context and Stakes. LF is currently making their professional stage debut playing a supporting lead role in a highly physical comedy theater production (spanning 2 acts over 2.5 hours), involving a cast of 7. Prior to this, LF had not worked as an actor nor used their voice extensively for 6 months. Rehearsals began a month prior to this evalu-

ation and involved 9 hours of scene work per day, 6 days a week, for a total of 14 days before moving to the theater for production week and then previews. The play opened a week ago and runs for a 3-month season, 8 shows per week over 5 days (with no shows on Monday and Tuesday). LF's role involves use of a loud character voice and regular shouting and raucous laughing with simultaneous high physicality. The theater's resident speech pathologist had undertaken a vocal injury risk assessment (Table 8–2), and the vocal load (quantity and manner of voicing)[36] and overall risk for developing an occupationally induced dysphonia was deemed high.[37,38]

Although the company employs an actor in a "swing" capacity (understudy), that actor is currently replacing another performer so cannot perform for LF if required. LF informed the clinician that there was an emergency contingency for the associate director to temporarily fill their role if imperative.

LF is from another Australian state and is staying on their own in company accommodations. They informed the clinician that they do not talk much outside of the show context and had undertaken complete voice rest the prior 2 Mondays. They noted that, although this had been useful, the voice had not returned to baseline by the subsequent Wednesday and had deteriorated significantly on both of the Saturday and Sunday double-show days. They reported that, in addition to the voice con-

Table 8–2. Ergonomic and Person-Factor Influences on Vocal Health (Phyland, 2005) in Relation to LF

Influence	Examples of Potential Influences (Positive and Negative)
Current Work Environment and Vocal Demands	
Place of Most Voicing	Moderately large theater without voice amplification
Vocal Dose	High intensity, frequency, and duration of voicing time
Manner of Voicing for Work	Loud speaking, character voice, Yorkshire accent required, high degree of concomitant physical effort

Table 8–2. *continued*

Influence	Examples of Potential Influences (Positive and Negative)
Voicing Schedule	Number of hours per day voicing (>5 hours), number of consecutive days (5), periods of performance voice rest (1/ wk), shows per week (8 + rehearsals × 1 = 9), double shows/ day (×2), weeks on/off (none)
Vocal Recovery	Short voicing turnaround times
Room Acoustics	Theater acoustics good but voicing over loud props and music at times
Use of Acoustic Support/Strategies	May have potential for sound tech to "ride mic" to amplify LF when talking over stage noise
Posture While Voicing	Various postures and high physicality including leaps, exercising, hanging upside down while shouting, etc.
Air Conditions	Humidity, quality, temperature, consistency, heating, odors, air conditioning and proximity to vents unknown
Work Stressors	Intimidated by director, found production week highly stressful, high workload, worried will lose the job because of voice. Employment status: contract
Voice Efficiency	Use of extrinsic laryngeal muscles to increase loudness and change pitch, audible inhalations, speaking on residual air, habitual use of hard glottal attacks, pressed phonation for character voice
Routine of Work Practices for Voice	Does 1-hour nonspecific vocal warm-up (too long!!!), no cool-down, no voice preparation prior to commencement of production
Manner of Voicing for Work	High intensity required, use of inefficient character voice, high degree of effort
Person Factors	
General	Age (not highly experienced stage performer), physical fitness: high, health: good, lifestyle and quality of life: unsure
Voice Training	Type and relevance to work (speaking), quantity, consistency and recency (minimal)
Vocal Fitness	Decreased vocal fitness leading up to rehearsals. Cumulative fatigue noted with decreased recovery times, recent high vocal activity (eg, rehearsal schedule)
Vocal Load Outside of Work	Low
Value Attached to Voice	Moderately high voice expectations for performance

374 Voice Therapy: Clinical Case Studies

cerns, they were also stressed about their performance in general and felt that the director was giving critical feedback to them more frequently than to the other performers.

Self-Evaluations of Current Physical Aspects of Vocal Function

1. An adapted Borg CR10 Perceived Phonatory Effort Scale[39] (PPE) was completed. The patient was asked to rate current vocal effort on a 0 to 10 scale where 0 = "extremely easy" to produce voice and 10 = "extremely hard" to produce voice. The patient rated vocal effort as 4/10 just prior to the evaluation but reported at the end of the last week of performances they would have rated themselves as 6/10.

2. The Evaluation of the Ability to Voice Easily (EAVE) scale was completed just prior to the laryngeal evaluation to assess current perception of their voice status.[40] LF presented with a total EAVE score of 29/48 (Figure 8–1) which placed them just above the cutoff point of 24 for risk of a perceived voice disorder for an occupational voice user. On the Level of Concern 2-item scale (scored separately from the total EAVE), they received the maximum score (8/8), indicating a high level of concern about their voice at that time.

Self-Reported Impact on Quality of Life

LF scored 3/40 on the VHI-10,[11] indicating minimal to low impact of voice concerns on overall quality of life; however, LF remarked that they found it difficult to answer, as today's voice was not typical and the questions did not seem relevant to the current voice issue nor to performance concerns.

Self-Reported Impact on Performance

LF reported that their performance was mildly impacted by their current voice issue, particularly by the end of 2 consecutive performances

in 1 day. Specifically, the director had given LF a note last week to "be more playful with their voice as they sounded pushed and were sometimes losing character." LF attributed this to the recent sense of needing more vocal effort to access the required pitch and loudness dynamics. They also wondered whether their concerns about throat discomfort and perceived reduction in voice reliability were distracting them from their usual acting processes.

Auditory-Perceptual Assessment

Perceptual voice evaluation of conversational speech and on specific vocal tasks (reading aloud, pitch glides, projected and soft speech) revealed a mild dysphonia. The aberrant perceptual features identified on the Perceptual Voice Profile[41] (Figure 8–2) were occasional phonation breaks, slight strain, and mild breathiness of voice quality; mildly high modal loudness; and slightly low modal pitch for age and gender. Maximum phonation times on vowel prolongation exceeded 25 seconds and pitch range was considered within normal limits, although increasing breathiness was noted on ascending pitch.

Additional Features:

1. **Conversational Speech.** Tendency toward hard glottal attacks in connected speech; audible inhalations but good subglottic control of respiration for loud voicing; normal resonance

2. **Character Voice With Yorkshire Accent.** Mild strain and/or pressed quality; accent required altered focus of resonance with backed tongue posture; laryngeal hyperfunction especially during loud phonation with visible recruitment of extrinsic laryngeal muscles

Stimulability

Therapeutic probes during initial perceptual evaluation (eg, forward placement with fronted vowels on ascending pitch glides, vocal

Name/ID :   Date: Time:

Evaluation of Ability to Voice Easily (EAVE) Score Sheet (version 1)

Please answer this in relation to your **speaking** voice and how you perceive your voice to be right **now**.

Today…..	Not at all	Mildly	Moderately	Extremely	Score	
1. My voice feels dry/scratchy	1	2	3	4	2	
2. My voice is husky	1	2	3	4	2	
3. I can project my voice*	4	3	2	1	2	
4. I can access the range of my voice easily *	4	3	2	1	3	
5. I am concerned about my voice	1	2	3	4		4
6. It takes effort to use my voice	1	2	3	4	2	
7. I feel good about using my voice	4	3	2	1	3	
8. My voice feels strained	1	2	3	4	2	
9. My voice feels strong*	4	3	2	1	2	
10. My voice is cutting out on some sounds	1	2	3	4	3	
11. My voice feels ready for work if it was required*	4	3	2	1	2	
12. I am worried about my voice	1	2	3	4		4
13. I am having difficulty speaking softly	1	2	3	4	3	
14. My voice is reliable*	4	3	2	1	3	
*reverse scored					29 /48	8 /8

Scoring instructions

Please note that the Total EAVE score does not include Voice Concern (VC) items 5 & 12 so report these as a separate score.

Maximum Total EAVE score = 48

Voice Concern (VC) items 5 & 12 = 8

© Phyland, D. (2020)

FIGURE 8–1. LF's completed EAVE.

Perceptual Voice Profile

Name: __LF__ Date: _____

Clinician: __DP__ U.R.: _____

	Pitch		Loudness			Quality										
Degree of Impairment	High	Low	Monotone	Loud	Soft	Monoloud	Breathy	Strained	Rough	Glottal Fry	Pitch Breaks	Phonation Breaks	Voice Arrests	Falsetto	Tremor	Diplophonia
Normal	X		X			X			X	X	X		X	X	X	X
Slight		X						X				X				
Mild				X			X									
Moderate																
Moderate Severe																
Severe																

From " A Sound Judgement " CD ROM © 1997 J.Oates & A.Russell

Please note Normal= an absence of the feature

FIGURE 8–2. LF's perceptual voice profile.

offloading with SOVT exercises) indicated high stimulability for change and improved voice quality. The perceptual quality showing the largest relative change was chosen to gauge the magnitude of improvement, with strain perceived to reduce by more than 80%, akin to the methodology proposed with the Vocal Plasticity Index.[42]

Laryngeal Imaging

Laryngeal videostroboscopy was performed transorally with a rigid videolaryngoscope as the client declined nasendoscopy. Findings included:

- Mildly hyperemic vocal folds and inter-arytenoid mucosa with frothy hypo-pharyngeal secretions and mucus stranding at anterior-mid third junctions of vocal folds
- Slight-mild asymmetric (right > left) but fully compressible edema localized to anterior-mid junctions of vocal folds

- Full mobility and symmetry of vocal fold abduction and adduction but with hyper-adduction on phonation onset
- Slightly incomplete glottal closure characterized by an hourglass pattern on high pitch with modal loudness
- Periodic and symmetric vibrations with mildly reduced mucosal waves and amplitudes bilaterally with a tendency toward a closed-phase predominance on low pitches

Summary of Findings and Recommendations

- Laryngeal imaging with videostroboscopy revealed mild generalized vocal fold inflammation, slight-mild focal edema at anterior-mid third junctions (right more than left but no discrete pathology diagnosed), and tendency toward hyperadduction on phonation.
- Laryngeal examination was consistent with the perceptual evaluation and client self-report of the physical aspects of vocal function with a good prognosis for favor-

able recovery and improved vocal efficiency for longevity.

- LF presented as highly motivated with a need for rapid turnaround of voice to avoid show cancellation.
- A formal Certificate of Capacity for Victorian Workcover purposes detailing voice activity restrictions was completed. (In Australia, this is a document completed by the treating medical practitioner that specifies a work-related injury/illness and details a person's capacity to work and any limitations to perform their regular work tasks.)

Diagnosis was specified as mild localized vocal fold edema and maladaptive laryngeal postures deemed as work related due to compounded phonotrauma and cumulative fatigue. The SLP prioritized voice therapy with subsequent collaboration with an on-site resident speech pathologist/voice consultant, a graduated return to normal performance schedule, and guidance on vocal health future-proofing for production season. She recommended a maximum of 1 show per day (6 shows in 1 week) followed by a return to full capacity, contingent on progress and under speech pathologist guidance. She also recommended minor lifestyle and diet modifications to mitigate any potential laryngopharyngeal reflux contributions.

Intervention

Overarching Goals

1. Restore LF's vocal health status to baseline
2. Help LF recognize the potential link between their current stress and vocal health and implement improved well-being and lifestyle measures
3. Empower LF to have full access to their vocal dynamics, strength, and ease of voice production so as to improve their global vocal performance[9] to meet their artistic expectations and that of the creative team

4. Enable LF to fully meet and sustain vocal performance demands for the entire production season of 8 shows per week with acceptable levels of fatigue and good recovery across performances
5. Establish regular vocal health practices including appropriate voice warm-up and cool-down routines tailored to LF's voice and specific performance demands

Session Voice Therapy Goals

1. Quickly and effectively resolve impairment symptoms (return to usual voice quality, pitch and loudness ranges, and stamina with minimal to no throat discomfort)
2. Decrease recruitment of extrinsic laryngeal muscles and increase subglottic control of airflow and supraglottic resonance for loud voicing (on and off stage) to minimize vocal fatigue
3. Identify aspects of their performance that may pose threats to their vocal longevity and ways to obviate these

"The Show Must Go On" Approach

In view of the expectation for LF to perform that night and the stimulability for immediate improvement in vocal quality, voice therapy was provided the same day as the assessment consultation. This session entailed informational and affective counselling (overarching goals #1, #2, and #5; session goal #3; explained in the Counseling section), as well as dynamic physiologic-orientated voice therapy techniques to directly modify voice production and improve interoception with fast transfer and generalization to the performance context (overarching goals #1, #4, and #5; session goals #1-#3; explained under Direct Voice Therapy below).

Counseling

The initial part of the session involved contextual discussion of the proposed role of a heavy vocal load and cumulative fatigue leading to maladaptive voicing patterns and likely phonotrauma-induced mild vocal fold tissue change. The clinician reassured LF that their voice symptoms were reversible based on the examination findings, variability of the symptom severity, and good immediate stimulability for change, so as to *decatastrophize*[36] the voice concerns (overarching goal #2) and align therapy goals. In addition, the SLP explored current vocal health practices and recommended ways to improve or better adhere to vocal health (overarching goals #1 and #4). Examples of these measures include increasing the time between eating before shows, and/or after shows and at bedtime, to mitigate any reflux effects; addressing the manner, timing, and usefulness of vocal warm-up and cool-down exercises; managing the vocal load outside of the performance context; avoiding self-medicating with prednisone; and managing stress and anxiety.

Direct Voice Therapy

The clinician subsequently provided a series of targeted voice exercises to reduce phonatory effort and hyperfunctional laryngeal behaviors, reduce hyperadducted vocal fold closure, increase supraglottic resonance, potentially reduce vocal fold edema and inflammation, and assist in vocal fold tissue recovery. Specifically, these comprised SOVT exercises including straw phonation, lip trills, raspberries and tongue trills, forward buzzy "woos," kazoos, and phonating /v/, /z/, and /dʒ/. (See Video 4 Labio-Lingual Trills [Raspberries] by Murphy Estes.)

These impedance tasks were produced over 5 to 10 minutes starting with (1) sustained sounds (at least 5 seconds) then progressing to (2) continuous gentle pulsing of loudness and (3) pitch glides. Modification of the sound production was cued where needed, focusing on initiation and maintenance of sound at the place of semi-occlusion/articulator, kinesthetic awareness of forward oral sensations, relative lack of involvement of extrinsic laryngeal muscles and the resultant ease of production, and improvement and continuity in voice quality. LF needed encouragement to let go of the "heaviness" and to maintain a resonant and flexible sound across all SOVT variants. Pitch and loudness were gradually extended for each exercise as LF created the target sound consciously and consistently. At the end of 7 minutes or so, LF remarked they felt as if they had "divorced their throat" and "had more space in their throat." They also perceived a reduction in strain and breathiness of vocal quality in connected speech. Using an adaptation of the Accent Method by Smith,[43] LF then the rhythmically accentuated the same voiced fricatives (/v/, /z/, /dʒ/) and forward vowels (/u/, /i/) by creating pitch and loudness changes with variations in subglottic airflow (Table 8–3). (See Video 25 Modified Accent Method by Phyland.)

The SLP highlighted the importance and ease of achieving these accents and changes primarily with thoracic and abdominal muscles and with minimal laryngeal effort, and continued the concept of maintaining the focus of forward oral resonance. In addition, while LF was focusing on respiratory/phonatory coordination, the SLP instructed them to eliminate audible inhalations and hard glottal attacks on initial vowel words and again focus on reduced laryngeal hyperfunction. (See Video 17 Contrasting Glottic Onset Types by Bond.) These exercises were then transferred into nasals and connected speech over a 5-minute period as LF mastered continuity and good vocal quality throughout. The SLP also briefly explored subglottic resonance via kinesthetic awareness of chest vibrations with the patient, with good effect. By the end of this period, LF was speaking with normal voice quality, pitch, and loudness, and they informed the clinician that their voice seemed back to normal.

The same voice production concepts were then trialed with LF speaking in their character voice, using various lines and contexts from the show. As soon as they commenced the Yorkshire accent, LF initially regressed to a more pressed, strained phonation type but

Table 8–3. Hierarchy of Sounds Using an Adaptation of the Accent Method (Kotby & Fex, 1998)

1. Production of sustained voiceless fricatives /s/, /ʃ/, /θ/ to promote awareness of abdominal/diaphragmatic involvement in the expiratory phase for speech

2. Sustained voiceless fricatives are then accentuated across varying rhythms and tempos. The clinician models the fricative, starting with an initial short soft segment, followed by an accentuated longer and stronger segment (with simultaneous light clapping or finger clicking), and client alternates in response with the sound in the same rhythm.

3. Voiced fricatives are then introduced in the same fashion with focus on airflow and continuous and effortless voicing on playful and increasingly faster rhythmic patterns.

4. Once these are consistently well produced with minimal strain and balanced airflow on phonation, vowels are introduced. Typically, these are performed with exaggerated breathiness and low modal volume to decrease laryngeal hyperfunction then gradually energized in intensity and resonance with clinician-client alternating rhythms in same fashion as the fricatives.

5. Other articulatory combinations are gradually introduced using the same accentuated method and transitioning to connected speech.

quickly self-corrected and was able to implement the same previous strategies to achieve good quality and balanced resonance.

LF then identified and demonstrated challenging parts of the show that required heightened emotion, shouting or speaking simultaneously with high physical demands (such as climbing a ladder). For each of these scenarios, LF achieved improved voicing efficiency with increased subglottic control of airflow for phonation, decreased laryngeal hyperfunction, and optimized resonance. At all times, care was taken not to alter the essence of line delivery, character, or dramatization, but to focus only on improving the voice aspects.

By the end of the 50-minute session, LF informally reported they felt more confident to perform that night with greater vocal flexibility and reliability. The speech pathologist noted perceptually that the vocal quality and continuity were essentially normal, there were no longer any audible inhalations, there were minimal episodes of hard glottal attacks on vowel-initial words, and there was demonstrable mastery and integration of principles of efficient voice production. LF repeated the adapted PPE[39] and EAVE[40] and rated themselves as 2/10 (2 points less than pre-therapy) for degree of phonatory effort in connected speech, and scored 19/28 (10 less) on the total EAVE and 4/8 on vocal concern (4 less).

Two days following the initial session, the company manager contacted the speech pathologist to inform her that, although LF had done their best performance ever the prior night, they had arranged a cover to do 1 of the 2 shows the next day, as recommended, so as to ensure LF did not overload their voice.

Session #2, Five Days Following the Initial Session

LF was seen for speech pathology follow-up 5 days later and reported their voice had returned to baseline status and that they were managing well vocally with their role with shorter recovery times between performances. In this session, the speech pathologist reviewed the exercises and recorded the SOVT sounds they produced best to be used as "vocal resets" and for recovery from vocal fatigue, if required. Specifically, LF's production of voiced lip trills, sustained "woo" and /v/ were perceived by the clinician and LF to create the best optimal resonance with the least laryngeal hyperfunction and by LF to "seem to keep my sound in a good place for the longest." LF was encouraged to use these sounds regularly as primers for 2- to 5-minute bursts to provide so-called "vocal unloading" (particularly by decreasing extrinsic laryngeal muscle recruitment) and vocal fold "massage" to achieve an optimal laryngeal posture for voicing. In addition, the importance of adopting a preventative approach to mitigate and reverse cumulative vocal fatigue was emphasized and strategies to facilitate this discussed. This included the early identification of key signs of fatigue, avoidance of under-recovery, and the implementation of extracurricular voice conservation measures, when needed.

LF was therefore discharged from the clinic, as no further intervention was deemed necessary, but they were encouraged to return if this situation changed. The Voice Clinic team subsequently purchased tickets to the show and enjoyed the performance immensely.

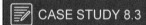

CASE STUDY 8.3

Myofascial Release for an Adult Touring Musical Theater Performer With Vocal Fatigue

Wendy LeBorgne

Voice Evaluation

Case History

Chief Complaints. Dysphonia and vocal fatigue. This patient self-referred to the voice center for evaluation of dysphonia following several weeks of vocal fatigue while performing 8 physically and vocally demanding shows per week.

History of Voice Complaint. Patient LM, a 31-year-old cisgender female, was a performer in town during a national Broadway tour and had been experiencing vocal fatigue following performances for several weeks. She found difficulty in maintaining "clarity" in her upper range and reported her singing voice was quite fatigued after a show. Additionally, she reported difficulty traversing her passaggio, but she did not believe that it was audible to her audience. She also reported a general tiredness in her voice after shows and a lack of desire to sing or speak. She had not perceived a change in the quality of her speaking voice. Upon further inquiry, she reported that as her vocal fatigue had increased, she noticed throat pain, neck and jaw discomfort, upper back tightness, and changes in her breathing patterns, resulting in near-panic attacks. Her costume consisted of a tight corset and restricted her normal breathing patterns. On the day of examination, a complete voice evaluation was conducted, including laryngeal videostroboscopy and laryngeal function testing, including aerodynamic and acoustic measures.

Because Patient LM traveled to a new city every 3 to 4 weeks, she was unable to see her regular otolaryngologist for this problem. However, she routinely saw her New York City-based otolaryngologist for annual vocal wellness visits and management of seasonal allergies. A thorough history was taken, and the videostroboscopic examination was reviewed by a local otolaryngologist and forwarded to her New York City-based ENT. Her case history revealed that 3 weeks prior to arrival in town, she had developed a mild upper respiratory infection, which was treated with 10 days of antibiotics as well as an albuterol inhaler. She reported that she continued to sing during the infection, although she was coughing significantly at the time. She reported that her cough subsided within 4 days of being placed on the antibiotics but that her voice had not felt "quite right" since that time.

Voice Use. Patient LM had a leading role in the touring show and performed that role 8 times per week. Her typical day included waking up around 11 AM, going to rehearsal from noon until 2 PM, relaxing or napping in the afternoon, and reporting back to the theater by 6 PM. Following the show, she typically went out to dinner with friends and returned to her hotel by 2 AM. The typical length of the show was approximately 2.5 hours. She had been performing professionally for 13 years and had rarely missed a performance due to illness or vocal problems. This was her sixth national tour of a Broadway show. With her last tour, she reported some cervical spine pain, which required several months of physical therapy following completion of the tour. She reported these issues to stem from costuming, microphone placement, and her wigs.

Patient LM was in excellent physical shape and had approximately 17 years of formal voice training and coaching. Early in her career, she reported having vocal fold nodules, which resolved with rest, therapy, and continued vocal training. She was concerned that the nodules may have recurred with the recent harsh coughing. She was a nonsmoker but was often exposed to passive smoke in restaurants and bars, and she also had to perform several scenes with fog on the stage. She had no complaints of gastroesophageal reflux (GERD) or dysphagia.

Current medications included Zoloft for treatment of mild depression and Allegra for seasonal allergies. Patient LM was well versed in vocal hygiene and was extremely compliant. She consistently drank 8 to 10 glasses of water per day and only 1 cup of coffee. She traveled with a steamer, which she kept backstage in her dressing room and used daily. Although she reported being a "vocally enthusiastic" person, she attempted to use her voice conservatively on days of shows and in noisy environments.

She was married, and her husband was living in New York, with the rest of her close friends scattered across the country. She engaged in daily FaceTime conversation with her spouse and friends but had decreased this recently due to her voice.

Laryngeal Imaging

Under direct light, this patient presented with grossly normal-appearing true vocal folds bilaterally. Some mild vascularity was noted on the superior surface of the vocal folds, but the medial edges appeared smooth and straight bilaterally. While sustaining the vowel /i/, stroboscopic lighting was employed, and it was observed that she presented with a small anterior glottal gap, which was present at all pitches tested. The amplitude of vibration and mucosal wave appeared mildly decreased bilaterally, but the overall system was quite flexible. The open phase of the vibratory cycle was slightly dominant, whereas the symmetry of vibration was irregular at low pitches only. No mass lesions, paralysis, or paresis were noted.

Auditory-Perceptual Evaluation

Perceptually, the patient rated her own voice as mildly dysphonic with increased vocal effort. She reported that she did not feel like she could take an unrestricted breath and that her neck felt tight. The voice therapist observed mild dysphonia characterized by roughness, breathiness, and increased vocal strain. The CAPE-V[15] was administered and the patient was determined to have an overall CAPE-V score of 17/100, indicating a dysphonia of a mild nature. Pitch of the voice was within normal limits for age and gender. Resonance was focused in the laryngeal region, with occasional denasal resonance noted. Physically, she presented with an asymmetrical stance with right shoulder elevation and forward head position. Her respiratory patterns were inconsistent, ranging from appropriate diaphragmatic breathing to shallow and clavicular with sighing.

382 Voice Therapy: Clinical Case Studies

Manual Palpation

Upon palpation of the larynx, this patient had significant tenderness with light touch in the thyrohyoid space, and the entire larynx was noted to rest in an elevated position with base of tongue tension.

Acoustic and Aerodynamic Analysis

The CAPE-V and the Rainbow Passage were recorded in a normal conversational voice. Her attempt at this task revealed a mean fundamental speaking frequency of 181.3 Hz (SD 21.3) on the CAPE-V and 185.3 Hz (SD 13.6) on the Rainbow Passage. She was asked to describe her voice problem, and her response was recorded and analyzed as conversational speech and revealed a mean fundamental frequency of 186.9 Hz and a standard deviation of 16.4 Hz. Both reading and conversational samples of speech were considered to be within normal limits.

The patient was asked to glide to her highest and lowest pitches in 2 separate attempts to attain her physiologic frequency range. She peaked at a frequency of 1244 Hz, and

her lowest tone was measured at 164 Hz. No audible pitch breaks were noted in her voice. She maintained an adequate range for her age and voice type (Table 8–4).

Patient LM had excellent dynamic control of her voice, with the exceptions of the extremes of her range and the passaggio into her head voice (at about 698.5 Hz). At that point, she was only able to achieve a dynamic difference of 18 dB. Unfortunately, the solos that she sang in the show were in that general area of her voice difficulty.

Following acoustic assessment, this patient completed aerodynamic tasks of vital capacity, mean airflow rates at maximum and comfortable sustained phonation, and voicing efficiency using the Phonatory Aerodynamic System (PAS) (Table 8–5).

Impressions

The clinician determined that Patient LM was experiencing vocal difficulties consistent with a mild laryngeal myasthenia, which most likely resulted from singing during an upper respiratory infection and severe coughing. At the

Table 8–4. Pretreatment Voice Range Profile for Patient LM

Semitone	Hertz	Minimum dB	Maximum dB
40	164.8	59	76
43.5	207.6	60	86
47	246.9	57	91
50.5	311.1	58	91
54	370	58	93
57.5	466.2	65	98
61	554.4	67	102
64.5	698.5	82	100
68	830.6	74	111
71.5	1046.5	77	113
75	1244.5	81	105

8. Performance Voice 383

Table 8–5. Pretreatment Aerodynamic Analysis for Patient LM

Frequency (Hz)	Flow Volume (mL)	Flow Rate (mL/s)	MPT
185	3220	102	33.3
165	3430	160	21.5
500	3370	102	33.1

time of the evaluation, the upper respiratory infection and the coughing had resolved completely, and the clinician advised this patient to enroll in a formal voice therapy program.

> *Laryngeal myasthenia* has been used as a clinical descriptor for laryngeal muscle weakness and imbalance, typically in reference to a clinical presentation that warrants rebalancing the voice after injury or surgery. This term is not to be confused with *myasthenia gravis*, a chronic neuromuscular disease.

Plan of Care

Long-Term Goal. The patient will eliminate vocal fatigue and remain free from laryngeal discomfort in the context of her occupational demands and social activities during continuous voice use for up to 2 hours.

Short-Term Goals:

1. The patient will report reduced laryngeal pain/discomfort by 85% following myofascial release (MFR).
2. The patient will complete Vocal Function Exercises (VFEs) 2 times per day, 7 days per week, with attention to optimal exercise technique with 90% accuracy and minimal verbal, tactile, or visual cues.
3. The patient will complete RVT at a conversational level with 90% accuracy and minimal verbal, tactile, or visual cues.

Decision Making

Based on the above information, the clinician determined this patient would benefit from a direct voice therapy program to rehabilitate her voice and return to meeting her daily functional communication needs.

Intervention

Over the course of 2 weeks (the length of time the patient was in town), 3 voice therapy sessions were completed, each approximately 50 to 55 minutes in length. Each session included MFR, VFEs, and RVT. The first session was approximately 15 minutes of MFR, 25 minutes of VFEs, and 20 minutes of RVT. The subsequent sessions resulted in 10 minutes of MFR and 15 to 20 minutes each on VFEs and RVT.

The voice therapy program included VFEs, designed to condition and balance the laryngeal musculature,[44,45] and modified RVT, designed to promote a frontal, oral, open focus during conversational speech, in conjunction with MFR to alleviate fascial restrictions, reduce fascial pain, and improve respiratory patterns.[46–49] Additionally, technical/physical reintegration into performance and coordination with stage management on costuming and amplification were implemented. Challenges included the short duration that the patient was in town, which did not allow for adequate treatment time, and the ongoing issues caused by her costume restrictions, which were not going to be altered by the production team.

Myofascial Release

Short-Term Goal #1. *The patient will report reduced laryngeal pain/discomfort by 85% following myofascial release (MFR).*

Due to the significant hyperfunctional voice patterns, laryngeal elevation, and inappropriate respiratory patterns, the initial therapy session consisted of 30 minutes of MFR followed by 30 minutes total of VFEs and RVT.

The patient was placed in a supine position and therapy began with assessment of fascial restrictions. Manual therapy of the larynx may include laryngeal massage, laryngeal reposturing, and/or MFR, which are all considered independent modalities and may be utilized differently. It is important to note that as of this writing, speech pathologists may consider manual laryngeal techniques as a part of (not exclusively) the entire voice therapy session because SLPs may not bill for manual therapy alone. Also, as manual therapy training is not a typical part of education for speech pathologists, it is important to note that the clinician treating this patient has had over 40 hours of additional training, resulting in Level I Certification of MFR.

> LeBorgne points out that MFR or other manual therapies are tools to be used as part of the entire treatment plan and not a single modality to use during an entire voice therapy session. She also discusses that use of these modalities is not typically taught in graduate training for SLPs, so additional training is needed for responsible implementation.

The most significant fascial restrictions were noted in the sternal/rib cage area, between her scapula, bilateral shoulders (right > left), bilateral jaw, and extrinsic laryngeal muscles. Full discussion of MFR techniques is beyond the scope of this chapter; however, references are provided for further reading at the conclusion of this case study. MFR began with an occipital condyle release. The clinician's hands were placed lightly under the patient's head, touching the base of the occipital bone (Figure 8–3). This was held for 60 to 90 seconds to allow for release. This patient was noted to have fascial restriction and contraction with each inspiration for the first several minutes, indicating patterning of pulling the base of the skull and "setting" her body with each breath. It is not uncommon during MFR work to note changes in breathing patterns. Within the first session, this patient's respiratory patterns changed from high/clavicular to broad-based, low, full, diaphragmatic patterns. Following the occipital-condyle release, a bilateral jaw release was accomplished. MFR continued to further address restrictions in the

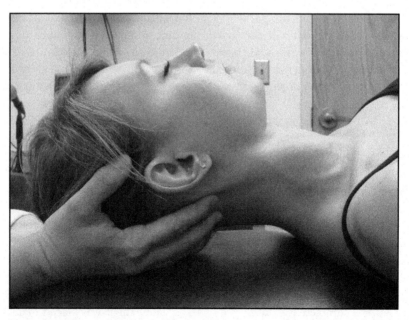

FIGURE 8–3. Myofascial release (MFR): occipital-condyle release.

infrahyoid (Figure 8–4) and thoracic regions (Figure 8–5). (See Video 26 Myofascial Release by LeBorgne.)

Immediately upon completion of MFR, this patient reported improved breathing ("as if she could finally take a deep breath") as well as improved vocal resonance and ease of production.

Following MFR, Patient LM was introduced to both VFEs and RVT. Patient LM was

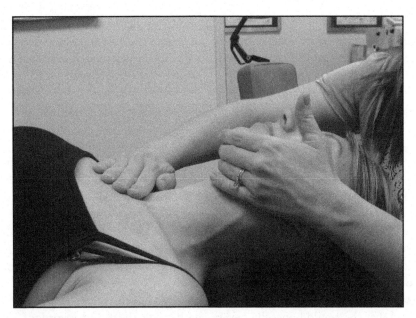

FIGURE 8–4. Myofascial release (MFR): infrahyoid release.

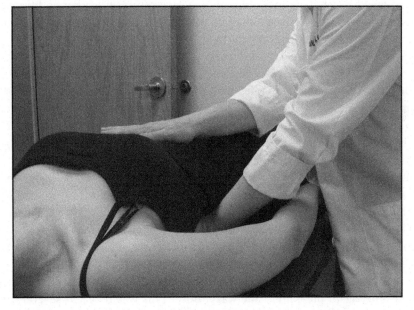

FIGURE 8–5. Myofascial release (MFR): thoracic region.

386 Voice Therapy: Clinical Case Studies

also counseled regarding vocal hygiene and the importance of recognizing when she needed to take a day off from singing during times of infections. Because of her skill as a singer, she easily assimilated proper technique for both exercise programs.

Vocal Function Exercises

Short-Term Goal #2. *The patient will complete VFEs 2 times per day, 7 days per week, with attention to optimal exercise technique with 90% accuracy and minimal verbal, tactile, or visual cues.*

The VFE program used for this singer included the musical notes C through G. In the first portion of the exercise program (warm-up), the clinician asked her to sustain the vowel /i/ on the musical note F for as long as possible. Special attention was drawn to the fact that the /i/ sound was to be produced in a nasal, overly forward-placed tone. Patient LM expressed concern that this was not the way she would sing an /i/ vowel. The clinician explained to her that these were not "singing exercises" and that she would hopefully never sing with the amount of nasality required for this exercise. The second part of the exercise program, designed to stretch the vocal folds to maximal length, was to have Patient LM glide from her lowest pitch to her highest pitch on the word "knoll" using an extremely forward focus. Her first attempt at this exercise resulted in a beautiful glide to her highest note, and then she started to glide back down again. This is a common mistake seen in many singers because it is similar to a vocalise often called the "siren," in which one glides from the lowest note to the highest note and back down again in one breath. The importance of stretching only to her highest note and then stopping was impressed on Patient LM. The SLP also reminded her to use proper abdominal breathing through all exercises. Step 3 of the exercise program was to glide from her highest note to her lowest note, again on "knoll." She was extremely proficient at this but needed a word

of caution not to initiate the tone with a hard glottal attack or go into glottal fry phonation at her lowest notes. Finally, the clinician taught her the exercises designed to build adductory efficiency and stamina of the intrinsic laryngeal musculature. These consisted of the patient sustaining the musical notes C, D, E, F, and G, on the word "old" without the /d/, for as long as possible and as softly as possible, but with an engaged tone. Special care was taken to ensure Patient LM began with a coup de glotte phonation, meaning that she initiated the phonation at the precise moment the vocal folds adducted and that the resonators were perfectly tuned to the vowel. It is important to be extremely precise with singers' onset of phonation and not allow them to cheat themselves on a less-than-optimal onset. The clinician made several attempts with this patient to ensure precise onset of the tone and breath. LM was an extremely astute patient and performed the exercises with accuracy after minimal instruction. VFEs were to be completed 2 times per day—no less, no more. The SLP provided her with a log sheet and recorded MP3s of the exercises to keep track of her phonation times on the exercises and asked her to bring it back to each return visit. (For additional information on VFEs, see Case Study 3.6 by Stemple.)

Resonant Voice Therapy

Short-Term Goal #3. *The patient will complete RVT at a conversational level with 90% accuracy level and minimal verbal, tactile, or visual cues.*

A modified regimen of RVT was employed with this patient as she progressed through the steps quickly. As with most singers, this patient had an excellent sense of vocal tract resonance. The first step of RVT was to have her hum on a comfortable pitch in her speech range using /molm-molm-molm/. The clinician asked her to note where she sensed vibrations while phonating. LM reported a general sense of "buzzing" in her cheeks and nose. This was repeated several times. Next, the SLP asked the patient to maintain this "buzz" while chanting, then doing a messa di voce (slow-soft, gradually increasing to loud-fast, and then gradually decreasing back to slow-soft), then overinflecting voiced syllables.

She was extremely proficient at this, and therapy continued into chanted sentences. Sentences used included frontal consonants and all-voiced phrases (eg, "No one knew Nanny," "My mom made money," "Now Nan knew Nelly," "One Monday morning"). The sentences were used to promote a frontal, oral, open focus during connected speech. The SLP asked the patient to first chant the sentences with a nasal, forward tone, then to overinflect them with the same tone, and then to speak them in a normal voice while maintaining the forward (not nasal) resonance. Minimal cues were required when performing this stage of RVT. LM reported that her voice "felt good" when doing RVT. She was advised to do these exercises at least twice a day.

During the second session, she was able to progress with the next stage of RVT, which entailed warming up with the initial steps of

RVT introduced in the first session and then moving to a list of voiced-voiceless syllables and then sentences. These were performed in the same fashion as the voiced exercises, over-inflected. The only difficulty that Patient LM had was during the speaking portion of the sentence level. She had the tendency to drop her voice at the last syllable into a glottal fry phonation pattern. When cued, she was able to immediately correct it. Patient LM found RVT easy to do on her afternoon break and was able to do the exercises 3 times daily.

Finally, during the third session, the patient was proficient enough in the RVT exercises that paragraph reading was added. The same principles of maintaining a frontal, oral, open focus were applied at this level. By this time, however, Patient LM was well aware of any glottal fry phonation and essentially was able to eliminate it from all reading and conversational speech. These strategies were applied to her lines and song text for daily practice.

Because of the limited amount of time she was in town, the patient was seen 2 times per

Table 8–6. Posttreatment Voice Range Profile for Patient LM

Semitone	Hertz	Minimum dB	Maximum dB
40	164.8	58	76
43.5	207.6	57	85
47	246.9	58	93
50.5	311.1	58	92
54	370	58	95
57.5	466.2	62	98
61	554.4	67	101
64.5	698.5	69	104
68	830.6	71	113
71.5	1046.5	77	112
75	1244.5	79	105

Table 8–7. Posttreatment Aerodynamic Analysis for Patient LM

Frequency (Hz)	Flow Volume (mL)	Flow Rate (mL/s)	MPT
185	3360	100	33.7
165	3410	103	33.3
500	3380	101	33.4

week for the 2 weeks that remained of her stay. She was extremely compliant with all recommendations, and rapid progression was noted with therapy. Her VFE maximum phonation time (MPT) improved from an average of 22.4 seconds at the initiation of therapy to an average of 35.2 seconds by the fourth therapy session. She particularly enjoyed doing RVT and found that her voice was "lighter and easier" after only a few days of doing it.

Therapy Results

At the end of the 2-week period of therapy, Patient LM felt her voice was markedly improved but opted to continue doing both VFEs and RVT. Posttherapy voice range profile and aerodynamic results may be seen in Tables 8–6 and 8–7, respectively. Note the marked improvement in her airflow rates at low pitches, as well as an increase in dynamic range at the 698.5-Hz frequency. A follow-up stroboscopic evaluation also was done, and it revealed only a small posterior glottic gap. No anterior glottic chink was present at any pitch on stroboscopic evaluation.

Summary and Concluding Remarks

Patient LM received word that, following the closing of this Broadway tour, she would begin rehearsing for the New York premiere of a new Broadway musical in a supporting role. Although we could not spend the ideal amount of time in therapy with her, she had such a strong underlying vocal mechanism that it only took minimal guidance to see dramatic improvement.

Suggested Readings Include:

- *The Myofascial Release Manual*[50]
- *Myofascial Release: The Search for Excellence—A Comprehensive Evaluatory and Treatment Approach*[51]
- *Fascial Release for Structural Balance*[52]

 CASE STUDY 8.4

Voice Recalibration With the Cup Bubble Technique for an Adult Country Singer With Chronic Phonotrauma

Jenny C. Muckala

Voice Evaluation

History of Voice Complaint

A 43-year-old professional male country singer first presented complaining of 1 year of chronic dysphonia, which had been worsening for 3 years. He had lost portions of his high range, singing was effortful, there was qualitative decline with limited use, and his speaking quality was fluctuating. He had been using Prevacid, a proton pump inhibitor (PPI), for 3 years with limited improvement in voice quality or other reported symptoms. A 3-week course of prednisone did not yield any improvement in voice quality or range. He was a baritone and lead vocalist in a country trio; however, he frequently sang in the tenor range for most of his performances. He sang 200 shows in the past year. He had no formal voice training and no regular voice warm-up regimen but was able to use his voice in a way he was pleased with. He reliably drank 4 glasses of water per day (32 oz/day) and 2 caffeinated sodas. He did not use tobacco, alcohol, or illicit drugs.

Perceptually, his voice was moderately dysphonic, characterized by consistent roughness, reduced habitual speaking pitch, consistent strain, and inconsistent glottal fry. He was unconcerned with the quality of his speaking voice. His singing voice limitations were his primary focus. Videoendoscopy with stroboscopy revealed vocal fold mobility within normal limits (WNL) and varices with erythema and irregular medial edges the length of the membranous vocal folds. Stroboscopic parameters were present but mucosal wave and amplitude were reduced bilaterally at modal pitch. He had complete closure pattern with a small posterior gap at modal pitch.

The laryngologist diagnosed him with dysphonia, chronic laryngitis, bilateral true vocal fold ectasias, and GERD, and referred him to the speech pathology team for speaking and singing voice rehabilitation to reduce mechanical trauma of sustained voice production and reduce risk for further vocal injury. He did not return and was lost to follow-up.

Three years later, this patient returned because there was no longer a way to work around his voice limitations. He had performed more than 250 shows that year. His voice was "passable" in quality and range at the beginning of each week, but never "normal," and declined with even limited use. He had difficulty speaking in competing noise, even with voice rest. He had tried addressing these issues with a vocal coach, implementing a myriad of vocal warm-ups including lip trills, tongue trills, "tongue forward" exercises (patient's words) without noticeable improvement, and "moving his belly when he breathes," which he found difficult to execute. Nothing helped.

Laryngeal Imaging

Following repeat stroboscopy, the laryngologist diagnosed the patient with a right true vocal fold (TVF) polyp with left TVF reactive changes, as well as persistent bilateral TVF ectasias. These benign vocal fold lesions are impact injuries, consistent with persistent and consistent loud voice use in a variety of contexts. Indirect and direct voice rehabilitation

addressing his speaking and singing voice use were strongly recommended, as before.

Auditory-Perceptual Assessment

Perceptually, the patient's voice was moderately dysphonic, characterized by consistent roughness, strain, and breathiness at the conversational level. His habitual respiratory pattern was primarily chest/clavicular elevation on inspiration, and the clinician observed pressured voicing because of breath holding during exhalation.

Acoustic Measures

The patient's MPT was only 6 seconds, severely limited for professional use, where the average expected is 25 to 32 seconds for males. His voice range was severely limited from 92 to 220 Hz, as his former range extended to 493 Hz for many of the songs in his set. His habitual speaking pitch was 92 Hz.

Manual Palpation

Gentle palpation revealed a reduced thyroid hyoid space and tenderness at a pain level of 6 (1 = "no pain," 10 = "severe pain"). There was visible recruitment of his anterior neck musculature with anterior chin extension, as well as a consistently elevated shoulder posture during all voice production.

Quality-of-Life Impairment

The patient's Voice Handicap Index (VHI) total score was 49 (Physical = 19; Functional = 12; Emotional = 16).[53] This outcome indicated a moderate degree of self-perceived voice handicap. He self-rated his voice limitation as severe. The VHI proved to be a helpful tool in monitoring patient perception of change from session to session.

Plan and Decision Making

Treatment goals were directed by current voice quality, observations of body stance and movement, and his stimulability for voice change.[54] The patient's phonotrauma was multivariate, and therefore the intervention would need to have a tiered approach to have a broad-spectrum effect and change in the patient's status. The patient was treated by a speech pathologist specializing in singing voice disorders. Adequate patient education, gauging the patient's readiness for change, frequent follow-up, and consistent communication between the speech pathologist and physician were all high-level priorities.[55] Of equal relevance were the patient-related factors that could have affected the success of intervention such as readiness for change, compliance with therapeutic recommendations, stimulability for target behaviors and voice change, and emotional and physical condition.[56]

Therapy attendance and compliance with recommendations were a challenge from the onset. The patient toured heavily, had heavy speaking voice demands on a daily basis, often in competing noise, and was unwilling to cancel performances. His family was entirely reliant on income from his touring. He also reported significant anxiety associated with his inability to meet the speaking and singing demands of his touring trio. The speech pathologist and the physician therefore worked closely to coordinate care that accommodated his heavy touring schedule. He got less than 6 hours of sleep nightly and had a reported low tolerance for this fatigue physically, but also experienced negative effects on cognition and psychomotor tasks consistent with research on fatigue.[57,58] He was easily overwhelmed with information, was difficult to physically get into therapy, and continuously reiterated his high stress, fatigue, and anxiety associated with his voice disorder.

Intervention

The patient had poor self-care habits that contributed to poor vocal hygiene, poor voice conservation, and low self-awareness of his body and movement. Therefore, the focus of his initial treatment session was vocal hygiene and voice conservation, with an introduction to efficiency in phonation using a SOVT facili-

tator. This was intended to establish contrast between the dysphonia and strain of his habitual voice use, with the ease of a balanced phonation using the cup bubble facilitator. Each treatment session was recorded on the patient's smartphone to assist in home replication of treatment targets and better generalization of gains.[59]

Acute vocal fold injury may be addressed through varied levels of voice rest, ranging from moderated use throughout the day to strict observance of silence, depending on the injury.[60] His recommended reduction in use was combined with clearly defined parameters for improving vocal hygiene, as vocal hygiene alone would not have yielded as dramatic of a result.[61] Vocal hygiene recommendations were to (1) hydrate adequately with approximately 2 liters of water daily since hydration and phonatory effort are inversely related,[62] (2) use topical hydration twice daily (steam his voice), (3) use a cool mist humidifier over his side of the bed at night, and (4) manage reflux through consistent and appropriate use of his PPI. Voice conservation recommendations were to (1) avoid speaking in competing noise, (2) implement a "60/10 rule" (where he would be silent for 10 consecutive minutes each hour), (3) stay within touching distance of his listeners at home and on the road, and (4) stop using the Bluetooth speaker in the car to eliminate his "cell yell" habit.

> "Cell yell" is a colloquial term used to describe the automatic increase in vocal intensity displayed by many people when talking on the phone, especially on speakerphone. The phenomenon is likely due in large part to the Lombard effect and a subconscious perception of distance from the communication partner, paired with a desire to ensure communication clarity. Ambient noise in a moving car is quite high, which contributes to the Lombard effect. Sustained high vocal intensity increases a person's overall vocal dose and can put them at greater risk for phonotrauma.

The Semi-Occluded Vocal Tract Facilitator

This patient's low self-awareness, lack of voice training, and high level of stress necessitated a concrete, simple treatment approach to create a higher likelihood of success. Subglottal air pressure and adductory forces are much greater in nonclassical, untrained singing typical of the country singing that this patient engaged in,[63] and therefore the potential for phonotrauma and strain during rigorous voice use was much greater. Trained classical singers create a louder sound with less subglottal air pressure than untrained singers.[63]

The goal in using an SOVT facilitator was to improve vocal economy in phonation with less mechanical trauma to the tissue.[1] The cup bubble facilitator provided a visual and auditory confirmation of the continuity of airflow during phonation, with low resistance from the water. Referentially, it was easy for him to use his voice with a bubble, which was gratifying and resulted in an immediate shift in tonal quality and provided a contrasting manner for voicing. The evidence of airflow movement was externalized, which was important for someone with low self-awareness. This tool was a redirection from what he *heard* to what he *felt* during phonation. He was supported with consistent sensory feedback to improve long-term compliance with recommendations and adherence.

He was cued to maintain spinal alignment with a neutral head position. Since country singing has been demonstrated to be most similar in respiratory support to speaking voice use,[64] little treatment focus was on breath intake to vital capacity. Instead, he was encouraged to breathe "with his ribs" on inspiration, starting with a relaxed abdomen, which would allow his rib cage to expand laterally, anteriorly, and posteriorly. All breathing involves the diaphragm (and is therefore diaphragmatic), *and* this allowance of rib cage expansion decreased rigidity in his respiratory system and provided novel, expanded awareness of his respiratory movement.

The clinician instructed him to touch his upper lip to the water but not to submerge it, inhale through his nose slowly, and start a bubble on exhale that was "as steady as a motorboat," not inconsistent rhythmically. (See Video 27 Cup Bubble Facilitator by Muckala.) The clinician modeled the target to provide the patient with an anchor for production. Targets were (1) continuous bubbles in the water during phonation, (2) clarity of tone also described to the patient as a "smooth" tone, and (3) no sensation of effort, tightness, or strain during phonation in the extrinsic or intrinsic muscles of the larynx and neck.

Self-awareness and self-monitoring tasks included reflection on the following 3 questions: How did it feel? How did it sound? Could you do that again? His perception of effort to produce sound was relative to his habitual production; initially only awareness of "difference" was salient and helpful as a reference. Contrasting qualitative improvement immediately from a rough, dysphonic production to a proportionally clearer, "smoother" tone was evident in more than 90% of productions with consistent subglottic airflow. Roughness was eliminated and a mild breathiness was present. This task was "easy for him" and not fatiguing; he generated more tone with less effort as his familiarity with this task and hierarchy increased.

A voiceless bubble at a consistent rate helped establish airflow rate and low effort prior to the addition of sound. It was a good referent for ease of phonation without strain, and he generated a steady, voiced bubble at a speaking voice pitch with immediate voice onset, tonal clarity that exceeded conversational speech, and no fatigue for a 5- to 6-second phonation window. This simple, repeatable task allowed the clinician to draw attention to the patient's slumped posture, anterior chin and neck posturing, and forward shoulder posture, which reduced his access to his vital capacity and a more efficient sound production.

Each repetition of the cup bubble exercise was a reiteration of success: tonal clarity and ease of phonation. There was no report of patient fatigue or deterioration in quality after 10 repetitions of this facilitator. This stimulability for immediate change in voice quality surprised the patient. The clinician and the patient discussed the need for motor memory, which could only be achieved through daily practice and consistency, for vocalization at greater vocal intensity with optimal efficiency and ease. Video recordings of the clinician modeling and the patient self-modeling of therapy tasks improved practice accuracy at home.

His next treatment session was 23 days later. His voice quality was worse, as he had continued the intensity of his touring schedule. He was unable to sing without his voice "cutting out" and he was severely dysphonic by the end of a 3-performance weekend. His VHI score was 89 that day. He reported vocal fatigue and strain with all levels of voice use, and significant fatigue and soreness in the strap muscle of his neck. He was visibly exhausted with a flat facial affect and was very verbal about how "he wasn't sure what he could do" to improve his voice. His right true vocal fold polyp had become hemorrhagic. His laryngologist and speech pathologist advised him to observe strict voice rest for 1 week based on stroboscopic findings.

Prognosis was only fair for a successful therapeutic outcome because of a long history of poor patient compliance with treatment recommendations; the complexity of his voice disorder; a high pressure, voice-dependent occupation; a high VHI score; and other complicating medical factors that have been demonstrated to be related to negative treatment outcomes.[55] Based on this data, he was at high risk for voice therapy dropout.[65] At this point, he was committed to "do whatever it took to get [his] voice back." He canceled all performances until further notice. Weekly treatment sessions functioned better to establish and maintain a higher level of accountability as well as to improve the patient's confidence in

his competence to effect change. He returned for his third treatment session 8 days later to assess his voice quality and compliance status and to discuss how to proceed with voice rehabilitation. The patient had strictly complied with voice rest, followed hydration recommendations, eliminated speaking in competing environments, and only spoke at a within-touching-distance volume. Voice quality was perceptually improved. Stroboscopic evaluation of his vocal folds revealed a decrease in erythema and a stable right true vocal fold lesion. He kept data daily on compliance with the 60/10 rule, hydration, and within-touching-distance volume, and brought all data back at his next appointment.

Ongoing complaints of fatigue, soreness in the strap muscles of his neck, and rapid deterioration in voice quality were used as the most salient references of inefficient production during reintroduction of the cup bubble as a recalibration exercise. After 10 iterations of the cup bubble in isolation, his voice was mildly breathy and mildly rough, but he had no complaints of strain during voice production. The patient produced 30 sustained cup bubbles at 110 Hz for 5 to 6 seconds each time and reported no fatigue, deterioration in voice quality, or sensation of effort during these 5 minutes of continuous use. Spontaneous speech was still characterized by a moderately severe roughness, mild breathiness, and strain during production with glottal fry at the ends of phrases. This was a helpful contrast for differences in voice function and assisted in increasing the patient's awareness of salient acoustic and sensory differences between the target production and his habitual, dysphonic production. His speaking pitch elevated from 92 to 110 Hz during the cup bubble, and he commented that this tone was "more pleasant" to listen to. High-frequency use of a low-impact voice facilitator with discrete therapy tasks yielded a voice with proportionately more clarity, consistency, and comfort during production without any change in ana-

Table 8–8. Cup Bubble Hierarchy

Cup Bubble Hierarchy Level		Target	Accuracy
Cup Bubble Alone		10 times	90%
• The regularity of the bubble sounds rhythmic, like a motorboat. The result is a clearer and more consistent tone held out to the end of a natural breath.			
• Make sure your upper lip meets the water and is not completely submerged. Use the water as a feedback tool.			
• Find the minimum amount of steady airflow necessary to initiate voicing with regularity, ideally calibrating to a lower level of effort in voice initiation and use.			
Cup Bubble + "ooo"		10 times	90%
• Hold this bubble for 2-3 seconds first for a clear and consistent tone with EASE, and then remove the cup, revealing the open vowel "ooo" for another 2-3 seconds.			
• There should be the same EASE of production during the "ooo."			
• For example: Bbbbbb + ooooooo			
Cup Bubble + "ooo" + Count		10 times	90%
• Bubble for 2-3 seconds again to get that smooth tone without effort. Recalibrate your effort level.			
• After consistent bubbling, remove the cup for the open vowel "ooo."			
• Coarticulate that vowel with a 1-word utterance you use frequently; vowel-initial words are easiest.			
• For example: Bbbbbb + oooooooo + ok (no break between ooo and word - all one sound)			
• For example: Bbbbbb + oooooooo + alright (no break between ooo and word—all one sound)			
Cup Bubble + "ooo" + Phrase For example:	**Phrase Level Hierarchy of Production**	3 times	90%
• What's for dinner?	**First time through** Long "ooooo" + phrase on monotone pitch		
• Where's the bathroom?			
• What did you want?			
• What time is it?	**Second time through** Long "ooooo" + phrase with intonation		
• What's the rush?			
• Where did you go?			
• What's your name?	**Third time through** Short "ooooo" + phrase with intonation		
• Why is it cold?			
• How are things?			
• Why did he go?			
• When do you close? Where is the car?			

tomical composition. Targets were simple enough for the patient to replicate accurately with minimal clinician assistance. Transfer of this calibrated tone to sustained phonation at each of the subsequent levels (sustained vowel, single word, and phrase length) yielded consistent tone clarity, ease of production, and no complaints of fatigue (Table 8–8). At home, the patient used MP4 recordings of himself from each session to meet his goals of increased patient awareness, independence, and transfer and to solidify and generalize gains.[59]

Patient compliance with recommendations for the next 3 sessions was exemplary. His countenance improved significantly and he reported that, despite the financial strain, this break from constant touring and performance had allowed him time to recuperate and reconnect with his family, which had all improved his overall quality of life. On his eighth session, his voice sounded *and* felt "the best it had been in ages." His VHI total score was 32, indicative of a mild rating of self-limitation. From his highest rating of 89, his overall improvement in VHI rating had been 53 points. An 18-point threshold shift is statistically significant.[53]

His vocal folds were visualized and the right TVF lesion had resorbed. Mucosal wave, vertical phase difference, and amplitude were all functionally efficient for sustained phonation. The patient wanted to return immediately to a full touring schedule. Since he had not been using his voice any more rigorously than at moderate intensities for speaking voice use for 1 month, detraining effects would risk returning to immediate performance-level rigor. It was recommended he complete 2 to 3 more therapy sessions to upregulate rigor of use and target his broader voice range. With better task specificity and dynamic, sustained voice use, he would be more likely to maintain his gains, further improve his fatigue resistance, and mitigate risk for reinjury.[64] The cup bubble hierarchy parlays well into resonant voice work. The patient agreed to this plan but never showed up for any of the subsequent sessions.

Once he became aware that his right TVF lesion had resolved, he had achieved his goals: the elimination of his hemorrhagic lesion, a physical barrier to vigorous voice use. Knowing voice therapy patients have a 65% dropout rate in compliance and adherence, clinicians have a sizable job to create a functional reset for individuals who have variable levels of self-awareness and compliance.[65] While optimizing his voice use at the performance level was a clinical long-term goal, when the patient had achieved his ends, he returned to performance satisfied. A structured approach for voice care and use, combined with his compliance with the plan, led to a successful treatment outcome, and the patient was very pleased.

> Adherence to voice therapy, like many behavior change therapies, is low. In this case, despite the importance of voice quality and vocal endurance being central to his occupational voice needs and the demonstrated benefit of voice therapy, this patient struggled with adherence. Barriers to attendance included financial strain, concern for loss of notoriety being away from the stage, and likely other factors not revealed to the clinician. This patient was lost to follow up, and there is no ultimate metric of successful therapy.

 CASE STUDY 8.5

Timing Multimodality Voice Therapy to Treat an Adult Singer With a Vocal Fold Polyp and Mild Atrophy

Juliana Codino

Voice Evaluation

Case History

Chief Complaint. Vocal fatigue, voice break in the first passaggio, loss of range (D5 and above), lack of volume, lingering cough since upper respiratory infection (URI), and pain in throat triggered by increased voice use and by cough. The patient was diagnosed with a small hemorrhagic polyp on the left vocal fold and mild vocal fold atrophy.

History of Present Illness and Voice Demands. LS is a 59-year-old cisgender woman who presents for a comprehensive voice and upper airway evaluation in the interprofessional laryngology clinic. She is a classically trained mezzo-soprano, has a master's degree in vocal performance, and works full-time as a middle school and high school choir teacher, where she conducts 3 choirs. Additionally, she sees 8 to 12 private voice students a week in her home studio. She does not use amplification in the classroom. She is not currently performing professionally, but she occasionally participates in musical theater productions at a local level.

The patient stated that she has had a persistent cough for the last 6 months that started after an URI. The coughing fits are usually not violent and last less than 1 minute. The cough used to be productive while she was sick but then it became a dry cough. She initially saw her primary care provider (PCP), who prescribed a Medrol dose pack, which helped with the cough while she was taking it. She was then placed on a steroid inhaler, which reduced the cough significantly. However, she stopped using the inhaler when it ran out, and the cough consequently returned. At that time, she had an important choir concert, and she recalled having very high singing and speaking voice demands for about 1 week. She stated it was particularly challenging to go through that week of rehearsals given the dry cough. She had continued to experience coughing episodes since then, particularly throughout the day and aggravated by voice use.

A few days after the concert, she noticed that she developed voice limitations that started as vocal fatigue and lack of volume by the end of the day. These symptoms were particularly evident whenever she had private lessons after a full day of teaching. Even though she was not performing at that time, she perceived a break in her first passaggio. She also reported a clear limit on the higher end of her singing range (D5 and above) that impaired her ability to model for students. A few weeks later, these symptoms were progressively getting worse and more frequent, and she developed intermittent throat pain triggered by singing or talking for extended periods of time. Since then, she had been trying to include more visual aids during her teaching but explained she had to continue to model with her voice for those private students that were just starting voice lessons. She has low voice demands at home. She lives with her husband and they have no children. Their social life is very active, but they have been avoiding going out socially because she felt it was "too much on her voice."

The patient reported classic GERD symptoms that included heartburn, chest pressure, excessive burping, and metallic taste in her mouth but that have been under control for over 2 years with a twice-daily PPI prescribed by her PCP. She reported no other medical comorbidities nor regular medications.

Laryngeal Imaging

Laryngeal videostroboscopy was performed with both a flexible distal chip scope and a rigid scope. Salient examination findings included: mild bilateral vocal fold (VF) atrophy, small hemorrhagic left VF polyp, right VF contact changes, bilateral symmetrical abduction and adduction of the VFs, glottic closure characterized by intermittent hourglass deformity, no supraglottic hyperfunction, normal arytenoid mucosa and mild posterior cobblestoning, equal vocal process height, and normal/regular vibratory capability of the VFs with symmetric phase and normal amplitude (Figure 8–6).

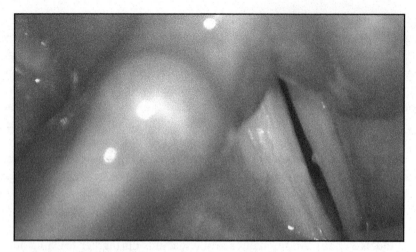

FIGURE 8–6. Rigid laryngoscopy still of patient LS before treatment.

In some practices, both flexible and rigid laryngoscopes are used. Flexible scopes allow imaging during speech and singing in addition to some non-speech tasks like sniffing and whistling. Some believe the use of flexible imaging during these tasks improves the assessment of the presence of motion asymmetries or movement disorders. Rigid laryngoscopy is believed to demonstrate improved quality and clarity of the image when looking for very subtle mucosal abnormalities. In singers, there is arguably considerable value in being able to assess dynamic voice production such as singing, as well as in obtaining the highest mucosal detail possible.

Vocal Effort and Patient-Reported Outcome Measures

The OMNI-Vocal Effort Scale was completed.[10] The patient rated vocal effort on a 0 to 10 scale where 0 = "extremely easy" to produce voice and 10 = "extremely hard" to produce voice. The patient reported that vocal effort was 6/10 during the evaluation and 10/10 at worst, occurring at the end of the days she taught private students.

Quality-of-Life Impairment:

1. VHI-10[11]: 16/40 (threshold = 11)[66]
2. Cough Severity Index[67]: 19/40 (cutoff = 3)
3. Reflux Symptom Index[68]: 31/45 (cutoff = 13)

Auditory-Perceptual Assessment

The GRBAS scale was administered. The patient was determined to have an overall grade of dysphonia score of 1/3, indicating a dysphonia of mild nature. Aberrant perceptual features identified in the voice include roughness (1/3) and strain (1/3). No breathiness or asthenia were noted. The pitch of the voice was within normal limits for age and gender. Resonance was intermittently focused in the laryngeal region. Respiration was primarily abdominal-thoracic.

Posture

Head posture was assessed as normal. Mildly elevated bilateral shoulder position during speaking was observed.

Manual Palpation Assessment

Muscle tension was assessed and rated on a 0 to 5 scale where 0 = "no tension" and 5 = "most tension."

Results Indicated:

1. 2/5 tension at the thyrohyoid space without report of pain
2. 1/5 tension at the base of tongue (BOT)/suprahyoid region without report of pain
3. 2/5 tension on left sternocleidomastoid (SCM); 2/5 tension on right SCM
4. Normal laryngeal elevation assessed by swallowing and vowel ascending glissando /i/
5. 1/5 restriction of lateralization of thyroid cartilage bilaterally

Acoustic Analysis

Acoustic analysis was completed pre- and posttherapy (Table 8–9).

Patient's Goals

LS's main goal after hearing the diagnosis was to "get rid of the polyp." She felt this was a "career-ending" problem given that she also had overlapping aging changes.

Stimulability

Determination of a patient's candidacy for voice therapy: The patient was found stimulable for no strain in voicing utilizing Flow Phonation[69] strategies and was able to easily transfer that to functional phrases and a short conversation, which immediately influenced her self-efficacy for behavioral changes.

Impressions and Decision Making

LS should benefit from voice therapy to target mild compensatory strain secondary to the VF polyp and mild VF atrophy. The polyp was likely the reason for the new break in her passaggio and other voice issues, possibly as a result of extensive coughing combined with high voice demands at the time of onset of vocal symptoms. The mild VF atrophy might have been contributing to her vocal fatigue, lack of volume, and range restrictions. If, after a trial of voice therapy, the polyp was not resolved, then VF surgery should be considered. Regarding the cough, the benefit of

steroids in the past with eventual return of the cough suggested a pulmonary etiology. LS was prescribed a 5-day course of prednisone by the laryngologist. If the cough got better while on the medication and then returned, she would need to go back to her PCP for more aggressive pulmonary management or be referred to a pulmonologist. If the steroids did not affect her cough, she should return to the laryngology clinic for trial treatment for neurogenic cough with behavioral cough suppression strategies implemented in therapy.

Plan of Care

Long-Term Goals:

- Be able to teach and participate in social and singing activities without subsequent vocal fatigue, voice breaks, lack of loudness, cough, and throat pain
- Incorporate specific vocal hygiene instructions tailored to vocal demands

Short-Term Goals:

- Decrease effort in phonation, improve vocal endurance, and increase pitch range without audible voice breaks through SOVT exercises,[1] Flow Phonation,[69] and Resonant Voice strategies[60]
- Reduce laryngeal tension and introduce circumlaryngeal massage[70]
- Implement cough suppression techniques during coughing fits while the nature of the cough is being evaluated

If/when a repeat laryngoscopy with videostroboscopy shows that the polyp has resolved:

- Incorporate VFEs,[44] which are proven effective in managing vocal symptoms secondary to mild atrophy

Intervention

LS was very motivated to start voice therapy, which was planned to be conducted in a hybrid model: Some sessions would be through a telemedicine platform and other sessions in person.

Table 8–9. Acoustic Assessment Pre- and Posttreatment

Pt LS	Pretreatment	Posttreatment	Norms
Spectrogram /a/ vowel			
Mean F0 Rainbow Passage	219 Hz	218 Hz	
Semitones Rainbow Passage	B2-C4	C3-F#4	
Mean dB Rainbow Passage	57 dB	63 dB	
Min-Max dB Rainbow Passage	35-62 dB	37-75 dB	
CPP (SD) /a/ vowel	8.52 dB (0.55)	11.52 dB (0.43)	11.46 dB (0.45) *Murton et al (2020)
CSID /a/ vowel	31.53	12.56	
CPP Rainbow Passage	4.89 dB	6.14 dB	6.11 dB *Murton et al (2020)
MDVP /a/ vowel		Indicated relatively within light gray circle per June 2008 norms MDVP Model 5105	

Dark gray area: pretreatment; Heavy black line: posttreatment

These were planned to last 45 minutes. After completing the evaluation and stimulability tasks and discussing the rationale for voice therapy and the plan of care with the patient, the clinician introduced vocal hygiene tasks and encouraged LS to start implementing them immediately.

1. After considering the dimensions of the classroom and choir concert hall, the clinician recommended a single amplification device that could benefit the patient in all the different rooms that she worked in.
2. To reduce the vocal load of teaching voice, the clinician presented different options to assist with modeling singing during lessons. These included changing octaves or using a musical instrument to model the sound.
3. The clinician presented replacement behaviors to reduce chronic cough and throat clearing, including alternating short sniffs with exhalation on prolonged fricative sounds like /s/ or /f/, taking frequent sips of water, sucking on nonmedicated and non-mint lozenges, and performing a hard swallow.

Session #1: Telemedicine

The patient reported that taking prednisone had significantly reduced her cough. Given this outcome and per the laryngologist's recommendation, she had already made an appointment with her PCP to continue pulmonary management of the cough. She also stated that she had been trying the throat clearing suppression techniques with good results. She was advanced with the use of Flow Phonation and practiced this while using her new voice amplifier in one of the music classrooms (she was in school for the telemedicine appointment). The amplifier gave her the loudness she needed to talk to a room full of 30 to 35 teenagers, and she could easily regulate the loudness with the volume knob. She reported awareness of reduced laryngeal and perilaryngeal tension. Through negative practice, she demonstrated the ability to discriminate between the target voice versus the uncoordinated voice production.

Session #2: In Person

One week later, LS reported she had not experienced as much vocal fatigue in the last week since she had been implementing the strategies mentioned above, and she admitted she found that in the past she had been modeling "more than what her students actually needed."

Circumlaryngeal massage was introduced and the patient was instructed in how to perform it on herself daily. Pressure in a circular motion was applied with the thumb and index finger in the thyrohyoid space. The procedure was repeated with the tips of the hyoid bone. The larynx was stretched downward and moved laterally. Focal tenderness was given more attention. Finally, gentle kneading on the sternocleidomastoids was used. Additionally, SOVT exercises with the use of a straw (0.5 cm diameter and 24 cm long)[71] in water were instructed. (See Video 28 Straw Phonation in Water Hierarchy by Codino.) Given that, as a singer, she had already been exposed to these exercises, she successfully completed the following protocol:

1. Sustain airflow only with the straw in water to develop awareness of lower laryngeal posture and feeling of "easy throat" with uninterrupted airflow for 5 to 10 seconds. Repeat 5 times.
2. Sustain one comfortable pitch with the straw in water for 5 to 10 seconds. Repeat 5 times.
3. Glide with the straw in water from a comfortable low pitch to a comfortable high pitch on an ascending glissando. Repeat 5 times.
4. Glide with the straw in water from a comfortable high pitch to a comfortable low pitch on a descending glissando. Repeat 5 times.

5. Alternate with the straw in water 3 to 4 glides up and down, imitating the sound of a siren, within a comfortable range. Repeat 5 times.
6. Sing the melody of a song into the straw in water for a minute.

She was reminded to develop awareness of an easy, open throat while performing each repetition and adjust if needed. She was instructed to conduct these exercises 4 to 6 times a day, particularly in between her classes as a warm-up/cool-down.

Session #3: Telemedicine

The next session was scheduled online 2 weeks later, and LS reported diligently practicing SOVT exercises with water resistance and performing circumlaryngeal massage daily. Her voice had an improved core tone and sounded less strained. She had been evaluated by pulmonology and was using an inhaler that she estimated had reduced her coughing fits "by 90% or more," and she was still applying the throat clearing suppression strategies. Resonant Voice strategies were introduced, starting with the basic training gesture: chanting the sound /m/ on a comfortable pitch and loudness with particular focus on feeling vibrations in the "mask" area (the patient was prompted to use the tip of her fingers cupped around her nose and mouth if needed for tactile feedback) while experiencing "no tension in the neck around the larynx." Once the patient was confident in the feeling of this forward focus, she was advanced on to the vowel, word, and phrase levels. Using short phrases that facilitated the feeling of forward focus (eg, "Maybe Monday morning"), the clinician introduced chanting following certain pitches in the piano starting on A3 and moving upward every half step and went above her first passaggio (which was located around F4) and stopped once she reached C5. With this phonetic material and chanting every phrase on one single note, there were no obvious breaks in the passaggio area. This break, LS admitted, was the most challenging symptom that she had been experiencing because she felt it indicated "something lost" in relation to her vocal technique.

Reevaluation With Physician and SLP

Repeat videostroboscopy was scheduled 6 weeks following the first appointment and 2 weeks following the last therapy session. Laryngeal imaging demonstrated that the polyp on the left VF was completely resolved and that she still had VF bowing at the mid-membranous level (Figure 8–7). The cough was being managed by pulmonary medicine. She was encouraged to continue with voice therapy.

Session #4: Telemedicine

LS continued work on vocal range and used SOVT exercises with ascending and descending fifths, starting with water resistance and advancing the hierarchy up to open vowels preceded by voiced fricatives within the A3 to D5 range (Table 8–10). At the limits of the high end of her range (around D5 per the patient's description), LS was instructed to continue with alternating major seconds (Figure 8–8). She was initially guarded and hesitant to sus-

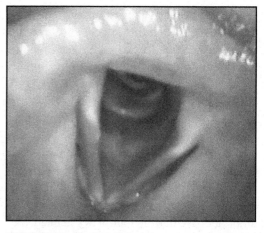

FIGURE 8–7. Flexible laryngoscopy still of patient LS at 6-week physician follow-up.

8. Performance Voice 401

Table 8–10. SOVT Protocol

SOVT with straw in water	A3 glide to E4 glide to A3
	A#3 glide to F4 glide to A#3
	. . . (continues ascending every semitone up to) . . .
	F#4 glide to C#5 glide to F#4
	G4 glide to D5 glide to G4
SOVT starting with straw in water and gradually removing the straw out of the water while doing a descending glide	D5 glide while fading the straw out of the water to G4
	C#5 glide while fading the straw out of the water to F#4
	. . . (continues ascending every semitone up to) . . .
	F4 glide while fading the straw out of the water to A#3
	E4 glide while fading the straw out of the water to A3
SOVT starting with straw (no water) and gradually removing the straw from mouth while doing a descending glide	D5 glide while fading the straw out the mouth to G4
	C#5 glide while fading the straw out the mouth to F#4
	. . . (continues ascending every semitone up to) . . .
	F4 glide while fading the straw out the mouth to A#3
	E4 glide while fading the straw out the mouth to A3
SOVT with fricative /v/ into vowel /u/	A3 glide to E4 glide to A3
	A#3 glide to F4 glide to A#3
	. . . (continues ascending every semitone up to) . . .
	F#4 glide to C#5 glide to F#4
	G4 glide to D5 glide to G4
SOVT with fricative /z/ into vowel /a/	A3 glide to E4 glide to A3
	A#3 glide to F4 glide to A#3
	. . . (continues ascending every semitone up to) . . .
	F#4 glide to C#5 glide to F#4
	G4 glide to D5 glide to G4

tain these alternating tones, particularly F5 though G#5, but with cueing of increased airflow and feeling of forward focus, she was more confident and successful in voicing those tones by the end of the practice. Helpful cues included examples such as, "Make sure the bubbles are steady" or "Do you feel the vibra-

tions in the mask area?" The clinician recommended that LS practice this exercise 3 to 4 times a week.

Session #5: In Person

LS returned 3 weeks later and reported being able to complete the exercises practiced on

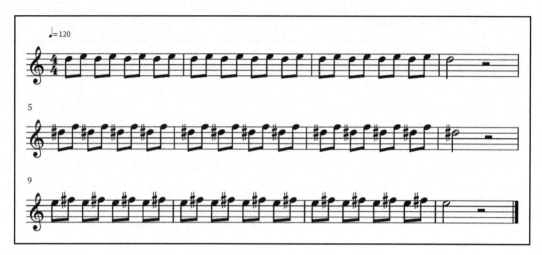

FIGURE 8–8. Notation of alternating major seconds.

the previous session up to A5 with no feeling of strain. She had been preparing a musical theater song for an audition with a tessitura of B3 to F5 with good outcomes. She reported that most of her initial concerns were resolved (vocal fatigue, voice break in the first passaggio, loss of range above D5, lack of volume, cough, and pain in throat), and the only concerns remaining were occasional lack of volume and mild feeling of effort to talk in specific social interactions. At this point in the therapy process and given the lack of complete closure/bowing observed at her 6-week return visit, the clinician recommended VFEs based on the premise that low-impact adductor exercises would improve glottic closure without triggering compensatory strain. (See Video 5 Vocal Function Exercises by Stemple.) LS recorded the exercises on her phone to facilitate practice and was instructed to practice them twice daily with the adductory power exercise between C4 and G4. She stated that she enjoyed doing SOVT exercises with water resistance throughout the day in between classes, since it provided relief throughout the day. She and the clinician agreed that she would continue to focus on resonant voice strategies in conversation and that she would use circumlaryngeal massage if she experienced throat pain or vocal fatigue.

Session #6: Telemedicine

LS was seen 2 weeks later and reported significant improvement in loudness and resolution of the feeling of effortful talking. She had been cast to participate in a local musical theater production and was starting rehearsals that day.

Concluding Remarks

This case demonstrates the importance of selecting the appropriate timing for interventions in a complex case of voice therapy. The initial diagnosis presented a lesion that would usually require surgical intervention, but the voice team considered a behavioral approach given the recent onset of voice symptoms and the small size of the polyp. The spindle-shaped closure was also contributing to the vocal symptoms, but the team decided to address the polyp first and to discuss with the patient a plan to address it following resolution of the polyp.

The positive outcome of this treatment plan is attributable to the patient's self-efficacy, which was probably influenced by the high stimulability and adherence, including excellent attendance, participation in therapy sessions, and practice between visits.

CASE STUDY 8.6

Perioperative Voice Therapy for an Adult Praise and Worship Leader With Phonotraumatic Lesions

Marina Gilman

Voice Evaluation

Case History

Chief Complaint. RR is a 45-year-old cisgender female Christian contemporary singer and praise team leader, presenting with a 3-year history of dysphonia.

History of the Voice Problem. RR reports gradually increased symptoms of hoarseness and reduced upper range with extended periods of voice use (speaking and singing) over the past few years. At first, she attributed her voice problems to stress, allergies, and reflux. Her primary care physician prescribed reflux medications. However, her voice continued to deteriorate to the point that she was often unable to lead worship or sing. At the time of her initial clinical voice evaluation, symptoms included rough, often strained vocal quality, vocal instability, reduced endurance, increased effort, and decreased range. Her overall medical history was unremarkable.

Voice Use History. RR worked successfully in the corporate world for 15 years. The high-pressure environment and family issues led her to leave the corporate world and focus more on her music. Her current day job environment is more relaxed, but no less vocally demanding.

RR has been singing since she was 5 years old, but never had formal training. On a talkativeness scale (1 = "quiet and reserved," 7 = "verbal and outgoing"), she rates herself as a 7+. Her vocal demands on the praise and worship team have steadily increased. She was recently appointed volunteer music director and a lay reader. Now, every Sunday for 2 services, she directs and is lead singer and keyboard player in the praise and worship band (consisting of electric guitar and bass, keyboard, percussion, and 2 to 4 backup singers). In addition, she reads scripture 2 Sundays per month. The band rehearses 1 or 2 times a week for several hours, as well as Sunday mornings before the first service.

RR has 2 children at home and is the "go-to" person within her extended family. RR reports no regular vocal warm-up routine, although she would "sing a bit" before rehearsals and on some Sundays. Recently, to "save her voice," she eliminated vocal warm-ups, especially on Sunday mornings.

Laryngeal Imaging

The referring laryngologist completed a laryngeal stroboscopic examination of the vocal folds. Movement of the vocal folds, phase symmetry, amplitude of excursion, and periodicity were within normal range. Significant findings included bilateral midmembranous edematous swellings resulting in an hourglass closure pattern with resultant air escape through anterior and posterior gaps. Mucosal wave was reduced at the site of the lesions, greater on the right than the left, resulting in differential vibratory patterns within and between each vocal fold. Lateral compression indicative of compensatory muscle tension was also observed.

Auditory-Perceptual Evaluation

The CAPE-V[15] was completed. The score was 46/100, indicating a dysphonia of a moderate nature. Aberrant features identified in the voice included breathiness, roughness, and mild strain.

Patient Self-Assessment

The Voice-Related Quality of Life (VRQOL)[72] self-assessment of the impact of the voice disorder on quality of life raw score was 19/50, converting to 77.5/100, suggesting that the patient's perception of the voice disorder has a moderate impact on her quality of life.

Voice Therapy: Clinical Case Studies

Acoustic and Aerodynamic Assessment

Acoustic and aerodynamic findings were consistent with the diagnosis of dysphonia. A primary finding of poor respiratory phonatory coordination was related to glottal inefficiency as evidenced by (1) equal reduction of duration in sustained voiced sounds /z/ and /a/, compared with the unvoiced sustained /s/,[73] and (2) lower mean F0 during running speech compared with sustained /a/. In addition, breath holding was noted during the running speech protocol (description of the cookie theft picture) as she spoke for up to 10 seconds without taking an adequate breath or without allowing for inspiration during pauses. Findings of reduced physiological pitch range with pitch breaks in the upper range were consistent with the medical findings of the laryngeal exam. Details are provided in Table 8–11 with normative data from Zraick et al (2013).[74]

Table 8–11. Acoustic and Aerodynamic Assessment

Measure	Results	Norms	Interpretation
Max Phonation Time: Voiced /a/, /z/	7 seconds each	21.24 seconds; SD 5.79; range: 5.79-29.46 sec on /a/	See narrative discussion
Max Phonation Time: Voiceless /s/	15 seconds	No norms specific to /s/ (usually taken as part of s/z ratio)	See narrative discussion
Speaking F0	194 Hz		
F0 on Sustained /a/	209 Hz	206.91 Hz; SD 22.22; range: 137.23-244.27 Hz	
Physiological Pitch Range	134-619 Hz C#3-D#5		Low overall range; limited ability to access head voice
Pitch Perturbation	3.5%	>1.05%	Increased
Intensity Perturbation	8.6%	≥3.85%	Increased
Mean Expiratory Airflow Rate (sustained /a/)	0.58 L/sec	0.14 L/sec SD 0.08	Increased
Mean Peak Expiratory Pressure Voicing Efficiency (/papapa/)	7.8 cmH$_2$O	5.76 cmH$_2$O SD 1.51	Increased
Mean airflow during voicing (/papapa/)	0.50 L/sec	0.13 L/sec SD 0.06	Increased
Running speech protocol (Cookie theft picture)	0.08 L/sec	No available norms	Breath-holding behavior noted

Plan of Care

Six weekly voice therapy sessions were recommended. Goals of therapy were to increase insight into postural and internal tensions impeding optimization of voice in all contexts, and to improve coordination of respiration and phonation.

Decision Making

Although RR had sung since she was a child, she had no formal training. A team meeting with RR, the laryngologist, and the SLP determined that, based on her dependence on her vocal intuition and native talent, an initial course of therapy would be the best option. If her goals were not met with the course of therapy, surgery was a further option.

Since RR was an "intuitive" singer, therapeutic exercises needed to have a strong sensory, experiential component. She needed to feel the differences. Many individuals, especially "natural singers," rely heavily on sensation and feeling when singing. Academic knowledge of the vocal mechanism is important but does not inform the internal "how do I do this." Therefore, it is incumbent upon the clinician to provide goals and strategies that stimulate change within the patient's internal organization. RR did not have a good sense of how to embody her theoretical knowledge, hence the consistent use of semi-occluded sounds throughout therapy.[1] Semi-occluded sounds such as lip trills; tongue trills (raspberry); and /z/, /v/, or /w/ on glides (sirens) demand optimal 3-systems coordination (one can't sustain the lip/tongue trill while breath holding).[1] Since they are nonaesthetic "noises," they do not activate the singer's self-criticism: "The voice needs to be ..." (*Note:* Many individuals have difficulty with some of these sounds. For many, the /w/ or "oo" sound with lips well rounded and the cheeks slightly filled with air are the easiest.)

In addition, the patient needed to pay attention to her physical organization (posture) in performance.[75,76] Playing and singing, while at the same time keeping the band together, demands split attention. To lead when singing and playing simultaneously, performers often "beat time with their voice." Even if the technique is good, since the hands are occupied playing, the only way to keep time is by nodding their head. In addition, the physical act of striking keys, plucking strings, or beating or shaking an instrument can stress the voice, due in part to the downward action of repeatedly pounding the instrument. These actions can impede breath support and exacerbate neck and laryngeal tension.

Intervention

Due to a busy schedule and the unpredictable nature of her job, RR was not always able to schedule regular weekly therapy appointments. She was, however, compliant with home practice.

The goals for this initial session included (1) conducting a brief assessment of the understanding of vocal production, breath support, resonance, and the functional differences between speaking and singing; and (2) creating a warm-up routine that RR could easily incorporate into her busy schedule. RR had a good academic understanding of vocal anatomy and the relationship of the 3 systems (respiration, phonation, and resonance), but not a somatic one. The embodiment of knowledge became the goal.

Semi-occluded sounds on sustained phonation were trained. In preparation for the lip trill, RR would lift the chest high on inhalation and then stiffen the abdominal muscles on the exhalation. Two strategies were used to bring awareness to the habitual pattern of not fully releasing the abdominal muscles:

1. Postural: Either sitting or standing, leaning forward from the hip joint while tensing and releasing the abdominal muscles. Leaning forward facilitates release of the abdominal muscles.
2. Sustaining the lip trill while simultaneously flexing and releasing the abdominal muscles. The release of the abdominal

muscles on inhalation, as the diaphragm contracts, allows the shoulders and chest to remain relaxed.

Once the lip trill became consistent on sustained phonation, the task was expanded to gliding easily through her midrange, followed by sustained phonation and glides on other semi-occluded sounds. As the task shifted to glides or another semi-occluded sound, RR was intermittently asked to notice what the belly was doing at the end of each utterance. With these cues, RR gradually became aware of habitual patterns of contracting the abdominal muscles and lifting the chest on inhalation and was able to release. Home practice was strongly recommended several times a day for 2 to 3 minutes each time using the same sounds trained during the session. This practitioner has found that incorporating short 2- to 3-minute daily warm-ups several times throughout the day promotes "vocal reset" as well as increased compliance. Since we take our body with us, patients can and will warm up "on the run."

Her second voice therapy session was 2 weeks later. RR reported reduced hoarseness at the end of the day. The clinician reviewed RR's home practice, consisting of glides and sustained phonation on lip trills with attention to a full release of the breath. Additional semi-occluded sounds were added for variation such as /w/ (oo) and /v/. To promote generalization, RR was trained to speak the vowels /a/, /e/, /i/, and /o/ while maintaining airflow on the semi-occluded sound of choice. There are 4 stages:

1. Speak the vowels clearly with attention to the movement of the tongue in the mouth.
2. Close the lips only, allowing free movement of the jaw, and speak the vowels again smoothly, without glottal stops.
3. Using the /w/ or "oo" semi-occluded sound, again speak the vowels while maintaining airflow (jaw is free to move, no glottal attacks).
4. Repeat slowly, releasing the semi-occlusion, ie, open the jaw while continuing

phonation. A smooth transition from one vowel to another is essential.

RR repeated each step several times before proceeding to the next step. RR initially found it difficult to isolate the movement of the tongue with lips closed and then while maintaining the semi-occlusion. The next challenge was the transition from semi-occlusion to open lips. The vowels would "pop out" when she opened her mouth and the resonance reverted to the habituated laryngeal resonance. Once RR was comfortable with this sequence, the vowels were replaced with short 1- to 2-syllable words beginning with the same semi-occluded sound; such as using the "oo" with puffed words such as "one," "wonder," "where," and "what." The complexity of the words was gradually increased as she became more proficient. By the end of the session, RR was able to speak 2- or 3-syllable words or phrases while maintaining the buzz of the semi-occlusion. The voice became spontaneously more resonant, as did the respiratory phonatory coordination.

By the third session, almost a month later, RR reported she was able to resume her daily vocal routine, including singing, without increased dysphonia. However, stamina was still a concern. Overall vocal quality was improved but continued to be somewhat dysphonic. Range was still limited. Her habitual use of glottal fry at the ends of utterances and the hard onset of vowel-initial words improved but were still an issue. To help her identify when and how she was holding her breath, she was trained in a simple exercise the clinician referred to as "the /s/ pulse." (See Video 29 /s/ Pulse and /wu/ Hierarchy by Gilman.) The exercise consists of short /s/ release repeated for 15 to 20 seconds. "Release" here relates to releasing the abdominal muscles AND any laryngeal or postural tension. It is important to give adequate pause time so the patient can internally "find" the tension and allow the inhalation to happen spontaneously. Actively breathing might promote hyperventilation and trigger their habitual pattern.

RR was cued to focus on the release of the abdominal muscles. After only 5 to 10 repetitions, she would spontaneously exhale, suggesting she was stacking her breath, using very little breath on phonation, then adding more with each inhale. The pace of the pause slowed with increased cues to fully release any holding. Gradually, she was easily able to increase the duration of the pattern. Frequently, patients will suddenly either gasp for air or release stacked air after only a few repetitions. Cueing is necessary at first to provide more time to determine and release the "holding" in the body (eg, knees, larynx, belly). If executed correctly, the breath is replenished during the release, when the vocal folds abduct and the abdominal muscles release, letting the air automatically fill the lungs. The /s/ was then changed to a voiced lip or tongue trill. Again, if the airflow is held, the lips and tongue will not vibrate. RR was encouraged to repeat the /s/ pulse exercise, both voiceless and voiced, several times throughout her day as part of her home practice. Sitting in traffic at a red light is an ideal time, as the traffic light will change after 10 to 20 seconds. She gradually became aware of her breath holding during conversation.

Between her third and fourth therapy sessions, she traveled to Los Angeles to visit a sister congregation. Over the course of the long weekend, she led services, worked with their praise team, and sang 4 services. Though her vocal demands during the weekend were greatly increased, she was pleased that her voice held up! This was a clear sign that she was improving! However, her frustration level remained high. Her voice was more predictable but still dysphonic, her range was still reduced, and she was expending effort in the process. A focus of this session was examination of her physical setup in church. Singing, conducting, AND playing the piano were a given. Alternative ways for her to play and sing without "beating time with her voice" were explored. Separating singing from playing, exploring her inner sensations of playing

alone, then singing alone, each with attention on musical/sound flow and ease (ie, "letting" rather than "making"), gave her some insight on when and how tension interfered when she both sang and played. This exploration was helpful, but not the solution.

Due to her continuing difficulties, the option of surgery was discussed in therapy and then in consultation with the laryngologist. On repeat laryngeal examination her vocal folds were no longer edematous; the bilateral mid-membranous fibrovascular lesions demonstrated reduced edema but were still present. Initially resistant to the idea of surgery, she eventually realized she had maximized her capabilities during therapy. The remaining vocal limitations were related to the pathology. At this point, she agreed to surgery. Preoperative counseling consisted of alerting family, friends, and colleagues that she would be on complete voice rest for 5 days minimum, communicating only by text/email, taking time off work, and finding substitutes for church.

Surgery to remove the lesions was performed. RR returned to the clinic on day 5 and was taken off of voice rest by the laryngologist. A brief initial voice therapy appointment reviewed the protocol for coming off voice rest—limited talking at a moderate dynamic level until return to therapy at 2 weeks postop.

Voice Therapy Post-Surgery

Therapy resumed 2 weeks following surgery. Goals of postop therapy were (1) to reinforce the respiratory/phonatory patterns developed preop and (2) to develop a new vocal warm-up routine that would also serve as a daily vocal check-in.

When RR arrived for the first postop therapy session, she was speaking softly and holding back or "protecting" her voice. Many patients, particularly singers, will "protect" their voice following surgery by speaking quietly but with reduced airflow. She reported being very compliant with home practice and voice use. She demonstrated the home practice exercises appropriately but had not generalized them to connected speech. Lip trills on sustained phonation at a comfortable pitch, and gentle glides (not full range) followed by tongue trills and /w/ with text at varying dynamic levels, were reviewed to facilitate generalization. She was very surprised at how "effortless" it became to speak!

The clinician encouraged RR to allow her range and loudness level to expand spontaneously using the semi-occluded sounds on vowels and using text within her comfort zone, maintaining resonance transitioning to regular speech. Full singing (performing) is not recommended for 4 to 6 weeks depending on healing. However, the line between singing and speaking is hard to define. Elements of both can involve sustained phonation, range, text, and resonance. It is important to gradually introduce these aspects in postop therapy by training transitions from speech to chant consisting of short bits of melody with, and then without, semi-occluded sounds over the 4- to 5-week postop period.

RR returned for the second postop visit 1 week later, somewhat frustrated. Singing and speaking were much easier and less effortful. But where was her voice? She had been struggling for so long with a voice that did not work, with low speaking F0, dysphonia, and increased effort, that she had no idea what her "real" voice was or how to find it. Following the warm-ups on glides and sustained phonation, her speaking F0 would spontaneously rise, but would drop back down to near glottal fry phonation within 3 syllables of speaking. This voice did not match her vocal self-image. It is important for the clinician to understand the connection between self and vocal self-image, based on both sensory and auditory feedback. RR's internal vocal self-image had gradually shifted to match the dysphonic voice. Now, the surgical intervention and therapy had eliminated the vocal fold characteristics that had resulted in the dysphonia. This new voice did not match her perceived vocal identity. For many, the sense of ease and improved flexibility postop are enough to accept their

"new" voice. However, this was not the case for RR.

The therapeutic challenge was to help RR become "friends" with the altered vocal quality and ease and realign her vocal self-image with this new reality. The postop goals were revised to reconcile the "new voice." Therapy shifted to integrating all the perceptual aspects of voice, such as range, resonance, function speaking, presenting, and singing. Vocal exercises to accomplish this included

1. Using a common phrase, "Good morning, how are you?" in a variety of contexts:
   a. spoken
   b. chanted on a single pitch
   c. chanted while varying the pitch
   d. sung while varying the pitch
2. Using "Good morning, how are you?" or another phrase in the same sequence as in exercise #1 but varying the resonance as well, such as using accents such as a country Western singer, classical singer, British accent, and Southern accent
3. Picking a phrase from a favorite song and:
   a. singing it
   b. speaking it in the contour of the pitches
   c. speaking and singing it again while exploring a variety of accents

Asking for a variety of vocalizations in both speaking and singing allowed RR to "discover" the voice using the wide range of resonances and pitch ranges available to her now. At the same time, these tasks reinforced efficient airflow and resonance. Linking speaking and singing allowed RR to reconnect to the voice in a nonjudgmental way. She now could choose which voice to use in what context.

By the third and final postop therapy session 2 weeks later, RR reported feeling comfortable with her voice. She maintained good, clear vocal quality throughout a conversation with only brief moments of glottal fry, which were quickly corrected. Vocal endurance was back to normal, and she was able to play and sing with a new awareness and with no vocal fatigue.

Results and Discussion

At this point about 5 weeks postop, RR was able to return fully to the praise team. She now had a better understanding of the voice. Vocal technique was fundamentally sound. Through therapy, RR now had the tools and awareness to fully and confidently resume her vocal life. She was encouraged to find a singing teacher who understood the vocal demands and style necessary for singing contemporary Christian music. She returned over the next 18 months once or twice for a wellness check and was given a clean bill of vocal health each time.

CASE STUDY 8.7

Perioperative Voice Therapy for a High School Music Teacher With a Vocal Fold Polyp

Maurice Goodwin

Voice Evaluation

Case History

Chief Complaint. Increased voicing effort, reduced vocal endurance, reduced overall voice range, worsening presence of breathy pitch breaks in singing voice

History of Voice Complaint. Diane, a 44-year-old cisgender woman, visited the clinic due to a gradual decline in her voice quality while speaking and singing. She works as a high school choral music teacher, a professional actress in local community theater productions, and a frequent soloist within her church choir program. Her symptoms began worsening about 6 weeks prior, halfway through the fall school calendar, without any specific triggering event. While she is accustomed to occasional hoarseness during busy seasons, this instance was different as it hasn't returned to normal and is getting worse. She experiences greater voice effort during various tasks, especially when singing, and her vocal endurance has decreased. Diane describes her speaking voice as "slightly more coarse," breathy, and lower in pitch. Although she can still sing, she encounters frequent pitch breaks in higher frequencies and a reduced overall pitch range. Diane has no history of diagnosed voice disorders, and a previous stroboscopy from a few years ago showed no abnormalities. She has seasonal allergies, managed with over-the-counter medications as needed, and occasional reflux symptoms related to spicy foods, which she avoids when possible. She is not experiencing premenopausal symptoms and has a close relationship with her primary care physician. There are no other significant medical history, surgeries, or comorbidities that could be contributing to her current voice issues.

Voice Use. Diane, a professional singer with extensive voice training, holds bachelor's degrees in music education and vocal performance. She maintains a long-standing relationship with her voice teacher of over a decade. In her daily role as a high school music teacher, Diane relies heavily on her voice, engaging in both high-frequency and high-intensity vocal tasks. Her responsibilities involve teaching multiple choral and general music classes daily, often requiring louder speaking volumes in large rehearsal spaces. Additionally, she participates as a soprano singer in her church choir twice a month and frequently takes on soloist roles within the same choir, performing at least every other month. Diane is also involved in an annual major production with a local theater group. Her vocal range typically spans from G3 to C6, and she excels in various singing styles, including choral, classical, musical theater, and gospel.

Patient-Perceived Vocal Quality and Effort

Diane self-assessed her voice quality using a 1 to 10 scale, with 1 indicating "low or no voice" and 10 representing "best or highest voice quality." Diane rated her speaking voice at 7/10 and her singing voice at 5/10. Furthermore, she completed the OMNI-Vocal Effort Scale,[10] which measures vocal effort on a 0 to 10 scale, with 0 signifying "extremely easy" production of voice and 10 indicating "extremely hard" production of voice. In speaking voice tasks, Diane reported a perceived vocal effort of 3 to 4/10; during most singing voice tasks, this effort increased significantly to 8/10, particularly with higher-frequency tasks.

Quality-of-Life Impairment
1. VHI-10: 17/40 (threshold = 11)[11]
2. Singing Voice Handicap Index–10 (SVHI-10): 29/40 (threshold = 20)[77]
3. Reflux Symptom Index: 9/45 (threshold = 13)[68]

Auditory-Perceptual Assessment
The CAPE-V[15] was administered and the patient was rated to have an overall CAPE-V score of 38/100, indicating a dysphonia of a moderate nature. Aberrant perceptual features in the voice include primary roughness, strain, intermittent breathiness, and pitch breaks. Vocal loudness was noted to be within normal limits. Pitch of the voice was within normal limits for age and gender; however, this sits in contrast to patient-perceived lowered pitch from her baseline. Resonance was balanced and within normal limits. Respiration was primarily abdominal with limited clavicle/chest elevation engagement.

Manual Palpation Assessment
Perilaryngeal palpation revealed mild clinician-perceived tension and moderate patient-perceived tenderness of the thyrohyoid space, as well as moderate tension and moderate tenderness of the suprahyoid area. When Diane engaged in speaking voice tasks, the clinician measured a sharp increase in perceived global laryngeal tension and elevation.

Acoustic and Aerodynamic Assessment
All data gathered for the assessment utilized Pentax Medical (Montvale, NJ) software

Analysis of Dysphonia in Speech and Voice (ADSV) and the Voice Range Profile (VRP). The protocols utilized are from the established American Speech-Language-Hearing Association Expert Panel to Develop a Protocol for Instrumental Assessment of Vocal Function (IVAP).[78] A handheld microphone was placed at a 90-degree angle at 3 to 5 inches from the mouth for data acquisition. Results of the assessment can be found in Table 8–12. Normative data were derived from Lewandowski et al and Pierce et al.[22,79]

Laryngeal Imaging
The laryngologist performed laryngeal videostroboscopy transorally with a rigid videolaryngoscope and the SLP was present. The examination found no supraglottal or hypopharyngeal masses. A right mid vocal fold edge lesion was observed, resulting in mildly reduced vibratory characteristics (mucosal wave and amplitude) of the right vocal fold. Evidence was present to support the potential for the early development of a contralateral lesion of the left vocal fold. There was full abduction and adduction of both vocal folds. Hourglass glottic closure was observed throughout all voicing tasks and range. Mild supraglottic hyperfunction and mediolateral compression were observed throughout the exam.

When assessing acoustic, aerodynamic, auditory-perceptual, or laryngeal examination findings, it is crucial to keep in mind that there are currently limited data available to establish a correlation between the severity of a vocal fold polyp and abnormalities (or stability) in voice characteristics.[80,81] This helps explain why individuals like Diane, as well as many other professional voice users with vocal fold lesions, can display objective voicing measures that are either typical or closely resemble typical values despite experiencing vocal limitations.

Postexam Decision Making
Diane presents with moderate dysphonia characterized by roughness, strain, and inter-

Table 8–12. Acoustic and Aerodynamic Assessment Results

	Rainbow Passage	Sustained Vowel	Norms	X Indicates Abnormal
Mean F0 (Hz)	187 Hz	175 Hz	158-229 Hz	
SD (Hz)	35.6 Hz	3.2 Hz	19.5-31.1 Hz	
Physiological Pitch Range (Hz)	130-739 Hz C3-F#5			

Sustained Vowel /a/	Results	Norms	X Indicates Abnormal
CPP (dB)	8.772 dB	8.6-14.9 dB	
CPP SD (dB)	0.503 dB	1.8 dB	
L/H Spectral Ratio (dB)	32.2 dB	30.8-44.6 dB	
L/H Spectral Ratio SD (dB)	1.06 dB	1.0-2.0 dB	
Mean CPP F0 (Hz)	175 Hz	160-305 Hz	
CPP F0 SD (Hz)	3.56 Hz	31.1 Hz	

Aerodynamic Measures	Results	Norms	X Indicates Abnormal
Mean Airflow During Voicing (L/sec): Rainbow Passage	2.3 L/sec	1.6 L/sec (SD 0.5)	X (abnormal high)
Duration (sec)	22 sec	23.15 sec (SD 2.67)	
Breaths (#)	6	4.72 (SD 1.73)	

mittent breathiness. Following laryngology evaluation, she was diagnosed with a right vocal fold polyp. During the evaluation, Diane responded well to voice therapy strategies. Flow phonation showed reduced laryngeal compression, and lip trills using a 1-3-5-3-1 pitch pattern demonstrated improved breath/voice coordination, especially in areas of her voice where she endorsed difficulty. Considering the examination findings and the impact on her daily functioning, both the laryngologist and speech pathologist recommended surgical removal of the vocal fold polyp to offer Diane the best chance of returning to her baseline vocal function. However, due to her ongoing teaching commitments in the middle of the fall semester, taking an extended leave from the classroom was not feasible. After thorough discussion and shared decision making with the voice care team, Diane opted for a different approach. She decided to undergo preoperative voice therapy to prevent further deterioration of the vocal fold lesion and improve her overall vocal function. This period of preoperative therapy would also help her prepare for the postoperative voicing and recovery expectations, aligning with her current situation and commitments.

Plan of Care

Diane's therapy plan included 1 session every 1 to 2 weeks until she could undergo microlaryngeal surgery (MLS) with the laryngologist to address the vocal fold polyp. After the surgery, it was advised that Diane continue therapy at the same frequency, with sessions occurring in person at the voice center, until she was discharged from the active care of the voice team.

Preoperative Therapy Goals

Long-Term Goal. Achieve balanced voicing in the context of a vocal fold lesion that results in reduced patient-perceived voice effort and fatigue

Short-Term Goals:

1. Integrate indirect therapeutic intervention into activities of daily voicing to reduce vocal load and increase overall voice hygiene
2. Independently apply series of SOVT exercises to daily warm-up routine at 80% of opportunities to help reestablish the patient's perceived baseline voicing effort

Intervention

Preoperative Therapy

Initial focus was placed on identifying Diane's essential voice requirements and personal voice-related goals. She needed to fulfill her duties as a high school music teacher and maintain vital social connections with family and friends. These were critical to her qual-ity of life, and the primary objective during preoperative therapy was to help her effectively manage these voice demands. This was achieved through a combination of direct and indirect intervention strategies.

Diane's indirect strategies included implementing a voice hygiene program emphasizing systemic and surface hydration, introducing voice conservation techniques, and incorporating planned periods of relative voice rest. Within the first session, these strategies were tailored to suit the demands of Diane's high-intensity teaching environment. Diane typically taught multiple choral classes daily, each with over 50 students, in a spacious rehearsal space. To address vocal intensity, the clinician focused on reducing the impact of vocal stress. Diane opted for a megaphone-like system over wearable amplification, allowing her to adjust volume as needed without relying on a wearable device. This choice offered versatility, as she could quickly remove the amplification for one-on-one student interactions. The next target for behavioral modification was how Diane conducted her choral rehearsals. Given her vocal strength, endurance, and wide vocal range before the vocal fold lesion, she was accustomed to modeling every voice part during rehearsals. To help her grasp the concept of vocal expenditure, the analogy of a "voice bank" was introduced, emphasizing the idea of managing vocal resources. By adjusting her classroom instructional style to rely more on spoken verbal cues and place greater emphasis on pitch from the piano, she significantly reduced the vocal effort required to meet her teaching needs.

One of Diane's primary goals was to reduce voice effort and fatigue. Although the use of surface electromyography (sEMG) was not conducted, palpable evidence of hyperfunction was observed during laryngeal endoscopy, closely aligning with Diane's perception of voice effort and fatigue. Diane had prior experience with straw phonation, a form of SOVT exercises known for improving breath and voice coordination, from her voice teacher. In the second and third therapy sessions, SOVT tasks were integrated into her daily warm-up routine. The hierarchy implemented is as follows:

1. Starting with single-pitch straw phonation, Diane selected the comfortable pitch Bb3. This involved repeating single-pitched tasks, emphasizing that voicing exercises need not be complex to be effective. This simple SOVT task allowed Diane to regain ease and reduce voice effort without added strain or fatigue, laying the foundation for more advanced exercises.

2. Diane progressed to voice glides within her speaking range, focusing on intensity modulation without specific pitch patterns. These glides covered Diane's typical speaking voice range (G3-E4), enabling her to adjust breath, phonation, and resonance based on her sensations and desired sounds. Diane could extend to higher pitches (around or above G4) when speaking more energetically. The goal remained vocal ease, and when faced with challenges or increased effort, Diane isolated specific pitches and reviewed strategies to alleviate strain.

3. Finally, the clinician introduced structured pitch patterns across a wider voicing range, paying attention to challenging areas or increased effort. Diane worked on small interval pitch patterns that grew in complexity as she gained confidence and comfort. Starting with a 1-3-1 pattern from A3 to G4, Diane identified these as "hot spots" in her speaking voice patterns. These structured patterns helped Diane fine-tune her strategies for specific pitches or groups across her vocal range. The patterns were extended to 1-3-5-3-1 or 1-3-5-6-5-3-1, with Diane reaching up to D5, resulting in tension release, ease in production, and improved voice quality.

It's worth noting that in the preoperative stage, the SLP largely acted as a facilitator. Through systematic work with straw phonation, Diane, a professional voice user, reflected on her voice effort and adjusted her voicing patterns as needed. The SLP's role as a facilitator empowered Diane as an expert in her voice function. Many indirect strategies, coupled with direct therapeutic intervention, reduced Diane's overall voicing effort and provided significant relief.

Pre- and Postoperative Evaluation

Between the initial therapy and preoperative reevaluation with the SLP and laryngologist, approximately 2 months elapsed. During this time, Diane attended 5 therapy sessions and identified behaviors contributing to the severity of her voice fatigue and effort. She reported an overall improved experience with her voice.

Following this period, Diane underwent microlaryngeal surgery (MLS) with the laryngologist and had a follow-up appointment with the voice care team 7 days postoperatively. During this 7-day postoperative phase, Diane was advised to observe complete voice rest. Stroboscopy at the follow-up appointment revealed mild edema on the right mid vocal fold at the procedure site, along with mildly reduced vibratory characteristics of the right vocal fold and incomplete glottic closure. The incomplete closure was likely attributed to Diane's expressed fear of causing harm to her voice or interfering with the procedure. Diane received positive feedback regarding the findings and expressed eagerness to commence postoperative therapy. Research has shown that a combination of MLS and postoperative voice therapy leads to improvements in both patient-perceived and clinician-measured vocal quality.[82]

Postop Therapeutic Intervention

In Diane's case, postoperative therapeutic intervention significantly differed from the functional target before the surgery, given the change in her laryngeal mechanism post-surgery. In total, Diane attended 6 postoperative therapy sessions. The treatment goals shifted from mitigating voice fatigue and effort to allowing time for postoperative healing, strengthening her voice, and gradually reintroducing complex voicing tasks at her comfort level. Understanding the postoperative healing stage remains a work in progress. A progressive therapy approach while monitoring ongoing improvement could look like:

- ▪ **Continued Postoperative Evaluation.** Regular check-ins with the laryngologist and speech pathologist to track progress and address any concerns
- ▪ **Returning to Pre-Lesion Function.** Aiming for Diane's self-perceived voice quality and effort to reach pre-lesion levels
- ▪ **Measurable Improvement.** Assessing improvements in both objective and subjective voicing function for speaking and singing tasks

The postoperative therapeutic process for vocal fold lesions can be broken down into stages:

- ▪ **Acute Phase (1 to 3 Weeks Post-Voice Rest).** This phase emphasizes understanding Diane's current limitations, addressing breathiness, and improving voicing ease. The focus is on coordinating breath and voice, mitigating vocal fold impact stress, and using resonant voice techniques. Exercises are unstructured, reducing emphasis on voice quality.
- ▪ **Postacute Phase (4 to 7 Weeks Post-Voice Rest).** The goal in this phase is to achieve improved voice quality, reduce breathiness, improve resonance, and naturally increase intensity. This phase highlights structured voicing exercises, often introducing small-interval pitch patterns. Diane, as a professional voice user, gradually extended exercise intensity and frequency, exploring speaking voice endurance and loudness.

- ▪ **Long-Term Rehabilitation and Maintenance (8+ Weeks Postsurgery).** This phase integrates all expected voicing tasks, including speaking and singing. Timed sessions help observe positive voicing behaviors and address factors contributing to perceived effort or fatigue. For singing, one might start with simple songs, progressively adding complexity. Techniques learned in earlier phases are applied to both speaking and singing.

This staged approach offers a structured framework for postoperative voice therapy, ensuring tailored care to support Diane's recovery and her pursuit of her voice goals.

> The author does an excellent job here of describing how postoperative voice therapy changes over time as the healing process advances. The reader is guided to learn more about post operative wound healing through a primer by Branski et al, 2006.[83]

Voice Teacher Handoff

The final phase of therapy involves transitioning Diane's care to her established voice teacher. This collaboration between the SLP and the voice teacher has been nurtured throughout the entire voice care journey. Diane's voice teacher has been kept informed of her progress at each stage with her consent. This collaboration enables Diane's voice teacher to continue guiding her after she is discharged. The SLP does not aim to replace the voice teacher but rather to complement their expertise. This established relationship allows the SLP and voice teacher to identify the specific skills needed for Diane to return to her baseline function. It also ensures ongoing communication with the voice care team in case of any future concerns or challenges in voicing function. In Diane's case, the voice teacher integrated learned therapeutic techniques into Diane's warm-up and cool-down routine. This included benchmarks such as rating voice quality, assessing voice effort, and fine-tuning auditory-perceptual qualities to enhance Diane's self-awareness of her voice.

Posttreatment Outcome and Reflection

At discharge, Diane noted a significant decrease in her perceived roughness, strain, and voice effort, and demonstrated improvement across her acoustic baseline measures. With an integration of singing voice tasks, she endorsed feeling significantly more prepared to meet the demand of her daily activities.[84,85] She was encouraged to follow up with the voice care team whenever needed. Given her high voicing demands as a teacher and performer, it would not be uncommon for her to encounter any level of voice challenge moving forward. It is not the goal of the voice care team to keep every professional voice user in constant care. However, keeping an open relationship where the voice care team exists as a resource during any time of voicing need is encouraged and should be established before discharge.

CASE STUDY 8.8

Perioperative Management for an Adult Jazz Singer With a Vocal Fold Cyst

Sarah L. Schneider and Mark S. Courey

Voice Evaluation

Chief Complaint. Voice changes in speaking and singing

DF was seen for a comprehensive voice evaluation in an interdisciplinary clinic with a voice-trained SLP and fellowship-trained laryngologist.

Case History

History of Voice Complaint. DF is a 39-year-old cisgender woman. She is a jazz singer and performs on and off in local and regional clubs. She is also a Hebrew teacher, both one-on-one and in a classroom setting. Her voice changes developed gradually over the last year without a specific inciting event. They impact her ability to teach and perform. Her singing is unreliable, with pitch breaks in her midrange and increasing difficulty accessing her head voice. Over the same period, her speaking voice has become rougher, with intermittent voice breaks and increased effort. Vocal fatigue and anterior neck discomfort are present with both speaking and singing. DF was diagnosed with a right vocal fold lesion and referred for voice therapy at an outside institution. After 2 sessions of therapy, surgery was recommended. She is seeking a second opinion.

DF is married with 2 children. She teaches about 5 private students per week, sings daily, and rehearses 2 to 3 times per month with her jazz trio. She sings a few gigs per month with amplification and an external voice monitor. She drinks 64 ounces of water and 2 cups of coffee per day. She smokes marijuana occasionally and drinks alcohol socially. She denies any breathing or swallowing concerns. She has no history of prior voice issues and no symptoms of reflux, sinusitis, nasal congestion, or nasal drainage.

Vocal History. DF obtained her undergraduate degree at a jazz conservatory and is an alto. She has studied with a voice teacher intermittently since college.

Patient-Reported Outcome Measures

Results of the provided patient-reported outcome measures are detailed in Table 8–13.[11,67,68,86–88]

Auditory-Perceptual Evaluation

Overall CAPE-V[15] was 52/100, indicating a moderate dysphonia, with roughness 34/100, breathiness 44/100, and strain 16/100. Aphonic voice breaks were noted during reading and spontaneous speech, with intermittent delayed voice onset. Resonance was focused posteriorly in the throat. Respiration was primarily thoracic and abdominal and not well coordinated with phonation. High shoulder placement was observed.

Laryngeal Palpation

Perilaryngeal muscle tension was assessed in the thyrohyoid and suprahyoid regions and rated on a visual analog scale from 0 (no tension) to 100 (most tension). The thyrohyoid region was 75/100 and suprahyoid region 75/100. The patient rated tenderness on the pain scale 0 (no pain) to 10 (worst pain) as 4/10 in the thyrohyoid region and 3/10 in the suprahyoid region.

Acoustic Assessment

Acoustic data were gathered remotely using Phonalyze by Cognizn, a web-based portal using Praat algorithms (https://phonalyze.com). Patients are sent a link via text message and record themselves with their phone positioned about 12 inches from their mouth. Normative data were derived from a literature review examining optimal norms for remote acoustic voice analysis.[88] Results are noted in Tables 8–14 through 8–17.

Stimulability Testing

Stimulability testing was completed using lip trills. There was a change in ease and quality at the phrase level in English and Hebrew. The patient identified changes in the sound and feel.

Laryngeal Imaging

Continuous Light. Using rigid endoscopy, a right vocal fold broad-based, yellow-appearing, subepithelial lesion at the junction of the anterior and middle third was observed and was surrounded by fresh blood.

Stroboscopic Light. Severe asymmetry of vibration developed with increasing pitch. Above 400 Hz, vibration was observed anterior to posterior around the lesion, which is referred to as teeter-totter vibration. Vertical phase difference and mucosal wave were moderately reduced over the right vocal fold lesion at low and modal pitches and absent at higher pitches (about 400 Hz). An asymmetric hourglass closure was noted.

Impression

This is a 39-year-old cisgender woman with a right vocal fold lesion (possible cyst), resolving right vocal fold hemorrhage, and secondary muscle tension dysphonia (MTD). She has moderate dysphonia with a breathy/rough quality, increased strain, and intermittent aphonic voice breaks in the setting of increased perilaryngeal tension and tenderness. She is stimulable for more balanced airflow and resonance with less strain to the phrase level; however, her voice remains breathy and rough,

Table 8–13. Patient-Reported Outcome Measures

Patient-Reported Measures	Preop	Postop
Voice Handicap Index–10 (VHI-10)	23/40	0/40
Reflux Symptom Index (RSI)	22/45	0/45
Dyspnea Index (DI)	8/40	0/40
Cough Severity Index (CSI)	1/40	0/40
Eating Assessment Tool–10 (EAT-10)	3/40	0/40
Singing Voice Handicap Index–10 (SVHI-10)	28/40	7/40

8. Performance Voice 417

Table 8–14. CPP in Sustained Vowel

	Preop	Postop	Norms
CPP	39.52	32.65	N/A
CPPS	14.3	8.29	F: 15.08 (2.04) / M: 17.18 (2.71)
Mean F0 (Hz)	251.55*	237.84*	F: 210.4 (22.7) / M: 110.91 (16.1)
Mean F0 SD (Hz)	5.95	28.55*	F: 2.37 (5.24) / M: 0.75 (0.28)

*indicates range out of normal value

Table 8–15. CPP in All-Voiced Sentence

	Preop	Postop	Norms
AVQI	1.64	**	F: 2.60 (0.67) / M: 2.28 (0.91)
CPP	26.03	**	N/A
Mean F0 (Hz)	221.23	**	F: 197.90 (16.70) / M: 133.1 (15.2)
Mean F0 SD (Hz)	30.21	**	F: 33.17 (5.82) / M: 51.34 (18.5)

*indicates range out of normal value. **not available

Table 8–16. CPP in the Rainbow Passage

	Preop	Postop	Norms
CPP	35.34	30.35	N/A
CPPS	8.34*	10.52*	F: 7.59 (0.73) / M: 7.22 (0.79)
Mean F0 (Hz)	223.95*	237.46*	F: 197.90 (16.70) / M: 133.1 (15.2)
Mean F0 SD (Hz)	36.63	41.37*	F: 33.17 (5.82) / M: 51.34 (18.5)

*indicates range out of normal value

Table 8–17. Physiological Pitch Range (Hz)

	Hertz	Notes	Semitone Range	Semitone Range Norms
Preop	200-466*	G3-Bb4*	16*	F: 37 (8) / M: 38 (13)*
Postop	187-886	F3-A5	29	F: 37 (8) / M: 38 (13)

*indicates range out of normal value

as expected given her diagnosis. She can identify the difference in the sound and feel and maintain it briefly in conversation following exercises. Given the cystic appearance of the vocal fold lesion,[89] high vocal demand, and limited ability to maintain necessary vocal function, expectations for recovery with voice therapy alone are low. However, voice therapy is recommended to observe for hemorrhage resolution and to work with the patient to optimize vocal hygiene and voice production patterns, followed by reevaluation and further consideration for surgical excision and postoperative voice rehabilitation.

Plan of Care

The patient was educated on the role of voice therapy. She was advised to begin practicing vocal exercises, 3 to 5 times per day for 2 to 3 minutes each time and to generalize the sensation of balanced phonation into all styles of voice production, even if it meant that her voice quality deteriorated. The goal was to eliminate ongoing trauma from secondary MTD and to promote healing if she underwent surgical excision. As there is a low likelihood that cystic lesions will resolve with therapy alone, a limited discussion of the risks, benefits, and alternatives for surgical excision of the lesion was undertaken. The discussion centered on the importance of resolving her secondary MTD to eliminate ongoing trauma and to promote postoperative healing. She was told that "pushing" voice postoperatively was thought to delay healing and increase the chance of postoperative stiffness, and could result in permanent vocal deterioration and/or developing a second or recurrent lesion. The patient, SLP, and laryngologist all agreed with the plan of care.

Goals of Preoperative Voice Therapy:

1. Optimize vocal hygiene and decision making by reducing phonotrauma, maintaining hydration, and balancing vocal on and off time to avoid vocal deterioration with use

2. Introduce voice exercises to optimize airflow and resonance while also increasing self-awareness of voice use patterns and self-efficacy to support postoperative recovery

3. Educate the patient regarding postoperative complete voice rest, modified voice use, and return to singing

Decision Making

In all voice users, the cost/benefit of conservative versus more aggressive behavioral or medical/surgical intervention is considered. Behavioral voice production patterns are involved in either the development or persistence of all non-neoplastic vocal fold lesions. Therefore, discussions exploring the patient's motivation and self-efficacy to modify methods of voice production are critical to support successful therapeutic and surgical outcomes. If a patient with increased vocal problems and mucosal changes is resistant to making vocal modifications, then their willingness and ability to follow postoperative guidelines promoting healing and reducing the risk of recurrent problems is questionable. A short trial of voice therapy is critical to learn more about the patient and their engagement in this process.

Intervention

Voice Therapy

The patient returned for 2 sessions of voice therapy, via video visit, over a 4-week period. At her initial session, she reported several vocal hygiene modifications and practiced established voice exercises several times daily. The exercises were helpful in reducing strain and feeling the sound in her mouth. However, her voice remained variable.

Meta-therapy, the conversations that help build a framework to modify a patient's knowledge, attitude, and awareness of the process of vocal improvement, was used throughout the sessions.[91] Indirect voice therapy included education on the anatomy and physiology of voice production, how vocal fold lesions impact voice use and vice versa, and how this relates to current concerns and vocal experiences. Managing vocal on and off time to avoid voice deterioration or fatigue/discomfort associated with voice use was explored.

The clinician advised the patient on recommended voice use schedules believed to promote healing. These included 1 week of complete voice rest followed by 3 weeks of modified voice use. Modified voice use is a gradual return to voice use based on the patient's progress in vocal quality, stamina/fatigue, and vocal effort. Typically, speaking voice use will return to normal about 1 month after surgery. Exploring range during voice exercises will begin 1 week after surgery, and limited singing may be resumed about 1 month postoperatively. Postoperative therapy is generally once every other week for 3 months, with exercises to practice and techniques to apply between sessions.

Direct voice therapy included laryngeal massage, tongue stretches, and lip trills. Perilaryngeal massage in the thyrohyoid and suprahyoid region were targeted. The patient was advised that massage could be used before or after periods of voice use to promote ease and reduce discomfort. She was advised to perform it 3 to 5 times per day for 1 minute in each location. Tongue stretches included:

1. Extend the tongue toward the chin, with the tongue wide, and hold. Observe a stretch at the back of the tongue, along the sides, and/or in the submandibular region.
2. Extend the tongue up toward the nose, release the jaw, and hold. Observe a stretch underneath the tongue.
3. Place the tongue tip behind the bottom teeth and arch the tongue up and out (like a "backbend"). Observe a stretch in the back of the tongue, along the sides, and/or in the submandibular region.

For all stretches, the jaw should release in a neutral position, and counterpressure at the temporomandibular joint can be applied as needed. Each stretch was to be performed 3 times each and held for about 2 breaths. (See Video 30 Tongue Stretches by Schneider.)

Lip trills, established during the evaluation, were reviewed. Three specific tenets were used to establish efficient voice production and promote patient independence with problem solving: (1) exhale consistent airflow during phonation, (2) maintain an easy throat (reduced effort/pressure), and (3) feel the sensation of voice in the mouth. Resonant voice production helps reduce the impact of vocal fold vibration to decrease inflammation and promote healing.[60] Ensuring patients understand this benefit can promote therapeutic "buy in" for practicing structured exercises and further for application of therapy techniques in daily speaking.

Over 2 sessions, lip trills were used to maintain ease and quality of voice production as complexity of tasks increased and then use of the trill faded. Reset words (eg, words used daily such as "yes," "no," "sure," "fine") were introduced and practiced with and without use of the lip trill. Practicing reset words to apply in day-to-day conversation without the use of a facilitator helps promote carryover and the ability to "reset" to the new voice use patterns during daily talking.

> "Reset words" that accentuate a sensation of anterior vibrations or forward resonance are an essential tool in voice therapy. Using a reset word helps remind the brain and body how to produce an easy, effortless voice. Encourage the patient to pick words with a strong resonant sensation, practice them daily, and use them in conversation to "reset" the voice back to comfortable baseline whenever they feel their voice becoming tense, fatigued, effortful, or uncomfortable.

Surgical Decision Making

Based on her demonstration of balanced phonation, resolution of the hemorrhage, and persistence of the cyst despite behavioral intervention, the patient was counseled on the risks and benefits of surgical cyst excision. Risks included persisting right vocal fold stiffness either due to the cyst or the surgical dissection, resulting in incomplete return of voice or further vocal decline due to loss of vocal flexibility, decrease in quality with roughness and strain, loss of range, and loss of ability to speak or sing in a meaningful manner. The clinician stressed the importance of postoperative therapy, training airflow, and resonant voice production. Vibratory rates of vocal fold fibroblasts have been shown to affect production of mRNA and extracellular matrix proteins that influence healing.[92] Therefore, balanced voice production during the immediate healing phase may affect overall healing and vocal fold vibratory function. In plain terms, surgery and lack of adherence to voice recommendations could result in vocal fold scarring with loss of the ability to speak or sing. Lastly, the clinician discussed the small probability that the lesion would reoccur.

Surgical Techniques

A microlaryngoscope was placed through the mouth to expose the vocal folds and allow direct access with microsurgical instruments. The vocal folds were closely inspected with 0- and 70-degree telescopes. A binocular microscope was used to view the vocal folds at high magnification for the surgery. Palpation revealed that the lesion was adherent to the deeper layers of the vocal fold. A surgical plan to approach the lesion through an area of normal mucosa was formulated. Once the normal structures were identified, sharp dissection with micro instruments was undertaken to identify and separate the lesion along with its supporting abnormal blood vessels from the surrounding normal tissues. Epinephrine was applied topically to control bleeding. The remaining normal mucosal structures were replaced over the surgical site to promote primary healing.

Postoperative Recovery and Voice Therapy

Weeks 1 to 4. Recent evidence suggests that surgically induced inflammation resolves by postoperative day 3 or 5[93] and that early mobilization of the vocal folds with efficient vibratory patterns may result in improved healing characteristics. Due to clinic scheduling, this patient was asked to observe 6 days of complete voice rest postoperatively to allow resolution of edema.

At 6 days postoperatively, auditory-perceptual evaluation revealed a mild to moderate breathy quality with mild to moderate strain, moderately reduced intensity, and mildly increased pitch.

Vocal fold stiffness is common following cyst excision and may manifest in the described vocal quality, especially after a week of voice rest. Stroboscopy confirmed erythema and stiffness of the right vocal fold. At low frequency, there was evidence of subtle vibration. The patient was advised to speak about 5 to 10 minutes per hour and to listen to her body. If she experienced increased vocal strain, fatigue, or a negative change in quality, she should rest her voice. She was counseled to maintain hydration, avoid loud voice use, and use alternatives to throat clearing. The patient asked if continued voice rest would be better for her voice to "maximize healing." However, the clinician encouraged her to use her voice to promote vocal fold vibration and healing and discussed recent studies on vocal fold wound healing indicate that balanced production of voice, limited short periods of voice rest, and low-impact vocal fold vibration promote healing.[94]

Lip trills were reinitiated with focus on balancing phonatory airflow and achieving oral resonance without strain on sustained sounds, glides, and sirens for about 2 minutes, 5 times per day. The patient was advised to stop voice exercises if they exacerbated strain, caused fatigue, or resulted in negative change in vocal quality. If there were several hours of quiet during the day, voice exercises should be completed in lieu of complete voice rest.

Experiencing intense sensations of oral resonance requires rapid and relatively complete vocal fold closure to produce a robust acoustic signal. Right vocal fold stiffness and incomplete glottic closure pattern result in a weaker vocal signal, and harmonics cannot be amplified by the shape of the vocal tract in the same way. The patient was educated and reassured that she would not feel the same vibration of sound that she felt previously during therapy. As vocal fold pliability and closure improve, the sensation associated with increased oral-nasal resonant voice production should return.

Postop week 2, during voice therapy via video visit, laryngeal massage and tongue stretches were resumed to address reported tightness and vocal fatigue. Lip trills were reviewed and then transitioned to resonant voice exercises using /m/, moving through the hierarchy of tasks from phonemes (exploring her pitch range in preparation to resume singing) to conversation, in both English and Hebrew. It is important to note that moving through an exact hierarchy is less important than supporting the patient to identify changes in voice production patterns related to airflow, resonance, ease, and quality. If the patient can reliably identify these changes, use conversation, and troubleshoot lapses, they can begin to reset their voice from habitual to target patterns.

Each week for the first month postoperatively, the patient's voice use time was gradually increased. By postoperative week 4, she had nearly resumed daily voice use patterns with continued regard for vocal awareness and self-monitoring.

Weeks 4 to 8. By 4 weeks postoperatively, stroboscopy revealed an increasing vertical phase difference on the right vocal fold at modal and low pitches with some increase in mucosal wave. DF's speaking voice was mildly breathy with more balanced airflow and oral resonance.

She had not returned to teaching but was feeling closer to normal in day-to-day speaking.

As speaking voice time increased, vocal exercises were increased. Lip trills and resonant voice exercises continued in speaking. High-level vocal tasks for singing were introduced. Vocalises (1-5-1, 1-2-3-4-5-4-3-2-1, 1-3-2-4-3-5-4-2-1) in a comfortable range, gradually extending her pitch range in both directions, were targeted (G3-F5), initially with lip trills and then tongue-out trills to help increase awareness of tongue tension, and then moved on to semi-occluded vowels as she progressed through her range.

Weeks 8 to 12. Stroboscopy continued to show improvement in vibratory parameters, but with continued reduction of vertical phase difference and mucosal wave on the right, especially with increasing pitch. Use of resonant voice production in spontaneous talking was reinforced, and singing voice became the primary focus. The patient reported her voice felt "small" and her range remained reduced. When beginning to move from SOVT exercises to open vowels, her voice became breathy and her middle voice (E4-C5) was unstable and weaker.

Keeping in mind how reduced vibratory parameters on the right vocal fold may impact vocal ease and quality, work continued to balance the transition from SOVT exercises to open vowels paired various consonants (eg, tongue-out trills to /m/ to vowels, /vui/, /via/,

> This patient is multilingual and uses her voice occupationally in English and Hebrew. It is important for the SLP to learn about language and dialectical differences in voice production when working with someone whose first language is not English. The reader is reminded that not all phonemes in the English language occur in other languages and resonant placements may differ; this may impact both perception and production of voice if the patient's first language is not English.

422 Voice Therapy: Clinical Case Studies

y-buzz to /ya/). This was completed on increasingly complex note patterns matched to her singing genre. Attention was paid to balancing thyroarytenoid versus cricothyroid activation, along with resonance, to optimize ease and quality while working toward the desired sound production. When DF began to maintain vocal consistency with less resistance in the anterior portion of the mouth, these techniques were incorporated into her repertoire. Her middle voice began to stabilize and slowly gain strength. With progress in both speaking and singing, at postop week 10 she felt confident to resume one-on-one Hebrew lessons with about five, 1-hour students per week.

Weeks 12 and Beyond. The patient maintained her one-on-one teaching and resumed classroom teaching with voice amplification about 4 months postoperatively. She also resumed rehearsals with her jazz trio. She used amplification and a monitor during rehearsals. She sang her first gig about 5 months postoperatively, a short performance with only 2 songs. It was an excellent goal to work toward because it increased her vocal confidence related to performance. Daily voice use patterns were consistent at this point. She generally did not experience vocal fatigue. Speaking voice quality was borderline breathy to normal and remained consistent regardless of the amount and type of voice use. As her vocal demand increased and she was maintaining therapeutic gains, the frequency of voice therapy sessions went from monthly to intermittent check-ins to ensure consistency, carryover, and opportunities to troubleshoot more athletic vocal tasks such as projected voice use and higher-impact voice use (eg, growling, belting). She resumed work with a voice teacher.

Postoperative Evaluation

Interval History

The patient returned 9 months after surgery for interdisciplinary evaluation. She reported intermittent vocal variability, mostly due to fatigue related to the level of vocal demand and life stressors. She managed without significant swings in vocal quality or long periods of voice rest. She could reset her voice with exercises and found ways to readjust her schedule. She maintained regular warm-up and cool-down routines and independent bodywork to manage personal tension and stressors. She worked with her voice teacher occasionally. She was mindful of vocal decisions, could meet all personal and professional vocal demands, and generally did not feel limited by her voice.

Patient-Reported Outcome Measures

Postoperative patient-reported outcome measures were completed. Results are in Table 8–13.

Auditory-Perceptual Evaluation

Overall CAPE-V score was 4/100, indicating inconsistent borderline dysphonia, roughness of 0/100, inconsistent breathiness of 4/100, and inconsistent strain of 4/100.

Laryngeal Palpation

Tension in the thyrohyoid region was rated 10/100 and suprahyoid region 28/100. The patient rated tenderness in the thyrohyoid region as 0/10 and in the suprahyoid region as 2/10.

Acoustic Assessment

Posttreatment acoustic measures are documented in Tables 8–14 through 8–17.

Laryngeal Imaging

Continuous Light. Symmetric vocal fold adduction and abduction. No vocal fold lesions.

Stroboscopic Light. Vibration was mostly regular. Vibratory parameters were mildly reduced on the right vocal fold at low and modal pitches and severely reduced at higher pitches. Closure was complete at higher intensity and slit-like at low intensity.

Impression

This is a 39 year-old cisgender woman who is a jazz singer and Hebrew teacher 9 months post-microflap excision of a mucous retention cyst. She reports improvement in vocal quality, range, and stamina/dependability. The patient attended 2 sessions of preoperative voice therapy over a 4-week period and 11 sessions postoperatively (twice per month for 4 months, then once per month for 2 months, then once every other month for 1 session). Perceptual and stroboscopic findings improved compared to the preoperative exam. The patient can meet all vocal demands with minimal fatigue or change in quality with use. She manages her voice well and will benefit from maintaining mindful vocal decision making, warming up and cooling down as established, and continuing work with her singing teacher. Further voice therapy is not recommended at this time.

Plan of Care

The patient is discharged from voice therapy. She will follow up with the interprofessional team in 3 months to assess progress 1 year postoperatively.

Decision Making

The patient reported and demonstrated vocal improvement after combined intervention. It is common after cyst excision to have some residual vocal fold stiffness from either the development of the cyst or the dissection to remove it. Given recent vocal variability, follow-up at 1 year postoperatively is required to assess sustained gains.

Summary: Clinician Reflections

Many factors need to be considered when evaluating and treating professional and performing voice users with vocal concerns. Cases such as this are multifactorial and require a multidisciplinary approach to be most successful. In addition to the typical medical and behavioral considerations, it is paramount that we understand the professional/performer's lifestyle, vocal demand, vocal expectations, and schedule. Preoperative voice therapy can often also be the best postoperative therapy. In some cases, voice therapy alone can help avoid surgical intervention. In the cases it does not, the goal is to provide the patient with the knowledge and skills necessary to achieve the best vocal outcome and avoid future voice problems.

 CASE STUDY 8.9

Multimodality Voice Therapy for a Prepubescent Singer With Vocal Nodules

Patricia Doyle and Starr Cookman

Voice Evaluation

Chief Complaint. Dysphonia, vocal fatigue associated with speaking and singing, vocal range restriction

History of Voice Complaint

Patient DH is a 9-year-old cisgender female semiprofessional actor and singer (since age 5) who presented to the clinic with a complaint of persistent hoarseness over the past 2 years. Onset of the problem occurred after she performed while dysphonic in a musical theater show at a residential summer performing arts camp. The day after, she was nearly aphonic. Although her voice improved somewhat with rest, it did not fully recover. In response, the patient's mother sought the assistance of a vocal coach, with whom DH worked for 6 months. DH's voice worsened during this period. When DH was 8 years old, her mother switched from a vocal coach to a voice teacher. This teacher focused on techniques and gave DH vocal hygiene recommendations. After 1 year of instruction, DH's voice continued to remain moderately dysphonic after singing. At this point, her pediatrician referred her to an otolaryngologist.

DH was born 2.5 weeks premature and spent 1 day in the NICU. She reached all developmental milestones on time. At age 8, she developed a whooping cough lasting 2 to 3 months. At the time of the assessment, she

424 Voice Therapy: Clinical Case Studies

was not taking any medications and reported no known allergies. DH's mother noted that she herself had been hoarse since childhood but had never sought a diagnosis. DH is not exposed to secondary smoke. She drinks approximately 1 caffeinated soda weekly and 50 to 60 ounces of water daily. The Reflux Symptom Index (RSI) score at the time of her assessment was 9, with 13 or greater being suggestive of reflux.

Voice Use

At home, DH lives with an older brother and her parents, where she talks frequently and yells at her brother an average of 2 or 3 times per day. DH's mother reported, "She is singing all the time." At school, DH participates in class and talks socially with her peers during lunch and recess. She also plays soccer 5 times per week, yelling frequently during practice and games. She participates in a singing lesson once a week for 1 hour. She auditions for voice-overs and commercials 2 to 3 times monthly (she has been cast 3 times in the past year) and sings in several local theater productions annually. DH described herself as an alto who sings in a contemporary belted musical theater style. Overall, she estimated singing for 2 to 4 hours on a typical day and for a maximum of 6 hours in her busiest vocal scenario.

Laryngeal Imaging

Laryngeal videostroboscopy was completed at the time of the otolaryngological evaluation with a rigid, 70-degree endoscope. The larynx was adequately visualized during sustained phonation at approximately 350 Hz. Laryngeal observations made at the time of the initial examination included bilateral, nontransparent vocal fold nodules at the midpoint of the vibrating portion of the true vocal folds. The base of the right nodule was broader than the left. An hourglass-shaped glottal configuration prevailed during vibratory cycles. Also observed were anterior-to-

posterior phase asymmetry, moderate decrease of the amplitude of vibration bilaterally, and slight decrease in mucosal wave propagation bilaterally. Periodicity of vocal fold vibration, arytenoid movement, and vocal fold elongation with elevated pitch were all within normal limits. No supraglottic compression was noted during phonation. There was no evidence of velopharyngeal insufficiency, allergic rhinitis, or laryngopharyngeal reflux. Management recommendations from her otolaryngologist included speech-language pathology assessment and treatment, temporary singing restriction, and a follow-up videostroboscopic evaluation at the completion of voice therapy.

> The authors mention that the bilateral midmembranous phonotraumatic lesions were diagnosed as nodules. Important to note, these lesions are described as "nontransparent," which might indicate they are more mature and perhaps fibrous in nature compared to early nodules.
> A classification system operationalized by Verdolini et al in the *Classification Manual of Voice Disorders–I*[94] noted the difference in expected healing of various lesions.

Auditory-Perceptual Assessment

The CAPE-V[15] was used for auditory-perceptual analysis of the patient's vocal quality. The patient presented with mild to moderate dysphonia (22/100) characterized by moderate roughness (27/100), mild breathiness (11/100), moderate strain (31/100), intermittently increased pitch (7/100), and intermittently increased loudness (6/100). Pressed glottal fry was heard on approximately 15% of words, usually, but not always, at the end of an utterance. Persistent sharp throat clearing was observed 7 times in 1 hour. The patient used harsh glottal attacks 41% of the time when reading the Towne-Heuer Reading Passage, which exceeds the expected average of 15%.[95]

She used a clavicular breathing pattern and appeared to have limited inhalation in preparation for speech, as evidenced by increased vocal strain at the ends of phrases. Excessive laryngeal movement was visible during speech.

Manual Palpation Assessment

Palpation of the perilaryngeal area by the clinician revealed laryngeal resistance to manual lateral displacement at rest and with phonation. Mild constriction of the thyrohyoid space as well as tightness in the submandibular sling were also present during phonation. The patient denied discomfort or tenderness during light palpation of the laryngeal complex.

Singing Assessment

Vocal range was assessed by having the patient sing 5-note ascending and descending major scales throughout her range. DH's singing range was from F#3 to Bb5 (185-932 Hz). Her ability to control vocal dynamic variation was assessed using a messa di voce task. In this task, the patient is asked to sing from soft to loud and back to soft on a single pitch in addition to additional pitches representative of reported problem areas and perceived register transitions (passaggio). Additional vocal tasks were used, including glissandos (sirens); short, staccato high-pitched repetitions; and a sample song to evaluate vocal quality and technique. DH exhibited overt clavicular displacement during preparatory inhalation. Delayed onset of phonation was also observed upward from F5 at moderate volume and from C5 at soft volume. Pressed vocal quality prevailed throughout her range. Pitch was intermittently and randomly flat with no vibrato. She exhibited tongue retraction and limited jaw excursion for higher pitches. Resonance was decreased orally throughout her range. Aphonic breaks were noted intermittently, particularly above C5. When singing a selection from her repertoire, vocal register use included modal register from F#3 to A4 and head voice from A#4 to Bb5. The shift from modal to head register was marked by an abrupt change from loud and pressed to light and breathy.

Quality-of-Life Indices

The VHI-10 was administered[11] and the patient scored 17/40, corresponding with a mild to moderate negative impact. The SVHI-10 was also administered with a patient score of 29/40, indicating a moderate to severe negative impact.

Laryngeal Function Studies

Aerodynamic data were collected using the Pentax Medical Phonatory Aerodynamics System (PAS) software. At the patient's medium volume, all measures were within normal limits compared to normative data for females aged 6 to 9.11 years, with average subglottal air pressures of 10.18 cmH$_2$O (norm = 10.08), mean airflow rate of 130 mL/sec (norm = 130) and mean glottal resistance of 78 cmH$_2$O/L/sec (norm = 92.77). Maximum phonation time was low normal at 9 seconds compared with a normative value for girls age 6 to 9.11 years of 11.3 seconds.[97] Maximum prolongation on /s/ was 21 seconds and on /z/ was 13 seconds with an s/z ratio of 1.6, which is considered increased.[97] Average fundamental frequency during connected speech was low normal at 233 Hz compared to the expected range for 9-year-old girls of 228 to 305 Hz.[98] Frequency range during speech was 141 to 376 Hz. Maximum frequency range was less than 2.5 octaves (A3-Bb5 or 223-932 Hz), which is decreased compared to the average maximum phonation frequency range of 6- to 11-year-old girls of 184 to 1587 Hz.[99]

Stimulability

The patient was stimulable for improvement at the time of the assessment using lip trills, which resulted in temporary improved flow phonation in conversation following the task, as well as using manual laryngeal manipulation by the clinician, which yielded some release of peri-laryngeal tension during sustained phonation.

Impressions

DH presents with a moderate dysphonia of the speaking voice and a moderate to severe dysphonia of the singing voice. Both DH and her mother appear motivated to fully engage in the therapeutic process necessary to eliminate vocal fold nodules. Prognosis for recovery of vocal function is good to excellent, while prognosis for complete elimination of mid vocal fold protrusions is somewhat guarded.

Plan of Care

Based on the findings of the assessment, it is recommended that the patient be seen for 10 to 12 sessions of individual in-person voice therapy, initially for 1 session per week and then decreasing in frequency over a period of 6 months.

Long-Term Goals:

1. Educate patient and caregiver regarding key factors suspected in the pathogenesis and maintenance of vocal fold nodules, optimal vocal hygiene, environmental modifications to promote healthy voice use, and normal laryngeal development through puberty
2. Improve voice efficiency and reduce vocal fold impact force through reduction of laryngeal hyperfunction, improved breath flow during speech, increased forward resonance, decreased use of harsh glottal attacks, and improved dynamic vocal flexibility
3. Achieve physiologic changes including lesion size, improved mucosal wave vibration, and improved glottal closure pattern (decrease the posterior musculo-membranous glottal gap and achieve the desired barely abducted glottal closure pattern described by Verdolini and colleagues)[100]

Short-Term Goals:

1. The patient (and her mother) will demonstrate improved understanding of current vocal overuse patterns and vocal conservation strategies as evidenced by patient report in her vocal log and discussion during therapy sessions. Educational handouts will be provided to reinforce this.
2. The patient will demonstrate a diaphragmatic/abdominal breathing pattern while maintaining perilaryngeal relaxation in contexts of increasing vocal complexity with 90% success by the end of treatment.
3. The patient will demonstrate sustained phonation with a reduction in pressed vocal quality while using SOVT techniques, then will transfer optimized glottic configuration during phonation to contexts of increasing vocal complexity with 80% success by the end of treatment.

Decision Making

Proceeding with therapy was straightforward. The patient's level of dysphonia, matched with her desire to be healthy enough to perform, provided good motivation for the patient and her mother. Furthermore, nodules are known to respond well to treatment. One of the main factors contributing to DH's vocal problem was the lack of a vocal health advocate at multiple levels, resulting in a 2-year time span between the onset of symptoms and seeking medical care. Key decision makers for this child (DH's mother, professionals at the performing arts camp, DH's vocal coach, and DH's singing teacher) did not refer her to otolaryngology despite persistent dysphonia. The length of time between onset and proper diagnosis resulted in DH's nodules being more developed and stiffer, and the patient's compensatory muscle tension more firmly rooted itself in her muscle memory, thereby lengthening the patient's path to recovery. This information guided the clinician's decision to make parent and child vocal education one of the main goals of voice therapy. Respiratory retraining was targeted due to the patient's use of a clavicular breathing pattern, which is inefficient for both speech and singing, as it can lead to increased tension in the perilaryngeal musculature. The clinician chose the full exhalation on /f/ with the hand on the stomach, as the release of the abdominal musculature at the end of the exhalation allows the patient to feel the stomach move out with inhalation to establish a diaphragmatic/abdominal breathing pattern. A voiceless lip or tongue trill was also selected to demonstrate valve mechanics and the need for sufficient breath flow to the end of an utterance. The clinician also reasoned that modifying the patient's vocal production to decrease vocal fold impact allows for reduction and/or resolution of the nodules. The use of SOVT exercises is well represented in the literature and in this book to decrease vocal fold impact stress, and therefore will not be expounded upon here. For DH, the clinician chose to use 3 types of SOVT exercises, with some overlap of purpose but with different specific subgoals.

1. Voiced tongue trills: Unlike with the vocal folds, the patient can easily feel and monitor the vibration at the tongue. Particularly when working with a child, having a task that is easily monitored (is the tongue vibrating or not?) is beneficial. The sustained trills are used to teach the patient to evenly distribute the breath to the end of the phrase.
2. The gliding trills introduce the changing breath demand required for higher and lower pitches.
3. The onset/offset trills train gentle onset of phonation. If the patient overengages the vocal folds at onset, the trill stops or the airflow noticeably changes.

The patient was able to use the trill to determine if she was providing adequate breath support as she explored different parts of her vocal range.

The clinician elected to add the "Eye Pop," which was originally developed as an educational toy to teach about aerodynamics (Figure 8–9), with the purpose of making the vocal exercises more fun for the patient and, hopefully, increasing home practice compliance. The visual feedback provided by the balls can also be both motivating and enlightening. If the ball drops with the addition of voicing, the patient can easily understand that they have hyperadducted at the level of the vocal folds. When they learn to maintain ball height with addition of voicing, they can surmise that they have increased transglottal airflow, likely decreasing vocal fold hyperadduction. The clinician monitors unwanted breathiness. (See Video 31 Ball Blower Semi-occluded Vocal Tract Exercise by Doyle.)

Stemple's VFEs were chosen to work on balancing the respiratory, phonatory, and res-

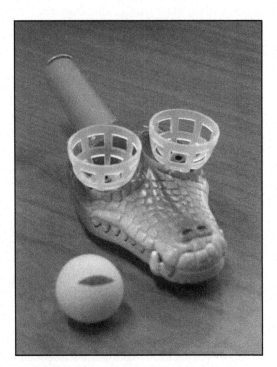

FIGURE 8–9. "Eye pop" ball-blower toy.

onatory subsystems; full description of these exercises can be found in Case Study 3.6. (See Video 5 Vocal Function Exercises by Stemple.)

Intervention

Goal #1. *The patient and her mother will demonstrate improved understanding of current vocal overuse patterns and vocal conservation strategies as evidenced by patient report in her vocal log and discussion during therapy sessions.*

DH and her mother were involved in educational discussions and provided with written handouts on vocal hygiene, including activities associated with vocal injury, vocal conservation strategies, identifying early signs of vocal deterioration and ways to modify behaviors accordingly, and child-appropriate vocal repertoire. DH was asked to keep a vocal log to document: (1) vocal status between treatment sessions; (2) compliance with home practice exercises and behavioral recommendations; (3) suspected factors influencing vocal changes; (4) emotional response to voicing issues; and (5) questions for the clinician. DH and her mother were provided with information about the ways in which the professional performing environment can threaten vocal health as well as ways to advocate for a performer's voice. Specific vocal conservation strategies included ways she could fight with her brother with reduced or no yelling, nonverbal ways for DH to cheer on her teammates at soccer games, and reducing loudness required to speak in class by sitting near the teacher. DH's mother was encouraged to provide visual and verbal reminders to the patient, encouraging vocal naps throughout the day. The clinician provided education regarding possible pubescent vocal changes, including a gradual lowering of vocal pitch, increase in breathiness, difficulty in register management, and difficulty projecting in her upper range.[101] DH was fully compliant and used the log to share her improved decision making and subsequent improvement in her vocal quality. Although DH's mother expressed interest in helping her daughter's voice and was pleased with her progress, she often balked at recommended vocal conservation measures and other restrictions. To convince her, the clinician delved deeper into the science and pathophysiology behind the connection between voice use and the development of vocal nodules.

Goal #2. *DH will demonstrate a diaphragmatic/abdominal breathing pattern while maintaining perilaryngeal relaxation in contexts of increasing vocal complexity with 90% success by the end of treatment.*

Relaxation exercises were chosen to target specific muscles identified during the speech pathology assessment as interfering with efficient voice production and/or breathing. These included neck/shoulder stretches, lateral laryngeal massage (gentle lateral rocking of the thyroid cartilage from side to side), and submandibular massage (thumb pressure applied to the area with gentle massage, used to improve pliability and monitor for unwanted engagement during respiratory or vocal tasks).

Through demonstration and tactile feedback, DH was introduced to easy exhalation on /f/. This was accomplished by asking her to place her hand on her abdomen and inhale gently. DH was then asked to exhale while sustaining an /f/, noticing the inward movement of the abdominal wall. At the end of the breath, the release of the abdominal musculature gives the patient the opportunity to feel the stomach move out with inhalation. Voiceless lip or tongue trills were added to demonstrate valve mechanics and the need for sufficient breath flow to the end of the utterance. DH mastered abdominal/diaphragmatic breathing at the exercise level after only 2 sessions. The correct pattern was incorporated into her speech work by session #3 and into her singing beginning at session #5. These exercises, when combined with the other exercises working on resonance and improved glottal efficiency, helped DH successfully increase her oral resonance, decrease tongue tension in speech, and decrease harsh vocal quality during treatment. However, she continued to have some submandibular engagement in singing above about D5.

Goal #3. *The patient will demonstrate sustained phonation with a reduction in pressed vocal quality while using SOVT techniques, then will transfer this glottic configuration to contexts of increasing vocal complexity with 80% success to generalization by the end of treatment.*

After learning the voiceless tongue trills, DH was asked to add sustained voicing at a comfortable pitch while sliding her pitch up and down within her speaking range and while completing a phonatory onset/offset exercise. In this exercise, DH was asked to transition back and forth between voiceless and voiced trills on one breath without any break in the trill or significant airflow change. She mastered the tongue trill exercises very quickly. Trill work was expanded to sung tongue trill scales used as a vocal warm-up.

For continued work on goal #3, the ball-blower toy was introduced. When using this tool, the patient blows into the tube, causing two foam balls to float. The patient is then asked to keep the balls afloat steadily with and without voicing. If the ball drops with the addition of voicing, the patient can easily understand that they have hyperadducted at the level of the vocal folds, thereby preventing adequate transglottal airflow. When they learn to maintain ball height with addition of voicing, they can surmise that they have increased transglottal airflow, likely decreasing vocal fold hyperadduction. The clinician monitors unwanted breathiness. When DH first added voicing to the ball-blower, the balls did not move, even though she had been able to get them to float for the voiceless task. This suggested that she was hyperadducting her vocal folds. With practice, she was able to figure out how to get the balls in the air while phonating. The clinician was having difficulty getting DH to establish the kazoo buzz sound used in VFEs. She asked DH to alternate from the ball-blower to the formation of the kazoo buzz for the Stemple exercises, and DH was then successful.

The clinician introduced and trained Stemple's VFEs[102] to balance the respiratory, phonatory, and resonatory subsystems. While doing the pitch glide exercises, DH initially would lose breath connection in her passaggio (vocal register transition) from middle to head voice (at about Eb5, or 622 Hz). This was evidenced by a loss of the vibratory buzz on her lips and by the loss of the feeling of breath on her hand. By therapy session #4, she could glide correctly to A5 (880 Hz), and by session #8, the range increased to D6 (1175 Hz). Her prolongation times increased from a starting average of 13 seconds to an average of 22 seconds at the time of discharge. These changes may be attributable to both improved efficiency of the vocal mechanism as well as improved vocal fold pliability.

Discussion

DH received a total of 12 sessions of voice therapy. At the time of discharge, she no longer experienced vocal deterioration and was happy with her vocal quality, range, and stamina. Her VHI-10 score reduced from 17/40 to 0/40, while her SVHI-10 score reduced from 29/40 to 12/40. Repeat laryngeal videostroboscopic examination revealed resolution of vocal fold edema, improved mucosal wave bilaterally, and reduced nodule size bilaterally. Her posterior glottal gap had reduced to within normal limits. Three years after discharge from therapy, the patient returned to the clinic for management of allergies. Laryngeal videostroboscopy revealed almost complete resolution of her nodules with no signs of any recent exacerbation. Dysphonia severity posttherapy was judged as borderline normal, improved from mild to moderate. Repeat CAPE-V scores were as follows: Overall dysphonia improved from 22/100 to 8/100; roughness improved from 27/100 to 0/100;

Table 8–18. Pre- and Posttreatment Measures

Measure	Pretreatment	Posttreatment
Subglottal Air Pressure (cmH$_2$O)	10.18	6.57
Airflow Rate (mL/sec)	130	130
Glottal Resistance (cmH$_2$O/L/sec)	78	50
s/z Ratio	21:13 (1.6)	15:13 (1.15)
Average Fundamental Frequency (Hz)	233	218

breathiness severity was unchanged at 11/100; strain improved from 31/100 to 12/100; and habitual speaking pitch and loudness normalized, improved from 7/100 and 6/100, respectively. Pre- and post-laryngeal function studies measures are detailed in Table 8–18.

References

1. Titze IR. Voice training and therapy with a semi-occluded vocal tract: Rationale and scientific underpinnings. *Hear Res.* 2006; 49(April):448-460.

2. Titze IR. Inertagrams for a variety of semi-occluded vocal tracts. *J Speech Lang Hear Res.* 2020;63(8):2589-2596. doi:10.1044/2020_JSLHR-20-00060

3. Iwarsson J. Facilitating behavioral learning and habit change in voice therapy—Theoretic premises and practical strategies. *Logop Phoniatr Vocol.* 2015;40(4):179-186. doi:10.3109/14015439.2014.936498

4. Johnson A, Sandage M. Exercise science and the vocalist. *J Voice.* 2021;35(3):376-385.

5. Crocco L, McCabe P, Madill C. Principles of motor learning in classical singing teaching. *J Voice.* 2020;34(4):567-581. doi:10.1016/j.jvoice.2018.12.019

6. Emerich KA. Nontraditional tools helpful in the treatment of certain types of voice disturbances. *Curr Opin Otolaryngol Head Neck Surg.* 2003;11(3):149-153. doi:10.1097/00020840-200306000-00003

7. Becker DR, Shelly S, Kavalieratos D, Maira C, Gillespie AI. Immediate effects of mindfulness meditation on the voice. *J Voice.* Published online November 22, 2022. doi:10.1016/j.jvoice.2022.10.022

8. Treinkman M. Focus of attention in voice training. *J Voice.* 2022;36(5):733.e1-733.e8. doi:10.1016/j.jvoice.2020.08.035

9. Schlinger M. Feldenkrais method, Alexander technique, and yoga—Body awareness therapy in the performing arts. *Phys Med Rehabil Clin N Am.* 2006;17(4):865-875. doi:10.1016/j.pmr.2006.07.002

10. Shoffel-Havakuk H, Marks KL, Morton M, Johns MM III, Hapner ER. Validation of the OMNI vocal effort scale in the treatment of adductor spasmodic dysphonia. *Laryngoscope.* Published online October 12, 2018. doi:10.1002/lary.27430

11. Rosen CA, Lee AS, Osborne J, Zullo T, Murry T. Development and validation of the voice Handicap Index-10. *Laryngoscope.* 2004;114(9 I):1549-1556. doi:10.1097/00005537-200409000-00009

12. Arffa RE, Krishna P, Gartner-Schmidt J, Rosen CA. Normative values for the voice Handicap Index-10. *J Voice.* 2012;26(4):462-465. doi:10.1016/j.jvoice.2011.04.006

13. Shoffel-Havakuk H, Chau S, Hapner ER, Pethan M, Johns MM. Development and validation of the Voice Catastrophization

Index. *J Voice*. 2019;33(2):232-238. doi:10
.1016/j.jvoice.2017.09.026

14. Castro ME, Sund LT, Hoffman MR, Hapner ER. The Voice Problem Impact Scales (VPIS). *J Voice*. 2024;38(3):666-673. doi:10
.1016/j.jvoice.2021.11.011

15. Kempster GB, Gerratt BR, Abbott KV, Barkmeier-Kraemer J, Hillman RE. Consensus Auditory-Perceptual Evaluation of Voice: Development of a standardized clinical protocol. *Am J Speech Lang Pathol*. 2009;18(2):124-132. doi:10.1044/1058-03
60(2008/08-0017)

16. Benninger M, Murry T, Johns M. *The Performer's Voice*. 2nd ed. Plural Publishing; 2016.

17. Goy H, Fernandes DN, Pichora-Fuller MK, Van Lieshout P. Normative voice data for younger and older adults. *J Voice*. 2013; 27(5):545-555. doi:10.1016/j.jvoice.2013.03
.002

18. Siupsinskiene N, Lycke H. Effects of vocal training on singing and speaking voice characteristics in vocally healthy adults and children based on choral and non-choral data. *J Voice*. 2011;25(4):e177-e189. doi:10.1016/j.jvoice.2010.03.010

19. Sanchez K, Oates J, Dacakis G, Holmberg EB. Speech and voice range profiles of adults with untrained normal voices: Methodological implications. *Logop Phoniatr Vocol*. 2014;39(2):62-71. doi:10.3109/1401
5439.2013.777109

20. Buckley DP, Abur D, Stepp CE. Normative values of cepstral peak prominence measures in typical speakers by sex, speech stimuli, and software type across the life span. *Am J Speech Lang Pathol*. 2023;32(4):1565-1577. doi:10.1044/2023_AJSLP-22-00264

21. Zraick RI, Smith-Olinde L, Shotts LL. Adult normative data for the KayPentax phonatory aerodynamic system model 6600. *J Voice*. 2012;26(2):164-176. doi:10.1016/j.j
voice.2011.01.006

22. Lewandowski A, Gillespie AI, Kridgen S, Jeong K, Yu L, Gartner-Schmidt J. Adult normative data for phonatory aerodynamics in connected speech. *Laryngoscope*. 2018; 128(4):909-914. doi:10.1002/lary.26922

23. Free N, Stemple JC, Smith JA, Phyland DJ. The immediate impact of targeted exercises on voice characteristics in female speakers with phonotraumatic vocal fold lesions. *J Voice*. 2024;38(5):1251.e33-1251.e52. doi:
10.1016/j.jvoice.2022.01.008

24. Yiu EML, Lo MCM, Barrett EA. A systematic review of resonant voice therapy. *Int J Speech Lang Pathol*. 2017;19(1):17-29. doi:
10.1080/17549507.2016.1226953

25. Steinhauer K, Klimek M, Estill J. *The Estill Voice Model: Theory & Translation*. Estill Voice International; 2017.

26. Gray R, Michael D, Hoffmeister J, et al. Patient satisfaction with virtual vs in-person voice therapy. *J Voice*. 2024;38(5):1088-1094. doi:10.1016/j.jvoice.2022.03.011

27. Alves M, Kruger E, Pillay B, van Lierde K, van der Linde J. The effect of hydration on voice quality in adults: A systematic review. *J Voice*. 2019;33(1):125.e13-125.e28. doi:10.1016/j.jvoice.2017.10.001

28. Tanner K, Roy N, Merrill RM, et al. Nebulized isotonic saline versus water following a laryngeal desiccation challenge in classically trained sopranos. *J Speech Lang Hear Res*. 2010;53(6):1555. doi:10.1044/1092-43
88(2010/09-0249)

29. Assad JP, Magalhães M de C, Santos JN, Gama ACC. Dose vocal: Uma revisão integrativa da literatura. *Rev CEFAC*. 2017; 19(3):429-438. doi:10.1590/1982-0216201
71932617

30. Lott J. The use of the twang technique in voice therapy. *Perspect Voice Voice Disord*. 2014;(1989):119-123.

31. Mills R, Hays C, Al-Ramahi J, Jiang JJ. Validation and evaluation of the effects of semi-occluded face mask straw phonation therapy methods on aerodynamic parameters in comparison to traditional methods. *J Voice*. 2017;31(3):323-328. doi:10.1016/j
.jvoice.2016.04.009

32. Guzman M, Acevedo K, Leiva F, Ortiz V, Hormazabal N, Quezada C. Aerodynamic characteristics of growl voice and reinforced falsetto in metal singing. *J Voice*. 2019;33(5):803.e7-803.e13. doi:10.1016/j
.jvoice.2018.04.022

33. Caffier PP, Ibrahim Nasr A, Del Mar Ropero Rendon M, et al. Common vocal effects and partial glottal vibration in professional non-classical singers. *J Voice*. 2018;32(3):340-346. doi:10.1016/j.jvoice.2017.06.009

34. Gartner-Schmidt J, Gillespie A. Conversation training therapy: Let's talk it through. *Semin Speech Lang*. 2021;42(1):32-40. doi: 10.1055/s-0040-1722751

35. Kamper SJ, Maher CG, Mackay G. Global rating of change scales: A review of strengths and weaknesses and considerations for design. *J Man Manip Ther*. 2009;17(3):163-170. doi:10.1179/jmt.2009.17.3.163

36. Phyland D. The measurement and effects of vocal load in singing performance. How much singing can a singer sing if a singer can sing songs? *Perspect ASHA Spec Interest Groups*. 2017;2(3):79-88. doi:10.1044/persp2.sig3.79

37. Phyland D, Miles A. Occupational voice is a work in progress: Active risk management, habilitation and rehabilitation. *Curr Opin Otolaryngol Head Neck Surg*. 2019; 27(6):439-447. doi:10.1097/MOO.0000000 000000584

38. Ferrari EP, da Trindade Duarte JM, Simões-Zenari M, Vilela N, Master S, Nemr K. Risk of dysphonia in theater actors: Proposal for a screening protocol. *J Voice*. 2023:1-7. doi:10.1016/j.jvoice.2023.04.015

39. Ford Baldner E, Doll E, Van Mersbergen MR. A review of measures of vocal effort with a preliminary study on the establishment of a vocal effort measure. *J Voice*. 2015;29(5):530-541. doi:10.1016/j.jvoice.20 14.08.017

40. Phyland DJ, Pallant J, Free N, Behlau M. On the EAVE: A new scale for self-evaluation of the physical aspects of speaking voice function. *IALP Voice Symp (preparing Publ.* 2021.

41. Oates J, Russell A. Learning voice analysis using an interactive multi-media package: Development and preliminary evaluation. *J Voice*. 1998;12(4):500-512. doi:10.1016/S0892-1997(98)80059-3

42. Dejonckere PH, Lebacq J. Plasticity of voice quality: A prognostic factor for outcome of voice therapy? *J Voice*. 2001;15(2):251-256. doi:10.1016/S0892-1997(01)00025-X

43. Kotby MN, Fex B. The accent method: Behaviour readjustment voice therapy. *Logop Phoniatr Vocol*. 1998;23(1):39-43.

44. Angadi V, Croake D, Stemple J. Effects of Vocal Function Exercises: A systematic review. *J Voice*. 2019;33(1):124.e13-124.e34. doi:10.1016/j.jvoice.2017.08.031

45. Wrycza Sabol J, Lee L, Stemple JC. The value of Vocal Function Exercises in the practice regimen of singers. *J Voice*. 1995;9(1):27-36. doi:10.1016/S0892-1997(05)80220-6

46. Roy N, Bless DM, Heisey D, Ford CN. Manual circumlaryngeal therapy for functional dysphonia: An evaluation of short- and long-term treatment outcomes. *J Voice*. 1997;11(3):321-331. doi:10.1016/S0892-19 97(97)80011-2

47. Roy N, Nissen SL, Dromey C, Sapir S. Articulatory changes in muscle tension dysphonia: Evidence of vowel space expansion following manual circumlaryngeal therapy. *J Commun Disord*. 2009;42(2):124-135. doi:10.1016/j.jcomdis.2008.10.001

48. Cardoso R, Meneses RF, Lumini-Oliveira J. The effectiveness of physiotherapy and complementary therapies on voice disorders: A systematic review of randomized controlled trials. *Front Med*. 2017;4(Apr):1-9. doi:10.3389/fmed.2017.00045

49. Mathieson L. The evidence for laryngeal manual therapies in the treatment of muscle tension dysphonia. *Curr Opin Otolaryngol Head Neck Surg*. 2011;19(3):171-176. doi:10.1097/MOO.0b013e3283448f6c

50. Manheim C. *The Myofascial Release Manual*. 3rd ed. Slack, Inc.; 2008.

51. Barnes JF. *Myofascial Release: The Search for Excellence—A Comprehensive Evaluatory and Treatment Approach*. Rehabilitation Services Inc.; 1990.

52. Myers T, Earls J. *Fascial Release for Structural Balance*. Lotis Publishing; 2010.

53. Jacobson BH, Johnson A, Grywalski C, et al. The Voice Handicap Index (VHI): Development and validation. *Am J Speech Lang Pathol*. 1997;6(3):66-69. doi:10.1044/1058-0360.0603.66

54. Behrman A. Common practices of voice therapists in the evaluation of patients. *J Voice*. 2005;19(3):454-469. doi:10.1016/j.jvoice.2004.08.004

55. Smith BE, Kempster GB, Sims HS. Patient factors related to voice therapy attendance and outcomes. *J Voice*. 2010;24(6):694-701. doi:10.1016/j.jvoice.2009.03.004

56. van Leer E, Hapner ER, Connor NP. Transtheoretical model of health behavior change applied to voice therapy. *J Voice*. 2008;22(6):688-698. doi:10.1016/j.jvoice.2007.01.011

57. Dawson D, Reid K. Fatigue, alcohol, and performance impairment. *Nature*. 1997;388:235-237.

58. Williamson AM, Feyer A. Moderate sleep deprivation produces impairments in cognitive and motor performormance equivalent to legally prescribed levels of alcohol intoxication. *Occup Env Med*. 2000;57:649-655.

59. van Leer E, Connor N. Use of portable digital media players increases voice therapy patient motivation and practice frequency in voice therapy. *J Voice*. 2012;26(4):447-453. doi:10.1016/j.jvoice.2011.05.006

60. Abbott KV, Ph D, Li NYK, et al. Vocal exercise may attenuate acute vocal fold inflammation. 2013;26(6):1-27. doi:10.1016/j.jvoice.2012.03.008

61. Behrman A, Rutledge J, Hembree A. Vocal hygiene education, voice production therapy, and the role of patient adherence: A treatment effectiveness study in women with phonotrauma. *J Speech Lang Hear Res*. 2008;51(2):350-366

62. Verdolini K, Titze IR, Fennell A. Dependence of phonatory effort on hydration level. *J Speech Hear Res*. 1994;37(5):1001-1007. doi:10.1044/jshr.3705.1001

63. Cleveland TF, Stone RE, Sundberg J, Iwarsson J. Estimated subglottal pressure in six professional country singers. *J Voice*. 1997;11(4):403-409. doi:10.1016/S0892-1997(97)80035-5

64. Hoit JD, Jenks CL, Watson PJ, Cleveland TF. Respiratory function during speaking and singing in professional country singers. *J Voice*. 1996;10(1):39-49. doi:10.1016/S0892-1997(96)80017-8

65. Hapner E, Portone-Maira C, Johns MM. A study of voice therapy dropout. *J Voice*. 2009;23(3):337-340. doi:10.1016/j.jvoice.2007.10.009

66. Arffa RE, Krishna P, Gartner-Schmidt J, Rosen CA. Normative values for the Voice Handicap Index-10. *J Voice*. 2012;26(4):462-465. doi:10.1016/j.jvoice.2011.04.006

67. Shembel AC, Rosen CA, Zullo TG, Gartner-Schmidt JL. Development and validation of the Cough Severity Index: A severity index for chronic cough related to the upper airway. *Laryngoscope*. 2013;123(8):1931-1936. doi:10.1002/lary.23916

68. Belafsky PC, Postma GN, Koufman JA. Validity and reliability of the Reflux Symptom Index (RSI). *J Voice*. 2002;16(2):274-277. doi:10.1016/S0892-1997(02)00097-8

69. Watts CR, Diviney SS, Hamilton A, Toles L, Childs L, Mau T. The effect of stretch-and-flow voice therapy on measures of vocal function and handicap. *J Voice*. 2015;29(2):191-199. doi:10.1016/j.jvoice.2014.05.008

70. Roy N, Ford CN, Bless DM. Muscle tension dysphonia and spasmodic dysphonia: The role of manual laryngeal tension reduction in diagnosis and management. *Ann Otol Rhinol Laryngol*. 1996;105(11):851-856. doi:10.1177/000348949610501102

71. Smith S, Titze I. Characterization of flow-resistant tubes used for semi-occluded vocal tract voice training and therapy. *J Voice*. 2017;31(1). doi:10.1016/j.jvoice.2016.04.001

72. Hogikyan ND, Sethuraman G. Validation of an instrument to measure voice-related quality of life (V-RQOL). *J Voice*. 1999;13(4):557-569. doi:10.1016/S0892-1997(99)80010-1

73. Gilman M. Revisiting sustained phonation time of /s/, /z/, and /ɑ/. *J Voice*. 2021;35(6):935.e13-935.e18. doi:10.1016/j.jvoice.2020.03.012

74. Zraick RI, Smith-Olinde L, Shotts LL. Erratum: Adult normative data for the KayPentax phonatory aerodynamic system model 6600. *J Voice*. 2013;27(1):2-4. doi:10.1016/j.jvoice.2012.10.003

75. Gilman M, Johns MM. The effect of head position and/or stance on the self-perception of phonatory effort. *J Voice*. 2017; 31(1):131.e1-131.e4. doi:10.1016/j.jvoice.2015.11.024

76. Gilman M. The influence of postural changes on extralaryngeal muscle tension and vocal production. *Perspect ASHA Spec Interest Groups*. 2018;3(3):82-87. doi:10.1044/persp3.sig3.82

77. Cohen SM, Statham M, Rosen CA, Zullo T. Development and validation of the Singing Voice Handicap-10. *Laryngoscope*. 2009; 119(9):1864-1869. doi:10.1002/lary.20580

78. Patel RR, Awan SN, Barkmeier-Kraemer J, et al. Recommended protocols for instrumental assessment of voice: ASHA expert panel to develop a protocol for instrumental assessment of vocal function. *Am J Speech Lang Pathol*. 2018;27(3):887-905

79. Pierce JL, Tanner K, Merrill RM, Shnowske L, Roy N. A field-based approach to establish normative acoustic data for healthy female voices. 2021;64(March):1-16.

80. Free N, Stemple JC, Smith JA, Phyland DJ. Variability in voice characteristics of female speakers with phonotraumatic vocal fold lesions. *J Voice*. Published online February 20, 2023. doi:10.1016/j.jvoice.2023.01.019

81. Öcal B, Tatar E, Toptaş G, Barmak E, Saylam G, Korkmaz MH. Evaluation of voice quality in patients with vocal fold polyps: The size of a polyp matters or does it? *J Voice*. 2020;34(2):294-299. doi:10.1016/j.jvoice.2019.04.009

82. Petrovic-Lazic M, Jovanovic N, Kulic M, Babac S, Jurisic V. Acoustic and perceptual characteristics of the voice in patients with vocal polyps after surgery and voice therapy. *J Voice*. 2015;29(2):241-246. doi:10.1016/j.jvoice.2014.07.009

83. Branski R, Verdolini K, Sandulache V, Rosen CA, Hebda RP. Vocal fold wound healing: A review for clinicians. *J Voice*. 2006;20(3):432-442.

84. Agarwal J, Wong A, Karle W, Naunheim M, Mori M, Courey M. Comparing short-term outcomes of surgery and voice therapy for patients with vocal fold polyps. *Laryngo-scope*. 2019;129(5):1067-1070. doi:10.1002/lary.27697

85. Dastolfo-Hromack C, Thomas TL, Rosen CA, Gartner-Schmidt J. Singing voice outcomes following singing voice therapy. *Laryngoscope*. 2016;126(11):2546-2551. doi:10.1002/lary.25962

86. Gartner-Schmidt JL, Shembel AC, Zullo TG, Rosen CA. Development and validation of the Dyspnea Index (DI): A severity index for upper airway-related dyspnea. *J Voice*. 2014;28(6):775-782. doi:10.1016/j.jvoice.2013.12.017

87. Belafsky P, Mouadeb D, Rees C, et al. Validity and reliability of the Eating Assessment Tool (EAT-10). *Ann Otol Rhinol Laryngol*. 2008;117(12):919-924. doi:10.1177/000348940811701210

88. Schneider SL, Habich L, Weston ZM, Rosen CA. Observations and considerations for implementing remote acoustic voice recording and analysis in clinical practice. *J Voice*. 2024;38(1):69-76. doi:10.1016/j.jvoice.2021.06.011

89. Shohet J, Courey M, Scott M, Ossoff R. Value of videostroboscopic parameters in differentiating true vocal fold cysts from polyps. *Laryngoscope*. 1996;106:19-26.

90. Helou LB, Gartner-Schmidt JL, Hapner ER, Schneider SL, Van Stan JH. Mapping meta-therapy in voice interventions onto the rehabilitation treatment specification system. *Semin Speech Lang*. 2021;42(1):5-18. doi:10.1055/s-0040-1722756

91. Wolchok JC, Brokopp C, Underwood CJ, Tresco PA. The effect of bioreactor induced vibrational stimulation on extracellular matrix production from human derived fibroblasts. *Biomaterials*. 2009;30(3):327-335. doi:10.1016/j.biomaterials.2008.08.035

92. Branski RC, Verdolini K, Rosen CA, Hebda PA. Acute vocal fold wound healing in a rabbit model. *Ann Otol Rhinol Laryngol*. 2005;114(1 I):19-24. doi:10.1177/000348940511400105

93. Titze IR, Hitchcock RW, Broadhead K, et al. Design and validation of a bioreactor for engineering vocal fold tissues under combined tensile and vibrational stresses. *J Bio-*

mech. 2004;37(10):1521-1529. doi:10.1016/j.jbiomech.2004.01.007

94. Verdolini K, Rosen CA, Branski RC. *Classification Manual of Voice Disorders-I.* 2nd ed. Psychology Press; 2012.

95. Heuer R, Towne C, Hockstein NE, Andrade DF, Sataloff RT. The Towne-Heuer Reading Passage—A reliable aid to the evaluation of voice. *J Voice.* 2000;14(2):236-239. doi:10.1016/S0892-1997(00)80031-4

96. Weinrich B, Brehm SB, Knudsen C, McBride S, Hughes M. Pediatric normative data for the KayPentax phonatory aerodynamic system model 6600. *J Voice.* 2013;27(1):46-56. doi:10.1016/j.jvoice.2012.09.001

97. Mendes Tavares EL, Brasolotto AG, Rodrigues SA, Benito Pessin AB, Garcia Martins RH. Maximum phonation time and s/z ratio in a large child cohort. *J Voice.* 2012;26(5):675.e1-675.e4. doi:10.1016/j.jvoice.2012.03.001

98. Sorenson DN. A fundamental frequency investigation of children ages 6-10 years old. *J Commun Disord.* 1989;22(2):115-123. doi:10.1016/0021-9924(89)90028-2

99. Ma EPM, Li TKY. Effects of coaching and repeated trials on maximum phonational frequency range in children. *J Voice.* 2017;31(2):243.e1-243.e8. doi:10.1016/j.jvoice.2016.05.013

100. Verdolini K, Druker DG, Palmer PM, Samawi H. Laryngeal adduction in resonant voice. *J Voice.* 1998;12(3):315-327. doi:10.1016/S0892-1997(98)80021-0

101. Wilson D. *Voice Problems of Children.* Williams and Wilkins; 1987.

102. Stemple JC, Lee L, D'Amico B, Pickup B. Efficacy of Vocal Function Exercises as a method of improving voice production. *J Voice.* 1994;8(3):271-278. doi:10.1016/S0892-1997(05)80299-1

9

Gender Affirming Voice Care

Introduction

Sandy Hirsch

Five decades ago, Joan Regnell, associate professor in the speech and hearing department at George Washington University, began working with transgender clients in the university clinic. Closely associated with the Johns Hopkins gender care program, a need for what was then known as transgender voice therapy was easily identified, and a program developed. In 1977 Kalra presented the first American Speech-Language-Hearing Association (ASHA) paper on gender affirming voice care (GAVC),[1] followed fairly closely by Oates and Dacakis in 1983.[2] It is an understatement to point out that GAVC has evolved in myriad ways since then. Further seminal papers by Oates and Dacakis[3] and Pausewang-Gelfer[4] followed soon thereafter.

Those early papers heralded a now deep and detailed hyperapplication of voice care to the multidisciplinary focus of gender affirming care. Adler especially is recognized as one of the earliest in the field, seeing transgender/gender nonconforming (TGNC) clients since the early 1980s, while Becklund Friedenberg's 2002 article[5] was referenced for many years as a guideline for how to develop a GAVC program. I have had the distinct honor and privilege of serving the transgender/gender nonconforming (TGNC) community since 1988 and, as such, have contributed to and watched history moving forward with other pioneers. We all strive to contribute to academic and clinical advancement in our field. As a contributor to the fifth edition of *Voice Therapy: Clinical Case Studies* in 2019, it has not slipped my attention that it was published the same year as the third edition of Adler et al's *Voice and Communication Training for the Transgender/Gender Diverse Client*,[6] further fortifying a canon of literature that began as a trickle of information in texts such as Andrews' *Manual of Voice Treatment: Pediatrics Through Geriatrics*[7] and Boone and McFarlane's sixth edition of *The Voice and Voice Therapy*.[8] Adler et al's 3 editions, beginning in 2006, have all included transgender/gender nonconforming (TGNC) authors—Marci Bowers (she/her), MD; singer/teacher Alexandros Constansis (he/him); actor Rebecca Root (she/her); and actor Delia Kropp (she/her)—but none of these contributors are speech-language pathologists (SLPs). SLP Josie Zanfordino (she/her), a transgender woman, began working with TGNC people in 2007, and Wynde Vastine (they/them) began working

438   Voice Therapy: Clinical Case Studies

with TGNC people as a voice trainer in 2007 before becoming an SLP in 2020. With these few exceptions, to date, SLPs working with TGNC people have largely been cisgender. That tide is finally turning. Indeed, most of the case studies on gender affirming care in this edition have been written by SLPs within the TGNC community.

Fifty years after SLPs began doing GAVC, the spectrum of genders in the field of GAVC is consistently widening. By extension, the depth and breadth of the cases presented here demonstrate the expansion of goals in GAVC. The fifth edition of *Voice Therapy: Clinical Case Studies* presented 2 transgender cases: one transfeminine case and one transmasculine. Since 2019, GAVC has moved from the presumption of a binary perspective in setting goals with a client to an assumption of training the full range of the vocal instrument to play in such a way to meet the needs and goals of the full gender and vocal spectrum—masculine, feminine, nonbinary, agender, and all gender. We are not engaged to tell a client how to sound; our task is to guide a person in finding a voice that affirms their gender, improves their quality of life, decreases dysphoria, and increases euphoria. The cases presented here cover a wide variety of goals: the needs of adolescents, as well as their navigation through the school system, (Case Study 9.5 by Goldberg); the needs of transmasculine speakers challenged with muscle tension dysphonia (MTD), which is common (Case Study 9.3 by François and Buckley); the various and creative approaches to working with nonbinary singers (Case Study 9.6 by Kapila); a transgender female who required a fast track to present as a bridesmaid at an upcoming family wedding (Case Study 9.1 by Hirsch); the initial challenges and ultimate success and euphoria of a nonbinary speaker (Case Study 9.4 by Gutierrez); and the importance of perioperative care for optimal pitch-elevation surgery outcomes (Case Study 9.2 by Vastine and Yung). A team approach is appropriately being recommended and recognized as the gold standard.

To support the varied goals of a range of genders, clinicians need to comprehensively and creatively integrate the art and science of voice work. Pitch changes must fully incorporate resonance manipulation and possibly inflection adjustments to optimally guide clients in playing their instrument. Goals were at one time based on "normative" values and are now guided by personal "gender-affirmation" within a looser "normative framework" to meet multiple vocal goals and needs. The client always leads; the clinician provides creative acoustic solutions through discovery. Solutions, though creative, must be based in voice and speech science and presented and taught within a healthy sustainable framework. I have had clients choose not to change inflection, which, as one of my clients stated, may have "too much personality tied up in it." People with binary goals no longer want to "pass" (widely, a term no longer accepted) but want to sound "cis-assumed."

It is now generally understood that the marriage of pitch and second formant (F2) changes appears to help the approximation of gender target goals. Hirsch's Acoustic Assumptions (HAA)[9–11] show anecdotal evidence that the combination of pitch changes with articulatory precision, oral shape, tongue position, and oral posture at the end of an utterance[11] appear to approximate some of the target male/female vocal tract configurations Peterson and Barney described in 1952.[12] Surgical interventions for GAVC are evolving rapidly as well. Even since the fifth edition of this book was published in 2019, the narrative around gender affirming voice surgeries—specifically pitch-elevation surgeries—has become more comfortable, fluent and, in many cases, less anxiety inducing for clients considering this option. Surgical and therapeutic voice team approaches and perioperative care are now nuanced in such a way that clients feel supported, informed, and free to make decisions that follow their unique needs, rather than as inflexibly dictated by the healthcare system.

Voice clinician Wynde Vastine and laryngologist Katherine Yung discuss this in detail in their surgical case.

How might these sixth edition cases be a call to action? Research in GAVC has proliferated in the past 20 or more years, but we still lack a healthy body of evidenced-based therapeutic study. We now have the beginnings of evidence for resonance modification, such as the HAA approach[9-11] mentioned in the transfeminine case. As indicated earlier, the approach supports an F2 shift in combination with pitch modifications that appear to lead to a shift in gender perception. Several studies have supported this notion.[11,13-16] The field increasingly hungers for further perceptual and acoustic therapeutic case studies and research. I invite clinicians to meet that challenge as they bring all of themselves to this marvelously varied table of our voice work. It requires, simultaneously, a laser-focused and lateral, out-of-the-box view.

Finally, before diving into the excellent cases presented in this sixth edition, it is important to consider the weight of language and terminology. We are, after all, speech-**language** pathologists—words matter. In general, voice care terminology has thankfully evolved from a language of blame, shame, and catastrophe to one focused on anatomy and function. Terms such as "abuse" and "misuse" have been replaced with "phonotrauma" or "vocal load," and "hoarse" with "dysphonia," to name but a few. Appropriately, the nuanced terminology for GAVC has also evolved, and continues to do so, at lightning speed. This topic deserves a chapter of its own. Suffice to say, it is crucial that we all regularly refresh our cultural responsiveness, language, and humility to remain current in our narrative and sensitive to the unique needs of every transgender or gender nonconforming person. We no longer live in a gender binary world. Truthfully, we never have—gender diversity has been part of human life since the beginning of time. Today it would be ignorant at best, and traumatizing at worst, to deny this diversity of person and language. Gender diversity is to be celebrated. It is human.

As a white, cisgender, heteronormative SLP who has been recognized in GAVC for over 3 decades, I am acutely aware of my responsibility to the TGNC community. I have worked to remain faithful to my own cultural responsiveness and humility. I have made mistakes and had to own and repair them. I invite and charge any clinicians or voice trainers new to GAVC, or indeed any clinical focus, to do the same. That is each of our work. Never presume to know enough. The landscape of gender changes every time we think we understand it. Blink, and the page has turned. Myriad resources are available and easily accessible. To name but one, Goldberg, who writes in this edition about working with adolescents, is an exceptional teacher and trainer in this realm. The Trans Voice Initiative, which includes Goldberg, Vastine, and Kapila, is also a rich resource. As Aaron Devor (he/him), transgender professor of sociology at the University of Victoria, BC, and holder of the world's first title of chair in transgender studies, says at the beginning of his course *Moving Trans History Forward*, "We have two eyes, two ears, and one mouth. Listen more than you speak." Be inquisitive, creative, kind, and learn. Let us all keep moving history forward.

Case Studies

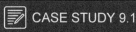

CASE STUDY 9.1

Using Acoustic Assumptions in Gender Affirming Voice Care for an Adult Transgender Woman

Sandy Hirsch

Voice Evaluation

Chief Complaint. Vocal dysphoria; communication misaligned with gender identity

History of Voice Complaint

SH is a 26-year-old, assigned male at birth (AMAB), transgender woman who began experiencing gender dysphoria in her early 20s. She was seen for her intake appointment seeking gender affirming voice guidance after a 2- to 3-year journey into gender transition. SH reported anxiety and dysphoria when using her voice and stated that the pitch of her voice was a significant barrier to her living as a woman and therefore to the quality of her life. She also reported she was less outgoing due to her voice. SH noted that her pitch range was limited; to her, she "sounded like a man" when she laughed, and it was cognitively and physically effortful trying to produce what she deemed a "feminine" voice. She reported she had not yet made a focused effort to modify her voice independently. At the time of intake, she was not out to her parents, but was out to one of her brothers. She was not yet out at work. SH reported she was presenting socially in her "true gender approximately 40% to 50% of the time" and planned on transitioning 100%.

Physical/Medical History

SH's hearing was within normal limits (WNL). She reported no significant illnesses or mental health challenges. SH reported ongoing cat allergies. She reported no reflux. Water intake was reported as "constant," and she reported consuming an average of 0 to 1 alcoholic beverage a week. SH enjoys exercise. She reported that she loves to hike, and jogs approximately 3 times per week. SH was taking the feminizing hormones estradiol and spironolactone (spiro). At the outset of therapy in late May, SH was receiving electrolysis for hair removal 2 to 4 appointments per month and was working with a psychotherapist regularly to address her gender dysphoria and overall mental health.

Voice Use

SH is a software engineer who uses her voice in meetings and socially. At the time of intake, her voice use was considered moderate. She

was not considered to be a "vocal athlete." She reported that she hoped to be able to sing with a rock band in the future. SH enjoys hiking as well as playing chess, guitar, and occasionally video games and the viola. SH is in a committed relationship with a partner who is supportive of her transition. Her brother and friends are also supportive.

Laryngeal Imaging

Laryngeal videostroboscopy was not completed. Many transgender people seeking GAVC do not present with a concern of vocal pathology or vocal qualities that would suggest the need for traditional voice therapy. If concerns emerge during the time of the acoustic or perceptual evaluation, the recommendation is to refer to a laryngologist for a comprehensive laryngological exam, including videostroboscopy, before proceeding with GAVC. If there are atypical findings at that time, GAVC could proceed, but should include appropriate training and therapeutic goals to address any findings of concern.

> There remain differing opinions about the importance of pretherapy laryngeal imaging when providing GAVC, and the literature can be vague about its use. The Standards of Care for the Health of Transgender and Gender Diverse People, Version 8, provides comprehensive guidelines for the treatment of transgender/gender diverse people and suggests the use of laryngeal imaging should be considered when the clinician notes a voice disorder or when the patient reports symptoms consistent with MTD or other voice concerns.[17] As indicated by the author of this case, these concerns were not present and laryngeal imaging was therefore deferred.

Vocal Effort, Fatigue, and Pain

SH reported mild effort when independently trying to produce a modified voice. She stated that her early efforts led her to realize this would require work and skilled training. At that time, she stopped trying on her own and sought skilled support.

Quality-of-Life Impairment

SH's Voice Handicap Index (VHI) score was 10/120 at the time of her evaluation, considered a rating of "minimal amount of handicap."[18] SH completed the Trans Woman Voice Questionnaire (TWVQ)[19] for self-perception of vocal function and participation in everyday life. The rating scale responses in the questionnaire are: 1 = "never or rarely," 2 = "sometimes," 3 = "often," and 4 = "usually or always." It is divided into vocal functioning and social participation questions. SH's total pretraining score was 93/120. She rated a 4 ("usually or always") on 17/30 items that address levels of anxiety, self-perception of vocal quality, perception of femininity and naturalness, and levels of confidence vocally. She rated 3 ("often") on 5/30 of items regarding the pitch range of her speaking voice, effort when modifying her voice, and overall confidence socially. SH rated 2 ("sometimes") on 2/30 of the items regarding voice quality and social confidence, and 1 ("never or rarely") on 6/30 of the items regarding vocal volume and confidence using her voice. Summarized, most of her responses reflected social discomfort with the sound of her current voice. She perceived it to be incongruous with her gender. SH provided an overall rating of her voice to be "somewhat male" and stated her ideal voice would sound "very female."

Auditory-Perceptual Assessment

Both SH and the clinician perceived SH's pitch and resonance to be masculine leaning. SH's voice quality was subjectively assessed to be clear (without dysphonia). Her vocal volume in conversation was deemed to be WNL for conversation. SH was not asked to repeat, nor was there a perception that she was "shouting" or speaking loudly. SH's conversational rate

was perceived as mildly rapid, possibly attributable to the fact that she reported she was somewhat anxious at the time of evaluation. This is often the case with new clients. SH and the clinician both perceived her nonspeech tasks, including laughter, cough, and throat clear, to sound "chesty" or "deep."

Oral Exam and Manual Palpation

Strength and range of motion of tongue and lips were WNL. Velar movement on /a/ was WNL. Thyroid cartilage and hyoid bone were without report of pain on palpation. Lateralization of thyroid cartilage and hyoid were WNL (without perceived stiffness or resistance). The thyrohyoid space was WNL. There was no noted tension on palpation at the base of tongue (BOT) and no report of pain in the suprahyoid region.

Aerodynamic and Acoustic Analysis

- **Maximum Sustained Phonation (MPT).** 19 seconds on /a/ and 20 seconds on /i/ (norms = 25-35 seconds for male speakers and 15-25 seconds for female speakers).[20] Anecdotally, untrained male speakers tend to have lower MPTs than the above norms.
- **s/z Ratio.** 0.88 (22/25) (norm = <1.25).[20] This measure is generally used as a "flag" measure only if there are suspected concerns about laryngeal function, but there were no overt concerns. In SH's case, it was used due to a report of mild vocal effort.
- **Pitch.** Habitual pitch (stating name and date) was 118 Hz (norms: male = 90-130 Hz[20] and female = 155-220 Hz[6,21]). Counting from 1 to 10 measured 121 Hz, reading of the first 3 sentences of the Rainbow Passage to "beyond the horizon" measured 123 Hz, and SH's spontaneous speech task (<1 minute) was 134 Hz. All pitch measures were assessed to be within a male-perceived mean of 90 to 130 Hz.[20]
- **Pitch Range.** SH's Hz range on a glissando was 82 to 485 Hz (E2-B4), with a mean of 247 Hz (B3). Semitone (ST) range was

442 Voice Therapy: Clinical Case Studies

31 and WNL.[20] SH's upper range of 485 Hz indicated enough ceiling in her upper frequencies for a comfortable, natural feminine speaking range.

- **Vocal Intensity.** SH was noted to be WNL at 70 dB during reading and 69 dB during spontaneous conversation.[20]
- **Resonance.** On a rating scale of brightness (0 = dark, 5 = bright), the clinician and SH agreed that her voice had a dark, chesty resonance, and rated her 1/5 for brightness.

Stimulability

SH was able to match pitch in 3/3 attempts and to match varying inflectional patterns given by the clinician in 3/3 attempts when provided both vocal and visual models. To achieve the visual model, the clinician demonstrated increasing semitone range for inflection in a simple phrase by stacking Duplos™ and having SH rise and descend in pitch while touching them. SH was able to discriminate between "dark" and "bright" resonance acoustic outputs when provided a model of the vowel sound /i/ produced with rounded and relaxed-smile postures that result in dark and bright resonances, respectively.

Decision Making

During the decision-making process, SH rated her motivation to change her voice as a 5/5 on a scale of 0 to 5. She also reported a 4/5 for commitment to taking responsibility for her voice exercises. SH stated a very busy work schedule and trepidation about "getting it right" were barriers to meeting her desired voice. She was considered an excellent candidate for GAVC.

Plan of Care

The clinician recommended 50-minute sessions of GAVC once a week for 8 to 12 sessions.

Client Goals. At the time of intake, SH stated that her personal goals were to:

1. Have her gender affirmed when speaking with strangers in 4/5 opportunities

2. Have her gender affirmed in voice-only interactions in 4/5 opportunities
3. Have a personal voice and communication confidence rating of 4 in 4/5 opportunities
4. Maintain confidence in her overall communication when giving professional presentations in 4/5 opportunities

Clinician Goals. SH will develop a healthy, sustainable voice within a normative feminine pitch range, maintaining a bright forward focus resonance and communication style that affirm her gender.

Intervention

GAVC encompasses modifying pitch and retuning resonance. In addition, it may include learning new inflectional patterns, a full range of nonverbal communication, and subtle changes in semantics.[6] Nonverbal communication will not be discussed in this case. A comprehensive explanation of approaches can be found in Adler et al (2019).

The author developed a rubric called Hirsch's Acoustic Assumptions (HAA)[9,11] for clients to develop tools that allow for communication agency. (See Video 32 Hirsch's Acoustic Assumptions by Hirsch.) The rubric is based on accepted voice and speech science concepts: source filter and coarticulation theories well known to clinicians, an understanding that the physiological gesture gives rise to the acoustic output, and knowledge that raising vowel formants appears to increase a perception of femininity.[15] A combination of resonant voice therapy (eg Lessac Madsen Resonant Voice Therapy [LMRVT])[22] to bring SH's resonance higher and more forward, HAA, and materials from the accent modification canon for inflection addressed SH's voice and communication goals.

Session #1

Following a comprehensive explanation of the anatomy and physiology of voice, the clinician trained SH in stretches to deactivate any muscle tension in the upper back, upper chest, rib cage, neck, facial, and oral muscles and gave her written instructions on how to do these daily before beginning her vocal warm-up. There are many appropriate stretches. Clinicians should feel comfortable training the best ones in their voice toolkit. (See Video 3 Physical Rolldown Stretch by Murphy Estes and Video 30 Tongue Stretches by Schneider for 2 examples.)

Sessions #2 and #3

Pitch and resonance training began with the basic training gesture (BTG) from the LMRVT program (see Case Study 3.7 by Orbelo, Li, and Verdolini Abbott for more details on LMRVT).[22] This includes a series of chants on a comfortable target pitch beginning with /mmm/ for a forward focus resonance sensation. To indicate forward focus, the client might feel a slight tickle at the alveolar ridge or on the upper lip. Targeting the same pitch, the exercise builds toward a multisyllabic chant (/mmmm/, /mi/, /mimi/, /mitmi/, "Meet me Peter, meet me") and finally a spoken "Meet me Peter, meet me" generalizing the forward focus resonance. LMRVT was initiated to establish a healthy and easily executed method of training her elevated pitch range and to introduce the sensation of forward focus. Using the iPhone™ app Tuna Pitch™, SH initially targeted a pitch of 185 Hz, a comfortably sustainable target that would allow for room at the top of her range for inflection training. SH was advised to practice the whole BTG, completing 2 sets of 10 at each level, twice a day. The clinician asked her to develop 20 everyday phrases of no more than 4 to 6 words, across her social and professional contexts, that she could begin integrating into her daily practice.

Following the establishment of her pitch elevation, SH was introduced to the use of 2-syllable and multisyllabic words for inflectional practice. To increase SH's semitone range for inflection, the clinician used Audacity™ for auditory feedback and Real-Time Pitch in Multispeech™ for visual feedback. This approach helped SH determine her optimal top and bottom pitches. The challenge was not in going too low, but in landing on a logical, resolved low. Too high at the bottom made the word or phrase sound unresolved, unfinished, "unnatural," or "hollow." SH had a good auditory memory and an acute awareness of motor planning and muscle memory, making her progress fluent. Within the first 3 sessions, SH grew comfortable with her higher pitch and new inflectional patterns, though she still needed modeling to remember to inflect in conversation. SH appeared ready for the introduction of the HAA resonance rubric and the beginning of self-efficacy, carryover, and maintenance. The clinician and client discussed that "We do not have the option of changing the vocal tract, so we need to use a series of acoustic workarounds to facilitate a trained higher pitch, still housed within an assigned male at birth (AMAB) instrument, to resonate like that of an assigned female at birth (AFAB) instrument and speaker." The clinician showed SH 2 cardboard tubes of different lengths and diameters—a toilet paper roll tube and a paper towel roll tube cut to size for this purpose. The clinician demonstrated the different resonances from varying tube length and diameters by saying, "Hi, my name's Sandy" into both tubes to illustrate different resonances. The clinician then changed oral configuration to a relaxed /i/ smile across the longer/wider tube to demonstrate how to brighten resonance. She gave SH a handout of HAA (Table 9–1) and explained the approach during her training session. SH was able to practice "playing her vocal and oral instrument" to meet her desired outcomes. Following is the approach as it is provided to clients. SH made a self-assessment flow chart to decide which variables needed attention at each recording. SH practiced changing configurations, recording, and solving for resonant challenges, as well as determining which variables overall (pitch, inflection, or resonance) needed attention until she was able to integrate these

444   Voice Therapy: Clinical Case Studies

Table 9–1. Hirsch's Acoustic Assumptions (HAA): Upper Range/Feminine/Nonbinary Feminine-Leaning Goal

---

Hirsch's Acoustic Assumptions (HAA): A Framework for Solving Resonance Challenges
Upper Range/Feminine/Nonbinary Feminine-Leaning Goal

How we articulate a sound affects our vocal tone. We can "play with" levels of pressure in articulation, change mouth shape, and change tongue position to adjust our tone for a "brighter" resonance.

Consonants are divided into voiced and voiceless sounds. Voiced means the vocal folds are vibrating. Voiceless means they are not. Place your fingers on the side of your throat to feel the difference between vvvv and fff. vvvv buzzes, but ffff does not, right? Below are the voiced and voiceless pairs (left set is voiced, right set is unvoiced/voiceless).

  b/p; d/t; v/f   z/s, j/ch, (**jar/ch**air) g/k   th/th (**the/th**ing) zh/sh
  (vi**s**ion/**sh**ore)

Voiced sounds have a darker tone than voiceless ones. Articulate the voiced sound with a lighter touch of tongue or lips to avoid a dark burst. Sometimes it helps to very lightly drum your fingers on top of your hand like raindrops to feel a light touch. Translate that feeling to your tongue. If 5 is maximum pressure, feel about a 3/5 for a brighter tone. Pressure at the constriction is approximate.

/m/, /n/, /ng/ (eg, "ing," "bong," "long"): /m/ is produced with a bit of a squishy, pressed feeling at the lips, /n/ with the tongue on the palate behind the top front teeth, and /ng/ with the back of the tongue to the palate. Lighten the contact as much as possible so that the sound blends fluently with other sounds in a word. Experiment with levels of articulation effort to find the brightness you want.

Liquids/glides: Sounds /l/ (**l**emon), /er/ (flow**er**), /y/ (**y**ellow), and /w/ (**w**hen) are all produced with articulation at the tongue or lips. Again, lighten the touch of articulation. You might think /h/ after /w/(h) but do not actually articulate it. Produce the "er" with a gentle mid mouth feeling, rather fully pressing toward the soft palate. If 0 is no pressure and 5 is maximum, feel pressure at the constriction as approximately a 3/5. Play with what gives you what you want.

Vowel sounds and diphthongs (ay, oy, eye, ow) in general produce a dark or low resonance, except for the ee ("Peter," "feet") sound. Produce all of these sounds with a bit of a lift/lip spread—just a light lift, almost as a "How wonderful!" smile. Or, slightly advance the tongue or "float" the tongue forward to mid mouth. It doesn't take much to brighten the tone. This is why telephone salespeople are told to smile when answering the phone! Play with what gives you what you want.

An open mouth at the end of a sentence keeps the sound alive and allows for a brightening of resonance. Maybe stretch vowels slightly where appropriate, eg, "Hi, how are yoooou?" "I know just what you meeean!" "I'll have suhhme"—remember the vowel shape formants that we discussed! If you end on a closed sound like in "some," open your mouth slightly again. Play with what gives you what you want.

9. Gender Affirming Voice Care   445

Table 9–1. *continued*

Steps for the approach: (1) Read one of your short phrases as though you're learning to read—sound by sound. (2) Identify any spots that might sound dark. (3) Identify your solution as above and code the solution above the sound (b, eg, = 2 or 3/5 pressure; vowels maybe get an ee mouth shape and a forward tongue float; the end of a phrase gets an open oral posture <). (4) Articulate the phrase silently at a normal rate with the articulation change to feel the motor planning changes. (5) Record multiple takes (max. 4), one at a time, and listen back after each recording as you feel comfortable and adjust the articulatory variables for each recording until you are satisfied. Take data after each recording! What is your satisfaction rating from 0-5? What is your auditory/visual cortex telling you regarding gender perception? Are you hearing who you want to hear? Do you need to adjust pitch, inflection, or resonance? Keep asking organized questions

---

approaches into conversation with personal satisfaction.

Progress and Ongoing Challenges: Sessions #4 to #18

By session #4, SH was living in her gender socially and professionally. She also reported that she had been asked to be a bridesmaid in her brother's wedding. This included making a short speech. SH had multiple hurdles before the event, but she was excited to meet the challenge. The clinician and SH both decided on an ambitious schedule of twice-a-week sessions for the following 2 months until the wedding, doubling their efforts. Her goal was to develop a sustainable, personal, cisgender-assumed voice and commensurate nonverbal behaviors.

In session #5, the clinician started to discuss and develop nonverbal communication such as walking, sitting, and standing to build SH's confidence in being in the wedding party. By session #10, SH was growing in confidence during conversation, but she realized it was still challenging to maintain all her vocal and speech parameters during high-effort cognitive tasks, such as meetings or in-depth conversations with her partner. The clinician introduced the use of a conversational pitch anchor and SH learned how to "hang" and reset her pitch on a vocal thought-pause such

as "and," "if," "um," "so," "but," or "well." This was the only exercise for which the clinician trained her to keep words at a specific pitch of 196 Hz (G3). She practiced these words repetitively using her Tuna Pitch™ app and then practiced blending them in short phrases, such as "Aaaand (196 Hz) if you want to do it that way you might consider . . . " or "Buuuut (196 Hz) the other option might be . . . " and so forth. She successfully integrated these hangers into professional presentations.

In session #18, SH worked on these skills in her wedding clothes. During this session, SH was also instructed in nonspeech tasks such as laughing, coughing, and clearing her throat. All these tasks involve practicing a gentle cough or clear with a slight anterior tongue posture and /i/ configuration. Laughter was practiced on a series of progressive /hi/ hi/s while pulsing her abdominal muscles until SH found her own laugh at her desired pitch. (See Video 33 Shaping Non-Speech Vocalizations by Hirsch).

Posttreatment Acoustic Analysis: 18th Session

SH's pitch and resonance were reassessed in reading and spontaneous speech. Her speaking fundamental frequency (SFF) during the first 3 sentences of the Rainbow Passage was 205 Hz, with a semitone range (STR) of 24. Her SFF in spontaneous speech was 207 Hz with an STR of 25. SH rated her resonance to be 4/5 for brightness. SH's intensive GAVC was completed at 18 sessions. She reported that she felt happy and confident. She was ready for the wedding. Her final session was spent fine-tuning her resonance and nonverbal nuances. All but 6 of her measures on the TWVQ[19] were recorded at a 1 ("never or rarely"). Her total score post-training was 37/120 (as a reminder, per this questionnaire, the lower the score, the higher the satisfaction rating). SH reported a rating of 2—that she still "needed to concentrate" when using her voice, that it wasn't as "perfectly feminine as [she] would like," and that she was still occasionally being misgendered. She reported that sometimes her voice still sounded "male" to her when she laughed and that her voice occasionally fell out of her desired range in conversation when she lost mental focus. Overall, SH rated her voice to be "somewhat female" just before the wedding.

Discussion and Reflections

SH reported that she was "elated, ecstatic, and confident" at the wedding. She was able to give a short speech, maintaining her voice. SH reported that her role as a bridesmaid was the most joyous occasion of her life and that her "gender was affirmed 100% of the time" during the occasion. Two months post-training at a follow-up check-in session, SH's reading was 199 Hz and SFF was 211 Hz with STRs of 25 for both. She was maintaining her targets.

It is not uncommon for people to have to continue nuancing and fine-tuning their instrument for some years after training. SH recognized that need and continues to check in via email on occasion to ask questions or send voice samples. She and the clinician both agreed her successful outcome was due to her hard work and focus, but perhaps also to their willingness together as a client/clinician team to be creative in their solutions and recognize there is not a one-size-fits-all approach to GAVC. Tools need to be applied uniquely and with gentle artistry to help each individual find their personal voice.

CASE STUDY 9.2

Pitch-Elevation Surgery and Perioperative Voice Care for an Adult Transgender Woman

Wynde Vastine and Katherine C. Yung

Voice Evaluation

Chief Complaint. Voice and gender incongruence, pitch-elevation surgery candidate

We had the pleasure of seeing VC for an interdisciplinary (speech-language pathology and laryngology) voice and upper airway evaluation. The physician diagnosed the patient with dysphonia, other voice and resonance disorders, and gender dysphoria. To facilitate gender affirming informed consent, the SLP and laryngologist discussed these diagnoses with the patient and obtained her consent prior to assigning these diagnoses in the evaluation.

History of the Complaint

VC is a 26-year-old transgender woman and curatorial assistant (a job with moderately high vocal demands) with complaints of voice and gender incongruence, and an interest in pitch-elevation surgery. She reports that distress from this incongruence has been present all her adult life but increased over the past 5 years. She describes her current voice as fatigued and "locked up," and notes that her average pitch tends to drop with prolonged periods of speaking. She clears her throat intermittently throughout the day. Rest improves the feeling of vocal strain, but anxiety exacerbates it. She also reports safety concerns if she "forgets" and uses a lower-pitched voice in situations of surprise or with reflexive sounds such as laughing or sneezing. VC notes that voice is her biggest trigger of gender dysphoria. Because of this distress, she limits her speaking in social and professional situations, which has prevented her from advancing in her career. She sings for fun to the radio but does not have any formal training, nor is singing a goal.

Auditory-Perceptual Assessment

The Consensus Auditory-Perceptual Evaluation of Voice (CAPE-V)[23] was administered. The patient had an overall score of 27/100, indicating a dysphonia of a mild-moderate nature. Aberrant perceptual features identified in the voice included mild-moderate strain and mild-moderate intermittent roughness (particularly at the end of phrases). Overall vocal intensity was noted to be WNL in a quiet environment. Her vocal pitch was intermittently low for voice/gender goals. The resonance focus was laryngeal, and respiration appeared to be primarily thoracic. There was frequent evidence of breath holding prior to phonatory onset.

Manual Palpation Assessment

Muscle tension was assessed and rated on a 0 to 5 scale where 0 = "no tension" and 5 = "most tension."

Results indicated:

1. 4/5 tension at the thyrohyoid space
2. 3/5 tension at the hyoid attachments
3. 4/5 tension at the sternocleidomastoid muscles
4. 4/5 tension at the base of tongue
5. 3/5 tension at the trapezius muscles
6. 4/5 tension on lateral laryngeal movement bilaterally

Patient Self-Assessment

1. Vocal Fatigue Index (VFI)[24]:
   a. Tiredness and avoidance: 19/44
   b. Physical discomfort: 0/20
   c. Improvement with rest: 2/12
2. VHI-10[25]: 8/40
3. TWVQ[19]: 90/120

VC noted, "Currently my voice is 'somewhat female.' My ideal voice would be 'very female.'" While the patient's self-rating on the VHI-10 was not clinically significant (<11), results on the VFI indicate significant impact of fatigue on daily voice use, and the TWVQ revealed significant negative impact of voice and gender incongruence on her communicative quality of life.

Laryngeal Imaging

When evaluating voice disorders, laryngeal videostroboscopy is essential to visualize the structure and health of the larynx.[26] In cases of gender affirming care, it may not always be indicated due to (1) avoidance of unnecessary medicalization of the trans experience as outlined in the gender affirming care model[27-29]; (2) screening for potential voice disorders indicates there is no suspicion of a voice, swallowing, or upper airway disorder; and (3) avoidance of unnecessary medical costs, thus reducing barriers to transition-related care. However, VC's interest in surgery and her complaints of fatigue combined with auditory-perceptual features of strain and roughness indicated the need for imaging.

Laryngeal videostroboscopy was performed transorally with a 70-degree telescope assessing glottal closure, mucosal wave, and mucosal lesions that cannot be assessed with a plain light examination. Results revealed that the laryngeal position in the neck was elevated and that mild-moderate lateral and mild-moderate anteroposterior supraglottic constriction were present with phonation. Utilizing stroboscopic light, the following functional parameters were noted: complete glottal closure; mucosal wave and amplitude of lateral vocal fold excursion WNL; symmetrical abduction and adduction; occasional aperiodicity; and both phase symmetry and vertical height WNL.

The authors discuss the use of laryngeal videostroboscopy in this case as necessary because of the patient's desire to be considered a candidate for pitch-altering surgery. They further discuss that if there is no suspicion for pathology, then laryngeal imaging like videostroboscopy may not be necessary. Even when seeking voice care for gender congruence rather than due to a change in voice quality, a benign or malignant vocal pathology can be present. It is the clinician's responsibility to complete a comprehensive risk profile to determine whether laryngeal imaging is indicated.

For example, a change in quality from the patient's baseline necessitates imaging, as it would for any other patient entering the voice clinic. Recurrent voice loss or substance use such as smoking or vaping are other issues that would necessitate laryngeal imaging. In the absence of any concerning features, many voice clinicians are comfortable initiating behavioral voice strategies without laryngeal imaging for gender affirming care. Throughout behavioral voice training or therapy, the clinician continually monitors whether there is a need for laryngeal imaging at any time.

Acoustic and Aerodynamic Assessment

While acoustic and aerodynamic values are typically indicated in a comprehensive voice evaluation, particularly for surgical cases, due to the COVID-19 lockdown these measures were not obtained for this patient. The fact that these measures were not obtained, but goals were still met, hopefully opens discussion in our field regarding if and when their inclusion is necessary. The mean F0 from her voice sample reading of the Rainbow Passage was 175 Hz, as recorded via the lapel microphone with the Olympus CL-S11 laryngeal videostrobsocopy system at a 30-degree angle, 6 inches below her mouth.

Patient Education

The clinician educated the patient on the role of voice therapy to balance the breathing, phonatory, and resonance systems to achieve efficient phonation and its role in sustaining gender affirming targets and optimizing surgical rehabilitation. Risks and benefits of different gender affirming voice options (voice therapy only or voice therapy plus surgery) were explained in detail. Since VC verbalized interest in pitch-elevation surgery, endoscopic glottoplasty for vocal fold shortening (Wendler glottoplasty described in detail later in the case) was described at length, including how

the procedure is performed, typical results, the expected course of recovery, and potential risks including decreased vocal loudness, loss of upper singing range, and inability to attain pitch goals.

Stimulability

VC was stimulable for improvement using the following strategies: She completed syllable /u/ and phrase-level flow resonance tasks using the tactile cue of detecting consistent airflow on her finger, which was held about 1 inch in front of her mouth. With moderate cueing for consistent airflow on her finger and attention to oral vibratory locus, she endorsed decreased vocal strain, decreased roughness, and improved gender congruence.

Impressions

VC is a 26-year-old transgender woman who presents with mild-moderate dysphonia accompanying significant voice and gender incongruence that limits communication in all aspects of life. Laryngeal videostroboscopy was significant for hyperfunctional supraglottic constriction with phonation, which correlates with the auditory-perceptual features of vocal strain and roughness, as well as with the significant tension with palpation of the larynx. She appears to be an excellent candidate for a combined gender affirming therapy and surgery approach, considering her high motivation and demonstrated stimulability, as well as the impact of voice on her personal safety and communicative quality of life.

Plan of Care/Recommendations

Treatment is recommended in the form of voice therapy and surgical intervention. The clinician explained the treatment options during the evaluation session. The patient has elected to undergo treatment. Therapy will be conducted for 7 to 12 sessions of 45 to 60 minutes each. Sessions will be conducted 1 to 3 times monthly. The patient's long-term goal is to achieve a healthy, sustainable feminine voice for daily occupational, social, and emotional needs.

Goals of therapy will be to attempt changes in vocal function through the following strategies:

1. Establish oral resonance through the use of balanced airflow and phonatory coordination to reduce vocal strain and vocal fatigue preoperatively, and to reduce inflammation and promote postoperative vocal fold healing
2. Eliminate throat clearing using behavioral replacement strategies to prevent postoperative phonotrauma and reduce hyperfunctional muscle tension with voice use
3. Use manual laryngeal therapy with accurate placement and duration to reduce physical discomfort with phonation
4. Shift resonance formants to achieve efficient resonance congruent with feminine gender in structured speech tasks, as evidenced by patient report and clinician data

Decision Making

Typically, individuals desiring gender affirming voice services opt for 1 of 2 routes: voice training alone or surgery in combination with voice therapy, with other possibilities including opting not to change their voice at all or working on their voice solely by themselves. Avoiding gatekeeping (the requirement of unnecessary medical or psychological validation to provide care) entails fully discussing the risks, benefits, and limitations of surgery, including the crucial role of voice therapy in facilitating surgical healing, and reviewing gender affirming voice targets not addressed through surgery. However, the amount and course of therapy is individually tailored to the person's baseline vocal health and goals and is provided with the individual's informed consent. Our role as providers is not to prescribe a specific voice and gender outcome, but to support the individual in making fully informed decisions about the services they pursue to address their individual voice goals.

Surgery is not simply a tool for someone who "fails therapy," nor is it the inevitable choice for all transgender people seeking a feminine voice. Anecdotally, Vastine and Yung have observed the following themes in people who ultimately opt for pitch-elevation surgery:

1. Some patients find that they simply are unable to achieve their desired voice through training alone. They may have a desired target pitch range that is outside of the capabilities of their larynx. Surgery may help them achieve this range without strain.
2. Others find that they can achieve their desired voice in training but fear the possibility of "forgetting" to sustain their target pitch, such as in situations of surprise or with reflexive sounds such as sneezing or laughing.
3. Some find that the act of changing their voice is distressing or dysphoria inducing, as if it calls into question the truth of who they are. This may also be true of those who opt for nonsurgical options, but for some people, surgery is the only way to eliminate this distress.

450   Voice Therapy: Clinical Case Studies

4. While many find they can generalize their target voice through training alone, some find that only surgery can eliminate the cognitive effort in sustaining their target voice.
5. Some people have simply done the research on the surgery and have decided this is what they want.

VC arrived in our clinic knowing that she wanted to undergo surgery, citing her voice as the biggest trigger of dysphoria and the fear of her pitch dropping in situations of surprise. Her report of vocal avoidance that is limiting professional advancement is just one way in which her voice and gender incongruence is negatively impacting her full participation in life. Equally important are her complaints of vocal strain and frequent throat clearing, the presentation of which is consistent with MTD. The MTD must be addressed prior to surgery. By eliminating strain and facilitating phonatory efficiency through resonant voice, she will optimize surgical wound healing. Maladaptive behaviors such as throat clearing can have phonotraumatic effects on the vocal folds and can slow healing postsurgically. Even for surgical candidates without a presentation of MTD, preoperative therapy can prepare them for efficient postoperative voice use. Other gender affirming targets can be addressed before or after surgery, depending on their timeline.

Outside of voice-related factors, additional considerations for surgical planning often include coordination of other gender affirming surgeries. Due to concern for intubation injury, patients are generally advised to allow a 4- to 6-month window after glottoplasty before undergoing additional elective procedures that require intubation. Also, thyroid cartilage reduction poses a potential risk to the vocal folds (anterior commissure detachment). If patients are considering thyroid cartilage reduction, they are generally advised to undergo this procedure prior to or at the same time as pitch-elevation glottoplasty.

VC's priority was her voice, and there were no scheduling conflicts. She desired thyroid cartilage reduction at the time of glottoplasty.

Intervention

Refer to Table 9–2.

Preoperative Therapy

Preoperative therapy was conducted over the course of 3 sessions. It addressed the MTD and the related throat clearing, introduced gender affirming formant resonance, and gave VC tools to prepare for the voice rest protocol. Myofascial release to the jaw and thyrohyoid, as well as tongue stretch training, supplemented simple to complex conversational-level resonant voice tasks targeting airflow-phonatory coordination. When cued for "increased airflow" that was "almost but not quite breathy" on a 3-sentence introduction, VC quickly realized that this "lighter" voice felt better physically and emotionally and eliminated the need to clear her throat. To facilitate generalization, she completed daily 5-minute conversational-level negative practice alternation between her self-described "lighter" versus "throat" voice, otherwise applying her "lighter" voice throughout the day. She was introduced to the use of vowel formant shifts through the application of the /i/ shape to all other vowels to further improve voice and gender alignment. Counseling was provided when VC reported heightened transgender-related stress and anxiety, noting its impact on her voice. She reported mental health support for the anxiety but a desire for improved community support. The gender-related stress and its impact on the voice were validated and resources were provided for local trans and queer events as a way of building community. VC reflected appreciation for being supported through this process by another trans person (author WV). Educational counseling was provided on the typical gradual return to voice use following surgery: 2 weeks of complete voice rest, followed by 5 to

Table 9–2. Voice Therapy Goals and Techniques

Goal	Therapy Techniques
Establish oral resonance through the use of balanced airflow and phonatory coordination to reduce vocal strain and vocal fatigue preoperatively, and to reduce inflammation and promote healing postoperatively	• Semi-occluded vocal tract exercises (straw phonation in water) • "hmm" resonant voice resets • Balance airflow/phonatory coordination across a hierarchy of speech tasks
Eliminate throat clearing through the use of behavioral replacement strategies to prevent postoperative phonotrauma and reduce hyperfunctional muscle tension with voice	• Liquid sip behavioral replacement strategy • Prevent urge to clear throat by eliminating vocal strain
Use manual laryngeal therapy with accurate placement and duration to reduce physical discomfort with phonation	• Tongue stretches • Thyrohyoid and jaw muscle myofascial release
Shift resonance formants to achieve efficient resonance aligned with feminine gender in structured speech tasks	• Use of /i/ vowel formants • Kinesthetic awareness of facial, sinus, and super head vibrations

10 minutes of voice use per hour during week 3, 10 to 20 minutes per hour during week 4, and 20 to 30 minutes per hour during week 5.

> Clinical protocols for voice rest and return to voicing are not standardized across surgeons. The clinician is generally guided by surgeon preference but can also go to the literature to review postsurgical voice rest protocols following Wendler glottoplasty.

Surgical Intervention

The patient underwent uncomplicated thyroid cartilage reduction and endoscopic glottoplasty for vocal fold shortening (Wendler glottoplasty) via cold-steel technique. The chondrolaryngoplasty was performed via a submental incision with a laryngeal mask airway (LMA). With the thyroid cartilage exposed, the vocal folds were localized with flexible laryngoscopy performed via the LMA. Once the level of the vocal folds was determined, the cartilage above this level was safely removed. After completion of the chondrolaryngoplasty, the patient was intubated with a 5-0 microlaryngoscopy endotracheal tube (MLT) and the glottoplasty was performed. Laryngeal exposure was achieved via a customized Ossoff-Karlan-Dedo laryngoscope (Pilling®). Under the operating microscope, the anterior one-third of the infraglottic epithelium was removed sharply from bilateral vocal folds, including the anterior subglottic mucosa. Two interrupted stitches were placed to close the anterior commissure. At the conclusion of the surgery, the new anterior commissure was set back approximately 50% of the previous length of the membranous true vocal folds.

Postoperative Visit

Session #4 was a joint visit with the clinician and laryngologist, 2 weeks after surgery. VC reported adherence to the 2 weeks of complete voice rest. Laryngeal videostroboscopy was performed with a 70-degree rigid laryngoscope. Bilateral vocal folds were noted to be mobile with full rotation of her vocal processes. The anterior commissure was set back about 50% of the membranous length with mild bilateral posterior vocal fold edge erythema and edema. Bilateral vocal folds had intact mucosal wave and vertical phase difference posterior to the newly constructed anterior commissure, with touch closure observed across elicited pitches.

During her initial recorded voice sample, her pitch was higher than typical for her gender, age, and vocal goals (averaging 350 Hz), and she had a moderately strained upper-register voice with mild-moderate roughness and mild breathiness. While some amount of strain and roughness is typical for this stage of vocal fold healing, this degree of strain and the high-pitched voice needed to be addressed immediately. Since VC already had the foundational tools from the preop therapy, she was able to achieve a more functional pitch range and eliminate strain in about 10 minutes. The previously trained semi-occluded vocal tract (SOVT) "cup bubbles" exercise with tongue protrusion was used to decrease strain while finding a more efficient mean F0, appropriate to her reduced vocal fold length. (See Video 10 Straw Bubbles by Braden.) Once a more comfortable pitch range was located, the airflow and phonation were coordinated with scaffolding from words to simple conversational-level tasks, thus decreasing the strain and roughness. Her voice sample was re-recorded with a mean F0 of 196 Hz. She cried tears of joy and said, "I can't believe this voice is possible. This feels so relaxed." To facilitate healing and functional use of relaxed resonant voice, the clinician advised her to complete daily SOVT tongue protrusion cup bubbles 3 times per day and the trained resonant voice scaffold once per day, and to implement "relaxed" oral resonance in functional communication tasks during her 5 to 10 minutes per hour of voice use.

VC was using excessive muscle tension that she had used to reach higher pitches preoperatively. The laryngeal videostroboscopy exam showed that she was healing well with the ability to achieve a smoother sound than what she demonstrated on her voice sample. Postoperative voice therapy with an experienced SLP was crucial in helping her to unload the strain, achieve a more efficient voice, and support favorable postsurgical healing. Without appropriate postoperative voice therapy, VC may not have been able to attain her voice goals, no matter how exceptional her surgical result might have been, supporting previously published results that vocal happiness is significantly improved when surgeons collaborate with voice-specialized SLPs for therapy.[30]

Postoperative Voice Therapy
The rest of the follow-up therapy was completed over the course of 4 more sessions, initially at biweekly frequency to support her through the healing process via the modified voice rest protocol until she returned to typical voice demands. Continued counseling was required regarding the avoidance of using a loud voice in social situations, with education provided on the role of loud environments (via the Lombard effect) and alcohol in limiting awareness of speaking loudly. During these sessions, the clinician continued to facilitate a resonant voice with the newly changed anatomy (shorter vocal folds) and to optimize healing. Throughout the therapeutic process, VC learned to use SOVT exercises in the morning to help warm up her voice into a functional pitch range (averaging around 190 Hz) and as a tool for navigating the self-reported impact of anxiety on her voice, as she had stated, "My voice becomes more throaty when I am anxious." Guided kinesthetic awareness and progressive relaxation techniques were used with the SOVT cup bubbles exercise, which helped her to further differentiate between efficient versus strained phonation in conversational level tasks, thus improving her self-efficacy.

She quickly demonstrated increasing independence and self-cueing for her new mean pitch range and higher formant frequencies as trained in the preoperative therapy.

At the end of the course of postoperative therapy, she was trained in the efficient use of increased volume. This was done through using a "bright" or "twang" forward resonance, which was initially performed on /ng - i/ tasks to achieve and build auditory and kinesthetic awareness of this sound. She learned to use different degrees of this bright quality at the sentence to conversational level, ultimately demonstrating the ability to over- and undershoot the sound until she found a level of brightness that aligned with her vocal identity but eliminated strain during sentence- to simple conversational-level tasks at different volumes. (See Video 34 Increasing Loudness After Pitch-Elevation Surgery by Vastine.) VC found that cueing for a "sneeze sensation" further helped her achieve a feeling of vibrations "in my nose, behind my eyes, and even outside of my head" during loud tasks, which she demonstrated without strain. At this point, VC felt she had fully met her goals and verbalized happiness with her voice, and she was discharged from therapy.

CASE STUDY 9.3

Manual Therapy in Gender Affirming Voice Care for a Transmasculine Adult on Hormone Replacement Therapy (HRT)

Daniel P. Buckley and Felicia A. François

Voice Evaluation

Chief Complaint. Voice-gender incongruence

Case History

History of Voice Complaint. Patient DG (he/him) is a 38-year-old transgender man with gradual onset of voice problems. He began biweekly intramuscular testosterone injections 7 months ago and began to notice changes to his voice 3 months ago. His pitch has become slightly lower, he has some pitch instability, and he notices voice breaks. He shares that despite his slightly lower pitch, he continues to be misgendered in person and particularly over the phone. He would like the pitch of his voice to be even lower. He reports strain and vocal effort when trying to reduce the pitch of his voice. He doesn't like the tone or resonance of his voice and would like a more masculine-sounding voice overall. In some instances where increased safety is a priority, such as while traveling across the country for work or while interacting with strangers, he would like an even more stereotypically masculine voice to ensure he is gendered correctly. In other parts of his life, such as socially and at work, he doesn't mind having a slightly less stereotypically masculine voice. He would like the ability to slowly incorporate his goal voice at work rather than suddenly. The patient has not received the services of an SLP for his voice in the past. The patient reports no significant medical history and does not take any prescription medications other than his biweekly testosterone injections.

Voice Use. The patient works in disability policy advocacy as an organizer and outreach event coordinator and reports significant voice demands for work. He has many Zoom meetings each day, as well as at least one in-person outreach event each week. He often travels to other states for events, where he gives speeches in front of crowds; he usually has a microphone for these events, but not always. He is a social person and goes to loud social gatherings at least twice per month. He lives with his partner, and they love to sing for fun while at home together.

Laryngeal Imaging

Laryngeal videostroboscopy was completed. The following parameters, documented in Table 9–3, were assessed using the Voice-

Table 9–3. VALI Ratings

1. Glottal Closure: Posterior gap
2. Amplitude: Right: 60%, Left: 60%
3. Mucosal Wave: Right: 60%, Left: 60%
4. Nonvibrating Portion: Right: 0%, Left: 0%
5. Supraglottic Activity: anteroposterior: 1/5, mediolateral: 2/5
6. Vertical Level: On plane
7. Free Edge Contour: Right: Normal, Left: Normal
8. Phase Closure: Nearly equal to closed-phase dominant
9. Phase Symmetry: 100%
10. Regularity: 90%

Vibratory Assessment of Laryngeal Imaging (VALI).[31]

Vocal Effort, Fatigue, and Pain

The OMNI Vocal Effort Scale[32] was completed. The patient rated vocal effort on a 0 to 10 scale where 0 = "extremely easy" to produce voice and 10 = "extremely hard" to produce voice. The patient reported the following vocal effort scale values within the corresponding situational voice demands:

1. Typical one-on-one conversational voice use: 3/10 (social use; somewhat easy) and 6/10 (work; somewhat hard).
2. Louder speaking demands: 7/10 (street canvassing; somewhat hard to hard) and 6/10 (presenting at work meetings; somewhat hard)
3. Other: 6/10 (in loud social environments; somewhat hard) and 6/10 (when upset or emotional; somewhat hard)

The patient reports some mild pain (gesturing to the general perilaryngeal area) and fatigue after using his voice for extended periods of time (beyond 3 hours), but he reports that this resolves with voice rest and sleep.

Quality-of-Life Impairment

1. VHI-10[25]: 16/40 (threshold = 11)[33]
2. Voice Catastrophization Index[34]: 24/52
3. Transgender Self-Evaluation Questionnaire[35]: 111/150 (scores range from 30-150, with higher scores indicating greater voice impact)

Auditory-Perceptual Assessment

The CAPE-V[23] was administered and the patient was determined to have an overall CAPE-V score of 23/100, indicating a dysphonia of a mild nature. Aberrant perceptual features identified in the voice included primary strain and secondary intermittent roughness. Overall vocal loudness was noted to be WNL. Pitch of the voice was elevated for age and gender, and intermittent pitch breaks were heard. Resonance was focused in the oral region. Respiration was primarily abdominal-thoracic. Intermittent breath holding was observed.

Manual Palpation Assessment

Manual palpation assessment results are detailed in Table 9–4.

Of note, the patient reported the thyrohyoid space and superior edge of the hyoid bone body bilaterally to be areas of heightened discomfort, which correspond to his negative sensations of vocal effort when speaking for prolonged periods. Both during sustained phonation and at rest, the larynx appeared to sit in a high position, with the hyoid bone body resting at times level with and above the ramus of the mandible.

Acoustic and Aerodynamic Assessment

All acoustic data were collected with a dynamic headset microphone (WH20XLR; Shure; Niles, IL) placed at a 90-degree angle at 6 cm from the corner of the mouth and analyzed using Praat

Table 9–4. Manual Palpation Assessment Results

Muscle/Muscle Group	Clinician's Perception of Tension	Patient's Report of Pain/Discomfort
Suprahyoid Muscle Group (mylohyoid, stylohyoid, geniohyoid, digastric muscle: anterior and posterior bellies)	Moderate	Moderate
Infrahyoid Muscle Group (sternohyoid, sternothyroid, omohyoid; do not consider thyrohyoid here)	None	Mild
Thyrohyoid Space	Moderately reduced	Moderate
Sternocleidomastoid (SCM)	Mild	None

software. See Table 9–5 for results with normative data derived from Goy et al (2013), Boone et al (2014), and Buckley et al (2023).[36–38]

Aerodynamic data were collected using the Phonatory Aerodynamic System (PAS) by Pentax Medical (Montvale, NJ). Norms for the aerodynamic and acoustic measures of transgender patients do not exist at this time; therefore, we cannot say if any measures taken today are abnormal. Norms presented are those for cisgender women and cisgender men within the patient's age range from Lewandowski et al (2018)[39] and Zraick et al (2012).[40] Refer to Table 9–6.

> Notice that laryngeal videostroboscopy and acoustic and aerodynamic assessment are included in this case, as the patient reported voice changes (eg, voice breaks), increased vocal effort, and physical discomfort while voicing, and the clinician noted mild dysphonia with palpably increased perilaryngeal muscle tension.

Stimulability

The patient was introduced to laryngeal manipulation (laryngeal depression via sustained inferior traction applied to the hyoid bone) during sustained phonation while speaking at the conversational level. The clinician perceived a lower mean pitch during voicing, with less strain and more consistent vocal registration via reduced register breaks. Intermittently, the patient reported some mild discomfort with manual depression but noted that the "lower-pitched voice and change in vocal color" was appealing to him.

> The term "vocal color" is used by singers to indicate the resonant quality of the sound. Another term for this concept is "timbre." "Bright," "warm," and "brassy" are examples of words used to describe vocal color.

Impressions

The patient presents with voice-gender incongruence and a mild dysphonia characterized by primary strain and secondary intermittent roughness with intermittent pitch breaks. During palpation, the patient identified various loci of reported discomfort, and the clinician observed increased perceived tension primarily in the suprahyoid musculature and reduced opening of the thyrohyoid space during phonation and at rest. Further, the clinician observed that the patient's larynx rested in a perceived

456 Voice Therapy: Clinical Case Studies

Table 9–5. Acoustic Assessment Results

Task/Measure	Normative Reference	Results
Reading (The Rainbow Passage)		
Fundamental frequency (mean)	Males: 98-140 Hz Females: 183-234 Hz	186.8 Hz
Fundamental frequency (standard deviation [SD])[6]	Males: 16-37 Hz Females: 27-57 Hz	28.2 Hz
Smoothed cepstral peak prominence (CPPS)	Males: >6.40 dB Females: >6.49 dB	8.2 dB
Spontaneous Speech Sample		
Fundamental frequency (mean)	Males: 98-140 Hz Females: 183-234 Hz	189.2 Hz
Fundamental frequency (standard deviation [SD])[6]	Males: 16-37 Hz Females: 27-57 Hz	30.0 Hz
Sustained Vowel /ɑ/		
Smoothed cepstral peak prominence (CPPS)	Males: >11.72 dB Females: >11.05 dB	13.85 dB
Pitch Range		
Minimum pitch	N/A	125 Hz
Maximum pitch	N/A	678 Hz
Pitch range in semitones (ST)	Males: Mean: 34.2; Range: 27-41 ST Females: Mean: 29.5; Range: 22.2-36.7 ST	29.3 ST

high position, with the hyoid body both level with and above the ramus of the mandible, and laryngeal videostroboscopy revealed increased mediolateral compression during phonation. Both findings suggest increased perilaryngeal muscle tension that may impact voice production. Via acoustic evaluation, the patient's mean fundamental frequency during spontaneous speech was 189.2 Hz, which rests at the bottom of reference values derived from those assigned female at birth. This aligns with the patient's reports of self-perception of a high pitch for his gender, alongside the high position of the larynx, which may contribute to higher vowel formant frequencies and to increased perception of vocal femininity. These factors and the patient's reported voice-gender incongruence limit communication and participation in all aspects of life and impact his feeling of safety and comfort when interacting with

Table 9–6. Aerodynamic Assessment Results

Aerodynamic Measures	Results	Norms: Cisgender Women Ages 18-39	Norms: Cisgender Men Ages 18-39	
Vital Capacity (L) (expiratory volume)	3.1	2.87 ± 0.69	4.14 ± 1.14	
MFR (L/sec): Vowel (mean airflow during voicing)	0.11	0.13 ± 0.06	0.13 ± 0.06	
Laryngeal Resistance (cmH$_2$O/L/sec)	77.8	68.2 ± 53.08	79.44 ± 120	
Psub (cmH$_2$O)	7.2	5.4 ± 1.37	6.65 ± 1.98	
		Norms: Cisgender Women	Norms: Cisgender Men	Norms: Cisgender Women and Men Ages 18-39
MFR (L/sec): Rainbow Passage	0.13	0.14 ± 0.05	0.16 ± 0.05	0.15 ± 0.05
Duration (sec)	22.9	22.62 ± .17	23.42 ± 3.23	20.95 ± 2.06
Breaths (#)	5	4.75 ± 1.76	5.08 ± 1.72	4.38 ± 1.44

others. His goal is to obtain a "deeper, more masculine" voice that is more physically comfortable and is associated with reduced vocal effort. He appears to be a good candidate for therapy. Prognosis for improvement is good given positive stimulability testing today (both via auditory-perceptual evaluation and patient reported outcomes) and the patient's motivation and readiness for change.

Plan of Care

Therapy is indicated and will be initiated following this evaluation. Therapy will be conducted once every 1 to 2 weeks and will consist of 6 to 8, 45-minute therapy sessions. This may be increased or decreased pending the patient's response to therapy and personal goals; to be reassessed monthly.

Long-Term Goals:

1. The patient will report improved voice-gender congruence in 80% of interactions with familiar and unfamiliar conversation partners in home, work, and social environments.
2. Decrease vocal effort and strain in conversational speech at the patient's target pitch as evidenced by lower self-reported scores on the OMNI-Vocal Effort Scale.

458 Voice Therapy: Clinical Case Studies

Short-Term Goals:

1. The patient will perform laryngeal massage and reposturing maneuvers independently without cues or visual models twice daily.
2. The patient will perform cup bubble exercises (straw phonation in water) including descending pitch glides in the target pitch range (about 130-150 Hz) with minimal cueing from the clinician 5 times within a session.
3. The patient will read short passages aloud with a mean fundamental frequency in the target pitch range (<140 Hz) with minimal cueing from the clinician 5 times within a session.
4. The patient will engage in spontaneous discourse aloud while maintaining a predetermined "back" and "dark" resonance, with limited report of vocal effort and with minimal cueing from the clinician, for 10 minutes within a session.

Decision Making

In this case, the patient presented with the primary concern of gender-voice incongruence and wished to obtain a voice that he feels is more masculine. However, his reports of intermittent vocal effort and fatigue with prolonged voice use (socially and professionally), as well as the sensation of straining his voice when trying to modulate his voice to a lower pitch, suggest an imbalance of the subsystems of phonation and underlying elements of MTD, which should also be addressed. It may be useful and encouraged to adapt intervention targets to consider the physiology and contributing factors of both the dysfunction and the patient's voice goals, and to fine-tune targets that may address both simultaneously. Without addressing these symptoms of vocal hyperfunction and by solely focusing on lowering of the pitch and/or addressing resonance, the underlying vocal hyperfunction may contribute to unsustainable vocal function, and DG's course of therapy and response to treatment may be delayed.

Incorporating goals that directly meet the patient's stated goals is a way to promote motivation and establish rapport and trust. Pitch goals were established, as this was self-identified as an area the patient wished to have more control over, and resonance goals were established after education with the patient on the impact of laryngeal height/vocal tract shape on voice quality. It may be useful for the clinician to briefly educate on what those terms mean and how they may sound, as patients often benefit from the opportunity to practice different vocal qualities and determine for themselves what qualities and characteristic shifts make up their ideal voice. When providing gender affirming voice care, it is especially crucial to let patients guide treatment targets, as clinicians should not be prescriptive of what certain voices "should" sound like to fit into a socially determined binary of masculine and feminine. Specifically, with this patient, the goals will simultaneously address vocal longevity, stamina, and resonance/pitch goals.

Therapeutic techniques for goals were chosen using an evidence-based practice model, including all 3 tenets: best available evidence, clinician expertise, and client/patient perspectives. To reduce excessive perilaryngeal tension, laryngeal massage was incorporated, as it has been shown to improve symptoms in individuals with vocal hyperfunction.[41] Additionally, laryngeal massage and reposturing has been shown to aid in reducing speaking fundamental frequency, increasing estimated vocal tract length, and perceiving gender as more masculine for transmasculine individuals.[42,43] To aid in optimal phonatory-respiratory coordination and reduction of hyperfunction during phonation, SOVT exercises were used.[44,45] Throughout the entire treatment process, decreasing vocal effort was a main focus, given DG's reported effort levels on the OMNI Vocal Effort Scale.[32] Treatment involved an eclectic therapeutic approach that addressed multiple voice characteristics, including lower pitch and back resonance, as it is important to address not only pitch but also other elements of voice that contribute to gender perception.[11,46]

Intervention

Intervention began with an initial exploration of voice and the ways one can alter different pieces of the "Voice Puzzle" with an in-person appointment. (See Video 35 The Voice Puzzle in Gender Affirming Voice Care by François.) Education provided on aspects such as pitch, resonance, intonation/melody, articulation, and word choice allowed DG to begin exploring different combinations of these variations. All intervention sessions were led with both long-term goals in mind.

The first session involved 20 minutes of laryngeal massage. (See Video 36 Laryngeal Massage and Resposturing to Lower Pitch by Buckley.) The clinician introduced laryngeal massage and resposturing as a method to "help the voice box sit in a lower, more relaxed position." The clinician performed laryngeal massage on the patient while he held a mirror to visualize and explained the maneuvers, which included:

- Thyroid cartilage/laryngeal pull-downs: The clinician applied pressure to the suprahyoid muscles with their pointer finger and thumb bilaterally and dragged down along the lateral aspects of the thyroid cartilage, yielding inferior traction while pressing inward to apply medial pressure.
- Hyoid pushbacks: The clinician applied medial pressure to the anterior aspect of the hyoid bone and pushed slightly posteriorly.
- Lateral thyroid stretches: The clinician applied pressure to the thyroid cartilage unilaterally and moved the larynx to the contralateral side, then repeated in the opposite direction. This was performed

both as dynamic stretches where the larynx was moved laterally without pause and as static, slow stretches to both sides, holding each side in a lateral stretch for up to 30 seconds.

As time progressed, the clinician perceived that the larynx could be lateralized slightly farther than at the start of the session. DG reported the massage felt relaxing and showed independence with the maneuvers quickly. Voicing during some maneuvers was incorporated to generalize the lower, relaxed laryngeal position to a phonatory context. The clinician asked DG to phonate on various stimuli, including /m/ and /o/, with the focus on feeling low effort, and provided exploratory cues to attend to any auditory-perceptual changes that DG could perceive. This was used to promote carryover to voice use and to plant the initial thought of attending to somatosensory cues, while addressing short-term goal #1.

Next, the clinician led the patient through the SOVT cup bubbles exercise to explore his pitch range. The clinician instructed him to place a straw into a cup of water and begin blowing bubbles. Once a steady, consistent flow of air was established (as evidenced by a consistent pulsing/rate of bubbles), he was asked to begin phonating an /u/ through the straw, first at whatever pitch he liked if it was low effort and comfortable. (See Video 10 Straw Bubbles by Braden.) Initially, the patient demonstrated some phonatory breaks, but with increased duration of practice, these lessened. The clinician instructed the patient to focus on producing a voice with low effort that elicited even, consistent bubbles. To promote carryover to conversation- and discourse-level voice use, the clinician told DG to speak spontaneously following a 1- to 2-minute session of phonating on the comfortable pitch in the straw and water. He was instructed to attend to somatosensory voice targets such as how his voice felt (ie, effort) and sounded (ie, any aspects of voice quality). The patient reported that his voice sounded "lower in pitch" and felt "more relaxed," both of which were positive experiences for him. The clinician observed an initial lowering of spontaneous pitch and decreased strain. As the first session concluded, he was told to practice laryngeal massage/reposturing at home, as well as the SOVT single-pitch exercise in the straw and water with attention to somatosensory experiences.

In subsequent sessions, he was introduced to descending pitch glides in the straw and water to explore his lower range in a manner that facilitates low-impact phonation. He was guided to perform descending pitch glides in the target pitch range that matched his preferred speaking range, in accordance with short-term goal #2. He was instructed to begin at a comfortable pitch around G4 (~196 Hz) and slowly descend to a lower pitch, all while maintaining the previously reported low vocal effort. To assist with target acquisition, the clinician intermittently played the pitches C3 (~130 Hz), D3 (~147 Hz), and E3 (165 Hz) as the bottom pitch targets the patient would glide down to. Intermittently, the patient reported sensations of increased vocal effort, and the clinician perceived strain. Cues to attend to "relaxing" and "think of yawning slightly" during the initial descent assisted the patient greatly in reducing the negative reported sensations and yielded a voice with increased loudness, lower pitch, and decreased strain around the C3 to F3 ranges.

In subsequent sessions, DG reported more ease and consistency in his lower range with daily home practice of laryngeal massage and cup bubbles. Sessions then focused on transfer of skills in his lower range using a hierarchical approach. The clinician led him through exercises including sustaining a lower pitch on a single phoneme (ie, /m/), then advancing to the syllable (ie, "ma"), word (ie, "morning"), phrase (ie, "Maybe on Monday"), and sentence levels (ie, "May I interest you in a beverage?"). Resetting with a resonant /m/ hum around D3 improved his ability to maintain this lower pitch at the phrase level and beyond. After 2 sessions with this hierarchy, he was led through short reading passages, during which he was cued to reset with his low hum as needed. Intermittently, the patient reported some increased vocal effort and noted intermittent voice breaks. He was encouraged to use quick implementations of SOVT exercises or laryngeal massage and reposturing when he noticed negative voice symptoms in this context. DG reported it was initially difficult to know if his voice was "low enough" on some of the sustained phrases, so he downloaded a free pitch tracking app on his phone, which he found to be intermittently helpful. This work addressed short-term goal #3.

Throughout the pitch-specific exercises detailed above, DG also explored resonance on a continuum from "very back" to "very forward" with opportunities to try each spot on the continuum. Cues for a yawn-sigh were utilized to explore back resonance qualities. Intermittently, the clinician encouraged him to utilize manual depression of the larynx via laryngeal pull-downs to assist with laryngeal lowering that helped him acquire the "back" resonances. He practiced this by repeating various words and phrases with and without manual depression of the larynx while maintaining the "back" resonance throughout. The patient found it helpful to attend to the concept of a "slight yawn," which visually demonstrated a lower laryngeal position during phonation without the use of any digital manipulation of the larynx. DG found that a resonance that was "just forward of very back" was most appropriate for his everyday speech, but that "very back" may be helpful for situations where his safety is in question. Other qualifiers such as "dark" (using cues for reducing oral embouchure, with cues to reduce labial articulatory movement) and "light" (maintaining a smile while speaking) were explored at the discourse level, and DG found the combination of "just forward of very back" and "dark" was most appropriate for his ideal, authentic voice. He practiced his ideal voice over the course of 3 sessions, with eventual generalization to spontaneous conversation while staying mindful of a relaxed, reduced-effort way of producing voice to address short-term goal #4. Some sessions were carried out remotely via telehealth when there was not a need for clinician manipulation of the patient's larynx.

The final sessions of his course of voice therapy included generalization of his ideal/goal voice to different contexts. Contrast practice was used to reinforce volitional alternation between the voice he will use most of the time and the "very masculine" voice he wants to use in certain situations. The SLP encouraged continued utilization of any SOVT exercises, resonant humming /m/ sounds, or laryngeal massage/reposturing maneuvers as needed. He was also encouraged to monitor his vocal effort throughout practice and to note any instances of increased voice breaks or other negative voice sensations. By the end of the seventh session, the patient reported that his vocal effort was very low to minimal, and he noted fewer voice breaks. Because patients often report difficulty maintaining their ideal or goal voice across various contexts, including those that induce heightened emotion or stress, different emotional and situational contexts were used throughout therapy (ie, emotional versus nonemotional prompts of conversation). In later sessions, he practiced making phone calls to his friends and random businesses (to introduce voice use with unfamiliar individuals), giving presentations/talks related to his work, and having spontaneous conversations with the clinician in therapy.

Posttreatment Outcome Measures and Clinician Reflections

Following the course of treatment, DG completed a short voice recording that was analyzed for average fundamental frequency in speech; this was measured to be 138 Hz, which was within his target range as established in therapy. Palpation performed by the clinician revealed improved ratings of perceived tension (albeit this is a subjective measure and prone to various levels of reliability) and patient report of reduced pain/discomfort.

Following completion of therapy, he continued to perform laryngeal massage to prevent and reduce vocal fatigue before and after speaking engagements for work. He reported that SOVT exercises remained an effective tool for him to "feel good" before and after long periods of voice use and to remind him that a low level of vocal effort and heightened voicing efficiency is possible. He reported he intermittently appreciated using the pitch tracking app to check in on his pitch, but he ultimately felt he required more conscious attention to his resonance than his pitch in day-to-day conversations. He reported being happy with the progress made in therapy. DG reported greater confidence while presenting at work, and he shared he is no longer held back socially. He found that switching to the "very masculine" voice in some situations is easier than he initially expected. He is considering attending a voice therapy group every so often to maintain his skills.

CASE STUDY 9.4

Developing a Gender Affirming Voice in a Nonbinary Adult

Desi Gutierrez

Voice Evaluation

Chief Complaint. Misgendered in person and on the phone, and voice is too high

Case History

History of Voice Complaint. XZ is a 28-year-old nonbinary adult who presents for a comprehensive voice evaluation by the SLP and the laryngologist. Their goal is to have a lower, "more ambiguous" voice. They do not

Voice Therapy: Clinical Case Studies

hate their voice, but they often get misgendered and people perceive them as a woman, which is very distressing for them. They have attempted some voice modification independently online, but they have had difficulty identifying a voice they like. They also have ADHD, which they specified makes it difficult for them to develop and maintain routines. They have no additional dysphonia, dyspnea, or dysphagia.

Transition History. They began their social and medical transition approximately 2 years ago and are now out 100% of the time. They have considered initiating testosterone, but not at this time. They are not familiar with any surgical intervention for their voice, but they are similarly not interested. They report they are well connected with mental health and social resources.

Voice Use. The patient reports high vocal demand as a marine biology PhD student. They describe their professional vocal demand to be high, as they teach 2 courses and have a student leadership position. Their personal and social vocal demand is moderate, regularly talking with friends and their wife and participating in biweekly Dungeons and Dragons sessions.

Laryngeal Videostroboscopy

Laryngeal videostroboscopy was performed transnasally with a flexible distal chip videolaryngoscope. The exam was overall unremarkable with no vocal fold lesions or masses throughout the pharynx and larynx. The clinician noted full abduction and adduction bilaterally with complete glottic closure across pitches.

Patient-Reported Quality-of-Life Impairment

1. VHI-10[25]: 15/40 (threshold = 11)[33]
2. Voice-Related Experiences of Nonbinary Individuals (VENI)[47]: 52/68 (higher scores indicate the patient's voice has a higher impact on their quality of life)
   a. Physical: 20/28; functional: 26/32; emotional: 6/8

Auditory-Perceptual Assessment

The CAPE-V[23] was administered and the patient was determined to have an overall score of 28/100, indicating mild dysphonia. Aberrant perceptual features identified in the voice include high pitch, mild strain, and inconsistent mild roughness. Vocal loudness was noted to be WNL and pitch variability was high. Reduced phonatory airflow and variable anterior-posterior tone focus, with intermittent vocal fry, was noted. Respiration was primarily abdominal-thoracic.

Manual Palpation Assessment

Muscle tension was assessed and rated on a visual analog scale where 0 = "no tension" and 100 = "most tension." Results indicated 0/100 tension at the thyrohyoid space, suprahyoid region, or submandibular region. Patient denied tenderness with palpation.

Acoustic and Aerodynamic Assessment

All data were gathered remotely using Phonalyze, a web portal that utilizes Praat software and that patients can access with their smartphones. Norms are derived from a literature review examining optimal norms for remote acoustic voice analysis.[48] Patients record themselves using their own smartphones, positioned 12 inches from their mouth. See Tables 9–7 through 9–10 for Patient XZ's results.

Stimulability

Stimulability testing was completed using resonant voice therapy (RVT) techniques, which revealed a change in pitch, quality, resonance, and airflow. Specifically, they benefited from humming on a sustained /m/ pitch and gliding throughout their pitch range. The patient was able to identify changes in the sound and feel.

Impressions

This is a 28-year-old adult with incongruence between voice, communication, and gender. Laryngeal examination is unremarkable. In relation to their goal of a lower and more

9. Gender Affirming Voice Care 463

Table 9–7. Physiological Pitch Range

Hertz	Notes	Semitone Range	Semitone Range Norms (SD)	Abnormal
152-727	Eb3-F#5	28	F: 37 (8); M: 38 (13)	NA

Table 9–8. CPP Sustained Vowel /a/

	Value	Female Norms (SD)	Male Norms (SD)	Abnormal
Mean F0 (Hz)	211.12	210.4 (22.7)	110.9 (16.1)	N/A
Mean F0 SD (Hz)	7.16	2.37 (5.24)	0.75 (0.28)	N/A
CPP	24.86	N/A	N/A	N/A
CPPS	15.59	15.08 (2.04)	17.18 (2.71)	N/A

Table 9–9. CPP Voiced Sentence: "We were away a year ago."

	Value	Female Norms (SD)	Male Norms (SD)	Abnormal
Mean F0 (Hz)	200.57	197.90 (16.70)	133.1(15.2)	N/A
Mean F0 SD (Hz)	32.87	33.17 (5.82)	51.34 (18.5)	N/A
AVQI	5.28	2.60 (0.67)	2.28 (0.91)	N/A
CPP	22.18	N/A	N/A	N/A

Table 9–10. CPP Rainbow Passage (Sentences 1-5)

	Value	Female Norms (SD)	Male Norms (SD)	Abnormal
Mean F0 (Hz)	206.38	197.90 (16.70)	133.1(15.2)	N/A
Mean F0 SD (Hz)	35.01	33.17 (5.82)	51.34 (18.5)	N/A
CPP	22.22	N/A	N/A	N/A
CPPS	10.88	7.59 (0.73)	7.22 (0.79)	N/A

ambiguous voice, they demonstrated increased pitch as well as high variability in pitch and resonance. They were stimulable for improved pitch, quality, resonance, and airflow. They seemed highly motivated to attend therapy and implement recommendations, which are good prognostic indicators for voice therapy. Voice therapy is recommended to address incongruence between voice, communication, and gender and to optimize voice use patterns.

464   Voice Therapy: Clinical Case Studies

Plan of Care

The SLP and laryngologist discussed the above findings and the role of voice therapy with the patient. The patient would like to proceed with voice therapy and will schedule 4 sessions to begin, with additional sessions as needed based on progress. The patient will begin to increase self-awareness of daily voice use patterns. The patient verbalized an understanding of the findings and plan.

Long-Term Goal (LTG). Demonstrate improved voice, gender congruence, and ease and quality of voice production with 80% accuracy in conversational speech in the target pitch range and inflection independently with self-corrections

Short-Term Goals (STGs):

1. Maintain a daily routine for voice practice in both individual and social contexts, measured by journaling and daily reporting to the clinician
2. Employ laryngeal massage and tongue stretches to promote laryngeal and extralaryngeal relaxation as measured by patient report and clinician observation
3. Demonstrate improved coordination of breathing and phonation with improved resonance in conversation with 80% accuracy in the target pitch range and inflection

Decision Making

Based on their goals and vocal presentation, the patient is an excellent candidate for voice therapy. Therapy will allow them to explore the capabilities of their vocal mechanism and find a voice that feels affirming. Although they have researched vocal masculinization, they have a limited understanding of the aspects of voice that contribute to the perception of gender or how these can be manipulated to address their goal of androgyny. Exploring these nuanced concepts in therapy allows them to meet their goals while avoiding testosterone, which they are not otherwise interested in. Testosterone

has several physical and mental effects, and it may not provide their desired voice, as the effects on pitch may be too small or too large.[49] Moreover, they demonstrate inefficient voice use patterns, so they may inevitably need therapy to optimize their voice and address other components of gender perception. The only notable barrier to progress is their stated concern for adherence. Strategies to improve adherence and establishing a daily routine will be a focus of therapy.

Like many patients seeking gender affirming voice care, XZ did not have a strong concept of how they wanted their voice to sound. The approach to therapy centered the patient by exploring their vocal abilities and encouraging them to develop opinions regarding their goals. As such, various parameters of the voice that relate to the perception of gender were introduced and modeled for them on a spectrum. The clinician then guided the patient through exploration and encouraged them to develop thoughts. The parameters were not introduced with gendered language (eg, increased intonation is correlated with the perception of femininity) unless the patient asked. Because this patient has several vocal traits that contribute to the perception of femininity and they have a goal of androgyny, the clinician initially introduced methods and parameters that can increase their perception of masculinity, but used other parameters as needed.

Intervention

Therapy began with a long conversation about the patient's perceptions of voice and gender, including a discussion about how they are always in control of the direction of therapy, how they should feel empowered to form and express their opinions, and how developing their voice is for them and not for others. Since they don't hate their voice, they shouldn't let people in their life convince them otherwise. With the tools of therapy, they should feel empowered to use their new voice 100% of the time or choose how and when they alter their voice based on the situation or desired gender presentation. They expressed understanding and appreciation.

Short-Term Goal #1

Short-Term Goal #1. Maintain a daily routine for voice practice in both individual and social contexts, measured by journaling and daily reporting to the clinician.

To address the patient's concern for low adherence, they emailed the clinician every time they practiced. The clinician and patient agreed that if they had not practiced in about 48 hours, they would receive an email reminder. Throughout therapy, they typically opted to simply say, "Done," but as they had additional exercises, they began noting completion by exercise (eg, "Individual," "A little; practice with wife," "70% of the day"). Their adherence fluctuated throughout the course of therapy, ranging from practicing 5/14 to 12/14 days. Each session began with a recount of how many emails they sent to the clinician, to highlight that the emails were being tracked. They stated that this form of accountability was very helpful for them to stay on track.

Motivational interviewing (MI) techniques[50,51] were also used throughout therapy to support adherence. For example, their first session began with a long conversation exploring their goals and motivations for undergoing therapy. MI strategies included asking open-ended questions (eg, "What are your goals and how can I help you achieve them?"), reflective listening (eg, "I get the sense that you don't have a target voice in mind"), and summarizing their goals. Throughout therapy, the clinician supported their progress by affirming their new skills while providing feedback to enhance their effectiveness (eg, "I like the way you implemented this technique. Maybe we try a slightly different way and see how the sound changes"). At the end of each session, they recited their homework to elicit change.

Short-Term Goal #2

Short-Term Goal #2. Employ laryngeal massage and tongue stretches to promote laryngeal and extralaryngeal relaxation as measured by patient report and clinician observation.

The clinician introduced perilaryngeal massage techniques to reduce extraneous muscle tension, increase awareness of tension holding patterns, and manually induce an enlarged pharyngeal area and decreased pitch. The patient was instructed on independent completion with visual cues and modeling. Stretches included (1) anterior-to-posterior palpation of the thyrohyoid space, (2) pulling down on the superior border of the thyroid cartilage, and (3) lingual extension. Following these stretches, they demonstrated slightly decreased pitch and felt "openness" and "relief" in their throat. These techniques were used at the beginning of their independent voice practice and therapy sessions as well as throughout the day to manage perilaryngeal tension.

Short-Term Goal #3

Short-Term Goal #3. Demonstrate improved coordination of breathing and phonation with improved resonance in conversation with 80% accuracy in their target pitch range and inflection.

Resonance and Pitch. Patient XZ was first introduced to RVT techniques to establish a target pitch and introduce a fuller feeling and sound. They began humming at a comfortable pitch (~230 Hz, Bb3), and with cues to open and relax their throat, they were able to feel vibrations on their lips. They maintained this relaxed feeling with lip vibration on gentle sirens and glides. These glides primarily explored notes lower than where they initially hummed, but they also explored slightly higher pitches to learn the sound and feel. They were prompted to stop humming at a pitch that felt comfortable in their mind and throat. This was their first target pitch (~195 Hz, G3), on which they began chanting vowels (eg, /mɑ/, /mu/, /mɛ/), words (eg, "man," "magic," "morning"),

466 Voice Therapy: Clinical Case Studies

and /m/-loaded sentences (eg, "Molly needed milk money"). However, after practicing at the sentence level, they reported that it felt like they were "acting" and "putting on a deep voice" rather than finding a voice that suits them. RVT was discontinued for now.

The clinician introduced techniques for modifying tongue height to alter resonance in a more natural context. (See Video 37 Modifying Tongue Height to Alter Resonance by Gutierrez.) To first explore the effects of tongue height on their voice, they were educated on how their tongue height can impact the resonance of their voice without modifying the pitch.

The clinician said, *"Some sounds have a naturally high tongue position and others have a naturally low tongue position. It's the difference between /i/ and /ə/. You may notice that even on the same pitch, the quality of the sound changes. Try it and let me know what you notice."*

After briefly experimenting with high /i/ versus low /ə/ tongue height, they noted the /ə/ sounded deeper and they wanted to practice with low tongue height. They were prompted:

"You can keep the same sound and feeling of the /ə/ into more regular speech by maintaining a low tongue height. Of course, you have to move your tongue to maintain normal articulation, but as we move forward, think about keeping the back of your tongue low and relaxed."

They were prompted to sustain a neutral vowel /ə/, then advanced to consonant-vowel syllables (eg, /mə/, /nə/, /lə/). To promote carryover to speech, the patient was prompted to replace vowel sounds with the "uh" sound in words. For example:

"Muhn" (/mən/) → "Man"

"Muh-guhc" (/mə.dʒək/) → "Magic"

"Muh-nuh" (/mə.nə/) → "Money"

"Muh-cruh-wuhv" (/mə.krə.wəv/) → "Microwave"

The patient then advanced to phrases and sentences. For example:

"Nuh muhn uhs uhn uhluhnd" (/nə mən əz ən ə.lənd/) → "No man is an island."

"Nuhthuhn nuhvuh ruhn uhguhn" (/nə.θən nə.və rən ə.gən/) → "Nathan never ran again."

They were able to continue the lower sound and relaxed feeling at this level. They then alternated between sentences replacing vowels with /ə/ and speaking them normally, with high accuracy in maintaining a more open sound. With guidance, the patient noticed that their pitch lowered and intonation flattened without specifically addressing these parameters. They liked this voice better than their previous voice but were overall unsure of the sound.

At their second session, they returned with several opinions regarding the exercise. They enjoyed the fuller sound but thought the pitch was too high. They revisited RVT concepts and were quickly able to achieve the open sound introduced in the previous session. As they hummed on glides, their voice was most comfortable at about 183 Hz (F#3), or about 12 Hz lower than their former target, which they had considered too low. They used this pitch to chant vowels, words, and sentences into conversation. They benefited from humming on their target pitch prior to chanting and occasionally listening to their target pitch. Without intermittent auditory cues of their target pitch, their voice began to drift lower, which introduced strain.

> The author uses the term "fuller voice." A "full voice" is a term often used in singing to mean use of a voice that is clear (without breathiness), has forward resonance, and is perhaps slightly louder.

Intonation. In the same session, they built on this lower pitch by introducing natural intonation. Similar to previous concepts, intonation was introduced on a spectrum from high pitch variability in both words and sentences to flatter intonation with slight downward contour. Initially, the patient was shocked that anyone would prefer flatter intonation. Therefore, they introduced their natural, highly variable intonation on previously practiced sentences, but attempted to maintain their target pitch (F#3) as an average frequency. However, their average pitch rose and vocal fry returned, despite humming their target pitch before and after the sentence and visually tracking their pitch on a smartphone app. They continued to practice at this level until the next session. To build awareness of intonation, they were encouraged to attend to the intonations of people in their life and those whose voices they like.

They arrived at their third session with several reflections about intonation. They noticed that their friends and family of all genders have high pitch variability, but androgynous voices from AFAB individuals they enjoyed often had lower pitch variability. Since the previous session, they felt somewhat comfortable with the ability to find their target pitch and were able to independently find it within 1 semitone at the beginning of the session. Using sentences they were already practicing, the clinician prompted them to attempt a more stable intonation pattern with a slight lowering at the end. They benefited from decreasing their speech rate, modeling by the clinician, and visualizing their pitch with a smartphone pitch monitor. At this point, their target transitioned from a single pitch to a range from 160 to 185 Hz in conversation. They were able to stay within this lower range in conversation, but they began introducing strain and pushing their voice down to achieve their lower notes.

Airflow. In the same session, the clinician introduced flow phonation to ensure the patient maintained adequate airflow to support the lower end of their vocal range. (See Video 7 Flow Phonation by Gartner-Schmidt.) Airflow was introduced on a spectrum from excessive breathiness to lack of breath, which causes roughness and/or strain. The patient was prompted to place their open hand 1 to 2 inches from their face, take a full breath, and gently blow on their hand. They noted "nothingness" in their throat and the gentle air on their hand. Patient XZ then turned on their voice to make an /u/ sound on their target pitch. They reported that this airflow made maintaining their target pitch easier. Tasks advanced to /w/-initial words (eg, "why," "wow," "when"), short sentences (eg, "What's your name?" "Where are you?"), and using /u/ to set their voice for regular sentences (eg, "/u/-Good morning," "/u/-I'm in California"). After a few minutes of practice at the sentence level, they removed the /u/ aid, prompting them to feel the airflow on their hand without it, then slowly lowering their hand. They had difficulty removing their hand, so they practiced at this level until their next session.

At their fourth session, Patient XZ was able to maintain airflow in short sentences only. The clinician provided them with sentences of increasing length to help them manage airflow in longer phrases. This series of sentences called "Why don't you?" began with a single word ("Why?") and increased in length until it reached 38 words.[52] They initially had difficulty maintaining their breath through 5 to 8 words, but after a few minutes of practice and reintroduction of the /u/ and hand aids, they were able to maintain their breath throughout all sentences.

Carryover. Discussions of carryover into the patient's daily life began at the first session and increased in frequency throughout therapy. Since day 1, Patient XZ felt socially comfortable implementing these concepts into their daily routine, because they were 100% out as nonbinary and they had supportive friends, including their Dungeons and Dragons group, who were primarily LGBTQ+. After the first session, they began implementing open, relaxed tongue resonance into short, low-stakes conversations with their friends and wife, which they felt they were able to maintain with fair accuracy. At the second session, the clinician discussed implementing vocal resets, including resonant communicators (eg, "mhm," "umm") in accordance with RVT techniques. As new concepts were introduced, they were encouraged to incorporate them into increasingly more complex conversations with people and situations in which they felt less comfortable. Because they were concerned about their ability to maintain their voice while teaching their class, they presented one of their lectures during their fourth session, complete with standing as they would during class. As they began using their voice with more strangers, this served as an opportunity for feedback on how people gender them with their new voice.

Posttreatment Outcomes

After therapy, Patient XZ reported that they enjoyed their voice and felt comfortable producing it on command. With their target voice, they are rarely gendered feminine. They do not regularly use their target voice with their wife or friends, but they have implemented it into their daily communication with students, colleagues, and professors. They did not have a follow-up with the laryngologist; rather, outcome measures were collected at their last therapy session. The patient was determined to have an overall CAPE-V score of 4/100, indicating WNL voice quality. Aberrant features included slight, inconsistent strain. They demonstrated decreased pitch and pitch variability compared to their initial evaluation, which was confirmed in both perceptual and acoustic measures (Rainbow Passage: F0 = 177 Hz; F0 SD = 16.5 Hz).

This patient's course of therapy was not linear. As the patient learned more about their vocal capabilities and developed preferences, the clinician weaved between concepts and approaches to meet their needs. They rarely asked about how each component presented related to the presentation of gender; rather, they gravitated toward whichever sound they liked the best. This included using their unmodified voice in circumstances in which they wanted to. Through therapy, they built the skills and confidence to choose and modify their sound as they pleased. Following this initial course of therapy, the patient was guided to return for a 6-month follow-up to ensure continued satisfaction and account for any evolution of their vocal preferences and needs.

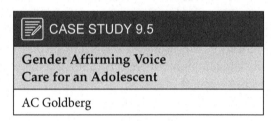

CASE STUDY 9.5

Gender Affirming Voice Care for an Adolescent

AC Goldberg

Introduction

No two individuals who seek out gender affirming voice care are the same, and no population is more outstanding in their individuality than adolescents. No other group of clients is more expansive with their identities, and no other patients require more clinical creativity and space for exploration. Therefore, treatment approaches must be highly individualized and uniquely flexible to adequately address the needs of this population. Regarding the myriad of factors related to endogenous, exogenous, or paused puberty, one must also account for how youth communicate their identities through their voices. Many adolescents are not simply seeking to align their voice with their gender, but are also seeking to explore their persona and how to communicate authentically on a multitude of levels. We must also consider language processing, and in this case specifically, the interplay of Gestalt Language Processing (GLP) with communication and treatment approach. Here, we look at one case as an example, remembering that no two nonbinary genders are the same, as we also explore how neurotype factors into communication style.

Trigger Warning. Mentions of self-harm and controversial clinical practices

Evaluation

Case History

BN is a 17-year-old autistic nonbinary adolescent who was assigned male at birth. They reported never being offered puberty blockers or gender affirming care, despite understanding and telling their providers and caregivers about their gender at a young age. From the ages of 6 to 13, they had a behavior incentive chart for which they earned "rewards" for acting in an "expected" manner. One of the items on this chart, which was a formal part of their Individualized Education Program (IEP) at school, reads: "Reduce scripting."

BN explained that the way they expressed their gender as a child was through scripting "My Little Pony" phrases and interactions. School professionals viewed this as a behavioral issue to intervene with and correct. When the clinician asked what impact this had on them and their communication, they said they had self-harmed and slowly became nonspeaking in school. They began using an augmentative and alternative communication (AAC) device intermittently to communicate 4 years after the introduction of the behavior plan.

BN's history is remarkable for trauma. Gender/neurodivergent trauma arises when people are exposed to therapies that deny their autonomy and instead force them to conform to seemingly arbitrary societal constructs. One treatment used with BN in the past was applied behavioral analysis (ABA). It is important to acknowledge that ABA has been the subject of debate among clinicians.[53,54] The Association of Behavioral Analysis International has recently published a position statement on the use of conversion therapies stating: "It is the position of the Association for Behavior Analysis International that conversion therapy and associated practices are fundamentally unethical and unjustifiable."[55]

> The editors encourage the reader to pursue further information on ABA to learn more about current perspectives and applications. With a primary focus on voice, further context is not provided in this text. Responsible, informed application of any therapeutic modality is critical to promote patient autonomy, well-being, and authentic communication.

BN reported anxiety and dysphoria that intensified as their endogenous puberty advanced and their voice began to change. This coincided with a family move to another state, where BN's IEP was adapted for high school and the behavior incentive plan was no longer used. In spite of this, BN reported feeling a deep shame associated with the scripts they used throughout their childhood to communicate about their gender experiences. During the interview, it became clear that BN, while identifying as nonbinary, might want to be read and gendered by listeners as a binary female speaker. Their shame and trauma associated with expressing femininity[56] plays a complex role in their identity, and they are aware of this. When the clinician first met BN, they were finishing their senior year of high school and preparing to move to college in the fall. They wanted to go to a new school feeling more confident about their gender expression and communication. BN reported that their pitch felt "too manly" and that this was interfering with their desire to communicate aloud. While in school, BN opted to use an AAC device full-time starting their sophomore year of high school. They reported that both the device and their discomfort with their vocal presentation significantly limited their social

470 Voice Therapy: Clinical Case Studies

opportunities and decreased their quality of life. BN's desired mode of communication is spoken, but the sound of their voice stopped them from wanting to access this communication set in front of everyone aside from immediate family for 2.5 years prior to the start of voice therapy. They reported having a small group of friends online, supportive parents, and 2 older siblings with whom they could practice communicating in a new voice.

Medical History. BN is autistic and diagnosed with anxiety and obsessive-compulsive disorder (OCD). At the start of services, BN had very recently gained access to gender affirming hormones estradiol and spironolactone (spiro). BN's medical history is also significant for encephalopathy, which was resolved via surgical shunt/repair when they were 3 years old. They reported remission of gastrointestinal symptoms and no formal diagnoses, though it is suspected that they have irritable bowel syndrome (IBS). Their health history is unremarkable for gastroesophageal reflux disease (GERD) or any underlying vocal pathology. Their hearing is WNL as per their most recent physical exam.

Therapy Goals

The words "feminine" and "femininity" are used throughout this text because they were used by the client; please note that the word "feminine" may be received as a microaggression by another nonbinary person and that each person's terms for themself should be honored.

Client Goals. BN's goals changed during therapy, as is typical for many transgender and nonbinary individuals, especially adolescents. At the time of intake, BN said their goals were:

- To be comfortable using their speaking voice at college (non-device-generated speech)
- To be accurately gendered while playing online video games

- To decrease social anxiety with strangers
- To be read as "female" whenever they want to be

Clinician Goal. To support BN in communicating confidently and authentically with a healthy voice and more congruent self-image

Initial Impressions

BN's voice, prosody, and inflection were all staccato with narrow pitch range and no variation of volume or resonance. The clinician believed that BN's GLP style and many years of primarily using an AAC device as their mode of communication had influenced the sound of their voice. That is to say, BN's language formulation and the sound of their voice were similar to that of device-generated speech. BN's pitch range on initial measures was restricted to 76 to 78 Hz across speech tasks, including sustained vowels, the Rainbow Passage (sentences 1-3), and back-and-forth conversation. Their clinician described their resonance as "anterior-cul de sac with twang," pitch as "flat," prosody as "monotone," and volume as "within normal limits." Because of BN's history of IEP-related services influencing their self-expression, they developed imposter syndrome around expressing their gender while communicating, something about which they were very forthcoming.

Voice Evaluation

This evaluation was completed with a 17-year-old whose expression and primary mode of communication fluctuated throughout care.

- Voice Quality: No dysphonia
- Average Pitch: 77 Hz across spoken tasks
- Maximum Sustained /a/: 31 seconds; pitch: 77 Hz; duration of /a/: WNL[57]
- Maximum Sustained /i/: 24 seconds; marginally reduced[57]
- Pitch Range: 76 to 78 Hz during reading and conversation; initially unable to produce pitch glides, with attempts result-

ing in steady increase in volume and no change in pitch

- Loudness: Able to vary loudness; 58 to 80 dB SPL
- Prosody/Inflection: Monotone; possible delayed echolalia (ie, influenced by or imitation of longer strings of speech from their AAC device)
- Resonance: Anterior-cul de sac with twang
- Tension: Self-reported Temporomandibular joint (TMJ) discomfort
- s/z Ratio: 1.33, WNL[57]
- Respiratory: WNL; diaphragmatic breathing
- Referrals: None; videostroboscopy not indicated as BN's vocal presentation did not contain signs or symptoms of traditional dysphonia or obvious underlying vocal pathology
- Related Services Without Interprofessional Collaboration: Psychotherapy, executive function coaching

Patient Questionnaires

TVQ[35]: Total score 84; moderate voice concern

BN indicated "usually or always" for 19/30 statements describing their actual experience "living as female." Items below most closely reflected their voice and communication goals outlined at the initiation of therapy:

- I feel anxious when I know I have to use my voice.
- The pitch of my speaking voice is too low (reiterated throughout course of care).
- When I speak, the pitch of my voice does not vary enough.
- I feel uncomfortable talking to friends, neighbors, and relatives because of my voice.
- My voice restricts my social life.
- My voice doesn't feel authentic to the "true me."
- I feel self-conscious about how strangers perceive my voice.

- I feel discriminated against because of my voice.

Other important factors:

- My voice makes me feel less feminine than I would like.
- My voice results in others misgendering me.
- I avoid using the phone because of my voice.
- I'm tense when talking with others because of my voice.
- I avoid speaking in public because of my voice.
- I feel frustrated with trying to change my voice.
- When I am not paying attention, my pitch goes down.
- When I laugh, my voice is too deep/ booming.
- My voice doesn't match my physical appearance.
- I am less outgoing because of my voice.
- It distresses me when I am misgendered because of my voice.

VHI total score: 62, severe concerns; scored "always" for 4 out of 10 statements in the functional domain, 0 out of 10 statements in the physical domain, and 9 out of 10 statements in the emotional domain.[18]

Initial Course of Care

BN initially had difficulty varying pitch without changing volume. Anterior-cul de sac resonance with twang was considered a positive prognostic quality, which enabled an increased brightness that BN would adopt as a desired vocal quality. BN's priorities included:

- A strong desire to move from using their AAC device to speaking
- A strong desire to be gendered in a feminine manner

472 Voice Therapy: Clinical Case Studies

- A strong desire to feel connected to their voice
- A strong desire to find an authentic voice that represented their gender *before* moving to college

The clinician and client decided on weekly meetings to address their vocal incongruence and began treatment with pitch-related tasks. It is important to note that BN did not have any priorities or goals addressing physical safety, but this was explored through various scripts to provide access to a hyperfeminine situational vocal set if needed, to prevent misgendering in a context that could lead to violence (such as speaking aloud in a restroom).

Navigating Identity, Terminology, and Self-Expression

While no two nonbinary genders are exactly the same, BN overtly disclosed their repressed femininity resulting from their behavior plan in elementary and middle school education. BN expressed the desire to communicate in a way that would result in others gendering them as female, but they expressed anxiety that others might tell them that these vocal/communication qualities were not desirable or authentic. The clinician encouraged BN to revisit their childhood scripts because they were a way of accessing a shift in pitch and reclaiming the femininity taken from them by behavior modification practices. During conversations related to these scripts, BN disclosed that while they felt "female," they would never call themself that, and had "settled on nonbinary" because their femininity would never be "real." This will be discussed further in the counseling section, relating to both trauma and imposter syndrome.[58]

Throughout the course of service, BN's pronouns shifted from they/them to she/her to she/they to fae/faer, and back to they/them. While their pronoun shifts were not clinically relevant because their gender remained feminine-nonbinary, conversations around pronouns influenced care by virtue of written documentation, counseling, and self-advocacy. As it is the role of the clinician to remain attentive to and supportive of changes in pronouns and identity language, each time BN's pronouns changed in their teletherapy name box, the clinician clarified identity language and documentation reflected those changes.[59] Additionally, the clinician used these opportunities to check in about goals and to determine if these changes in identity language would result in different short- or long-term voice and communication goals.

Progression

BN's course of therapy was 17 months long. Sessions fluctuated between weekly and biweekly due to scheduling. The first 5 sessions with BN focused on assessment, discussion around desired vocal qualities, and stimulability trials. By session #6, BN was able to alter their pitch in 50% of all highly structured trials with maximal prompting (eg, models for ascending modified scales, mimicking car alarm, imitating familiar people's voices) at F#3 (185 Hz) for open vowels, single words, and short phrases. BN's confidence grew and they asked to raise their pitch further. During session #10 (month 4), they were able to alter their pitch to G#3 (208 Hz) in 75% of all highly structured instances at the open vowel, word, and phrase levels. Once they were able to transition to G#3 in structured conversation, they began speaking to their family in their affirmed pitch some of the time. It became evident to the clinician that BN was more adept at reaching their target pitch in phrases and sentences due to their GLP. Strategies for carryover included imitation of scripted language from TV characters in the target pitch range, anchoring for the target range from previously memorized material, and methodical transition from imitation to formulation.

Between sessions #14 to #17, care transitioned to counseling-only to support generalization outside of treatment and to reducing social anxiety related to perceived fear of what others might say. At session #20, BN reported speaking to their family in their affirmed pitch 100% of the time. Around month 7 (session #21), the clinician began layering in other desired vocal qualities: breathiness, prosody, and legato. BN required visual cues for prosody and legato. Using screen sharing during teletherapy, the clinician used color and symbol coding as well as linear approximations of intonation patterns superimposed over text. The client and SLP collaborated to find representative voice samples containing the desired level of breathiness for BN to approximate imitation. Sessions #24 and #25 were joint sessions with BN and their parents, who initiated a conversation about OCD, which will be further discussed in the section on parent involvement. At this point, BN had decided to take a gap year before starting college and had secured a job at a local library. Sessions #31 to #37 were dedicated to sustaining pitch, desired level of breathiness, prosody, loud/confidential voice, and creating/practicing scripts for their new job. At session #38, BN self-discharged due to gender voice alignment, social success, work success, and alleviation of social anxiety when speaking to strangers. At this point, BN had not used their AAC device in over a year.

Counseling and Comorbidities

The following counseling practices were implemented or attempted: motivational interviewing, exposure/desensitization, trauma-informed practices, and management of anxiety and imposter syndrome. These practices are reflected in the narrative below.

When trauma impacts the brain, it cannot be contained, dialed back, or compartmentalized. The past intrudes on the present and the nervous system reacts accordingly.

Working with BN, trauma around repressing their feminine vocal qualities as a child (scripting "My Little Pony") was a consistent counseling topic as well as an access point for them to move into a pitch that represented their femininity. They were previously conditioned to mask this form of self-expression, which they described as "nonconsensual surgical removal." This forced them to keep these language-rich gestalts, *which also represented their gender*, private. They reported that they slowly became secretive about watching "My Little Pony" and even engaged in self-harm (head banging) when a script from the show became stuck in their head. This form of conditioned masking required targeted unlearning of negative associations during voice sessions for BN to gain comfort in expressing their femininity through their voice.[60] When the clinician inquired about communicating with their therapist, they explained that their therapist was helping them with issues related to compulsive behaviors, and they did not wish to disrupt their progress by addressing this, as it was unrelated. BN reported that they no longer self-harmed due to repression of "My Little Pony" scripts, so no contact seemed clinically necessary (or desired) with their outside providers, and their parents agreed. Another clinical consideration was BN's diagnosis of OCD, which will be addressed further in the parental involvement section.

To change BN's associations with these formerly beloved scripts, BN and the clinician listened to video samples on YouTube, imitated them, and discussed the positive messaging they contained. The clinician encouraged BN to repeat their favorite scripts when their mood was elevated and to begin to use the scripts again (even if not aloud). Slowly, BN reclaimed their scripts. They became animated and excited when talking about "My Little Pony." They used their favorite pony's voice as a pitch access point. BN, no longer needing these specific scripts to communicate, began

474 Voice Therapy: Clinical Case Studies

accessing them to induce gender euphoria when communicating.

Self-Advocacy and Accommodations

BN required long, uninterrupted processing and formulation time during their sessions. The clinician provided them with notes and recorded voice memos as needed to reinforce strategies and allow them access to the clinical space on their own time, when they could process uninterrupted by our interactions. Accommodations used included: transcripts of sessions, repetition of questions/prompts, typing in the chat as a form of communication, unlimited processing and formulation time, verbal and written session schedule outlines (developed jointly), unlimited repetitions/demonstrations, turning the camera off on their screen, turning the microphone off while they tried new vocal techniques, and flexible rescheduling if exhaustion made them unable to participate. The clinician also encouraged BN to revisit their insistence on no longer using their AAC device, as using a device should not be stigmatized and can often be a form of accommodation.

The clinician discussed self-advocacy at length with BN, who felt unsuccessful in their attempts to gain access to gender affirming care until recently. The clinician and BN created and rehearsed self-advocacy scripts to ask for sensory accommodations at their new workplace. They also wrote scripts related to self-advocacy for spaces such as the doctor's office, their future needs at college, and even their neighborhood. The importance of working with adolescents on self-advocacy cannot be overstated.

Parental Involvement

Around 9 months (session #24) after voice sessions began, BN's parents contacted the clinician without their knowledge or consent to discuss an uptick in perceived OCD-related behaviors. The clinician encouraged BN's parents to include BN in a conversation about

their health, and created a plan to discuss this at the next meeting. BN's mother expressed concerns around whether the voice work was intensifying BN's OCD symptoms, which they described as pacing, scripting, picking of skin, and carrying around the AAC device. BN's parents initiated a conversation around the AAC device to reinforce BN's goal of discontinuing use and were supportive and affirming in their statements. At this point in care, BN was consistently using an affirmed voice at home and in sessions but had still been unable to transfer their voice outside of the home. BN's parents were concerned that the uptick in these behaviors would lead to a backslide in progress, resulting in a return to using an AAC device, and that using the device, subsequently, would limit their employment opportunities. The clinician reminded BN and their parents that using an AAC device is a perfectly valid form of communication that would not take away any vocal progress but would rather make communication more accessible if needed. BN sat with their head down and did not speak during this session. The clinician checked in again about communicating with their counselor, who, at that time, was on parental leave. The following week the clinician, BN and their parents met again to discuss the same concerns. During this session, BN asked their parents to leave the room so they could practice job interview scripts. Within a week, they obtained a job where they were able to use their affirmed voice throughout the day with everyone they encountered. There was no further parental engagement with services.

Outcome

BN's story is one of great success. They benefited from services that respected their intersectional autistic and transgender identities through trauma-informed practices. BN had supportive parents who affirmed their gender and encouraged self-actualization. BN was able to revisit past traumas related to gendered scripting of "My Little Pony" and use those experiences to access an authentic voice. At the onset of sessions, BN was using an AAC device, anxious about using their voice, and limiting their social interactions. Upon discharge, BN was able to speak in an affirmed voice 100% of the time, gained employment, made friends, and has since entered college.

Further Thoughts

When thinking about BN's case, it is vital that clinicians consider the complex nature of a person's communication history. BN's GLP communication profile necessitated a conscientious approach, shifting vocal presentation from approximating that of their AAC device to a historically echolalic production of a beloved character. Validation of their echolalia allowed them to access an affirmed voice, something which they had previously been denied. Given the plethora of voices now available to AAC users, BN may have benefited from client-led consultation around selected device-generated vocal presentation. Finally, the importance of appropriately recognizing and responding to trauma cannot be overstated.

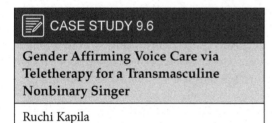

CASE STUDY 9.6

Gender Affirming Voice Care via Teletherapy for a Transmasculine Nonbinary Singer

Ruchi Kapila

Voice Evaluation

Client AG (he/they) is a Latine, Spanish-English bilingual, 21-year-old transmasculine nonbinary individual (disclosed AFAB) who presented to a teletherapy evaluation with complaints of intermittent hoarseness, laryngeal tension, and strain following introduction of testosterone hormone replacement therapy (HRT) 12 months prior to the visit. He is also a choral singer and avocational solo vocalist, reporting concerns with "accessing low notes" and pitch breaks in their passaggio.

Case History

Voice History. AG began singing choral music in church when he was 10 years old, which they continued until they left the church shortly before disclosing their gender and pronouns to immediate family at age 15. He concurrently sang in school choirs during middle school and high school from ages 12 to 17 and participated in solo and ensemble competitions. Their high school choral director (who AG disclosed to) was supportive of AG singing in their desired voice placement sections, encouraging him to "float" between alto and tenor lines during choral rehearsals and performances. However, AG reported feeling pressured to sing in traditional soprano or mezzo-soprano range for solo competitions due to the director's concerns regarding vocal injury, lack of experience working with trans and nonbinary singers, and uncertainty of how AG would be scored in classical voice contexts.

Given that AG lived in a small town and did not have ample financial resources for individual voice training, the choir director served as AG's voice teacher after school throughout his high school experience. He encouraged AG to consider moving toward a countertenor repertoire after high school to facilitate greater gender congruence without having to "risk voice changes" by receiving HRT. However, AG reported finding classical voice "limiting," and while they wanted to continue to develop classical technique, he also wanted to explore singing contemporary commercial music (CCM) and songwriting. Currently, AG participates in group voice classes at his community college and is seeking a mixed-voice chorus that is LGBTQ+ friendly, in addition to avocational songwriting and wanting to sing CCM samples on social media again.

Medical History. AG reported a medical history of depression, anxiety, seasonal allergies, childhood history of asthma with no recent episodes or exacerbation, and recent diagnosis of ADHD. Medications include topical testosterone 20% (40 mg), Wellbutrin/bupropion XL (150 mg) once per day, Abilify/aripiprazole (2 mg) once per day, and an over-the-counter (OTC) antihistamine taken as needed. Following graduation from high school, they sought gender affirming care through an LGBTQ+ clinic specializing in transgender health, where he works with a gender therapist, care coordinator, and psychologist. AG reported they have no history of intubation but are actively pursuing further gender affirming procedures. He denied any history of signs or symptoms of traditional dysphonia, dysphagia, GERD, and laryngopharyngeal reflux (LPR). AG does not smoke, drinks socially (1-2 drinks/week), takes edible forms of marijuana 3 to 4 times a year, and drinks approximately 64 to 108 ounces of water per day.

AG reported experiencing the aforementioned voice concerns during vocal warm-ups and rehearsals in his group voice class approximately 3 months after initiating testosterone. Given their online community-based research on expected voice changes and challenges with exogenous testosterone, AG felt reluctant to seek local medical intervention to assess their voice changes, especially given the dearth of gender affirming providers in their immediate area. However, when his group voice instructor noted inconsistencies in their vocal performance week to week, she strongly recommended going to the ear, nose, and throat physician (ENT) to rule out any abnormalities.

AG saw a general ENT approximately 1 month later, with no local laryngologist available. The videostroboscopy report per AG's care visit summary stated the exam was unremarkable with intermittent mild supraglottic constriction for higher pitches, likely consistent with recent HRT intervention. The ENT referred AG to an SLP within their insurance network for gender affirming voice intervention. AG attended an initial evaluation with this SLP, reporting that she provided introductory voice education, including vocal hygiene considerations, diaphragmatic breathing, and limited SOVT exercise introduction. AG reported feeling disappointed that the SLP had limited experience working with TGNC individuals, particularly singers, and that intervention focused on reinforcing a stereotypical cis-assumed male voice presentation. AG decided to continue working with community-based resources and attempting to vocalize regularly with brief warm-ups and cool-downs on 5-note scales per online video resources, but he admitted "avoiding practicing for days and weeks" when they felt discouraged.

Social History. AG lives in a small town approximately 100 miles away from the SLP in a rental house with 3 roommates they are disclosed to. He is currently employed as a barista full-time at a local coffee shop and attends community college for an associate's degree in electrical engineering. AG's father and 2 siblings are highly supportive of their gender journey and singing, but he reports a strained relationship with his mother, who frequently misgenders them and uses his deadname despite reminders. AG is not disclosed yet to extended family and is not frequently in contact. AG reports that, outside of his roommates and some coworkers, his primary supports are through online social media interactions.

Auditory-Perceptual Evaluation

The CAPE-V[23] protocol was employed to assess AG's voice and speech presentation. Overall, he presented with anticipated voice changes given HRT intervention with concern for mild dysphonia-like presentation. During conversational speech and sentence reading tasks, he presented with mild intermittent vocal fry. For sustained vowel tasks, AG presented with minimal strain and roughness not presented in connected or continuous speech tasks. CAPE-V ratings are summarized in Table 9–11. While resonance quality appeared

9. Gender Affirming Voice Care 477

Table 9–11. CAPE-V Scores

Consensus Auditory-Perceptual Evaluation of Voice (CAPE-V)	Preintervention		Postintervention	
Overall Severity	11/100 mm	Inconsistent	3/100 mm	Consistent
Roughness	9/100 mm	Inconsistent, vowels only	0/100 mm	Consistent
Breathiness	0/100 mm	Consistent	0/100 mm	Consistent
Strain	13/100 mm	Inconsistent, vowels only	0/100 mm	Consistent
Pitch	0/100 mm	Consistent	0/100 mm	Consistent
Loudness	0/100 mm	Consistent	0/100 mm	Consistent
Vocal/Glottal Fry	17/100 mm	Inconsistent, intermittent during reading and spontaneous speech	5/100 mm	Inconsistent, intermittent during reading and spontaneous speech
Resonance	Normal		Normal	

WNL, AG exhibited moderate forward focus throughout voice tasks, and he confirmed wanting to explore a "darker" timbre or more back-focused resonance quality for speech and singing.

Manual Palpation Assessment With Respiratory Observation

During a teletherapy clinician-led assessment, AG exhibited appearance of mild-moderate shoulder and neck tension, moderate base-of-tongue tension, and mildly reduced jaw excursion. Tasks for this assessment included lateral stretch of sternocleidomastoid (SCM) muscles, shoulder range of motion (ROM) elevation and rotation, lingual protrusion/retraction and palpation of suprahyoid muscle groups, mandibular ROM and manipulation, and palpation of temporomandibular joint (TMJ) with self-rating on the Likert scale (ie, 1-5) for tension, mobility, and discomfort (eg,

1 being "no discomfort" and 5 being "maximum discomfort or pain"). Moderate tongue retraction during ascending pitch tasks was also noted. AG demonstrated manual lateralization of the thyroid cartilage with ease. His breathing pattern was marked by moderate chest elevation, minimal shoulder elevation, and moderate abdominal expansion with occasional audible inhalation. At this time, AG self-disclosed he was not using a binder, but does use one at work and occasionally during voice classes.

Objective and Acoustic Assessment

With AG's consent, the SLP obtained immediate, albeit limited, objective and acoustic data as listed in Table 9–12 with video visit audio through Loopback software and Praat software for analysis on the SLP's computer. For vocal intensity values, limited values were obtained using a mobile app SPL meter called Decibel X

478 Voice Therapy: Clinical Case Studies

Table 9–12. Pre- and Postintervention Measures

Objective Measures	Preintervention	Postintervention
Maximum Phonation Time (MPT)	22.34 sec (within functional limits for AFAB individuals, but decreased for vocal performers)	27.58 sec
S/Z Ratio	0.91 (within functional limits)	0.94 (within functional limits)
Laryngeal Diadochokinetic Task (DDK)	5.67 syllables/sec (within functional limits)	5.83 syllables/sec (within functional limits)
Mean Fundamental Frequency (F0)	Sustained /a/: 155.9 Hz Sustained /i/: 149.2 Hz Rainbow Passage: 145.0 Hz Spontaneous speech: 146.8 Hz	Sustained /a/: 138.4 Hz Sustained /i/: 140.3 Hz Rainbow Passage: 129.4 Hz Spontaneous speech: 127.6 Hz
Mean Intensity (dB SPL)	Sustained /a/: 71.08 dB SPL Spontaneous speech: 73.54 dB SPL	Sustained /a/: 75.23 dB SPL Spontaneous speech: 72.47 dB SPL
Maximum Phonation Frequency Range (Hz)	116.3-637.8 Hz (B♭2 to D#5 on keyboard) 29.49 semitones (ST) Aphonic break: 282.1-502.3 Hz on initial ascending glissando	103.2-784.3 Hz (Ab2 to G5) 35.11 semitones (ST) Continuous
Minimum and Maximum Vocal Intensity Range (dB SPL)	57-85 dB SPL	52-94 dB SPL

with understanding that readings without calibration may be unreliable. The SLP demonstrated how to use the app and perform voice tasks to complete concurrently with other acoustic measures. Given AG's gender and participation in HRT, the SLP provided caveats that norms obtained for presumably cisgender males and cisgender females may have limitations when compared to the client's obtained values. Formant measures were not reported from live video visit-obtained recordings given documented unreliability[61] as compared to phone recordings.

Per recommendations outlined by Zhang et al,[62] the SLP also provided education and demonstration via a video visit "screenshare" function on how to obtain free voice recording software (eg, Audacity for computer, AVR X app on mobile phone), record .wav files with headset, and upload audio files to the electronic health record (EHR) system online for more representative acoustic analysis. However, AG reported via secure message to the SLP following the initial assessment that he felt dysphoric during attempts to record voice samples independently and was unable to upload files despite education and counseling. AG also self-reported executive functioning difficulties with initiating voice tasks for recording given work and school demands, stating he understood if the SLP could not provide services given these limitations.

While measures may be consistent with "normal" voice presentation for nonperformers, both MPT and phonation frequency range appear reduced given AG's performance voice goals, even if documented as anticipated for those taking testosterone following endogenous puberty.[63] Both decreased maximum fundamental frequency range and aphonic break from 282.1 to 502.3 Hz on the initial glissando task (approximately C$^#$4 to B4) could be of concern for potentially dysphonic voice presentation or consistent with anticipated voice presentation with exogenous testosterone as described by Agha and Hynes[64] and Cler et al[65] in their study of a transmasculine singer. However, AG reported weekly inconsistencies in range and performance in warm-ups depending on time of day, vocal task, and ascending versus descending scales.

Voice Quality-of-Life Measures

Given that no current validated voice questionnaire exists specifically for transmascu-line individuals,[6] the SLP provided AG with a link to electronic versions of the VHI-10[25] and Singing Voice Handicap Index–10 (SVHI-10)[66] to complete in their EHR chart. Pre- and post-intervention scores are listed in Table 9–13.

For the VHI-10, the items AG self-rated 3 ("almost always") or 4 ("always") were: "I feel as though I have to strain to produce voice," "The clarity of my voice is unpredictable," and "My voice problem upsets me." For the SVHI-10, the items AG self-rated 3 ("almost always") or 4 ("always") were: "It takes a lot of effort to sing," "I am unsure of what will come out when I sing," "My singing voice upsets me," "I have no confidence in my singing voice," "I have trouble making my voice do what I want it to," "My singing voice tires easily," and "I feel something is missing in my life because of my inability to sing." Consistent with AG's interview, his overall concern and functional impact appeared secondary to his singing voice performance as compared to speaking voice.

Stimulability Testing

Per AG's request, the SLP deferred the remainder of singing voice assessment tasks to the next session. The SLP provided education and demonstration with use of visual supports (eg, SLP models, internet resources such as GIFs and YouTube videos) regarding diaphragmatic breathing technique and remapping. The SLP also described and demonstrated progressive relaxation techniques and stretching as related to shoulders (eg, rolling forward and back, stretching upward, stretching toward

Table 9–13. Patient-Reported Outcome Measures

Patient-Reported Outcome Measures (PROMs) for Vocal Quality of Life	
Preintervention	Voice Handicap Index–10 (VHI-10): 13/40
	Singing Voice Handicap Index–10 (SVHI-10): 26/40
Postintervention	VHI-10: 7/40
	SVHI-10: 13/40

feet while seated), neck (eg, head movement in gentle half-circles), jaw, and tongue (eg, anterior lingual stretch with tongue blade behind lower incisors or with blade protrusion) with integrated yawn-sigh on descending modified glissandos. AG benefited from intermittent self-administered tactile feedback (eg, hand or thumb on chin with gentle pressure for increased jaw excursion) and visual feedback (eg, use of camera to assess tongue position) during structured voice tasks. AG was stimulable for easeful phonation and flow phonation targets without vocal fry on /h/-vowel syllables and during chant talk on pitch F3 for limited functional phrases, but presented with intermittent fry when bridging to speech-like intonation pattern. AG did not have a straw available to assess straw phonation this session, but the SLP assessed stimulability for other SOVT exercises with lip trills, sustained /v/, and "blowfish" (phonation with consistent buccal inflation with steady stream of air as described by Rosenberg and LeBorgne)[67] on modified glissandos and sustained phonation. (See Video 8 Lip Trills by Braden.)

Impressions and Decision Making

Because there were no known gender affirming voice care providers local to AG offering in-person services for acoustic and aerodynamic assessment, especially with singing voice specialty, the SLP elected to initiate a telehealth plan of care for singing and speaking voice habilitation and rehabilitation based on AG's behavioral voice evaluation and limited acoustic assessment in the interest of harm reduction for a particularly vulnerable client (ie, a trans, neurodivergent, avocational voice performer who was taking testosterone and had limited formal voice education).

AG presented with very mild dysphonia characterized by roughness and strain likely secondary to HRT. Given the client's motivation and performance in stimulability testing, AG was considered an appropriate candidate with a good prognosis for improvement with voice intervention. Due to anticipated priority regarding singing voice intervention, speech voice goals formulated with AG's observations focused on techniques overlapping with singing voice needs, including decreasing vocal fry and pressed phonation presentation with use of flow phonation, SOVT exercises, breathing remapping, resonant voice applications, and increased awareness of and techniques to address areas of tension. Given voice demands at work in addition to voice performance needs, the clinician also included education and implementation of vocal hygiene tasks. While not written as an explicit goal area, counseling and motivational interviewing regarding voice goals and intervention were important to include in AG's care.

Plan of Care

Behavioral voice intervention was scheduled as 4 to 6 weekly sessions, followed by 4 biweekly sessions if appropriate.

Long-Term Goal (LTG). The client will independently use flow phonation and resonant voice targets in approximating self-identified gender affirming voice configuration (eg, lower mean fundamental frequency, perceived lower formant shifting) at least 80% to 90% of the time in naturalistic conversation and when singing a familiar piece transposed to an appropriate key within 12 weeks.

Short-Term Goals (STGs):

1. The client will participate in an informal singing voice assessment to establish singing voice goals within 1 session.
2. The client will approximate flow phonation and resonant voice targets in self-identified preferred pitch range during structured conversational tasks at least 80% of the time given minimal to no cues within 6 weeks.
3. The client will verbalize and implement vocal hygiene recommendations as appropriate at least 80% of the time independently within 6 weeks.

Voice Intervention

Session #1 (Informal Singing Voice Assessment, STG #1)

For the initial telesession, the SLP initiated an informal singing voice assessment by asking AG to hum at a comfortable starting pitch of his choice, which was approximately F3. For each voice task, the clinician obtained intermittent confirmation of consent (eg, "How does that feel?" "Do you need to pause?") and confirmation of registration terms (eg, lower/higher register, passaggio, avoidance of traditional *fachs*) to ensure the client's sense of comfort and safety. AG was cued to sing a descending 5-note scale on /mu/ to approximate a darker timbre with occasional SLP models for increased jaw excursion and increased flow phonation for legato. AG approximated pitches on this voice task until C#4, where he exhibited a potential aphonic break consistent with the initial glissando task in evaluation.

> The German word *fach* is used to refer to the classification of different voice types in singing, such as dramatic soprano, lyric soprano, contralto, and lyric tenor.

Given the likelihood of registration challenges, the SLP cued AG to use an easeful, higher-pitched hum (eg, "dog whine") to approximate a higher register where the client could sustain pitch (approximately C5). From C5, AG was instructed to sing /hu/ for repeated descending and ascending glissandos over third intervals or 4 semitones on a slow tempo. AG exhibited mild tremulous quality but consistent phonation until attempting to descend to F4, where he demonstrated an aphonic break. During this session, AG was not stimulable for phonation from C#4 to F4. With the use of a descending glissando over thirds ascending on the keyboard, he was stimulable for phonation up to E5. AG agreed that their functional range was from B2 to D5, whereas prior to exogenous testosterone, his functional range was C3 to C6. AG denied wanting a traditional or stereotypical cis-masculine singing voice presentation. The plan of care was adapted to include short-term goal (STG) #4: "The client will sing a familiar piece transposed to an appropriate key for their range using flow phonation and resonant voice techniques at least 80% of the time with minimal to no cues within 6 weeks."

In a task adapted from Christie Block as delineated by Adler et al,[6] the SLP shifted focus to sensory mapping for resonance targets with increased oral opening while approximating lower modal pitch on /ma/ and /mo/ bridging to counting. The SLP cued AG to identify, via self-palpation and observation, sensory targets for resonance (eg, "buzzing nose and mouth versus buzzing toward lower jaw and chest"). AG used self-palpation for tactile feedback during chanting and speech tasks with client-formulated functional phrases and sentences, and with occasional models and visual cues with minimal to no vocal fry presentation. AG confirmed voicing was "much easier to produce" with flow phonation and resonant voice target awareness based on tactile feedback.

Weekly Sessions #2 to #4 (Flow Phonation and Resonant Voice Targets for Speech and Singing With Introductory Vocal Hygiene Education, STGs #1, #3, and #4)

AG requested to focus primarily on singing voice targets with some conversational practice toward the end of sessions. AG remembered to bring a cup and straw to sessions, and the SLP demonstrated use of straw phonation with cup bubbles to facilitate flow and easeful phonation for both tasks. (See Video 28 Straw Phonation in Water Hierarchy by Codino) AG was instructed to maintain a tight oral labial seal around the straw without additional facial tension, include some buccal inflation if helpful during sustained phonation tasks on F3, and incorporate modified ascending-descending glissandos starting on D3 to A3 (fifth intervals or 7 semitones) into his vocal warm-ups. AG benefited from cues to use pursed-lip breathing when approximating increased abdominal movement during respiration for singing warm-up tasks following repeated attempts to onset on residual breath instead of "resetting" with a full diaphragmatic breathing pattern.

AG initially required reminders and encouragement to bring song samples and excerpts within a 1- to 1.5-octave range (C3-C4, C3-G4) to target approximation of phonation within his passaggio. Given lyric sheets for cueing, AG approximated easeful phonation when attempting melodies for familiar choruses with use of cup bubbles and /mu/ but demonstrated increased vocal effort and mild strain when moving to lyrics despite cues and demonstration for light articulatory contacts. However, during structured conversational practice where the SLP instructed AG to script bullet points to minimize cognitive load, he effectively used resonant voice interjections or "fillers" (eg, "hmm," "um") to facilitate resonant focus and flow phonation targets with intermittent visual cues from the SLP. The SLP provided education and handouts on specific concerns for vocal hygiene, including implementing low-impact vocal warm-ups and cool-downs, taking 15- to 30-minute vocal "naps" or rest periods on working days or heavy voice use days, and using gestures and written/text communication as appropriate in noisy environments. AG agreed with these recommendations and applicability.

Biweekly Sessions #5 and #6 (Resonant Voice and Flow Phonation for Speech and Singing Incorporating Circumlaryngeal Massage, STGs #2 and #4)

AG reported consistent use of SOVT exercises and resonant voice targets during warm-up with consistent phonation in C4 to F4 range when in their "head voice." SLP incorporated *messa di voce* tasks to vary vocal volume dur-

ing singing on ascending glissandos for fifth intervals near his passaggio and higher register. Since AG initially demonstrated mild strain on ascending glissandos, the SLP demonstrated circumlaryngeal massage adapted from protocol descriptions in Dahl et al,[43] with focus on thyroid cartilage pull-downs during ascending glissandos. (See Video 36 Laryngeal Massage and Resposturing to Lower Pitch by Buckley.) Following the SLP models, AG self-administered thyroid cartilage pull-downs in isolation and during ascending glissandos over a 2- to 3-minute duration with no reported discomfort and reduced strain/effort, per client report. During subsequent structured singing tasks (eg, a capella and singing of verse accompanied by MP3 music files), the client demonstrated increased ease of phonation in the B2 to G5 singing range with minimal to no strain noted by both the SLP and the client. In naturalistic conversational tasks, AG demonstrated use of flow phonation and resonant voice targets with minimal to no vocal fry in the self-identified target pitch range uncued with at least 80% accuracy. AG declined recording singing and speech voice targets within the session, but he reported he had downloaded the VoiceAnalyst app and began using a mobile voice recording app for playback and self-assessment as able.

> The Italian term *messa di voce* is used to describe gradually increasing and decreasing vocal intensity on a single sustained pitch. The term translates to "placing of the voice." The technique is used in both singing lessons and in voice therapy, as it requires precise control of laryngeal and respiratory mechanics to modulate intensity while maintaining a steady pitch.

Given AG's improvements in approximating easeful phonation in conversational speech and limited singing voice tasks, alongside their reported financial challenges, the SLP referred him to 2 transmasculine singing voice teachers who had experience teaching CCM and classical voice and who offered sliding-scale services. The SLP also provided links to online social support groups for transmasculine singers. AG agreed with the plan and scheduled a follow-up, session #7, in 1 month.

Session #7 (Assessing Carryover of Flow Phonation, Resonant Voice Techniques, and Vocal Hygiene Information, LTG #1 and STG #3)

AG reported favorable outcomes when working with their chosen voice teacher on transposing and adapting his own songs to support their voice needs and strengths. During counseling and motivational interviewing regarding voice changes, AG reported continued use of flow phonation and resonant voice targets across conversational contexts and implementation of vocal hygiene considerations at work and in group voice class. He stated they would prefer to follow up with the SLP in 3 to 6 months in case of any significant voice changes. Overall, AG demonstrated improvement in auditory-perceptual measures on the CAPE-V for roughness, strain, and vocal fry with lower mean fundamental frequency across voice tasks and increased continuous maximum phonation frequency range on glissandos (see Tables 9–11 and 9–12). AG's self-reported measures for the VHI-10 and SVHI-10 (see Table 9–13) also demonstrated significant improvement, reporting 2 ("sometimes") or 1 ("almost never") for most statements.

Given AG's report and improvement in these measures for gender affirming voice considerations, the SLP recommended discharge with follow-up in 3 to 6 months if AG reported or experienced voice or respiratory changes following a procedure or change in testosterone dosage. The SLP also provided him with education (verbal and e-handout) regarding signs and symptoms of dysphonia and when to consult an ENT.

References

1. Kalra M. Voice therapy with a transsexual. In: Gemme R, Wheeler C, eds. *Progress in Sexology. Perspectives in Sexuality.* Springer; 1977. pp. 77-84

2. Oates J, Dacakis G. Speech pathology considerations in the management of transsexualism: A review. *Br J Disord Commun.* 1983; 18(3):139-151.

3. Oates J, Dacakis G. Voice change in transsexuals. *Venereol Interdiscip Int J Sex Heal.* 1997;10:178-187

4. Pausewang-Gelfer M. Voice treatment for the male-to-female transgendered client. *Am J Speech Lang Pathol.* 1999;32(3):201-208.

5. Becklund Friedenberg C. Working with male-to-female transgendered clients: Clinical considerations. *Contemp Issues Commun Sci Disord.* 2002;29:43-58.

6. Adler R, Hirsch S, Pickering J. *Voice and Communication Therapy for the Transgender/Gender Diverse Client: A Comprehensive Clinical Guide.* 3rd ed. Plural Publishing; 2019.

7. Andrews Moya L. *Manual of Voice Treatment: Pediatrics through Geriatrics.* Singular Publishing Group; 1995.

8. Boone D, McFarlane S. *The Voice and Voice Therapy.* Allyn & Bacon; 2000.

9. Hirsch S. Combining voice, speech science and art approaches to resonant challenges in transgender voice and communication training. *Perspect ASHA Spec Interest Groups.* 2017;2(10):74-82. doi:10.1044/persp2.sig 10.74

10. Beaton F, Ayers A, Pickering J, Kayajian D. Thud-tempters and mockingbirds: A cognitive–linguistic approach to acoustic assumptions. *Perspect ASHA Spec Interest Groups.* 2021;6(2):344-355. doi:10.1044/2021_persp-20-00279

11. Hardy TLD, Rieger JM, Wells K, Boliek CA. Acoustic predictors of gender attribution,

masculinity–femininity, and vocal naturalness ratings amongst transgender and cisgender speakers. *J Voice*. 2020;34(2):300.e11-300.e26. doi:10.1016/j.jvoice.2018.10.002

12. Peterson G, Barney H. Control methods used in a study of the vowels. *J Acoust Soc Am*. 1952;24:17-184.

13. Hillenbrand J, Clark M. The role of f0 and formant frequencies in distinguishing the voices of men and women. *Atten Percept Psychophys*. 2009;71(5):1150-1166. doi: 10.3758/APP.71.5.1150

14. Lee S-H, Yu J-F, Hsieh Y-H, Lee G-S. Relationships between formant frequencies of sustained vowels and tongue contours measured by ultrasonography. *Am J Speech Lang Pathol*. 2015;24(4):739-749. doi:10.1044/2015_AJSLP-14-0063

15. Kawitzky D, McAllister T. The effect of formant biofeedback on the feminization of voice in transgender women. *J Voice*. 2020;34(1):53-67. doi:10.1016/j.jvoice.2018.07.017

16. Leyns C, Daelman J, Adriaansen A, et al. Short-term acoustic effects of speech therapy in transgender women: A randomized controlled trial. *Am J Speech Lang Pathol*. 2023;32(1):145-168. doi:10.1044/2022_AJSLP-22-00135

17. Coleman E, Radix AE, Bouman WP, et al. Standards of care for the health of transgender and gender diverse people, Version 8. *Int J Transgend Health*. 2022;23(S1):S1-S259. doi:10.1080/26895269.2022.2100644

18. Jacobson BH, Johnson A, Grywalski C, et al. The Voice Handicap Index (VHI): Development and validation. *Am J Speech Lang Pathol*. 1997;6(3):66-69. doi:10.1044/1058-0360.0603.66

19. Dacakis G, Davies S. The Trans Woman Voice Questionnaire. Accessed October 4, 2023. https://www.latrobe.edu.au/__data/assets/pdf_file/0010/1393363/TGV-Resources.pdf

20. Kent SAK, Fletcher TL, Morgan A, Morton M, Hall RJ, Sandage MJ. Updated acoustic normative data through the lifespan: A scoping review. *J Voice*. Published online March 18, 2023. doi:10.1016/j.jvoice.2023.02.011

21. Gelfer MP, Schofield KJ. Comparison of acoustic and perceptual measures of voice in male-to-female transsexuals perceived as female versus those perceived as male. *J Voice*. 2000;14(1):22-33. doi:10.1016/S0892-1997(00)80092-2

22. Verdolini Abbott K. *Lessac-Madsen Resonant Voice Therapy Clinician Manual*. Plural Publishing; 2008.

23. Kempster GB, Gerratt BR, Abbott KV, Barkmeier-Kraemer J, Hillman RE. Consensus Auditory-Perceptual Evaluation of Voice: Development of a standardized clinical protocol. *Am J Speech Lang Pathol*. 2009;18(2):124-132. doi:10.1044/1058-0360(2008/08-0017)

24. Nanjundeswaran C, Jacobson BH, Gartner-Schmidt J, Verdolini Abbott K. Vocal Fatigue Index (VFI): Development and validation. *J Voice*. 2015;29(4):433-440. doi:10.1016/j.jvoice.2014.09.012

25. Rosen CA, Lee AS, Osborne J, Zullo T, Murry T. Development and validation of the Voice Handicap Index-10. *Laryngoscope*. 2004;114(9 I):1549-1556. doi:10.1097/00005537-200409000-00009

26. Patel RR, Awan SN, Barkmeier-Kraemer J, et al. Recommended protocols for instrumental assessment of voice: ASHA expert panel to develop a protocol for instrumental assessment of vocal function. *Am J Speech Lang Pathol*. 2018;27(3):887-905.

27. Edwards-Leeper L, Leibowitz S, Sangganjanavanich VF. Affirmative practice with transgender and gender nonconforming youth: Expanding the model. *Psychol Sex Orientat Gend Divers*. 2016;3(2):165-172. doi:10.1037/sgd0000167

28. Hidalgo MA, Ehrensaft D, Tishelman AC, et al. The gender affirmative model: What we know and what we aim to learn. *Hum Dev*. 2013;56(5):285-290. doi:10.1159/000355235

29. Vastine W, Gillespie AI, Hatcher JL, Hseu AF. Out of committee: Voice/gender affirming voice care defined and in practice. American Acadamy of Otolaryngology Head and Neck Surgery Bulletin. June 10, 2022. https://bulletin.entnet.org/home/article/22236751/out-of-committee-voice-genderaffirming-voice-care-defined-and-in-practice

30. Nolan IT, Morrison SD, Arowojolu O, et al. The role of voice therapy and phonosurgery

in transgender vocal feminization. *J Craniofac Surg.* 2019;30(5):1368-1375. doi:10.1097/scs.0000000000005132

31. Poburka BJ, Patel RR, Bless DM. Voice-Vibratory Assessment With Laryngeal Imaging (VALI) form: Reliability of rating stroboscopy and high-speed videoendoscopy. *J Voice.* 2017;31(4):513.e1-513.e14. doi:10.1016/j.jvoice.2016.12.003

32. Shoffel-Havakuk H, Marks KL, Morton M, Johns MM III, Hapner ER. Validation of the OMNI Vocal Effort Scale in the treatment of adductor spasmodic dysphonia. *Laryngoscope.* Published online October 12, 2018. doi:10.1002/lary.27430

33. Arffa RE, Krishna P, Gartner-Schmidt J, Rosen CA. Normative values for the Voice Handicap Index-10. *J Voice.* 2012;26(4):462-465. doi:10.1016/j.jvoice.2011.04.006

34. Shoffel-Havakuk H, Chau S, Hapner ER, Pethan M, Johns MM. Development and validation of the Voice Catastrophization Index. *J Voice.* 2019;33(2):232-238. doi:10.1016/j.jvoice.2017.09.026

35. Dacakis G, Davies S, Oates JM, Douglas JM, Johnston JR. Development and preliminary evaluation of the transsexual voice questionnaire for male-to-female transsexuals. *J Voice.* 2013;27(3):312-320. doi:10.1016/j.jvoice.2012.11.005

36. Goy H, Fernandes DN, Pichora-Fuller MK, Van Lieshout P. Normative voice data for younger and older adults. *J Voice.* 2013;27(5):545-555. doi:10.1016/j.jvoice.2013.03.002

37. Boone D, McFarlane SC, Von Berg S. *The Voice and Voice Therapy.* 7th ed. Pearson; 2014.

38. Buckley DP, Abur D, Stepp CE. Normative values of cepstral peak prominence measures in typical speakers by sex, speech stimuli, and software type across the life span. *Am J Speech Lang Pathol.* 2023;32(4):1565-1577. doi:10.1044/2023_AJSLP-22-00264

39. Lewandowski A, Gillespie AI, Kridgen S, Jeong K, Yu L, Gartner-Schmidt J. Adult normative data for phonatory aerodynamics in connected speech. *Laryngoscope.* 2018;128(4):909-914. doi:10.1002/lary.26922

40. Zraick RI, Smith-Olinde L, Shotts LL. Adult normative data for the KayPentax phonatory aerodynamic system model 6600. *J Voice.* 2012;26(2):164-176. doi:10.1016/j.jvoice.2011.01.006

41. Mathieson L. The evidence for laryngeal manual therapies in the treatment of muscle tension dysphonia. *Curr Opin Otolaryngol Head Neck Surg.* 2011;19(3):171-176. doi:10.1097/MOO.0b013e3283448f6c

42. Buckley DP, Dahl KL, Cler GJ, Stepp CE. Transmasculine voice modification: A case study. *J Voice.* 2020;34(6):903-910. doi:10.1016/j.jvoice.2019.05.003

43. Dahl KL, François FA, Buckley DP, Stepp CE. Voice and speech changes in transmasculine individuals following circumlaryngeal massage and laryngeal reposturing. *Am J Speech Lang Pathol.* 2022;31(3):1368-1382. doi:10.1044/2022_AJSLP-21-00245

44. Titze IR. Voice training and therapy with a semi-occluded vocal tract: Rationale and scientific underpinnings. *Hear Res.* 2006;49(April):448-460.

45. Meerschman I, Van Lierde K, D'Haeseleer E, et al. Immediate and short-term effects of straw phonation in air or water on vocal fold vibration and supraglottic activity of adult patients with voice disorders visualized with strobovideolaryngoscopy: A pilot study. *J Voice.* 2024;38(2):392-403. doi:10.1016/j.jvoice.2021.09.017

46. Leung Y, Oates J, Chan SP. Voice, articulation, and prosody contribute to listener perceptions of speaker gender: A systematic review and meta-analysis. *J Speech Lang Hear Res.* 2018;61(2):266-297. doi:10.1044/2017_JSLHR-S-17-0067

47. Shefcik G, Tsai PT. Voice-related Experiences of Nonbinary Individuals (VENI) development and content validity. *J Voice.* 2023;37(2):294.e5-294.e13. doi:10.1016/j.jvoice.2020.12.037

48. Schneider SL, Habich L, Weston ZM, Rosen CA. Observations and considerations for implementing remote acoustic voice recording and analysis in clinical practice. *J Voice.* 2024;38(1):69-76. doi:10.1016/j.jvoice.2021.06.011

49. Ziegler A, Henke T, Wiedrick J, Helou LB. Effectiveness of testosterone therapy for

masculinizing voice in transgender patients: A meta-analytic review. *Int J Transgend.* 2018;19(1):25-45. doi:10.1080/15532739.2017.1411857

50. Miller, WR, Rollnick S. *Motivational Interviewing: Preparing People for Change.* Guilford Press. 2002.

51. Sobell L, Sobell M. *Group Therapy for Substance Use Disorders A Motivational Cognitive-Behavioral Approach.* Guilford Press; 2011.

52. Behrman A. Chapter 5.10: Why don't you? In: Behrman A, Haskell J, eds. *Exercises for Voice Therapy.* Plural Publishing; 2020:103-104.

53. Conine DE, Campau SC, Petronelli AK. LGBTQ+ conversion therapy and applied behavior analysis: A call to action. *J Appl Behav Anal.* 2022;55(1):6-18. doi:10.1002/jaba.876

54. Comer JS, Georgiadis C, Schmarder K, et al. Reckoning with our past and righting our future: Report from the behavior therapy task force on sexual orientation and gender identity/expression change efforts (SOGIECEs). *Behav Ther.* 2024;55(4):649-679. doi:10.1016/j.beth.2024.05.006

55. Statement on conversion therapy and practices. Association for Behavioral Analysis International (ABAI). 2022. https://www.abainternational.org/about-us/policies-and-positions/policy-statement-on-conversion-therapy-and-practices,-2021.aspx

56. Adler R, Hirsch S, Mordaunt M. *Voice and Communication Therapy for the Transgender/Transsexual Client: A Comprehensive Clinical Guide.* Plural Publishing; 2012.

57. Ferrand C. *Speech Science: An Integrated Approach to Theory and Clinical Practice.* Allyn and Bacon; 2001.

58. Bravata DM, Watts SA, Keefer AL, et al. Prevalence, predictors, and treatment of impostor syndrome: A systematic review. *J Gen Intern Med.* 2020;35(4):1252-1275. doi:10.1007/s11606-019-05364-1

59. Telepractice. American Speech-Language-Hearing Association. Accessed September 28, 2023. https://www.asha.org/Practice-Portal/Professional-Issues/Telepractice/

60. Kupferstein H. Evidence of increased PTSD symptoms in autistics exposed to applied behavior analysis. *Adv Autism.* 2018;4(1):19-29.

61. Hancock AB, Childs KD, Irwig MS. Trans male voice in the first year of testosterone therapy: Make no assumptions. *J Speech Lang Hear Res.* 2017;60(9):2472-2482. doi:10.1044/2017_JSLHR-S-16-0320

62. Zhang C, Jepson K, Lohfink G, Arvaniti A. Comparing acoustic analyses of speech data collected remotely. *J Acoust Soc Am.* 2021;149(6):3910-3916. doi:10.1121/10.0005132

63. Block C. Making a case for transmasculine voice and communication training. *Perspect ASHA Spec Interest Groups.* 2017;2(3):33-41. doi:10.1044/persp2.sig3.33

64. Agha A, Hynes L. Exogenous testosterone and the transgender singing voice: A 30-month case study. *J Sing.* 2022;78(4):441-455.

65. Cler GJ, McKenna VS, Dahl KL, Stepp CE. Longitudinal case study of transgender voice changes under testosterone hormone therapy. *J Voice.* 2020;34(5):748-762. doi:10.1016/j.jvoice.2019.03.006

66. Cohen SM, Statham M, Rosen CA, Zullo T. Development and validation of the Singing Voice Handicap-10. *Laryngoscope.* 2009;119(9):1864-1869. doi:10.1002/lary.20580

67. Rosenberg M, LeBorgne W. *The Vocal Athlete: Application and Technique for the Hybrid Singer.* Plural Publishing; 2014.

Index

Note: Page numbers in **bold** reference non-text material.

A

Abbott, Verdolini, 48, 53, 289, 443
Abdominal breathing, 427–428
Abdominal tension, 334
Abductor type laryngeal dystonia
  description of, 15, 36, 221
  teletherapy without medical management for,
    236–242
  vocal tremor and, 236–242
Accessory nerve, **14**
Acoustic assessment
  aerodynamic assessment versus, 23
  in voice evaluation, 21–22
Adductor type laryngeal dystonia
  botulinum toxin injection for, 229–231
  description of, 15, 36, 221–222
  interprofessional practice for, 224–225
  medical and behavioral management for,
    224–232
  voice therapy without medical management
    for, 232–236
Adolescent
  exercise-induced laryngeal obstruction in,
    EILOBI techniques for, 346–353
  gender affirming voice care for, 468–475
  primary muscle tension aphonia in, flow
    phonation for, 120–127
  puberphonia in, intensive voice therapy for,
    133–140
ADSV. *See* Analysis of Dysphonia in Speech
  and Voice
"Adventures in Voice," dysphonia in child
  treated using concepts from, 55–61
Aerodynamic assessment
  acoustic assessment versus, 23
  description of, 12, 22–23
Aging Voice Index, 170
ALERT profile, 336, **337**
Alternate motion rate, 14–15

American Academy of Otolaryngology--Head
  and Neck Surgery, 7
American Academy of Speech Correction, 1
American Speech-Language-Hearing
  Association
  history of, 1
  Instrumental Voice Assessment Protocol, 227
  resources of, 34
Amitriptyline, 318
AMR. *See* Alternate motion rate
Analysis of Dysphonia in Speech and Voice,
  121, 171, 308, 410
Anchoring, 205–206
Apraxia of speech, 13
ASHA. *See* American Speech-Language-
  Hearing Association
Ataxic dysarthria, **17**
Auditory-perceptual assessment, 11–12
Augmentative treatments, 40
AVI. *See* Aging Voice Index

B

Back breathing, 338
BCST. *See* Behavioral cough suppression
  therapy
Behavioral cough suppression therapy
  for chronic cough
    adherence to, 283–284
    components of, 283
    description of, 281–282
    goals of, 282–283
    respiratory disease and, 297–305
    self-efficacy, 283
  for chronic refractory cough
    case study of, 284–290
    neuromodulators and, 316–322
    SLN injection and, 305–315
  neuromodulators and, 316–322
  SLN injection and, 305–315

Behavioral management, for exercise-induced laryngeal obstruction, 341–346
Behavior substitution strategies, for cough suppression, 319–320
Belting, 369
Benign midmembranous lesion, conversation training therapy for, 48–55
BI. *See* Bowing Index
Biofeedback, 327
BoNT. *See* Botulinum neurotoxin
Boot camp voice therapy
    definition of, 118, 136
    for functional dysphonia, 116–120
Botulinum neurotoxin
    laryngeal dystonia treated with, 31, 37, 222, 229–230
    secondary effects of, 258
    voice therapy and, 37
Bowing Index, 162–163
Box breathing, **303**
Breathing control strategies, for cough suppression, 320
Breathing recovery therapy, 324, 345
Brodnitz, Friedrich, 1

C

CaHA. *See* Calcium hydroxyapatite
Calcium hydroxyapatite, 36
CAPE-V. *See* Consensus Auditory-Perceptual Evaluation of Voice
Case history, 7, **8**
Casper-Stone flow phonation, **251**
CC. *See* Chronic cough
"Cell yell," 390
Central sensitivity syndrome, 323, 333–341
Cepstral peak prominence, 49, **50,** 163
Cepstral-Spectral Index of Dysphonia, 49, **50,** 114, 121, 192, 208
Children, "Adventures in Voice" concepts for dysphonia in, 55–61. *See also* Adolescent
Chronic cough
    behavioral cough suppression therapy for
        adherence to, 283–284
        components of, 283
        description of, 281–282
        goals of, 282–283
        respiratory disease and, 297–305
        self-efficacy, 283
        SLN injection and, 305–315

causes of, 281
    clinical checklist for, 290–297
    definition of, 281
    description of, 2, 6
    irritant-induced, 290–297
    mental health affected by, 281
    neurogenic causes of, 315
    respiratory disease and, 297–305
    urge to cough, 282, 284
Chronic habit cough, 2
Chronic refractory cough
    behavioral cough suppression therapy for
        case study of, 284–290
        neuromodulators and, 316–322
        SLN injection and, 305–315
    description of, 2, 281–282
    irritant-induced, 294
CHS. *See* Cough hypersensitivity syndrome
Circumlaryngeal massage
    manual, for primary muscle tension dysphonia, 109–115
    for vocal fatigue, 131
Classification Manual for Voice Disorders, 30
Clavicular breathing pattern, 427
CLE. *See* Continuous laryngoscopy with exercise
Cognate pairs, 125–126
Cognition, 32
Communicative Participation Item Bank, **9,** 268
Confidential Voice Therapy, 125
Consensus Auditory-Perceptual Evaluation of Voice, 11, 49, 120, 163, 170, **180,** 186, 226, 256, 307, **477**
Continuous laryngoscopy with exercise, 19, 348
Conversation Training Therapy, 68
    benign midmembranous lesion treated with, 48–55
    case studies of, 51–52, 69, 126
    description of, 24, 32
Coordinated voice onset, 339
Cough
    chronic. *See* Chronic cough
    productive, 12
    refractory chronic. *See* Refractory chronic cough
    strength assessment of, 12
    suppression strategies for, **303,** 319–321
Cough-control breathing, 300
Cough hypersensitivity syndrome, 282–283, 300, 302

Cough Severity Index, **9,** 170
CPIB. *See* Communicative Participation Item Bank
Cranial nerve examination, 13, **14**
CRC. *See* Chronic refractory cough
CSI. *See* Cough Severity Index
CSID. *See* Cepstral-Spectral Index of Dysphonia
Cup bubble technique with voice recalibration, for chronic phonotrauma in adult country singer, 388–394
CVO. *See* Coordinated voice onset

D

DBS. *See* Deep brain stimulators
Deep brain stimulation for vocal tremor, SLP's role in, 261–267
Deep brain stimulators, 37
Deep tendon reflexes, 226
DI. *See* Dyspnea Index
Diaphragmatic breathing, 320, 427–428
Diplophonia, 159
Dysarthria
    characteristics of, 13
    in Parkinson's disease, 224
    types of, **17,** 224
Dysphagia, muscle tension, 147–154
Dysphonia
    in children, "Adventures in Voice" concepts used to treat, 55–61
    description of, 3
    functional, boot camp voice therapy for, 116–120
    laryngeal imaging for, 19
    muscle tension. *See* Muscle tension dysphonia
Dysphonia International, 232, 235
Dyspnea
    episodic, 19
    with exertion, 12
    fragrance triggers for, 21
    with speaking, 12
Dyspnea Index, **9,** 170
Dystonic tremor, 223

E

Ear-cough reflex, 298
EBM. *See* Evidence-based medicine
EILO. *See* Exercise-induced laryngeal obstruction

EILOBI. *See* Exercise-Induced Laryngeal Obstruction Biphasic Inhalation breathing techniques
EMST. *See* Expiratory muscle strength training
Environmental fume exposure, paradoxical vocal fold motion from, 325–333
Episodic dyspnea, 19
Essential tremor, 264
Essential voice tremor, 37, 223, 263–264
Estill Voice Model, 369
Estill Voice Training, 206
Evidence-based medicine, 33
EVT. *See* Essential voice tremor
Exercise (dose) prescription, 40
Exercise-induced laryngeal obstruction
    behavioral management for, 341–346
    breathing recovery therapy for, 324
    definition of, 322
    differential diagnosis of, 343
    Exercise-Induced Laryngeal Obstruction Biphasic Inhalation breathing techniques for, 346–353
    historical description of, 2
    inspiratory stridor associated with, 12
    pulmonary function testing for, 306
Exercise-Induced Laryngeal Obstruction Biphasic Inhalation breathing techniques
    description of, 324
    exercise-induced laryngeal obstruction treated with, 346–353
Exercise-induced vocal cord dysfunction, 347
Exercise science, 37–38
Exercise specificity, 37
Exertion, dyspnea with, 12
Expiratory muscle strength training
    description of, 39
    phonation resistance training exercises and, for presbyphonia, 179–185
Expiratory wheeze, 12
Exuberant therapies, 38–40, **39**

F

Facial nerve, **14**
Factitious asthma, 2
Falsetto voice, mutational, 133–140
FEES. *See* Flexible endoscopic evaluation of swallowing
FITT Principle, 40

Flaccid dysarthria, 17
Flexible endoscopic evaluation of swallowing, 285–286
Flexible laryngoscopes, 396, **400**
Flexible videolaryngostroboscopy, 114
Flow phonation
  Casper-Stone, **251**
  for primary muscle tension aphonia, 120–127
  skills for, 123–125
Focal laryngeal palpation, 111
4-cycle breath pattern, 350, **350**
Frailty syndrome, 32
Fröschels, Emil, 1
Functional dysphonia, boot camp voice therapy for, 116–120

G

GA. *See* Geste antagoniste
Gargling technique, 123
Gastroesophageal reflux disease, 7, 281, 334, 336, 343
Gender affirming voice care
  for adolescent, 468–475
  gender affirming voice in nonbinary adult, 461–468
  gender spectrum for, 438
  Hirsch's Acoustic Assumptions in
    case study of, 439–446
    description of, 438–439
  laryngeal imaging for, 440
  manual therapy in, for transmasculine adult on hormone replacement therapy, 453–461
  overview of, 437–439
  pitch-elevation surgery and perioperative voice care, in transgender women, 446–453
  resonance modification in, 439
  surgical interventions for, 438
  teletherapy for, in transmasculine binary singer, 475–483
  in transgender women
    Hirsch's Acoustic Assumptions for, 439–446
    pitch-elevation surgery and perioperative voice care for, 446–453
  in transmasculine adult
    on hormone replacement therapy, 453–461
    teletherapy for, 475–483
Gender diversity, 439

GERD. *See* Gastroesophageal reflux disease
Geste antagoniste, 227, 229, 235
GFI. *See* Glottal Function Index
Gliding trills, 427
Glossopharyngeal nerve, **14**
Glottal dysfunction
  classification scheme for, **160**
  voice therapy for, 160–161
Glottal Function Index, **10,** 163
Glottal gaps, 159–214
Glottal incompetence, 12, **160,** 161, **213**
Glottal insufficiency
  definition of, **160**
  phonation resistance training exercises for, 160, 175
  from presbyphonia, 40, 175
Glottal mislearning, **160**
Grade, Roughness, Breathiness, Asthenia, and Strain, 11, 72, 114
Grandfather Passage, 13
Granulomas, vocal process, 79–85
GRBAS. *See* Grade, Roughness, Breathiness, Asthenia, and Strain
Guidelines for the Treatment of Hoarseness: Dysphonia, 6

H

HA. *See* Hyaluronic acid
HAA. *See* Hirsch's Acoustic Assumptions
Habitual pitch, 441
Hard glottal attack, 137
Hirsch's Acoustic Assumptions
  case study of, 439–446
  description of, 438–439
Hormone replacement therapy in transmasculine adult, gender affirming voice care for, 453–461
HPV. *See* Human papilloma virus
Human papilloma virus, 142
Hyaluronic acid, 36
Hyaluronic acid-based injectables, 188
Hyperkinetic dysarthria, **17**
Hypoglossal nerve, **14**
Hypokinetic dysarthria, **17,** 224

I

ILO. *See* Inducible laryngeal obstruction
ILS. *See* Irritable larynx syndrome

IMST. *See* Inspiratory muscle strength training
Indirect and augmentative therapies, 38–40, **39**
Indirect laryngoscopy, 6
Inducible laryngeal obstruction
    breathing recovery therapy for, 324
    definition of, 322
    description of, 2, 300
    inspiratory stridor associated with, 12
    irritant-induced, 323
    management of, 323
    medical conditions presenting with, 323
    psychogenic causes of, 323
    pulmonary function testing for, 306
Injection augmentation
    description of, 191, 197, 212
    for vocal fold paralysis, 35–36
    voice therapy after, 270
Inspiratory muscle strength training
    description of, 39
    vocal function exercises and, for
        presbyphonia, 161–169
Inspiratory stridor, 12
Instrumental Voice Assessment Protocol, 227
Intensive voice therapy
    description of, 40–41
    for teenager with mutational falsetto,
        133–140
Interarytenoid muscle, 159
Interprofessional model of care, 3
Interprofessional practice, for adductor type
    laryngeal dystonia, 224–225
Irritable larynx syndrome, 334, 340
Irritant-induced chronic cough, 290–297
IVAP. *See* Instrumental Voice Assessment
    Protocol

L

Labio-lingual drills, 68
Laryngeal diadochokinesis, 15
Laryngeal diagnosis, 4–5
Laryngeal dystonia
    abductor type
        description of, 15, 36, 221
        teletherapy without medical management
            for, 236–242
        vocal tremor and, 236–242
    adductor type
        botulinum toxin injection for, 229–231
        description of, 15, 36, 221–222

interprofessional practice for, 224–225
    medical and behavioral management for,
        224–232
    voice therapy without medical
        management for, 232–236
    botulinum neurotoxin injections for, 31, 37,
        222, 229
    dystonic tremor and, 222–223
    epidemiology of, 221
    mixed, 221–222
    muscle tension dysphonia versus, 222
    patient-reported outcomes for, 222
    phonemically loaded sentences for
        differential diagnosis of, **15,** 237
    respiratory, 323
    signs and symptoms of, 234
    subtypes of, 221
    testing for, **15,** 15–16
    treatment options for, 36–37, 222
    voice therapy for, 222
Laryngeal imaging
    for gender affirming voice care, 440
    scope used in, 18–19, 21
Laryngeal massage, 37, 459
Laryngeal Palpation Pain Scale, 18
Laryngeal reposturing, for cough suppression,
    320
Laryngeal videostroboscopy
    case study of, 285, 447–448
    description of, 18–19, 234
    history of, 2
    parameters of, **20–21**
    tasks for, 19
Laryngopharyngeal reflux, 7, 305, 344–345
Larynx
    focal palpation of, 111
    hypersensitivity of, 310, 321
    irritation to, 320–321, 333–341
Lateral cricoarytenoid muscle, 159
LCQ. *See* Leister Cough Questionnaire
Leister Cough Questionnaire, 298, 304
Lessac-Madsen Resonant Voice Therapy
    description of, 53, 129–130, 209, 289
    vocal communicator in, 122
    vocal fold nodules treated with, 93–101
    voice care education in, 96
    voice training in, 96–97
Lewy pathology, 223
Lip bubbles, 124–125
Lip trills, 68, 419–421

LMRVT. *See* Lessac-Madsen Resonant Voice
    Therapy
Lombard effect, 390
LPPS. *See* Laryngeal Palpation Pain Scale
LPR. *See* Laryngopharyngeal reflux
LSVT-LOUD, 40, 224, 268

M

Manual circumlaryngeal techniques, for
    primary muscle tension dysphonia,
    109–115
Manual therapy
    for gender affirming voice care in
        transmasculine adult on hormone
        replacement therapy, 453–461
    for vocal fold pseudocyst, 69
Maximum phonation time, 23
MDVP 6600. *See* Multi-Dimensional Voice
    Program 6600
Medical examination
    in upper airway evaluation, 5–7
    in voice evaluation, 5–7
Medicare, 34
Meta-therapy, 38, 41–42, 418
MFR. *See* Myofascial release
Microflap excision, 30, 74
Mixed dysarthria, **17**
Models of care, 3
Moses, Paul J., 1
Motor learning, 32, 48, 145
Motor planning, 13
Motor relearning, 287
Motor speech assessment, 13–16, 226
MPT. *See* Maximum phonation time
MTD. *See* Muscle tension dysphonia
Multi-Dimensional Voice Program 6600, 171
Multimodality teletherapy, for unilateral vocal
    fold paresis, 199–207
Multimodality voice therapy
    for translucent polypoid lesion in adult voice
        actor/singer, 363–371
    for vocal fatigue, 127–133
    for vocal fold polyp and mild atrophy in adult
        singer, 394–402
    for vocal fold pseudocyst, 61–71
    for vocal nodules in prepubescent singer,
        423–430
    for vocal tremor, 255–261

Murray Secretion Scale score, 286
Muscle tension aphonia, flow phonation for,
    120–127
Muscle tension dysphagia, interprofessional
    assessment and treatment of, 147–154
Muscle tension dysphonia
    description of, 107
    laryngeal dystonia versus, 222
    muscle tension dysphagia and, 151
    primary
        definition of, 107
        description of, 34–35, 40
        episodic swelling associated with, 111
        glottic and supraglottic contraction
            patterns associated with, 109
        manual circumlaryngeal techniques for,
            109–115
        sources of, 107
        vocal fold posturing in, 117
    secondary
        definition of, 107
        episodic breathing problems as cause of,
            328
        treatment of, 35
    in transmasculine speakers, 438
    treatment options for, 34–35
    vocal function exercises for, 328
Mutational falsetto
    description of, 108
    teenager with, intensive voice therapy for,
        133–140
Myofascial release, for vocal fatigue in adult
    touring musical theater performer,
    380–388

N

Nasal breathing, 338
Nasoendoscopy, 223
National Association of Teachers of Speech, 1
National Spasmodic Dysphonia Association,
    232, 235
Neurological examination, 5
Neuromodulators and behavioral cough
    suppression therapy, for chronic
    refractory cough, 316–322
Neuromuscular disease, 5
Nonbinary adult, gender affirming voice in,
    461–468

Index **493**

NSDA. *See* National Spasmodic Dysphonia
Association

O

OMNI-VES. *See* OMNI Vocal Effort Scale
OMNI Vocal Effort Scale, 10, 80, 170, **176,** 292,
307, 396, 458
Omohyoid muscle, inferior bellies of, 108
Onset/offset trills, 427
Oral hydration program, 89–92
Otolaryngologist, 4
Oxygen saturation, 19

P

Paradoxical vocal fold motion
breathing recovery therapy for, 324
description of, 2, 322
from environmental fume exposure,
long-term management of, 325–333
Paralaryngeal musculature, 16
Parkinson's disease
characteristics of, 223
diagnosis of, 223–224
dopaminergic medications for motor
symptoms of, 224
idiopathic, 224
Lewy pathology associated with, 223
neurologic examination for, 223
speech therapy for communication deficits
in, 224
tremor in, 224
voice disorder in, 4
voice therapy gains in, SpeechVive for
maintaining of, 267–274, **271**
PAS. *See* Phonatory Aerodynamic System
Patient-reported outcome measures
auditory-perceptual assessment, 11–12
definition of, 7
list of, **8–10**
PD. *See* Parkinson's disease
Peak cough flow, 23
Peak expiratory flow, 23
Peak flow, 23
Peak flow meters, 23
Pediatric Voice Handicap Index, 55, 60
PEP breathing. *See* Positive expiratory pressure
breathing

Perceptual Voice Profile, 374, **376**
Performance voice
multimodality voice therapy
for translucent polypoid lesion in adult
voice actor/singer, 363–371
for vocal fold polyp and mild atrophy,
394–402
for vocal nodules in prepubescent singer,
423–430
onsite voice therapy for adult theater actor
with vocal injury, 371–380
overview of, 361–363
translucent polypoid lesion in adult voice
actor/singer, multimodality voice
therapy for, 363–371
vocal fatigue, myofascial release for adult
touring musical theater performer with,
380–388
vocal fold cyst, perioperative management of,
415–423
vocal fold polyp
mild atrophy and, multimodality voice
therapy for, 394–402
voice therapy for, 409–415
voice recalibration with cup bubble technique
for chronic phonotrauma in adult
country singer, 388–394
Perilaryngeal tension, 108–109, 190
PFTs. *See* Pulmonary function tests
PGS. *See* Posterior glottal stenosis
Phonanium, 22
Phonation resistance training exercises
description of, 4–5, 39
expiratory muscle strength training and, for
presbyphonia, 179–185
glottal insufficiency treated with, 160, 175
presbyphonia treated with, 169–179, 179–185
voice therapy exercises, **177**
Phonatory Aerodynamic System, 23, 56, 121,
163, 425
Phonemically/phonetically loaded sentences,
15, 237
Phonotrauma
benign midmembranous lesion, conversation
training therapy for, 48–55
dysphonia in child treated using concepts
from "Adventures in Voice," 55–61
overview of, 47–48
surgical therapy for, 35

Phonotrauma *(continued)*
  undifferentiated, vocal function exercises for, 85–92
  vocal folds
    cyst, perioperative therapeutic care for, 71–79
    nodules, Lessac-Madsen Resonant Voice Therapy for, 93–101
    pseudocyst, multimodality voice therapy for, 61–71
    vocal process granulomas after traumatic brain injury, multidisciplinary treatment for, 79–85
    voice recalibration with cup bubble technique for, in adult country singer, 388–394
    voice rest for, 47
    voice therapy for lesions caused by, in adult praise and worship leader, 403–409
PhoRTE. *See* Phonation resistance training exercises
Physical rolldown stretch, 66, **66**
Physician, communication with, 170
Physiotherapy, speech, and language therapy intervention, 281
Pitch, lower, 138–139
Pitch-elevation surgery and perioperative voice care, in transgender women, 446–453
Pitch matching, 190
Platelet-rich plasma, 31
Plosives, 38
pMTD. *See* Primary muscle tension dysphonia
Positive expiratory pressure breathing, 308
Posterior glottal stenosis, 12
Postsurgical voice therapy, for recurrent respiratory papillomatosis and ventricular phonation in child, 140–147
Pratt, 22
Pregabalin, 318
Presbyphonia
  expiratory muscle strength training and phonation resistance training exercises for, 179–185
  glottal insufficiency from, 40
  inspiratory muscle strength training and vocal function exercises for, 161–169
  phonation resistance training exercises for, 5, 169–179, 179–185
Primary muscle tension dysphonia
  definition of, 107

description of, 34–35, 40
episodic swelling associated with, 111
glottic and supraglottic contraction patterns associated with, 109
manual circumlaryngeal techniques for, 109–115
sources of, 107
vocal fold posturing in, 117
Productive cough, 12
PROMs. *See* Patient-reported outcome measures
PRP. *See* Platelet-rich plasma
PSALTI. *See* Physiotherapy, speech, and language therapy intervention
Pseudocyst, vocal fold
  appearance of, 64–65
  multimodality voice therapy for, 61–71
Puberphonia, intensive voice therapy for teenager with, 133–140
Pulmonary function tests, 6, 305–306
Pursed-lip breathing, 327, 338
pVHI. *See* Pediatric Voice Handicap Index

R

RCC. *See* Refractory chronic cough
Recalibration therapies, 38–39, **39**
Recurrent respiratory papillomatosis and ventricular phonation, postsurgical voice therapy for child with, 140–147
Refractory chronic cough
  behavioral cough suppression therapy for, 284–290
  description of, 281–282
  irritant-induced, 294
REFS. *See* Reported Edmonton Frail Scale
Rehabilitation Treatment Specification System, 38
Relaxed-throat breathing, **303**
Reported Edmonton Frail Scale, 170
Rescue breathing, 308, 311, 325
Reset words, 419
Resonant voice, 95, 97, 132, 240
Resonant voice therapy
  case studies of, 66, 69, 148, 289, 368
  Lessac-Madsen. *See* Lessac-Madsen Resonant Voice Therapy
  in stimulability testing, 24
  for vocal fatigue in adult touring musical theater performer, 386–388

Respiratory disease and chronic cough, behavioral cough suppression therapy for, 297–305
Respiratory laryngeal dystonia, 323
Respiratory muscle strength training, 166
Respiratory patterns, 12–13
Respiratory-phonatory coordination, 66, 68, 210–211
Restrictive lung diseases, 297
Rigid laryngoscopes, 396
Rigid videolaryngostroboscopy, 114
RTSS. *See* Rehabilitation Treatment Specification System
Ruler exercise, 309, **310**
RVT. *See* Resonant voice therapy

S

Secondary muscle tension dysphonia
  definition of, 107
  episodic breathing problems as cause of, 328
  treatment of, 35
Self-advocacy, 474
Self-Determination Theory, 41
Self-efficacy, 57, 118, 122, 283
Semi-occluded vocal tract therapy
  case studies of, 66, 68–69, 145, 391–394
  protocol for, **401**
Sequential motion rate, 14–15
SGS. *See* Subglottic stenosis
Shared decision-making process, 258
Sibilants, 38
"Silent know how," 41
Singing Voice Handicap Index, **9, 94**
Singing Voice Handicap Index-10, **10**
SLN injection and behavioral cough suppression therapy, for chronic refractory cough, 305–315
SLPs. *See* Speech-language pathologists
SMR. *See* Sequential motion rate
Sniff/hiss strategy, 327
Sniffing, 338
Sodium oxybate, 230
Sound level meter, 22
SOVT. *See* Semi-occluded vocal tract therapy
Spasmodic dystonia. *See* Laryngeal dystonia
Spastic dysarthria, **17**
SPEAK OUT!, 40
Specificity of exercise, 37

Speech deterioration, 13
Speech-language pathologists
  assessment by
    auditory-perceptual, 11–12
    case history, 7, **8**
    cranial nerve examination, 13, **14**
    manual, 16, 18
    motor speech, 13–16
    patient-reported outcome measures. *See* Patient-reported outcome measures
    visual-perceptual, 12–13
  in deep brain stimulation for vocal tremor, 261–267
  informed decision making by, 34
  referrals to, 3–4
  as "right" clinician, 33–34
  on upper airway care team, 3
Speech rate, 13
Speech therapy, for Parkinson's disease-related communication deficits, 224
SpeechVive, for maintaining voice therapy gains in Parkinson's disease, 267–274, **271**
Stimulability testing
  description of, 23–24
  manual laryngeal reposturing techniques for, 111–112
"Strap" muscles, 16
Stridor, inspiratory, 12
Subglottal pressure, 22–23
Subglottic stenosis, 7
Sulcus deformity, of vocal folds, 209–210, 214
Sulcus vocalis, 160, 207–214
SVHI. *See* Singing Voice Handicap Index
SVHI-10. *See* Singing Voice Handicap Index-10
s/z ratio, 23, 441

T

TBI. *See* Traumatic brain injury
Teenager. *See* Adolescent
Telehealth, 293
Telemedicine, 399–401
Teletherapy
  for abductor laryngeal dystonia and vocal tremor, 236–242
  gender affirming voice care via, in transmasculine binary singer, 475–483
TGNC. *See* Transgender/gender nonconforming clients

Therapeutic alliance, 41–42, 57
Throat-clearing behaviors, 82, 88–89
Thyroarytenoid muscle, 136–137, 166
Thyroplasty, for vocal fold paralysis, 36
Tissue immobilization, 48
Tongue trills, 427, 429
Transgender/gender nonconforming clients, 437–438
Transgender women, gender affirming voice care in
  Hirsch's Acoustic Assumptions for, 439–446
  pitch-elevation surgery and perioperative voice care for, 446–453
Transmasculine adult, gender affirming voice care in
  on hormone replacement therapy, 453–461
  teletherapy for, 475–483
Transtheoretical model, of behavior change, 171
Trans Voice Initiative, 439
Trans Woman Voice Questionnaire, 441
Traumatic brain injury, vocal process granulomas after, 79–85
Treatment decisions. *See also specific treatment*
  differential diagnosis used in, 4
  laryngeal diagnosis used in, 4–5
Tremor
  description of, 12
  vocal. *See* Vocal tremor; Voice tremor
Trigeminal nerve, **14**
TTM. *See* Transtheoretical model
Twang technique, 369
TWVA. *See* Trans Woman Voice Questionnaire

U

Undifferentiated phonotrauma, vocal function exercises for, 85–92
Unilateral upper motor neuron dysarthria, **17**
Unilateral vocal fold paralysis, postsurgical voice therapy for, 185–192
Unilateral vocal fold paresis
  interprofessional treatment for, 192–199
  multimodality teletherapy for adult avocational singer with, 199–207
Upper airway disorders
  breathing in, 11–12
  cough in, 11–12. *See also* Cough
  history of clinical work in, 2

Upper airway evaluation
  components of, 5–24, **6**
  documentation of, 24
  history of, 1–3
  laryngeal imaging in, 19
/u/ prolongation, 123–125
Urge to cough
  assessment of, 299
  description of, 282, 284
UTC. *See* Urge to cough

V

Vagus nerve, **14**
VALI. *See* Voice-Vibratory Assessment With Laryngeal Imaging
VCI. *See* Voice Catastrophization Index
Ventricular phonation and recurrent respiratory papillomatosis, postsurgical voice therapy for child with, 140–147
VFI. *See* Voice Fatigue Index
VFSS. *See* Videofluoroscopic swallow study
VHI. *See* Voice Handicap Index
VHI-10. *See* Voice Handicap Index-10
Videofluoroscopic swallow study, 147
Videolaryngostroboscopy, 114
Visual-perceptual assessment, 12–13
Vocal color, 455
Vocal cord dysfunction, 2, 322
Vocal effort
  manifestations of, 10
  subglottal pressure and, 23
Vocal fatigue
  manifestations of, 10
  multimodal voice therapy for, 127–133
  myofascial release for adult touring musical theater performer with, 380–388
Vocal fold(s)
  adduction of, **178**
  aerodynamic assessment of, 22–23
  closure mechanisms for, 159, 270
  injection augmentation of, 191, 197, 212
  mucosa of, 18
  phonotraumatic lesions of, 47
  recovery from injury by, 47
  stiffness of, 420
  sulcus deformity of, 209–210, 214
  throat clearing effects on, 88
  valving action of, 159

Vocal fold cysts
perioperative management of, in adult jazz
singer, 415–423
perioperative therapeutic care for, 71–79
treatment of, 30
voice therapy for, 30
Vocal fold lesions
microflap excision of, 30, 74
voice therapy for, 30
Vocal fold motion
assessment of, 18–19
paradoxical, 2, 322, 324
Vocal fold motion impairments
paralysis. *See* Vocal fold paralysis
paresis. *See* Vocal fold paresis
treatment options for, 35–36
Vocal fold nodules
Lessac-Madsen Resonant Voice Therapy for,
93–101
multimodality voice therapy for, in
prepubescent singer, 423–430
Vocal fold paralysis
cough strength affected by, 12
definition of, 35
injection augmentation for, 35–36
postoperative voice therapy for, 185–192
thyroplasty for, 36
treatment options for, 35–36
unilateral, 185–192
voice therapy for, 35–36
Vocal fold paresis
definition of, 35
treatment options for, 36
unilateral
interprofessional treatment for, 192–199
multimodality teletherapy for adult
avocational singer with, 199–207
Vocal fold phonation, 144
Vocal fold polyps
mild atrophy and, multimodality voice
therapy for, 394–402
perioperative voice therapy for, in high
school music teacher, 409–415
treatment of, 30
true, 389
voice therapy for, 30, 394–402, 409–415
Vocal fold pseudocyst
appearance of, 64–65
multimodality voice therapy for, 61–71

Vocal fold scar and sulcus
surgeries for, **213**
voice therapy for, 31
Vocal function exercises
case study of, 89–90
description of, 48, 427
as exuberant therapy, 40
inspiratory muscle strength training and, for
presbyphonia, 161–169
muscle tension dysphonia treated with, 328
undifferentiated phonotrauma treated with,
85–92
for vocal fatigue in adult touring musical
theater performer, 386
Vocal health and hygiene
description of, 40
recommendations for, 390
terminology to describe, 62
Vocal hyperfunction, 108
Vocal injury, onsite voice therapy for adult
theater actor with, 371–380
Vocalises, 369, 421
Vocal pacing, **67**
Vocal process granulomas after traumatic brain
injury, multidisciplinary treatment for,
79–85
Vocal strain, 83–84
Vocal Tract Discomfort Scale, **10**
Vocal tract shaping, 205
Vocal tremor. *See also* Voice tremor
abductor laryngeal dystonia and, teletherapy
without medical management for,
236–242
characteristics of, 222
compensatory muscle tension for, 257
deep brain stimulation for, SLP's role in,
261–267
dystonic, 223
multimodality voice therapy for adult
classical singer with, 255–261
reducing voicing duration to treat, 242–255
visual-perceptual ratings of, **246–247**
voice therapy for, 223, 255–261
vowel phonation for detecting, 16
Voice
performance. *See* Performance voice
pubertal changes in, 137
resonant, 95, 97, 132, 240
Voice Assessment for Laryngeal Imaging, 307

498   Voice Therapy: Clinical Case Studies

Voice behaviors, 33
Voice breaks, 229
Voice care
  gender affirming. *See* Gender affirming voice
    care
  history of, 1
Voice care education, 96, 130–131
Voice care team
  history of, 1
  otolaryngologist on, 4
Voice Catastrophization Index, **9**
Voiced fricatives, 126, **379**
Voiced gargle, 125
Voiced lip bubbles, 125
Voice EvalU8, 22
Voice evaluation
  acoustic assessment in, 21–22
  aerodynamic assessment in, 22–23
  components of, 5–24, **6**
  comprehensive, **6**
  documentation of, 24
  history of, 1–3
  instrumental assessment in, 18–23
  medical examination in, 5–7
  stimulability in, 23–24
Voice Fatigue Index, 10, **10**, 128, 187
Voice Handicap Index, **8,** 78, 134, 187, **245,** 248,
    389, 441
Voice Handicap Index-10, **8,** 128, 163, **180, 184**
Voiceless bubble, 391
Voiceless fricatives, 124, 126, 232, **379**
Voiceless phrases/conversation, 124
Voice Problem Impact Scales, **9,** 170
Voice Puzzle, 459
Voice quality, 11
Voice Range Profile, 410
Voice-Related Quality of Life, **8,** 86, 403
Voice rest
  description of, 30
  indications for, 48
  postoperative, 76
Voice stimulability testing, 23–24
Voice Symptom Scale, **95**
Voice therapy
  adductor type laryngeal dystonia treated
    with, 232–236
  adherence to, 32, 394
  after injection augmentation, 270
  barriers to, 32–33
  botulinum neurotoxin injection and, 37

candidate for, 31–33
components of, 37
decision making in, 37–42
definition of, 37
direct, 38, 131–132, 378, 419
discharge from, 41
essential voice tremor treated with, 37
exuberant therapies, 38–40, **39**
glottal dysfunction treated with, 160–161
glottal incompetence treated with, 160–161
goals of, 29–30, **451**
indications for, 29–31
indirect, 131, 146–147, 418
indirect and augmentative therapies, 38–40,
    39
intensive, 40–41, 133–140
laryngeal dystonia treated with, 232–236
multimodality
  for vocal fatigue, 127–133
  for vocal fold pseudocyst, 61–71
  for vocal nodules in prepubescent singer,
    423–430
  for vocal tremor, 255–261
muscle tension dysphonia treated with, 35
onsite, for adult theater actor with vocal
    injury, 371–380
in Parkinson's disease, SpeechVive for
    maintaining of gains in, 267–274, **271**
for phonotraumatic lesions in adult praise
    and worship leader, 403–409
postsurgical
  for recurrent respiratory papillomatosis
    and ventricular phonation in child,
    140–147
  for unilateral vocal fold paralysis, 185–192
recalibration therapies, 38–39, **39**
Rehabilitation Treatment Specification
    System application to, 38
resonant voice in, 97
self-efficacy in, 57
session-based tasks for, **251–254**
strategies for, 38, **39**
structured program for, 84
techniques for, **451**
in treatment paradigm, 33
variables in, 41–42
vocal fold paralysis treated with, 35–36
vocal fold polyp in high school music teacher
    treated with, 409–415
vocal tremor treated with, 223

Index   **499**

Voice tremor. *See also* Vocal tremor
    essential, 37, 223, 263
    severity of, 16
    testing for, 15–16
    treatment options for, 36–37
Voice Tremor Scoring System, 16, 262, **262, 266**
Voice-Vibratory Assessment With Laryngeal
        Imaging, 19, **20–21,** 162, 227, 237, 454
Voicing duration reductions, for vocal tremor,
        242–255
VoiSS. *See* Voice Symptom Scale

VPIS. *See* Voice Problem Impact Scales
VRP. *See* Voice Range Profile
VRQOL. *See* Voice-Related Quality of Life
VTSS. *See* Voice Tremor Scoring System

W

Wheeze, expiratory, 12
Whispering, 16, 124
Wound healing, 47